# Hematologic Malignancies

**Series Editor**

Martin Dreyling
München, Germany

This series of professional books provides in-depth information on all aspects of the diagnosis and treatment of different hematologic cancers, including clinical evaluation, imaging diagnosis, staging, current treatment strategies, novel targeted approaches, and evaluation of treatment response. Readers will also find coverage of methodological and research issues and factors that influence treatment outcome. Each volume is designed to serve both as a quick reference and as a comprehensive source of knowledge that will be invaluable in improving management of the malignancy under consideration. The volume editors and authors have been selected for their international reputations and acknowledged expertise. The series will appeal to hematologists and oncologists in hospitals or private practices, residents, and others with an interest in the field.

More information about this series at http://www.springer.com/series/5416

Christoph Röllig • Gert J. Ossenkoppele
Editors

# Acute Myeloid Leukemia

Springer

*Editors*
Christoph Röllig
Medizinische Klinik und Poliklinik I
University Hospital Carl Gustav Carus
Dresden
Germany

Gert J. Ossenkoppele
Department of Haematology
Amsterdam University Medical Center
location VUMC
Amsterdam
Noord-Holland
The Netherlands

ISSN 2197-9766 ISSN 2197-9774 (electronic)
Hematologic Malignancies
ISBN 978-3-030-72675-1 ISBN 978-3-030-72676-8 (eBook)
https://doi.org/10.1007/978-3-030-72676-8



This Springer imprint is published by the registered company Springer Nature Switzerland AG
The registered company address is: Gewerbestrasse 11, 6330 Cham, Switzerland

# Preface

It is an exciting era to be involved in the care of AML patients. Numerous new developments concerning all aspects from bench to bedside of this myeloid disorder justify a comprehensive review. This book provides in-depth information on all aspects of the biology, diagnosis, and treatment of AML. Dedicated AML experts from all over Europe and overseas have contributed to the various high-quality chapters of this book and address the most burning questions that always come up at meetings on AML.

This book offers you the possibility to read it from cover to cover, but in this age of "surfing" and "hyperlinks" you can also select topics of your specific interest, for example, in relation to a clinical problem or situation. We have tried to cover the total spectrum of topics of importance for the disease ranging from epidemiology, biology, diagnosis, and classification to treatment including supportive care issues. Special emphasis has been given not only to the pathogenic relevance of the genomic aberrations underlying the biological and clinical complexity of AML but also in relation to inform treatment decisions. The complex discussion on who is fit to receive intensive chemotherapy and chapters on measurable residual disease and the rapidly evolving field of new drugs are an important source of information.

This book is not only for hematologists, hematologists in training, oncologists but also for specialized nurses and other healthcare workers interested in AML. Also employees of pharmaceutical companies will find relevant information.

We hope that you really enjoy the content of this book; we at least had a lot of pleasure in composing, editing, and reading it.

Dresden, Germany — Christoph Röllig
Amsterdam, The Netherlands — Gert J. Ossenkoppele

# Contents

# 1 Epidemiology and Etiology of AML

Gunnar Juliusson, Sören Lehmann, and Vladimir Lazarevic

## 1.1 Incidence of AML by Age and Year

Acute myeloid leukemia (AML) (Döhner et al. 2015) is a grave disease, resulting in 85,000 deaths and 2.6 million years of lost life globally in 2016 (Foreman et al. 2018), and these numbers are expected to rise to over 150,000 deaths and 3.8 million years of lost life in 2040. This increase is mainly caused by a growing and aging global population. For 2020, 20,000 new cases per year are expected in the USA (SEER 2020) and 3100 in the UK (Cancer Research UK 2020).

In addition to the human loss, there is a substantial cost of treatment, care, and disability, calculated to €170,000 per patient younger than 60 years for the first 5 years in Sweden, with somewhat lower costs for older patients (Hernlund et al. 2019).

AML may strike at any age, from newborn to very elderly. However, the incidence rises sharply during middle age and peaks in ages 75–85 years (Fig. 1.1). The reported median age ranges from 68 years in the USA, Denmark, and Switzerland (SEER 2020, Østgård et al. 2015, Schnegg-Kaufmann et al. 2018) to over 70 in Japan, France, the UK, and Sweden (Maynadie et al. 2011; Ohnishi et al. 2014; Roman et al. 2016; Juliusson et al. 2009).

The overall crude incidence in the Scandinavian countries 2012–2016 is according to NORDCAN 2.9 per 100,000 males (M) per year and 2.6 for females (F) (NORDCAN 2020), 2.5 in Burgundy, France (M 2.8, F 2.2; Maynadie et al. 2011), 3.8 in Switzerland (M 4.1; F 3.4; Schnegg-Kaufmann et al. 2018), 4.26 in Kagawa, Japan (Ohnishi et al. 2014), 4.39 in the UK (M 4.9; F 3.9; Roman et al. 2016), and 4.31 in the United States in 2016 (M 5.4, F 3.5, according to SEER 2020). Age-adjusted incidences have significant variation due to the choice of standard population. In the UK, the adjusted standardized incidence during 2004–2013 ranged from 2.58 through 5.06 per 100,000 a year with different standard reference populations (Roman et al. 2016).

Age-adjusted incidence rates by year in the USA (SEER 2020), and by year, age, and sex in the Nordic countries (NORDCAN 2020) are shown in Fig. 1.2. In contrast to the slightly decreasing trend for age-adjusted incidence, the crude incidence in Sweden increased from 4.7 in 1997–2006 to 5.3 in 2007–2015, that is, an annual increase of 1.2% (Nilsson et al. 2020).

G. Juliusson (✉) · V. Lazarevic
Department of Hematology, Skåne University Hospital, Lund University, Lund, Sweden
e-mail: Gunnar.juliusson@med.lu.se

S. Lehmann
Department of Medical Sciences, Uppsala University, Uppsala, Sweden

Department of Medicine, Karolinska Institute, Stockholm, Sweden



C. Röllig, G. J. Ossenkoppele (eds.), *Acute Myeloid Leukemia*, Hematologic Malignancies,
https://doi.org/10.1007/978-3-030-72676-8_1

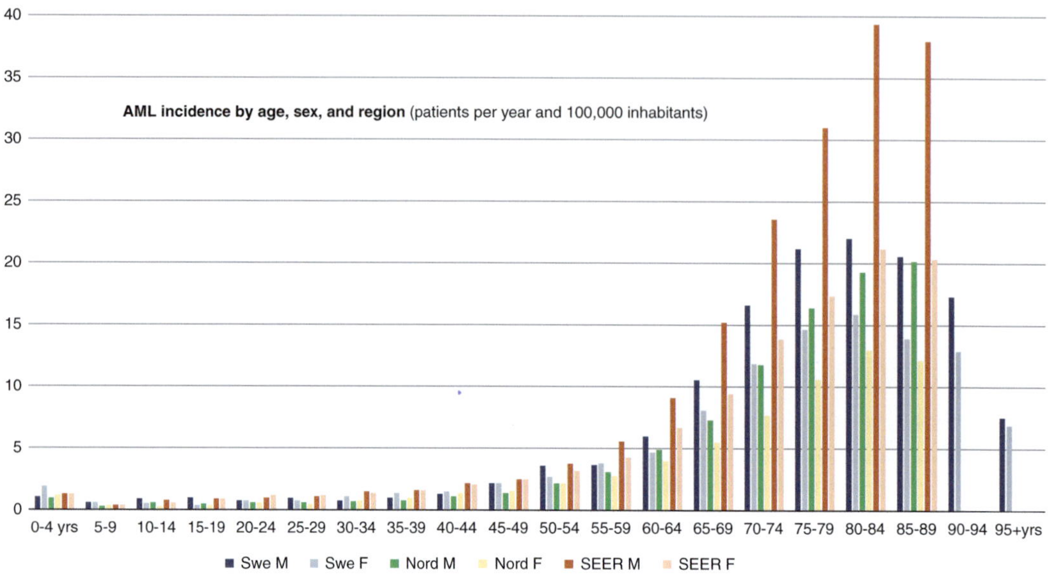


**Fig. 1.1** Incidence of AML (number of patients per 100,000 inhabitants and year) by age at diagnosis, sex and region (Swe, Swedish AML Registry 1997–2013; Nord, NORDCAN i.e., Nordic countries 2001–2016; SEER, US registry 2012–2016). *M* males, *F* females

AML in children is most common in newborns up to age 4 (Fig. 1.1), and SEER data for 1975–2014 indicates a rising incidence from 0.7 through 1.2 per 100,000 a year (Chen et al. 2019).

As with most hematologic malignancies, AML is more common in males than in females, which is most clearly seen in the age group 60–90 years. However, there are AML subsets that are more common in females, such as AML with *FLT3* internal tandem duplication (ITD) and/or *NPM1* mutation (Juliusson et al. 2020) and therapy-related AML (t-AML) (Hulegardh et al. 2015; Nilsson et al. 2020).

## 1.2 Prevalence

The number of people living after a diagnosis of leukemia overall in the USA is estimated to be 400,000 (SEER 2020), over 60,000 of them with AML, with a prevalence of 19 per 100,000, according to SEER (Shallis et al. 2019). The prevalence of AML patients in Scandinavia 2016, according to NORDCAN, is 13.9 per 100,000 (M 13.1, F 13.9), and the age distribution of prevalent Swedish patients in 2014 is shown in Fig. 1.3 (Juliusson et al. 2017), with a skewing toward younger people due to the strong effect of age on survival (Juliusson et al. 2009).

## 1.3 Evaluating Incidence

Most AML patients are previously healthy and have de novo disease (Juliusson et al. 2009), but one-third have previously received chemoradiotherapy for another malignant or non-malignant disease (t-AML), or have transformed from another hematologic disease (Fig. 1.4), typically myelodysplastic syndrome (MDS) or myeloproliferative neoplasia (MPN) (Chap. 2). The epidemiology of AML, including incidence and outcome, is therefore dependent on diagnostic criteria (Arber et al. 2016), which have changed.

Biologically and clinically, there is a continuum between high-risk MDS and AML with myelodysplasia-related changes, according to WHO (Swerdlow et al. 2017). These entities have genetic features in common (Lindsley et al. 2015), and whereas some genetic markers, such

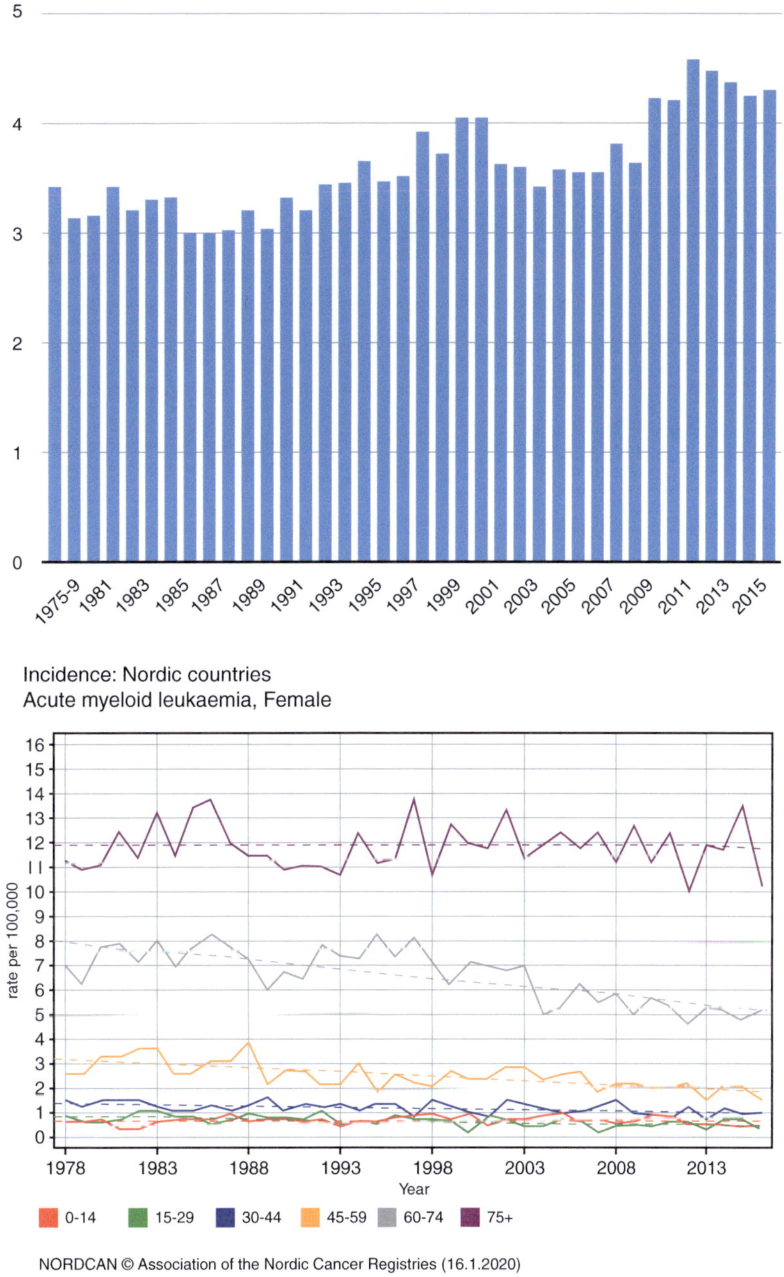


**Fig. 1.2** Top: Incidence rates per 100,000 and years 1975–2016 from SEER, age-adjusted to the 2000 US standard population (SEER 2020). Middle and Bottom: Incidence rates by age and year 1978–2016 in the Nordic countries (NORDCAN 2020). Middle: females. Bottom: males

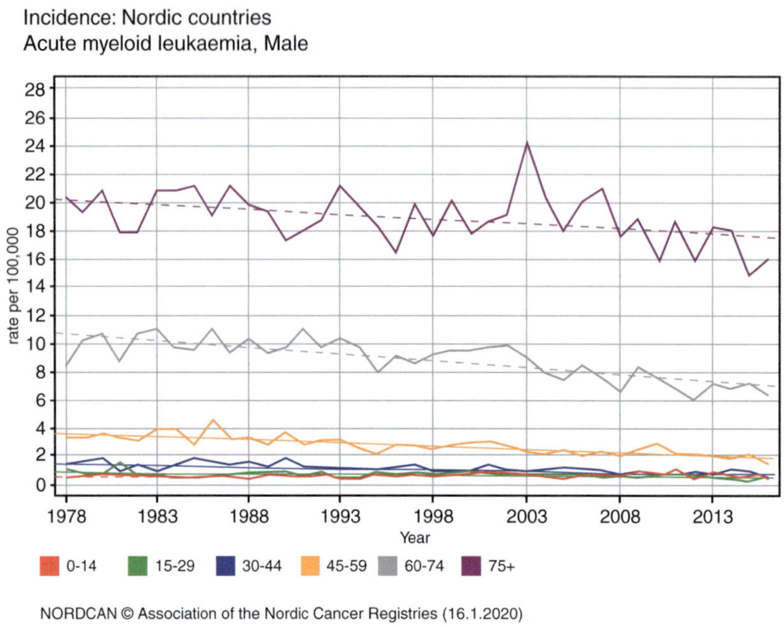


**Fig. 1.2** (continued)

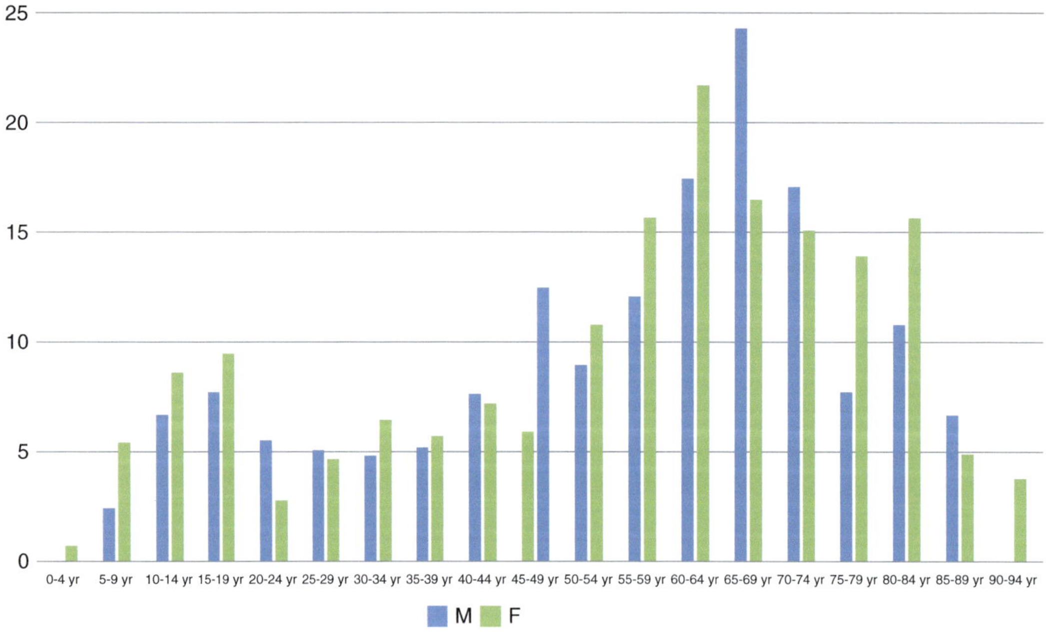


**Fig. 1.3** Prevalence in 2014 of people in Sweden diagnosed with AML 1997–2013 by age and sex

as *FLT3*-ITD and *NPM1*-mutations, present late in the development of AML and therefore indicate de novo AML (Abelson et al. 2018), others are common in both AML and MDS. Historically, the boundary between MDS and AML have been the percentage of leukemic blasts in blood and/or bone marrow. Up to 2002 patients with less than 30% blasts were diagnosed as MDS, but this bor-

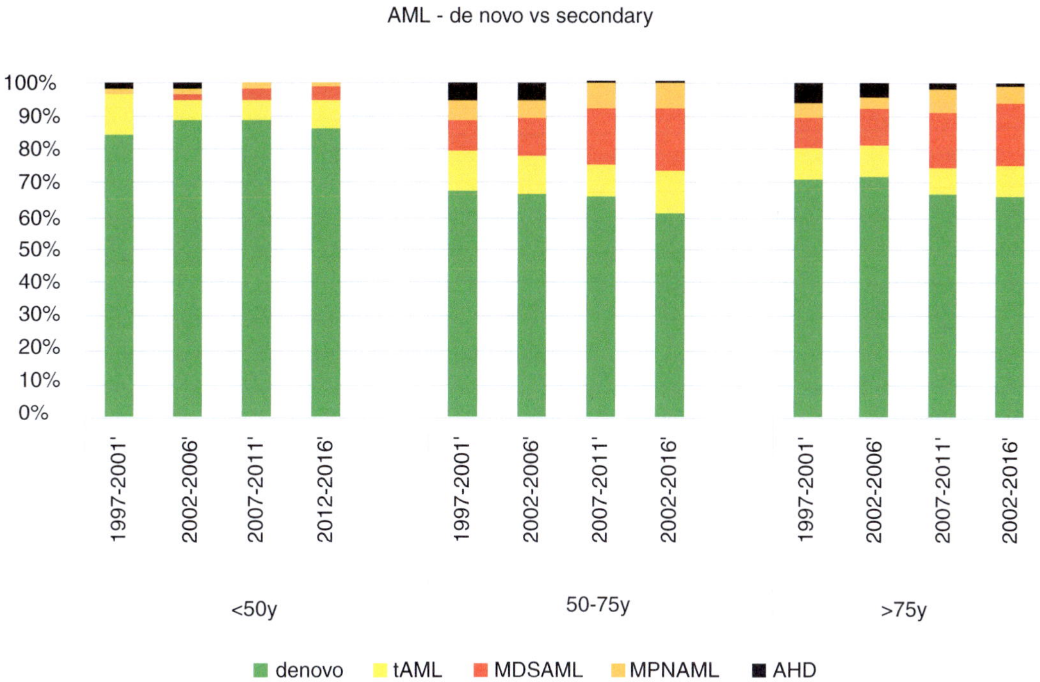


**Fig. 1.4** Proportion of de novo and secondary subtypes of AML in Sweden by age and time period. *tAML* therapy-related AML, *MDSAML* AML with previous myelodysplastic syndrome, *MPN* AML with previous myeloproliferative neoplasia, *AHD* AML with undefined antecedent hematologic disease

derline was subsequently lowered (Vardiman et al. 2002), so AML became defined by 20% blasts or more, with some exceptions. However, WHO states: "It is important to recognize that the threshold of 20% blasts distinguishing AML from MDS does not reflect a therapeutic mandate to treat cases with ≥20% blasts as acute leukemia" (Swerdlow et al. 2017, page 98). In Sweden, one fourth of the AML patients are now reported with <30% marrow blasts at diagnosis. This change of diagnostic criteria penetrated gradually into the clinic, and no clear-cut rise in the incidence was seen in the early 2000s, but it adds to the complexity of interpreting incidence data. Furthermore, secondary AML has often been excluded from clinical trials and was not reported to SEER before 2010 (Polednak 2014).

Another epidemiologic hazard is to distinguish if high-risk MDS patients actually have fulfilled criteria for AML transformation. It is common that late-stage MDS patients deteriorate with or without increasing white blood cell counts and appearance of circulating blasts, and abstention of full diagnostics in patients not eligible for specific treatment is common and clinically relevant. The variation of median ages at diagnosis of AML in different countries with similar life expectancy of the general population might also be due to different clinical routines among the very elderly (Lazarevic et al. 2018).

Secondary AML is rare in younger patients. Since MDS is most common among older males, a transformation of MDS to AML is also more common in males. In contrast, t-AML is more common in females, since chemoradiotherapy for breast cancer is a common background (Hulegardh et al. 2015; Nilsson et al. 2020). The incidence of t-AML is dependent on the type and intensity of chemoradiotherapy given, the number of such patients treated, and their long-term survival. In the 1970s, Hodgkin's lymphoma was treated with multiple alkylating agents (including nitrogen mustard) and large-field radiotherapy, leading to frequent cures of lymphoma but a high risk of therapy-related myeloid neoplasia (t-MN). With improved Hodgkin therapy, this risk decreased considerably already in the 1980s. Today, successful treatments of lymphomas and advanced breast cancer that still include alkylating agents and topoisomerase II-inhibitors seem to induce an increased proportion of t-AML (Nilsson et al. 2020).

## 1.4 Incidence of Special Genetic Subtypes

AML can be associated with a large number of different driver mutations, with different clinical impact. AML patients with rearrangement of *KMT2A* (previously named *MLL*) at 11q23 are younger (median age 20 years) and have poor prognosis, whereas those with core-binding factor AML [t(8;21)(q22;q22.1), *RUNX1-RUNX1T1*; and inv(16)(p13.1q22), *CBFB-MYH11*] also are young (median 45 years) (Roman et al. 2016) but have better prognosis. In contrast, those with MDS-related abnormalities [del(5q); monosomy 7, complex karyotypes, and more] are older and have poor prognosis. The concept of age-related clonal hematopoiesis (ARCH), with certain gene mutations in hematopoietic stem cells that when expanded with age may predispose to AML (Shlush 2018; Abelson et al. 2018), is an important development shedding light on AML pathophysiology.

A rare specific AML subtype is acute promyelocytic leukemia (APL) (Chap. 6), characterized by the *PML-RARA* hybrid gene, leading to AML with impaired hemostasis. Due to the high sensitivity of APL cells to the differentiating agents all-trans retinoic acid (ATRA) and arsenic trioxide (ATO), the long-term clinical outcome is favorable, with minimal need for chemotherapy and usually no indication for stem cell transplantation. Of interest is the great variation in incidence of APL between European countries, from 0.26 per 100,000 a year in Spain and Iceland to tenfold less in other countries, many of them in Eastern Europe (Dinmohamed and Visser 2019); in Sweden, the crude incidence of APL is 0.2 per 100,000 a year. The median age of APL is lower than that of most other AML subsets, in Sweden 58 years (quartile range 43–69 years), but still the incidence increases with age (Fig. 1.5). Despite therapeutic improvements, the early death rate

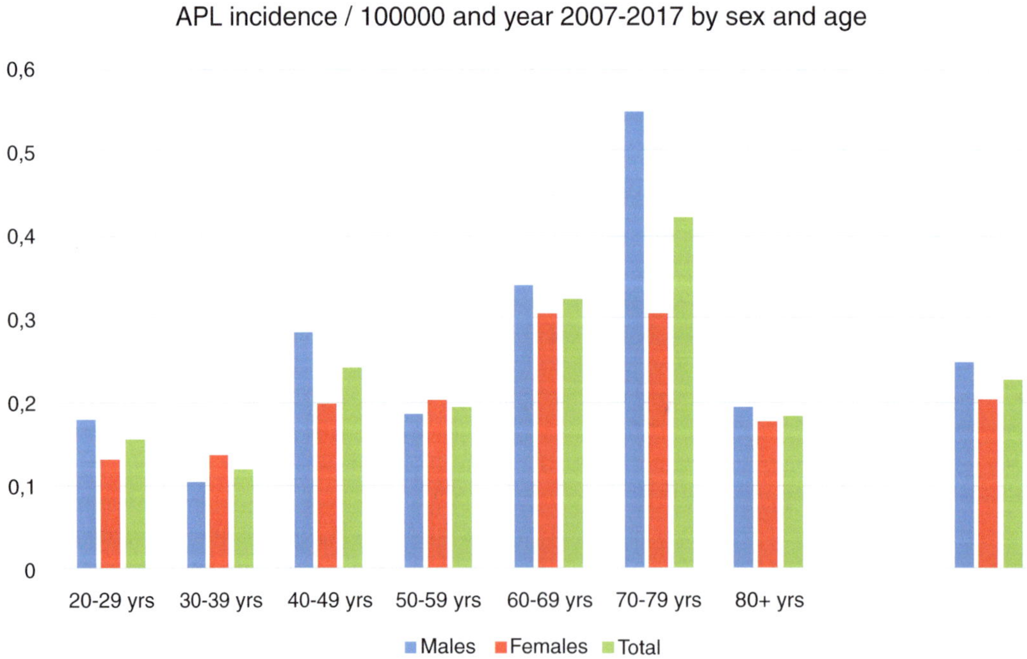


**Fig. 1.5** Incidence of APL in Sweden by age and sex

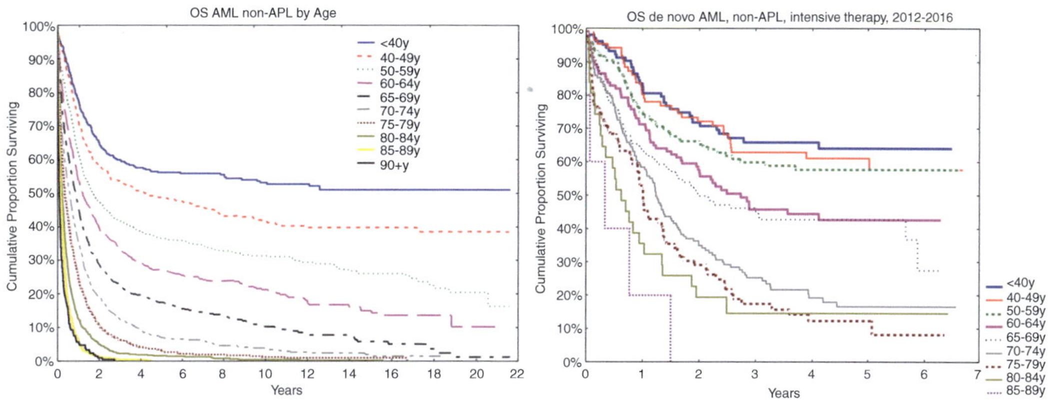


**Fig. 1.6** Overall survival by age in Sweden. Left: total cohort excluding APL 1997–2016. Right: de novo AML non-APL patients receiving intensive chemotherapy 2012–2016

remains high in older patients (Lehmann et al. 2017). It seems likely that still not all APL patients are diagnosed and reported properly.

## 1.5 Survival

Survival of AML patients is highly dependent on age (Fig. 1.6), genetic subtype (Döhner et al. 2015, Chap. 5), performance status (Juliusson et al. 2009), comorbidity, and previous diseases (Hulegardh et al. 2015). Survival has improved during recent decades, mostly for males in ages 50–75 years (Juliusson et al. 2019), in part due to greater use of allogeneic stem cell transplantation. Females have longer survival in most populations, both overall and with various cancer diseases, but currently the survival of AML in Sweden is independent of sex (Juliusson et al. 2019).

## 1.6 Etiology

Genomic instability is a hallmark of cancer (Hoffman et al. 2018). So far, the reason for this instability is largely unclear, but it is generally assumed that aberrations simply arise in a stochastic manner. The "two-hit hypothesis" of leukemogenesis implies that AML is the consequence of two or more mutations, one conferring a proliferative advantage (class I mutations) and another impairing hematopoietic differentiation (class II mutations) (Reilly 2005). Class I mutations include those of *FLT3*-ITD, *KRAS,* and *KIT* mutations, while fusions involving core binding factors (CBF) and mutations in *CEBPA* are class II abnormalities (Bachas et al. 2010). However, this model does not account for the wide spectrum of more recently described somatic alterations, nor do all patients carry class I and class II mutations.

The pathogenesis of AML is characterized by the serial acquisition of somatic mutations, and several genes are recurrently mutated (Jaiswal and Ebert 2019). Most mutations are inconsequential, and some passenger mutations may have neutral effects, while others clearly give rise to proliferative advantage, thereby increasing the risk of malignant transition (Cypris et al. 2019). Furthermore, aging is associated with a steady increase in the number of somatic mutations in nearly all tissues (Blokzij et al. 2016).

In contrast to genomic changes, epigenetic aberrations do not involve alterations in the DNA sequence. Dynamic modification of DNA and DNA-binding proteins play a crucial role in the regulation of gene expression, chromatin accessibility, and nuclear architecture, and it is postulated that age-related epigenetics can trigger leukemogenesis (Bocker et al. 2011; Jaiswal and Ebert 2019). Causes and risk factors for developing AML are listed in Table 1.1.

**Table 1.1** Causes and risk factors for developing AML

| |
|---|
| *External physical and chemical exposures* |
| Benzene |
| Cigarette smoking |
| Pesticides |
| Embalming fluids |
| Accidental or professional radiation exposure |
| Radiotherapy |
| Radioiodine (I-131) therapy |
| *Chemotherapy agents* |
| Alkylating agents (e.g., melphalan, cyclophosphamide) |
| Topoisomerase-II inhibitors (e.g., etoposide, doxorubicin) |
| Other drugs (e.g., azathioprin) |
| *Myeloid neoplasms with germline predisposition without a preexisting disorder or organ dysfunction* |
| AML with germline *CEBPA* mutation |
| Myeloid neoplasms with germline *DDX41* mutation |
| Myeloid neoplasms with germline predisposition and preexisting platelet disorders |
| Myeloid neoplasms with germline *RUNX1* mutation |
| Myeloid neoplasms with germline *ANKRD26* mutation |
| Myeloid neoplasms with germline *ETV6* mutation |
| Myeloid neoplasms with germline predisposition and other organ dysfunction |
| Myeloid neoplasms with germline *GATA2* mutation |
| Myeloid neoplasms associated with BM failure syndromes |
| Myeloid neoplasms associated with telomere biology disorders |
| JMML associated with neurofibromatosis |
| Noonan syndrome or Noonan syndrome-like disorders |
| Myeloid neoplasms associated with Down syndrome |
| *Other inherited diseases with predisposition to AML* |
| Klinefelter's syndrome |
| Fanconi anemia |
| Ataxia telangiectasia (AT) |
| Li-Fraumeni syndrome |
| Blooms syndrome |
| Nijmegen breakage syndrome |
| Constitutional mismatch repair deficiency syndrome |
| Werner syndrome |
| Severe congenital neutropenia |
| Dyskeratosis congenita |
| Shwachman-Diamond syndrome |
| Diamond-Blackfan anemia |
| Congenital amegakaryocytic thrombocytopenia and thrombocytopenia with absent radii |
| *Clonal hematopoiesis* |
| CHIP (Clonal hematopoiesis of indeterminate potential) |
| CHOP (Clonal hematopoiesis of oncogenic potential) |
| *Other risk factors for developing AML* |
| Higher age |
| Obesity |
| Autoimmune disease |
| Previous hematologic disease (MDS, MPN) |

### 1.6.1 External Physical and Chemical Exposures

Occupational exposures have decreased substantially in developed countries during the last decades due to increased awareness of chemical and mutagenic hazards and new regulations reducing exposures at workplaces. Thus, the role of occupational exposure as a reason for AML etiology has decreased but may still play a role in many parts of the world.

Benzene is probably the strongest carcinogen associated with leukemogenesis (Snyder 2012; Zhu et al. 2013). In a recent laboratory study, hydroquinone, the major metabolite of benzene in humans, increased expression of the p53 protein, increased apoptosis, and induced DNA double-strand breaks in human bone marrow stem cells as well as decreased stem cell differentiation and proliferation (Fircanis et al. 2014). A limited list of the toxic agents found in cigarette smoke includes benzene, formaldehyde, polonium 210, arsenic, lead, and ammonia. Interestingly, in this study, yolk sac stem cells seemed to be especially sensitive to the effects of hydroquinone, which is supported by evidence that exposure to smoking during pregnancy increases the risk of leukemia during childhood (Mucci et al. 2004).

A positive association between domestic pesticide exposure and childhood leukemia is confirmed, with statistically significant increased risks observed for all types of leukemia, and specifically for exposure during pregnancy, indoor exposure, prenatal exposure to insecticides and whatever the age at diagnosis. The maximum increase in risks were observed for AML among children aged 2 years or less, as well as for unspecified leukemia type observed after prenatal indoor exposure. The literature provides moderate- to low-quality of evidence, but still these new results justify the need of limiting the use of household pesticides during pregnancy and childhood (Van Maele-Fabry et al. 2019).

Excess mortality from lymphohematopoietic malignancies, in particular myeloid leukemia, and brain cancer has been found in surveys of anatomists, pathologists, and funeral industry workers, all of whom may have worked with formaldehyde (Hauptmann et al. 2009).

Ionizing radiation (Bizzozero et al. 1966) and alkylating agents share the ability to induce DNA damage, usually through double-strand breaks that may cause the mutations, deletions, or translocations required for hematopoietic stem cell transformation. A recent meta-analysis found an increased risk of leukemia among workers receiving protracted exposure to low-dose gamma radiation (Daniels and Schubauer-Berigan 2011). On the other hand, a study in radiology technologists identified an increased risk of leukemia among workers employed before 1950, when radiation exposures were higher. However, there was no convincing evidence of an increased risk of leukemia in medical radiation workers exposed to current levels of radiation (Yoshinaga et al. 2004). In a cohort of 308,297 radiation-monitored workers employed for at least one year by the Atomic Energy Commission, AREVA Nuclear Cycle, or the National Electricity Company in France, the Departments of Energy and Defence in the USA, and nuclear industry employers included in the National Registry for Radiation Workers in the UK showed strong evidence of positive associations between protracted low-dose radiation exposure and leukemia (Leuraud et al. 2015). Patients developing a therapy-related myeloid neoplasm (t-MN) after radioiodine treatment usually present with biological characteristics similar to those seen in patients with t-MN following other cytotoxic treatment modalities, associated with a low response rate to induction chemotherapy and poor prognosis. Karyotype was abnormal in 68% of patients, with chromosomes 7 (30%), 5 (26%), 8 (26%), and 3 (17%) being most frequently affected (Schroeder et al. 2012). t-MN after radiotherapy alone bears striking clinical and cytogenetic similarities to alkylator-associated t-MN, with frequent clonal abnormalities of chromosomes 5 and 7, relatively long latency, and poor outcomes even with intensive therapy (Nardi et al. 2012). However, some patients who develop t-MN after radiotherapy alone have recurring, balanced chromosomal translocations or normal karyotypes, and they have a better response to antileukemia treatment and longer survival. Thus, both cytogenetics and previous therapies determine the outcome of t-MN (Kayser et al. 2011).

### 1.6.2 Chemotherapy Agents

The development of MDS and AML following chemotherapy for a variety of malignancies (e.g., breast cancer, Hodgkin's lymphoma) is an unfortunate complication of curative treatment strategies, such as dose-intensive therapy with or without hematopoietic cell transplantation and growth factor support (Stone et al. 1994). This identification of an increasing incidence of t-AML in an attempt to improve cure rates emphasizes the critical importance of understanding the underlying pathogenetic mechanisms for development of t-AML (Seedhouse and Russell 2007). t-AML typically develops following alkylating agent-induced damage, at a median of 3–5 years following therapy for the primary malignancy, and is usually associated with an antecedent myelodysplastic disorder (Le Beau et al. 1986). This latency period suggests that multiple mutational events are involved in the development of the malignant phenotype (Schanz et al. 2018). However, increasing evidence points to the importance of selection pressure by chemotherapy conferring survival advantage of preexisting minimal mutated clones (such as *TP53* mutations) present already at the start of the treatment for the primary disease (Wong et al. 2015). Clonal chromosomal abnormalities have been reported in the majority of cases of t-AML. The most frequently reported abnormalities involve complete loss or interstitial deletions of the long arm of chromosomes 7 and/or 5. Other therapy-related leukemias are associated with rearrangements of the *MLL* (*KTM2A*) gene in chromosome band 11q23 (Thirman et al. 1993). AML associated with 11q23 often develops after treatment with drugs that target DNA-topoisomerase II (e.g., epipodophyllotoxins, anthracyclines) with a short latency of 12–18 months following treatment, and typically not associated with an antecedent MDS (Pedersen-Bjergaard and Philip 1991). Typical lesions are reciprocal translocations, such as t(9;11)(p21;q23) and t(11;19)(q23;p13); other translocations that do not involve the *MLL* locus have also been described, including the t(15;17), t(8;21), and inv(16) rearrangements. The risk of t-AML varies based on the chemotherapy dosing schedule, cumulative dose received, additional cytotoxic agents, and underlying disease characteristics, but generally does not exceed 5% of patients treated with topoisomerase II inhibitors. Accelerated telomere loss may precede the development of t-MN after autologous hematopoietic cell transplantation resulting in genetic instability and thereby contributing to the leukemic transformation (Chakraborty et al. 2009). Genetic polymorphisms of a number of drug-metabolizing enzymes may alter the risk of t-AML. As an example, polymorphisms in genes that encode glutathione S-transferases (GST), which detoxify potentially mutagenic chemotherapeutic agents, may increase susceptibility to t-AML as well as MDS. In one study, relative to de novo AML, the GSTP1 codon 105 Val allele occurred more often among patients with t-AML with prior exposure to chemotherapy, particularly those with exposure to known GSTP1 substrates (odds ratio 4.3; 95% CI 1.4–13), and not among t-AML patients with prior exposure to radiotherapy alone (Allan et al. 2001). DNA-damaging chemotherapy carries ~1% risk of t-MN, often harboring complex karyotypes and *TP53* mutations (Gillis et al. 2017). Preexisting clonal hematopoiesis (CHIP) at the time of start of chemotherapy for a primary malignancy significantly increases the risk of developing t-MN (Takahashi et al. 2017). CHIP after chemotherapy is likely related to a competitive advantage of pre-existing (possibly multiple) clones after the stress of chemotherapy or an altered immune microenvironment, rather than a direct mutagenic effect. Previously treated patients have increased rates of clonal hematopoiesis (CH), with enrichment of mutations in DNA Damage Response (DDR) genes (*TP53, PPM1D, CHEK2*). Exposure to radiation, platinum, and topoisomerase II inhibitors have the strongest association with CH with evidence of dose-dependence and gene-treatment interactions. In patients who progressed to t-MN, the clone at CH demarcated the dominant clone at t-MN diagnosis (Bolton et al. 2019).

There is some evidence of association between AML and treatment with other drugs. In a large population with primary autoimmune diseases, azathioprine exposure was associated with a sevenfold risk for myeloid neoplasm (Ertz-Archambault et al. 2017). There are still controversies if the use of taxanes, for example, paclitaxel, increases the risk of AML as well as the use of G-CSF for severe congenital neutropenia (SCN) (Lyman et al. 2010; Rosenberg et al. 2010) or low-dose of methotrexate for rheumatoid arthritis (RA) (Bhatnagar et al. 2016). The high frequency of CH in cancer patients suggests that screening for CH prior to the initiation of oncologic therapy may be feasible and may represent an avenue for molecularly based early detection and interception (Bolton et al. 2019).

### 1.6.3 Myeloid Neoplasms with Germline Predisposition

**Germline *CEBPA* mutations** are inherited in an autosomal dominant fashion and highly penetrant. The age of onset for AML with germline *CEBPA* mutations is lower than that for sporadic AML, with a median of 24.5 years (range 1.75–46 years) in 10 affected families (Tawana et al. 2015). AML patients with *CEBPA* mutations have a favorable clinical outcome that is limited to those with double mutations. Interestingly, individuals with germline *CEBPA* mutation-associated AML may recur with a different somatic *CEBPA* mutation, whereas in sporadic

AML, the *CEBPA* mutation appears stable throughout the disease course. Although the recurrence is triggered by independent clones, the patients can still achieve a durable response to therapy and favorable long-term outcome.

**Myeloid neoplasms with germline *DDX41* mutation**. Similar to AML with biallelic *CEBPA* mutations, the presence of *DDX41* germline mutation predisposes the acquisition of additional *DDX41* somatic mutation on the other allele. Detection of biallelic *DDX41* mutations is strongly supportive of a predisposing germline *DDX41* variant. The most common acquired somatic mutation is *DDX41* c.G1574A (p. R525H), which occurs in a highly conserved C-terminal motif, affecting ATP-binding site. The p.R525H mutation has also previously been reported at the time of progression to MDS or AML. The p.R164W mutation is associated with a predisposition to lymphoproliferative neoplasms, particularly follicular lymphoma. Lewinsohn et al. (2016) reported that three of their nine families with *DDX41* germline mutations had granulomatous immune disorder, raising the possibility of *DDX41* functions in immune response and their potential link to the lymphoid malignancy in affected pedigrees. In contrast to other myeloid neoplasms with germline predisposition, patients with *DDX41* germline mutation have long latency to develop myeloid neoplasm, with a mean age at diagnosis of 62 years, more similar to that of patients with sporadic AML/MDS. *DDX41* mutations are relatively common in adult MDS/AML (2.4%), often without known family history. Salient features of *DDX41*-related myeloid malignancies include male preponderance (79%), frequent preexisting cytopenia, additional somatic *DDX41* mutation, and relatively good outcome (Sébert et al. 2019).

**Myeloid neoplasms with germline *RUNX1* mutation** are reported in families with platelet disorder that was previously called familial platelet disorder with propensity to myeloid malignancies. These patients are characterized by a lifelong history of mild to moderate thrombocytopenia, mild bleeding tendency, and an increased lifetime risk of developing MDS or AML. The familial platelet disorder is inherited in an autosomal dominant fashion. There is also a mild platelet aggregation defect with collagen and epinephrine, similar to abnormalities caused by aspirin. Carriers of germline *RUNX1* mutations have an increased lifetime risk (35–40%) of developing MDS or acute leukemia, with an average age at diagnosis of 33 years (range, 6–76 years). However, there is clinical heterogeneity in the degree of platelet disorder, as well as the varying risks of developing MDS and AML manifested with a large range of prevalence of myeloid malignancy among affected families. In addition to myeloid neoplasm, development of T-lymphoblastic leukemia/lymphoma has also been reported in the context of familial platelet disorder with *RUNX1* mutation. AML secondary to familial platelet disorder has a high frequency of biallelic alteration in the *RUNX1* gene, indicating the acquisition of additional genetic events involving the other nonmutated *RUNX1* cooperative genes during progression to AML. There is no clear association of *RUNX1* mutational status with morphologic subtype of AML. Cytogenetic analyses have reported trisomy 21, monosomy 5, and 5q deletion in AML in the context of familial platelet disorder (Gao et al. 2019).

**Myeloid neoplasms with germline *ANKRD26* mutation** present with thrombocytopenia, previously called thrombocytopenia 2 and are characterized by moderate thrombocytopenia with normal platelet size, no or very mild spontaneous bleeding, and predisposition to developing myeloid neoplasm. It is inherited in an autosomal dominant manner. All individuals reported to date have an affected parent. Each child of an individual with *ANKRD26*-related thrombocytopenia has a 50% chance of inheriting the *ANKRD26* pathogenic variant. Once the *ANKRD26* pathogenic variant has been identified in an affected family member, prenatal testing for a pregnancy at increased risk and preimplantation genetic diagnosis are possible; however, phenotypic variability (due to variable expressivity) within families is observed. Recognition of this insidious form of inherited thrombocytopenia and its associated risk for myeloid neoplasm is important, to avoid that it be inappropriately managed as idiopathic thrombocytopenia pur-

pura and treated with steroids or splenectomy or misdiagnosed as MDS (Gao et al. 2019).

**Myeloid neoplasms with germline *ETV6* mutation** are another autosomal dominant familial thrombocytopenia, previously referred to as thrombocytopenia 5. The *ETV6* gene is located on the short arm of chromosome 12. *ETV6* encodes a transcriptional repressor critical for hematopoiesis, megakaryopoiesis, and embryonic development. Germline *ETV6* mutations are typically located in the DNA binding ETS domain and result in autosomal dominant inhibition of *ETV6* function through dimerization. Individuals carrying germline *ETV6* mutations have increased risks for hematologic malignancies, including AML, MDS, chronic myelomonocytic leukemia, B-lymphoblastic leukemia, and myeloma. Data are scant on disease penetrance. Thus far, the numbers of total patients reported is too small to ascertain associated syndromic features (Kennedy and Shimamura 2019).

**Myeloid neoplasms with germline *GATA2* mutation** have a broad phenotypic spectrum and may present with MonoMac syndrome or Emberger syndrome. However, germline *GATA2* mutations may also present with isolated neutropenia or bone marrow failure without syndromic features or family history. The bone marrow histology in *GATA2* deficiency is typically hypocellular and may manifest characteristic megakaryocyte dysmorphologies with micronuclei or splayed nuclei. Additional findings include monocytopenia and immunologic abnormalities. MDS with germline *GATA2* mutations is frequently associated with monosomy 7/del(7q) or trisomy 8, particularly in children and younger adults. A study of 426 cases of pediatric MDS identified germline GATA2 mutations in 37% of patients with primary MDS with monosomy 7 and in 16% of MDS cases with trisomy 8. Germline GATA2 mutations were identified in 72% of adolescents with MDS and monosomy 7 (Kennedy and Shimamura 2019).

**Myeloid neoplasms associated with bone marrow failure syndromes**. These entities include dyskeratosis congenita, Diamond-Blackfan anemia, Fanconi anemia, Shwachman–Diamond syndrome, and severe congenital neutropenia (Wilson et al. 2014, see below). These conditions are often diagnosed in childhood, if classical physical findings are absent diagnosis in adulthood is often delayed due to decreased awareness among practitioners (Gao et al. 2019).

**Myeloid neoplasms associated with telomere biology disorders**. Telomere disorders with germline *TERC* and *TERT* mutations have an autosomal dominant inheritance pattern with variable clinical presentations. The *TERT* and *TERC* mutation carriers may present with essentially normal complete blood cell count with only subtle abnormalities, such as elevated mean corpuscular volume or thrombocytopenia, before developing bone marrow failure. Some patients may have idiopathic pulmonary fibrosis or liver fibrosis. The co-occurrence of aplastic anemia and idiopathic pulmonary fibrosis is considered quite predictive for germline telomerase gene mutation. Bone marrow biopsy may show moderately increased reticulin fibrosis, notable myeloid dysplasia, and megakaryocytic lineages characterized by predominantly small, hypolobated, dysplastic-appearing forms. The affected families may have anticipation with progressive shortening of the telomeres in passing generations and show worsening phenotype. In addition to predisposition to MDS/AML, the telomere disorders may be associated with a variety of solid tumors, including squamous cell carcinoma and stomach, lung, esophageal, and colon cancers. Patients are sensitive to toxicities from chemotherapy and radiation and warrant specially tailored transplant regimens.

**JMML associated with neurofibromatosis**. Neurofibromatosis type 1 (*NF1*) is a hereditary condition commonly associated with multiple café-au-lait spots on the skin. About 10–25% of the general population has café-au-lait spots; *NF1* is suspected when a person has six or more. People with *NF1* also tend to develop varying numbers of neurofibromas, meaning benign (noncancerous) tumors on the covering of the nerves. The association between hematologic malignancies and germ-line mutations of *NF1* has been established in the pediatric setting. Children with neurofibromatosis 1 have a 500-fold increased risk of developing a rare form of leukemia, known as juvenile myelomonocytic leukemia (JMML); a higher incidence of non-Hodgkin's lymphoma and acute lymphoblastic leukemia has also been reported. *NF1* is a tumor suppressor gene localized on 17q11.2. It encodes neurofibromin, a negative regulator of proto-oncogene RAS. The loss of neurofibromin promotes RAS activity leading to constitutive downstream signaling and increased uncontrolled cell growth. Hyperproliferation is a mechanism that involves every organ system leading to the predisposition for both cancerous and non-cancerous disorders. It is at the base of the so-called RAS-opathies, a group of inherited disorders that share a germ-line mutation of the RAS-MAPK pathway, to which *NF1* belongs. Given the incidence of neurofibromatosis type 1 in the population (1/3000), and that of AML, more studies are needed to establish a direct connection between the AML and Neurofibromatosis type 1.

**Noonan syndrome or Noonan syndrome-like disorders**. Noonan syndrome (NS) is an autosomal dominant developmental disorder characterized by short stature, facial dysmorphisms, and congenital heart defects. Six cancer types have previously been reported in the literature in patients with NS and a *PTPN11* mutation, that is, JMML, neuroblastoma, ALL, non-Hodgkin lymphoma, glioma, and breast cancer. A JMML-like myeloproliferative disorder has been described in neonates with NS and the PTPN11 mutation. The disorder often regresses spontaneously, but fatal complications may occur. Other mutations that can cause hematological malignancies are *SOS1, RAF1, KRAS, NRAS, BRAF*, and *MAP2K1*. CBL syndrome (more formally known as "Noonan-syndrome-like disorder with or without JMML") has overlapping features to Noonan syndrome with significant variability. CBL syndrome and other RASopathy disorders, including Noonan syndrome, neurofibromatosis 1, and Costello syndrome, are important to recognize as these are associated with a cancer predisposition. CBL syndrome carries a very high risk for JMML (Jongmans et al. 2011).

**Myeloid neoplasms associated with Down syndrome**. Down syndrome is caused by trisomy 21 and is associated with an approximately 10–20-fold elevated relative risk of AML and MDS compared with the general population, and in particular an increased risk for acute megakaryocytic leukemia, FAB M7 (Shand 2017). Infants with Down syndrome may experience transient abnormal myelopoiesis (TAM), where circulating peripheral blood blasts are seen and may be accompanied by hepatic dysfunction, effusions, and rash; this occurs in approximately 10% of these patients. The majority of TAM cases harbor somatic mutations in *GATA1*, resulting in altered function of this transcription factor that plays an important role in hematopoietic cell maturation, particularly in the megakaryocyte lineage. Decreased *GATA1* expression results in megakaryocyte proliferation. Indeed, up to 30% of persons with TAM will progress to AML, commonly acute megakaryocytic leukemia. The development of AML in patients with Down syndrome likely relates both to acquired somatic mutations, such as *GATA1*, and also the presence of additional copies of genes on chromosome 21 that facilitate leukemogenesis, such as the oncogenes *RUNX1*, *ERG*, and *ETS2* (Brunner and Graubert 2018).

Newly discovered hereditary predisposition syndromes include, for example, *SAMD9* and *SAMD9L* mutations, which give rise to myeloid malignancies with chromosome 7 involvement in combination with neurological symptoms; in severe case, they manifest as MIRAGE syndrome (myelodysplasia, infection, restriction of growth, adrenal hypoplasia, genital phenotypes, enteropathy). Patients with germline *SAMD9* or *SAMD9L* mutations have a propensity to develop clones that have lost or inactivated the mutant SAMD9/SAMD9L allele. The mechanisms of this adaptation can be through truncating or loss of function mutations in cis with the mutant *SAMD9* or *SAMD9L* allele, or through genetic reversion through duplication of the wild-type allele. Improvement in blood counts has been observed to accompany this somatic inactivation of the mutant *SAMD9/SAMD9L* allele. A second strategy to eliminate the mutant gene is to delete all or part of chromosome 7 carrying the mutant *SAMD9/SAMD9L* allele. Although this is predicted to result in improved cell growth, this comes at the cost of promoting development of MDS with monosomy 7 (Tesi et al. 2017).

### 1.6.4 Other Inherited Diseases with Predisposition to AML

**Klinefelter's syndrome** is characterized by an extra chromosome X in boys/men; the 47,XXY karyotype associated with hypogonadism and infertility, and an increased risk for developing breast cancer, non-Hodgkin lymphoma, and lung cancer. Despite claims that Klinefelter's syndrome (KS) (Deschler and Lübbert 2006; Keung et al. 2002; Jalbut et al. 2015) increases the risk of having ALL, MDS, and AML, studies to date have not definitively established an epidemiological link. Intriguingly, almost half the cases of AML with KS occurred in the pediatric population ($\leq$18 years old at diagnosis), and no cases were diagnosed over the age of 64, in contrast to AML in general. These observations raise the question of whether KS, like certain other constitutional abnormalities, may predispose to an earlier onset of AML.

**Fanconi anemia** (FA) is the most common inherited bone marrow failure disorder and is caused by germline mutations in factors involved in DNA repair. FA is characterized by physical abnormalities present in 60–75% of affected individuals, most often presenting with short stature and skeletal abnormalities, bone marrow failure, and a propensity to develop malignancy. FA mutations are inherited generally in an autosomal recessive manner, or as an X-linked trait for pathogenic variants in *FANCB*. Causative mutations in at least 21 genes are responsible for the FA complementation groups. The estimated cumulative incidence of bone marrow failure is 50–90% by age 40, and the cumulative incidences of MDS, AML, and solid tumor malignancies are 30%, 10%, and 30%, respectively (Godley and Shimamura 2017).

**Li-Fraumeni syndrome** (LFS) is a rare cancer predisposing condition caused by germline mutations in *TP53*, the gene encoding the p53 transcription factor. LFS is typified by the development of a wide spectrum of childhood and adult onset malignancies, which includes, among others, the lymphoid and myeloid leukemias, myelodysplastic syndrome and, to a lesser extent, lymphoma. The distribution of *TP53* germline mutations in LFS is similar to those identified in tumors, with the majority clustered within the DNA binding domain where there are six recurrent "hotspot" mutations involving different codons. The published literature as to whether the presence of a germline *TP53* mutation confers a poorer prognosis in patients with hematopoietic cancers is limited. Similarly, there is little information regarding the optimal treatment approaches for primary or therapy-related disease in germline *TP53* mutation carriers. At present, it is not clear whether treatment regimens should be altered to avoid or reduce exposure to DNA damaging chemotherapeutic agents, as is done with patients who have FA or Ataxia Telangiectasia (Swaminathan et al. 2019). In addition, t-MN including MDS and AML are common in patients with LFS and portend a dismal prognosis with standard therapies and even allogenic SCT (Valdez et al. 2017).

**Bloom syndrome** (BS) is a rare genetic disorder characterized by short stature, increased skin sensitivity to ultraviolet rays from the sun (photosensitivity), multiple small dilated blood vessels (telangiectasia) over the nose and cheeks resembling a butterfly in shape, mild immune deficiency with increased susceptibility to infections, and most importantly, a markedly increased susceptibility to many types of cancer, especially leukemia, lymphoma, and gastrointestinal tract tumors. Bloom syndrome is a prototype of a group of genetic conditions known as chromosome breakage syndromes. The genetic abnormality in Bloom syndrome causes problems with DNA repair, resulting in a high number of chromosome breaks and rearrangements. The abnormal DNA repair is responsible for the increased risk for cancer. Bloom syndrome is inherited as an autosomal recessive genetic trait. The causative gene has been mapped to chromosomal locus 15q26.1 and is responsible for encoding a protein known as BLM. A single mutation, known as *BLMAsh*, is responsible for almost all cases of Bloom syndrome among Ashkenazi Jews. Analogous to Fanconi anemia, a preferential occurrence of monosomy 7 or del(7q) was found in bone marrow cells from Bloom syndrome patients with MDS or AML.

**Nijmegen breakage syndrome** (NBS) is a rare genetic disease presenting at birth with microcephaly and dysmorphic facial features that become more noticeable with age, growth delay, and later-onset complications such as malignancies and infections. NBS is caused by mutations in the *NBN* gene (8q21-q24), which lead to partially functional truncated fragments of fibrin, the gene product involved in repairing DNA double-strand breaks. There is no specific treatment for NBS. Subjects should be evaluated for immunodeficiency and treated as appropriate. Parents and caregivers should be counseled about the presenting signs of lymphoma and other malignancies. Radiation therapy should be avoided, if possible. Hematopoietic cell transplantation (HCT) is an option for select patients.

**Constitutional mismatch repair deficiency syndrome** (CMMRD) refers to patients and families with a germline mutation in one of the DNA mismatch repair genes (*MLH1, MSH2, MSH6, PMS2*) or the *EPCAM* gene. It is the most common cause of inherited colorectal cancer. While leukemia is not a typical malignancy seen in Lynch syndrome, there is a variant of this disorder that presents with similar features to *NF1* called mismatch repair deficiency syndrome, which is caused by homozygous mutations in one of four mismatch repair genes: *MLH1, MSH2, MSH6,* or *PMS2*. Café-au-lait spots, brain tumors, colorectal cancer, osteosarcoma, and other solid tumors are some clinical characteristics. Lifetime risk for myeloid malignancies is unknown; there is a risk of ~30% for developing lymphoma/ALL.

**Ataxia telangiectasia** (AT) is an autosomal recessive neurodegenerative disorder characterized by progressive ataxia, ocular telangiectasias, immune dysregulation, and a predisposition to lymphoreticular malignancies. Associated features include pulmonary disease, an increased incidence of malignancy, radiation sensitivity, growth retardation, and diabetes mellitus caused by insulin resistance. Patients with AT are either homozygous or compound heterozygotes for mutations in the gene ataxia telangiectasia mutated (*ATM*) located on 11q22.3 that results in truncated proteins in the majority of families with AT. The greatest risk, however, is in patients with biallelic germline mutations who are at increased risk of developing lymphoma and leukemia with observed/expected ratios of between 50 and 750. When treating leukemia in patients with AT, it is important to remember that ionizing radiation can carry exquisite toxicity in these patients owing to their impaired DNA repair pathway (Brown et al. 2017).

**Werner's syndrome** (WS) is an autosomal recessive genetic disease that is mainly characterized by scleroderma-like skin changes, juvenile cataracts, short stature, and signs of premature aging. The mutated gene is called *WRN (RECQL2)* located at chromosome 8p12, but the risk of developing AML is still unknown (Seiter et al. 2005).

**Severe congenital neutropenia** (SCN) encompasses a diverse range of disorders, including Kostmann syndrome, which is generally manifest in infants with recurrent infections (Kostmann 1956). The most common form of the disease is autosomal dominant and is related to *ELA2*, which encodes for neutrophil elastase, a serine proteinase involved in neutrophilic function. Recently, several other mutations in genes including *HAX1, G6PC3, GFI1, GATA2*, and *WASP* have all been implicated in SCN. The latest data on the long-term risk of developing a myeloid malignancy in this population is 2.3% per year after the first decade (Dale et al. 2000; Klein 2011).

**Dyskeratosis congenita** (DKC) is a bone marrow failure syndrome characterized by inherited mutations in the telomere maintenance pathway. DKC can be inherited in an autosomal-dominant, autosomal-recessive, or X-linked recessive pattern. Mutations in *TERT, DKC1, TERC*, or *TINF2* account for most cases. Typical findings among patients with DKC include the "triad" of skin hyperpigmentation, nail dystrophy, and oral leukoplakia, and these patients will typically develop bone marrow failure by 20–30 years of age. As a result of the underlying mutation, patients have markedly shortened telomeres, which contribute to bone marrow failure, as well as damage to other organs including pulmonary fibrosis and hepatic cirrhosis. Compared with the normal rate of telomere shortening in unaffected individuals of approximately 60 bp per year, individuals with telomere disorders lose telomeric DNA at approximately 120 bp per year. Transformation to AML occurs in approximately 10% of patients and is thought to occur via genomic instability related to shortened telomeres and associated DNA damage, resulting in dysplasia and an increased risk of hematopoietic malignancy (Brunner and Graubert 2018).

**Shwachman-Diamond syndrome** (SDS) is an autosomal recessive disorder caused by mutations in the *SBDS* gene, located on the long arm of chromosome 7 (7q11.21). The exact function of *SBDS* is unknown but involvement in RNA processing and building of ribosomes is suggested. Hematopoietic manifestations of SDS most often include isolated neutropenia, although many patients will eventually develop pancytopenia, which may progress to aplastic anemia. AML or MDS occurs in up to a third of patients by 30 years of age and is thought to relate to chromosomal instability and accelerated rates of apoptosis, which may be due to the role of *SBDS* in stabilizing the mitotic spindle during mitosis. Common cytogenetic abnormalities include monosomy 7, isochromosome 7, and deletion of 20q. Mutations of the tumor suppressor gene, *TP53*, may contribute to the development of MDS and AML in SDS. Hematopoietic cell transplantation should be discussed when clear evidence of progressive myelodysplasia is present and before AML develops (Brunner and Graubert 2018).

**Diamond-Blackfan anemia** (DBA) is characterized by red cell aplasia and typically spares the leukocyte and platelet lineages. DBA is typically inherited in an autosomal dominant fashion and is associated with mutations in a number of ribosomal proteins. The gene encoding ribosomal protein 19 (*RPS19*), located at 19q13.2, is mutated in 25% of patients with DBA. Disease-causing mutations in genes encoding the large (*RPL35A, RPL5, RPL11, RPL27*) and small (*RPS24, RPS17, RPS7, RPS10, RPS26, RPS27, RPS29*) ribosomal subunits have been described. Defects in ribosome function result in anemia early in life and patients with DBA may have characteristic skeletal anomalies, including craniofacial defects, and at times the classic triphalangeal thumb; this anemia is often steroid responsive, but many eventually require chronic transfusional support and hematopoietic cell transplantation. AML can occur in up to 20% of patients and typically occurs after 40 years of age. Although an HLA-matched sibling is the preferred donor for a patient with DBA requiring HCT, one must ensure that the donor does not also carry the same DBA defect as the patient (Brunner and Graubert 2018).

**Congenital amegakaryocytic thrombocytopenia** (CAMT) and **thrombocytopenia with absent radii** (TAR) syndrome are both characterized by hypoplastic thrombocytopenia. CAMT is inherited in an autosomal recessive manner via mutations in the *MPL* gene, which encodes the receptor for thrombopoietin (TPO). Patients have concomitant elevations in serum TPO levels, and thrombocytopenia from birth, which typically progresses to aplasia. CAMT is associated with an increased incidence of AML, typically in the second decade of life. While CAMT does not have phenotypic manifestations outside of thrombocytopenia, TAR syndrome is also associated with thrombocytopenia at birth, as well as a characteristic absence of the radii. TAR syndrome has been associated with mutations in *RBM8A*, which is involved in messenger RNA (mRNA) splicing. The thrombocytopenia in TAR syndrome often improves over time; both acute lymphoblastic leukemia and AML have been reported among patients with this rare disorder (Brunner and Graubert 2018).

### 1.6.5 Clonal Hematopoiesis

Clonal hematopoiesis (CH) has a role as a predisposition factor to AML. CH can be defined as the presence of clonal leukemia-associated somatic mutations in leukocytes from apparently healthy individuals that increases the risk to transform into malignant myeloid disease and is frequently related to stem cell depletion or exhaustion in the elderly (>65 years) (Babushok et al. 2016; Valent et al. 2019). CH of indeterminate potential (CHIP), alternatively named age-related CH (ARCH) (Shlush 2018), is a clinical entity defined by the presence of a cancer-associated clonal mutation in at least 4% of nucleated blood cells of individuals without frank neoplasia. However, these somatic clones do not always lead to overt disease, and instead can remain dormant in a preleukemic state. Mutations in genes involved in epigenetic regulation (*DNMT3A*, *TET2*, *ASXL1*) account for the majority of mutation-driven CH in humans. These mutations are rare in the young but highly prevalent in the elderly, with between 10 and 20% of those older than age 70 harboring a clone of appreciable size (Genovese et al. 2014). Two recently published retrospective studies have dealt with the question whether one can predict the onset of AML within the general population. A predictive AML "prodrome" could be identified by molecular genetic screening and the laboratory parameter of red cell distribution width (Abelson et al. 2018; Desai et al. 2018; Shlush 2018). To reflect this, a new model has been proposed that differentiates CH into CH of indeterminate potential (CHIP) and CH of oncogenic potential (CHOP), based on the type and function of the acquired somatic variants and their subsequent risk to transform into AML (Valent et al. 2019). Thus, CHIP mutations create a background conducive to the development of malignancy, but patients harboring these variants have only a slightly elevated risk of myeloid transformation compared to controls (Genovese et al. 2014; Steensma et al. 2015; Sperling et al. 2017; Valent et al. 2019). On the other hand, CHOP mutations are associated with disease progression playing a role in differentiation and/or proliferation of neoplastic cells, and many individuals with these mutations will develop a myeloid malignancy in their lifetime after a variable latency period (Valent et al. 2019). CHOP mutations are indicative of a high risk of malignant transformation with variable outcome determined by secondary driver lesions, the prognostic impact of CHIP mutations depends on the type and number of acquired mutations, their variant allele frequency (VAF), and the dynamics of clonal evolution. For example, isolated CHIP mutations may indicate clonal stability and are associated with relatively good prognosis, whereas co-occurrence with CHOP mutations or the presence of multiple CHIP mutations is often indicative of adverse outcome (Lin et al. 2016; Bullinger et al. 2017; Rose et al. 2017; Sallman et al. 2017; Valent et al. 2019). The appropriate management of individuals with CHIP is debatable but monitoring for hematological changes to detect signs of disease progression is certainly warranted (Steensma 2018). Prospective studies will be necessary to determine whether screening for AML will be feasible and clinically meaningful.

### 1.6.6 Other Risk Factors for Developing AML

**Age.** AML is more common in older people (Fig. 1.1). Historically, DNA damage was thought to be the main factor responsible for hematopoietic stem cell (HSC) aging. However, in the last few years, many new findings have defined an increasing number of biological processes that are intrinsically changing with age in HSCs. Epigenetics and chromatin architecture, together with autophagy, proteostasis, and metabolic changes, and how they are interconnected to each other gain growing importance for understanding the intrinsic aging of stem cells (Mejia-Ramirez and Florian 2020). Mechanistic understanding of why these variants are positively selected during aging is lacking in most cases. Further complicating the picture, CH has been observed in the absence of any known driver mutation. What causes apparent clonal expansion in these cases is unknown, but clonal expansion could be due to mutations in genes not previously queried in surveys of CH, mutations in the noncoding genome, or even genetic drift due to accelerated constriction of the stem cell pool (Jaiswal and Ebert 2019).

**Obesity** is a risk factor for cancer. Molecular changes during adipose tissue dysregulation can result in oxidative stress and subsequent DNA damage. This represents one of the many critical steps connecting obesity and cancer since oxidative DNA lesions can result in cancer-associated genetic instability. In addition, the byproducts of the oxidative degradation of lipids (e.g., malondialdehyde, 4-hydroxynonenal, and acrolein) and gut microbiota-mediated secondary bile acid metabolites (e.g., deoxycholic acid and lithocholic acid) can function as genotoxic agents and tumor promoters. Obesity is also a risk factor for hematologic malignancy, and there is evidence that the association remains regardless of timing of obesity (Poynter et al. 2016). A recent meta-analysis of prospective studies yielding an adjusted relative risk (RR) for AML of 1.53 (95% CI, 1.26–1.85) for individuals with a BMI >30 kg/$m^2$ compared to individuals with a BMI <25 kg/$m^2$. Obesity in adulthood is a modifiable risk factor for both MDS and AML (Castillo et al. 2012).

**Autoimmune diseases** (ADs) are associated with an increased risk, not only of lymphoproliferative disorders, but also of myeloid malignancies. The excess risk of myelodysplastic syndromes and/or acute myeloid leukemia is observed across several AD types, including systemic lupus erythematodes, rheumatoid arthritis, inflammatory bowel disorders, multiple sclerosis, among others. There appears to be an excess risk of MN risk in AD, independent of cytotoxic exposure, as suggested by occurrence of MNs early in the treatment course and among patients with no prior therapy (Boddu and Zeidan 2019). Certain drug classes, such as thiopurines (azathioprine), alkylating agents (cyclophosphamide), and topoisomerase inhibitors (e.g., mitoxantrone), should be carefully considered due to their well-documented leukemogenic potential and preferably substituted with safer treatment alternatives. On the contrary, a population-based study from Denmark showed that AD and infections were associated with an increased AML risk only in subjects with prior hematological disease and/or cytotoxic treatment. These observations suggest that inflammation plays a minor role in the development of de novo AML (Østgård et al. 2018). Other epidemiological data showed that chronic immune stimulation acts as a trigger for AML/MDS development (Kristinsson et al. 2011). The underlying mechanisms may also be due to a common genetic predisposition or an effect of treatment for infections/AD. However, survival data lend support to the notion that AML in patients with ADs appears to have characteristics and outcome more analogous to de novo AML than t-AML (DiNardo et al. 2013).

**Previous hematologic disease (MDS, MPN, CML).** Other myeloid malignancies, mainly MDS and MPNs, carry a risk of disease evolution to secondary AML (sAML). The risk of transformation varies depending on the underlying disease and may be facilitated by certain exposures, including genotoxic chemotherapy. Patients with MPN have an approximately 10% risk of evolution to AML over 10 years, which varies according to the underlying disease. The risk is lowest in essential thrombocythemia and as high as 20% for myelofibrosis (Cerquozzi and Tefferi 2015). There is a clear association between therapies used in treating MPN, specifically alkylating agents and radioactive phosphorus, and AML evolution; treatment with these agents results in a three to fourfold increase in the incidence of AML. Another mechanism that may contribute to clonal evolution and disease progression may be a chronic inflammatory state related to the underlying MPN (Gillis et al. 2017). Sequencing of secondary AML cases developing in the background of an MPN has identified recurrent mutations in *TET2*, *JAK2*, *IDH*, *IKZF1*, and *ASXL1*. Moreover, a number of patients with a *JAK2*-mutated MPN may develop *JAK2* wild-type AML, thought to arise either from a common pre-*JAK2* founding clone or due to parallel expansion of a distinct hematopoietic clone (Theocharides et al. 2007). Post-MPN AML with mutated *JAK2* typically proceeds through an accelerated myelofibrosis phase, while post-MPN AML that no longer harbors a *JAK2* mutation tends to arise from the chronic phase disease and may be associated with the use of cytotoxic therapies (Iurlo et al. 2019).

Prior to the introduction of tyrosine kinase inhibitors (TKI) for chronic myeloid leukemia (CML), patients with CML typically progressed from chronic phase to the blast phase within 5 years, at a rate of over 20% per year. Most cases of blast phase CML have a myeloid phenotype, while approximately 30% of patients have a lymphoid phenotype. Additional mutations may occur during transformation of CML, and approximately 80% of patients have additional cytogenetic abnormalities, such as duplication of the Philadelphia chromosome, and trisomies that are recurrent in de novo AML. Up to one-third of patients with CML in the myeloid blast phase harbor mutations in the tumor suppressor gene *TP53* (Hehlmann 2012). Additionally, *BCR-ABL* signaling upregulates transcription factors implicated in AML pathogenesis, for example, *EVI1*, which may contribute to leukemic transformation. Underscoring the continued requirement for *BCR-ABL1* signaling in CML evolution, the rate of transformation to blast phase CML in the TKI era has decreased markedly to approximately 1% per year (Jain et al. 2017).

Approximately one-third of patients with MDS progress to secondary AML, although this varies significantly according to the underlying MDS subtype and disease characteristics, including the percentage of bone marrow blasts, presence of characteristic cytogenetic abnormalities, and degree of cytopenia and fibrosis in the bone marrow. Progression to AML is associated with the acquisition of additional somatic mutations as well as epigenetic alterations within the MDS clone. Mutations in transcription factors and cytokine signaling genes, including *RUNX1*, *NRAS*, and *ETV6*, are more common at progression to sAML, compared with the frequency of these mutations at MDS diagnosis. Mutations in *RUNX1* are enriched in populations with tAML and other forms of sAML. Epigenetic modifications of the MDS genome appear to also play a significant role in AML progression, particularly through DNA methylation-mediated silencing of tumor suppressor genes (Brunner and Graubert 2018).

## References


Abelson S, Collord G, Ng SW et al (2018) Prediction of acute myeloid leukaemia risk in healthy individuals. Nature 559(7714):400–404

Allan JM, Wild CP, Rollinson S et al (2001) Polymorphism in glutathione S-transferase P1 is associated with susceptibility to chemotherapy-induced leukemia. Proc Natl Acad Sci U S A 98(20):11592

Arber DA, Orazi A, Hasserjian R et al (2016) The 2016 revision to the World Health Organization classification of myeloid neoplasms and acute leukemia. Blood 127(20):2391–2405

Babushok DV, Bessler M, Olson TS (2016) Genetic predisposition to myelodysplastic syndrome and acute myeloid leukemia in children and young adults. Leuk Lymphoma 57(3):520–536

Bachas C, Schuurhuis GJ, Hollink IH et al (2010) High-frequency type I/II mutational shifts between diagnosis and relapse are associated with outcome in pediatric AML: implications for personalized medicine. Blood 116(15):2752

Bhatnagar UB, Singh D, Glazyrin A, Moormeier J (2016) Paclitaxel induced MDS and AML: a case report and literature review. Case Rep Oncol Med 2016:8308179

Bizzozero OJ Jr, Johnson KG, Ciocco A (1966) Radiation-related leukemia in Hiroshima and Nagasaki, 1946–1964. I. Distribution, incidence and appearance time. N Engl J Med 274(20):1095

Blokzij F, de Ligt J, Jager M et al (2016) Tissue-specific mutation accumulation in human adult stem cells during life. Nature 538:260–264

Bocker MT, Hellwig I, Breiling A et al (2011) Genome-wide promoter DNA methylation dynamics of human hematopoietic progenitor cells during differentiation and aging. Blood 117(19):e182–e189

Boddu PC, Zeidan AM (2019) Myeloid disorders after autoimmune disease. Best Pract Res Clin Haematol 32(1):74–88

Bolton KL, Ptashkin RN, Gao T, et al (2019) Oncologic therapy shapes the fitness landscape of clonal hematopoiesis. https://www.biorxiv.org/content/10.1101/848739v1, https://doi.org/10.1101/848739

Brown AL, Churpek JE, Malcovati L et al (2017) Recognition of familial myeloid neoplasia in adults. Semin Hematol 54(2):60–68

Brunner AM, Graubert TA (2018) Genomics in childhood acute myeloid leukemia comes of age. Nat Med 24(1):7–9. https://doi.org/10.1038/nm.4469

Bullinger L, Dohner K, Dohner H (2017) Genomics of acute myeloid leukemia diagnosis and pathways. J Clin Oncol 35:934–946

Cancer Research UK 2020. https://www.cancerresearchuk.org/

Castillo JJ, Reagan JL, Ingham RR et al (2012) Obesity but not overweight increases the incidence and

mortality of leukemia in adults: a meta-analysis of prospective cohort studies. Leuk Res 36(7):868–875
Cerquozzi S, Tefferi A (2015) Blast transformation and fibrotic progression in polycythemia vera and essential thrombocythemia: a literature review of incidence and risk factors. Blood Cancer J 5:e366
Chakraborty S, Sun CL, Francisco L et al (2009) Accelerated telomere shortening precedes development of therapy-related myelodysplasia or acute myelogenous leukemia after autologous transplantation for lymphoma. J Clin Oncol 27(5):791
Chen X, Pan J, Wang S et al (2019) The epidemiological trend of acute myeloid leukemia in childhood: a population-based analysis. J Cancer 10(20):4824–4845. https://doi.org/10.7150/jca.32326
Cypris O, Božić T, Wagner W (2019) Chicken or egg: is clonal hematopoiesis primarily caused by genetic or epigenetic aberrations? Front Genet 10:785
Dale D, Person R, Bolyard A et al (2000) Mutations in the gene encoding neutrophil elastase in congenital and cyclic neutropenia. Blood 96:2317–2322
Daniels RD, Schubauer-Berigan MK (2011) A meta-analysis of leukaemia risk from protracted exposure to low-dose gamma radiation. Occup Environ Med 68:457–464
Desai P, Mencia-Trinchant N, Savenkov O et al (2018) Somatic mutations precede acute myeloid leukemia years before diagnosis. Nat Med 24(7):1015–1023
Deschler B, Lübbert M (2006) Acute myeloid leukemia: epidemiology and etiology. Cancer 107:2099–2107
DiNardo CD, Ogdie A, Hexner EO et al (2013) Characteristics and outcome of acute myeloid leukemia in patients with a prior history of autoimmune disease. Leuk Lymphoma 54(6):1235–1241
Dinmohamed AG, Visser O (2019) Incidence of acute promyelocytic leukemia across Europe: results of RARECAREnet—a population-based study. Stem Cell Invest 6:37. https://doi.org/10.21037/sci.2019.10.03
Döhner H, Weisdorf DJ, Bloomfield CD (2015) Acute myeloid leukemia. N Engl J Med 73:1136–1152
Ertz-Archambault N, Kosiorek H, Taylor GE et al (2017) Association of therapy for autoimmune disease with myelodysplastic syndromes and acute myeloid leukemia. JAMA Oncol 3(7):936–943
Fircanis S, Merriam P, Khan N, Castillo JJ (2014) The relation between cigarette smoking and risk of acute myeloid leukemia: an updated meta-analysis of epidemiological studies. Am J Hematol 89(8):E125–E132
Foreman KJ, Marquez N, Dolgert A et al (2018) Forecasting life expectancy, years of life lost, and all-cause and cause-specific mortality for 250 causes of death: reference and alternative scenarios for 2016-40 for 195 countries and territories. Lancet 392:2052–2090
Gao J, Gong S, Chen YH (2019) Myeloid neoplasm with germline predisposition: a 2016 update for pathologists. Arch Pathol Lab Med 143(1):13–22
Genovese G, Kahler AK, Handsaker RE et al (2014) Clonal hematopoiesis and blood-cancer risk inferred from blood DNA sequence. N Engl J Med 371:2477–2487
Gillis NK, Ball M, Zhang Q et al (2017) Clonal haemopoiesis and therapy-related myeloid malignancies in elderly patients: a proof-of-concept, case-control study. Lancet Oncol 18(1):112–121
Godley LA, Shimamura A (2017) Genetic predisposition to hematologic malignancies: management and surveillance. Blood 130(4):424–432
Hauptmann M, Stewart PA, Lubin JH et al (2009) Mortality from lymphohematopoietic malignancies and brain cancer among embalmers exposed to formaldehyde. J Natl Cancer Inst 101(24):1696
Hehlmann R (2012) How I treat CML blast crisis. Blood 120(4):737–747
Hernlund E, Redig J, Paulsson B et al (2019) Cost per treatment phase for AML patients receiving high-dose chemotherapy in Sweden. Blood 134(suppl):abstract #2154
Hoffman R et al (2018) Chapter 58—Pathobiology of acute myeloid leukemia. In: Hematology, 7th edition basic principles and practice, p 913–923
Hulegardh E, Nilsson C, Lazarevic V et al (2015) Characterization and prognostic features of secondary acute myeloid leukemia in a population-based setting: a report from the Swedish acute leukemia registry. Am J Hematol 90:208–214
Iurlo A, Cattaneo D, Gianelli U (2019) Blast transformation in myeloproliferative neoplasms: risk factors, biological findings, and targeted therapeutic options. Int J Mol Sci 20(8):1839
Jain P, Kantarjian HM, Ghorab A et al (2017) Prognostic factors and survival outcomes in patients with chronic myeloid leukemia in blast phase in the tyrosine kinase inhibitor era: cohort study of 477 patients. Cancer 123(22):4391–4402
Jaiswal S, Ebert BL (2019) Clonal hematopoiesis in human aging and disease. Science 366:6465
Jalbut MM, Sohani AR, Dal Cin P et al (2015) Acute myeloid leukemia in a patient with constitutional 47, XXY karyotype. Leuk Res Rep 4(1):28–30
Jongmans MC, van der Burgt I, Hoogerbrugge PM et al (2011) Cancer risk in patients with Noonan syndrome carrying a PTPN11 mutation. Eur J Hum Genet 19(8):870–874
Juliusson G, Antunovic P, Derolf A et al (2009) Age and acute myeloid leukemia: real world data on decision to treat and outcomes from the Swedish acute leukemia registry. Blood 113(18):4179–4187
Juliusson G, Abrahamsson J, Lazarevic V et al (2017) Prevalence and characteristics of survivors from acute myeloid leukemia in Sweden. Leukemia 31(3):728–731. https://doi.org/10.1038/leu.2016.312
Juliusson G, Hagberg O, Lazarevic V et al (2019) Improved survival of men 50 to 75 years old with acute myeloid leukemia over a 20-year period. Blood 134(18):1558–1561. https://doi.org/10.1182/blood.2019001728
Juliusson G, Jädersten M, Deneberg S, et al (2020) The prognostic impact of FLT3-ITD and NPM1-mutation in adult AML is age-dependent in the population-based setting. Blood Adv 4(6):1094–1101.

https://doi.org/10.1182/bloodadvances.2019001335. PMID: 32203582
Kayser S, Dohner K, Krauter J et al (2011) The impact of therapy-related acute myeloid leukemia (AML) on outcome in 2853 adult patients with newly diagnosed AML. Blood 117:2137–2145
Kennedy AL, Shimamura A (2019) Genetic predisposition to MDS: clinical features and clonal evolution. Blood 133(10):1071–1085
Keung YK, Buss D, Chauvenet A et al (2002) Hematologic malignancies and Klinefelter syndrome. A chance association? Cancer Genet Cytogenet 139(1):9–13
Klein C (2011) Genetic defects in severe congenital neutropenia: emerging insights into life and death of human neutrophil granulocytes. Annu Rev Immunol 29:399–413
Kostmann R (1956) Infantile genetic agranulocytosis; agranulocytosis infantilis hereditaria. Acta Paediatr Suppl 45:1–78
Kristinsson SY, Björkholm M, Hultcrantz M et al (2011) Chronic immune stimulation might act as a trigger for the development of acute myeloid leukemia or myelodysplastic syndromes. J Clin Oncol 29(21):2897–2903
Lazarevic VL, Bredberg A, Lorenz F et al (2018) Acute myeloid leukemia in very old patients. Haematologica 103(12):e578–e580. https://doi.org/10.3324/haematol.2018.196691
Le Beau MM, Albain KS, Larson RA et al (1986) Clinical and cytogenetic correlations in 63 patients with therapy-related myelodysplastic syndromes and acute nonlymphocytic leukemia: further evidence for characteristic abnormalities of chromosomes no. 5 and 7. J Clin Oncol 4(3):325
Lehmann S, Deneberg S, Antunovic P et al (2017) Early death rates remain high in high-risk APL. Update from the Swedish acute leukemia registry 1997-2013. Leukemia 31(6):1457–1459. https://doi.org/10.1038/leu.2017.71
Leuraud K, Richardson DB, Cardis E et al (2015) Ionising radiation and risk of death from leukaemia and lymphoma in radiation-monitored workers (INWORKS): an international cohort study. Lancet Haematol 2(7):e276–e281
Lewinsohn M, Brown AL, Weinel LM et al (2016) Novel germ line DDX41 mutations define families with a lower age of MDS/AML onset and lymphoid malignancies. Blood 127(8):1017–1023
Lin Y, Zheng Y, Wang ZC, Wang SY (2016) Prognostic significance of ASXL1 mutations in myelodysplastic syndromes and chronic myelomonocytic leukemia: a meta-analysis. Hematology 21:454–461
Lindsley RC, Mar BG, Mazzola E et al (2015) Acute myeloid leukemia ontogeny is defined by distinct somatic mutations. Blood 125(9):1367–1376
Lyman GH, Dale DC, Wolff DA et al (2010) Acute myeloid leukemia or myelodysplastic syndrome in randomized controlled clinical trials of cancer chemotherapy with granulocyte colony-stimulating factor: a systematic review. J Clin Oncol 28:2914–2924
Maynadie M, Girodon F, Manivet-Janoray I et al (2011) Twenty-five years of epidemiological recording on myeloid malignancies: data from the specialized registry of hematologic malignancies of Côte d'Or (Burgundy, France). Haematologica 96(1):55–61. https://doi.org/10.3324/haematol.2010.026252
Mejia-Ramirez E, Florian MC (2020) Understanding intrinsic hematopoietic stem cells aging. Haemato logica 105(1):22–37. pii: haematol.2018.211342
Mucci LA, Granath F, Cnattingius S (2004) Maternal smoking and childhood leukemia and lymphoma risk among 1,440,542 Swedish children. Cancer Epidemiol Biomark Prev 13:1528–1533
Nardi V, Winkfield KM, Ok CY et al (2012) Acute myeloid leukemia and myelodysplastic syndromes after radiation therapy are similar to denovo disease and differ from other therapy-related myeloid neoplasms. J Clin Oncol 30(19):2340–2347
Nilsson C, et al (2020) Manuscript in preparation
NORDCAN (Association of the Nordic Cancer Registries) (2020). http://www-dep.iarc.fr/NORDCAN.htm
Ohnishi H, Imataki O, Kawachi Y et al (2014) Age is an independent adverse prognostic factor for overall survival in acute myeloid leukemia in Japan. World J Hematol 3(3):105–114
Østgård LSG, Nørgaard JM, Sengeløv H et al (2015) Comorbidity and performance status in acute myeloid leukemia patients: a nation-wide population-based cohort study. Leukemia 29:548–555. https://doi.org/10.1038/leu.2014.234
Østgård LSG, Nørgaard M, Pedersen L et al (2018) Autoimmune diseases, infections, use of antibiotics and the risk of acute myeloid leukaemia: a national population-based case-control study. Br J Haematol 181(2):205–214
Pedersen-Bjergaard J, Philip P (1991) Two different classes of therapy-related and de-novo acute myeloid leukemia? Cancer Genet Cytogenet 55(1):119–124
Polednak AP (2014) Recent improvement in completeness of incidence data on acute myeloid leukemia in US cancer registries. J Registry Manag 41(2):77–84
Poynter JN, Richardson M, Blair CK et al (2016) Obesity over the life course and risk of acute myeloid leukemia and myelodysplastic syndromes. Cancer Epidemiol 40:134–140
Reilly JT (2005) Pathogenesis of acute myeloid leukaemia and inv(16)(p13;q22): a paradigm for understanding leukaemogenesis? Br J Haematol 128(1):18–34
Roman E, Smith A, Appleton S et al (2016) Myeloid malignancies in the real-world: occurrence, progression and survival in the UK's population-based Haematological Malignancy Research Network 2004-15. Cancer Epidemiol 42:186–198
Rose D, Haferlach T, Schnittger S et al (2017) Subtype-specific patterns of molecular mutations in acute myeloid leukemia. Leukemia 31:11–17
Rosenberg P, Zeidler C, Bolyard A et al (2010) Stable long-term risk of leukaemia in patients with severe congenital neutropenia maintained on G-CSF therapy. Br J Haematol 150:196–199

Sallman DA, Komrokji R, Cluzeau T et al (2017) ASXL1 frameshift mutations drive inferior outcomes in CMML without negative impact in MDS. Blood Cancer J 7:633

Schanz J, Cevik N, Fonatsch C et al (2018) Detailed analysis of clonal evolution and cytogenetic evolution patterns in patients with myelodysplastic syndromes (MDS) and related myeloid disorders. Blood Cancer J 8(3):28

Schnegg-Kaufmann A, Feller A, Baldomero H et al (2018) Improvement of relative survival in elderly patients with acute myeloid leukaemia emerging from population-based cancer registries in Switzerland between 2001 and 2013. Cancer Epidemiol 52:55–62. https://doi.org/10.1016/j.canep.2017.11.008

Schroeder T, Kuendgen A, Kayser S et al (2012) Therapy-related myeloid neoplasms following treatment with radioiodine. Haematologica 97(2):206–212

Sébert M, Passet M, Raimbault A et al (2019) Germline DDX41 mutations define a significant entity within adult MDS/AML patients. Blood 134(17): 1441–1444

Seedhouse C, Russell N (2007) Advances in the understanding of susceptibility to treatment-related acute myeloid leukaemia. Br J Haematol 137(6):513

SEER (2020) Cancer statistics review 1975-2016. https://seer.cancer.gov/csr/1975_2016/browse_csr.php?sectionSEL=13&pageSEL=sect_13_table.08

Seiter K, Qureshi A, Liu D et al (2005) Severe toxicity following induction chemotherapy for acute myelogenous leukemia in a patient with Werner's syndrome. Leuk Lymphoma 46(7):1091–1095

Shallis RM, Wang R, Davidoff A, Ma X, Zeidan AM (2019) Epidemiology of acute myeloid leukemia: recent progress and enduring challenges. Blood Rev 36:70–87. https://doi.org/10.1016/j.blre.2019.04.005

Shand JC (2017) Looking up for AML in Down syndrome. Blood 129(25):3273–3274

Shlush LI (2018) Age-related clonal hematopoiesis. Blood 131(5):496–504

Snyder R (2012) Leukemia and benzene. Int J Environ Res Public Health 9:2875–2893

Sperling AS, Gibson CJ, Ebert BL (2017) The genetics of myelodysplastic syndrome: from clonal haematopoiesis to secondary leukaemia. Nat Rev Cancer 17:5–19

Steensma DP (2018) Clinical consequences of clonal hematopoiesis of indeterminate potential. Hematology 2(22):3404–3410

Steensma DP, Bejar R, Jaiswal S et al (2015) Clonal hematopoiesis of indeterminate potential and its distinction from myelodysplastic syndromes. Blood 126:9–16

Stone RM, Neuberg D, Soiffer R et al (1994) Myelodysplastic syndrome as a late complication following autologous bone marrow transplantation for non-Hodgkin's lymphoma. J Clin Oncol 12(12):2535

Swaminathan M, Bannon SA, Routbort M et al (2019) Hematologic malignancies and Li-Fraumeni syndrome. Cold Spring Harb Mol Case Stud 5(1):a003210

Swerdlow SH, Campo E, Harris NL et al (2017) WHO classification of tumours of haematopoietic and lymphoid tissues. International Agency for Research and Cancer, Lyon

Takahashi K, Wang F, Kantarjian H et al (2017) Preleukaemic clonal haemopoiesis and risk of therapy-related myeloid neoplasms: a case-control study. Lancet Oncol 18(1):100–111

Tawana K, Wang J, Renneville A et al (2015) Disease evolution and outcomes in familial AML with germline CEBPA mutations. Blood 126(10):1214–1223

Tesi B, Davidsson J, Voss M et al (2017) Gain-of-function *SAMD9L* mutations cause a syndrome of cytopenia, immunodeficiency, MDS, and neurological symptoms. Blood 129(16):2266–2279

Theocharides A, Boissinot M, Girodon F et al (2007) Leukemic blasts in transformed JAK2-V617F-positive myeloproliferative disorders are frequently negative for the JAK2-V617F mutation. Blood 110:375–379

Thirman MJ, Gill HJ, Burnett RC et al (1993) Rearrangement of the MLL gene in acute lymphoblastic and acute myeloid leukemias with 11q23 chromosomal translocations. N Engl J Med 329(13):909

Valdez JM, Nichols KE, Kesserwan C (2017) Li-Fraumeni syndrome: a paradigm for the understanding of hereditary cancer predisposition. Br J Haematol 176(4):539–552

Valent P, Kern W, Hoermann G et al (2019) Clonal hematopoiesis with oncogenic potential (CHOP): separation from CHIP and roads to AML. Int J Mol Sci 20(3):789

Van Maele-Fabry G, Gamet-Payrastre L, Lison D (2019) Household exposure to pesticides and risk of leukemia in children and adolescents: updated systematic review and meta-analysis. Int J Hyg Environ Health 222(1):49–67

Vardiman JW, Harris NL, Brunning RD (2002) The World Health Organization (WHO) classification of the myeloid neoplasms. Blood 100:2292–2302

Wilson DB, Link DC, Mason PJ, Bessler M (2014) Inherited bone marrow failure syndromes in adolescents and young adults. Ann Med 46(6):353–363

Wong TN, Ramsingh G, Young AL et al (2015) Role of TP53 mutations in the origin and evolution of therapy-related acute myeloid leukaemia. Nature 518(7540):552–555

Yoshinaga S, Mabuchi K, Sigurdson AJ et al (2004) Cancer risks among radiologists and radiologic technologists: review of epidemiologic studies. Radiology 233:313–321

Zhu J, Wang H, Yang S et al (2013) Comparison of toxicity of benzene metabolite hydroquinone in hematopoietic stem cells derived from murine embryonic yolk sac and adult bone marrow. PLoS One 8(8):e71153

# Diagnosis and Classification of AML: WHO 2016

# 2

Maria Teresa Voso, Eleonora De Bellis, and Tiziana Ottone

## 2.1 Introduction

Acute myeloid leukemia (AML) is the most common acute hematological malignancy in adults, with an estimated annual incidence rate of 4.2/100000 persons/year (5.2 in males and 3.5 in females) (data from SEER 2016) (Arber et al. 2016; Papaemmanuil et al. 2013). AML is a disease of the elderly, with a median age of 68 years at diagnosis. Recently, significant improvements have been made in the understanding of AML biology and genetics, and in 2016, the World Health Organization (WHO) published an update of the classification of myeloid neoplasms and acute leukemias, integrating clinical features, morphology, immunophenotype, and cytogenetics with new molecular genetic alterations to better define disease entities (Arber et al. 2016). The complete 2016 WHO classification of AML is reported in Table 2.1.

In the last few decades, efforts have been made to study the genomic landscape of AML: the result is a progressive shift from a morphologic classification, to one based on genetic/cytogenetic profiles, also taking into consideration the impact of genetic lesions on prognosis (Papaemmanuil et al. 2013). On this basis, first in 2010 and later in 2017, an international working

M. T. Voso (✉) · E. De Bellis · T. Ottone
Department of Biomedicine and Prevention, University of Tor Vergata, Rome, Italy
e-mail: Voso@med.uniroma2.it

**Table 2.1** The 2016 revision of WHO classification of acute myeloid leukemia and acute leukemias of ambiguous lineage (Arber et al. 2016)

| Acute myeloid leukemia with recurrent genetic abnormalities | Myeloid sarcoma |
|---|---|
| AML with t(8;21)(q22;q22.1);*RUNX1-RUNX1T1* | **Myeloid proliferations related to Down syndrome** |
| AML with inv(16)(p13.1q22) or t(16;16)(p13.1;q22);*CBFB-MYH11* | Transient abnormal myelopoiesis (TAM) |
| APL with *PML-RARA* | Myeloid leukemia associated with Down syndrome |
| AML with t(9;11)(p21.3;q23.3);*MLLT3-KMT2A* | **Blastic plasmacytoid dendritic cell neoplasm** |
| AML with t(6;9)(p23;q34.1);*DEK-NUP214* | **Acute leukemias of ambiguous lineage** |
| AML with inv(3)(q21.3q26.2) or t(3;3)(q21.3;q26.2);*GATA2, MECOM* | Acute undifferentiated leukemia |
| AML (megakaryoblastic) with t(1;22)(p13.3;q13.3);*RBM15-MKL1* | Mixed-phenotype acute leukemia with t(9;22)(q34.1;q11.2);*BCR-ABL1* |
| AML with mutated NPM1 | Mixed-phenotype acute leukemia with t(v;11q23.3); *KMT2A*-reananged |
| AML with biallelic mutations of *CEBPA* | Mixed-phenotype acute leukemia, B/myeloid, NOS |

(continued)



C. Röllig, G. J. Ossenkoppele (eds.), *Acute Myeloid Leukemia*, Hematologic Malignancies,
https://doi.org/10.1007/978-3-030-72676-8_2

**Table 2.1** (continued)

| Acute myeloid leukemia with recurrent genetic abnormalities | Myeloid sarcoma |
|---|---|
| Provisional entity: AML with *BCR-ABL1* | Mixed-phenotype acute leukemia, T/myeloid, NOS |
| Provisional entity: AML with mutated *RUNX1* | Mixed-phenotype acute leukemia, NOS, rare types |
| **Acute myeloid leukemia with myelodysplasia-related changes** | Acute leukemias of ambiguous lineage, NOS |
| **Therapy-related myeloid neoplasms** | |
| **Acute myeloid leukemia, not otherwise specified (NOS)** | |
| AML with minimal differentiation | |
| AML without maturation | |
| AML with maturation | |
| Acute myelomonocytic leukemia | |
| Acute monoblastic/monocytic leukemia | |
| Pure erythroid leukemia | |
| Acute megakaryoblastic leukemia | |
| Acute basophilic leukemia | |
| Acute panmyelosis with myelofibrosis | |

**Table 2.2** Risk stratification of AML, based on genetic/cytogenetic profile (European Leukemia Net 2017), adapted from Dohner et al. (Dohner et al. 2017)

| Risk category | Genetic abnormality |
|---|---|
| Favorable | t(8;21)(q22;q22.1); *RUNX1-RUNX1T1* |
| | inv(16)(p13.1q22) or t(16;16)(p13.1;q22); *CBFB-MYH11* |
| | Mutated *NPM1* without *FLT3*-ITD or with *FLT3*-ITD$^{\text{low}}$[a] |
| | Biallelic mutated *CEBPA* |
| Intermediate | Mutated *NPM1* and *FLT3*-ITD$^{\text{high}}$[a] |
| | Wild-type *NPM1* without *FLT3*-ITD or with *FLT3*-ITD$^{\text{low}}$[a] (without adverse-risk genetic lesions) |
| | t(9;11)(p21.3;q23.3); *MLLT3-KMT2A*[b] |
| | Cytogenetic abnormalities not classified as favorable or adverse |
| Adverse | t(6;9)(p23;q34.1); *DEK-NUP214* |
| | t(v;11q23.3); *KMT2A*-rearranged |
| | t(9;22)(q34.1;q11.2); *BCR-ABL1* |
| | inv(3)(q21.3q26.2) or t(3;3)(q21.3;q26.2); *GATA2,MECOM(EVI1)* |
| | −5 or del(5q); −7; −17/abn(17p) |
| | Complex karyotype,[c] monosomal karyotype[d] |
| | Wild-type *NPM1* and *FLT3*-ITDhigh[a] |
| | Mutated *RUNX1*[e] |
| | Mutated *ASXL1*[e] |
| | Mutated *TP53*[f] |

[a]Low, low allelic ratio (<0.5); high, high allelic ratio (≥0.5)

[b]The presence of t(9;11)(p21.3;q23.3) takes precedence over rare, concurrent adverse-risk gene mutations

[c]Three or more unrelated chromosome abnormalities in the absence of one of the WHO-designated recurring translocations or inversions, that is, t(8;21), inv(16) or t(16;16), t(9;11), t(v;11)(v;q23.3), t(6;9), inv(3) or t(3;3); AML with *BCR-ABL1*

[d]Defined by the presence of 1 single monosomy (excluding loss of X or Y) in association with at least 1 additional monosomy or structural chromosome abnormality (excluding core-binding factor AML)

[e]These markers should not be used as an adverse prognostic marker if they co-occur with favorable-risk AML subtypes

[f]*TP53* mutations are significantly associated with complex and monosomal karyotype AML

group, on behalf of the European Leukemia Net (*ELN*), drew a risk-stratification model based on genetic and cytogenetic characteristics, that divided AML in three categories: favorable, intermediate, and adverse (Table 2.2) (Dohner et al. 2017). The 2017 update was required by the advancements in the definition of the mutational landscape in AML (Fig. 2.1), as well as by the development of novel antileukemic agents (Stone et al. 2017; Heuser et al. 2019; Döhner et al. 2010). Correct patient and disease stratification requires an integrated diagnostic process, including evaluation of morphology, immunophenotype, cytogenetics, and molecular changes. This is particularly important in the context of a modern personalized medicine approach, which is facilitated by the recent identification of targeted treatments. This applies also in cases of relapsed or refractory AML, where the same diagnostic algorithm must be used, due to the possibility of clonal evolution and emergence of "new" genetic alterations. Often, these alterations may be present at the time of initial diagnosis at the subclonal

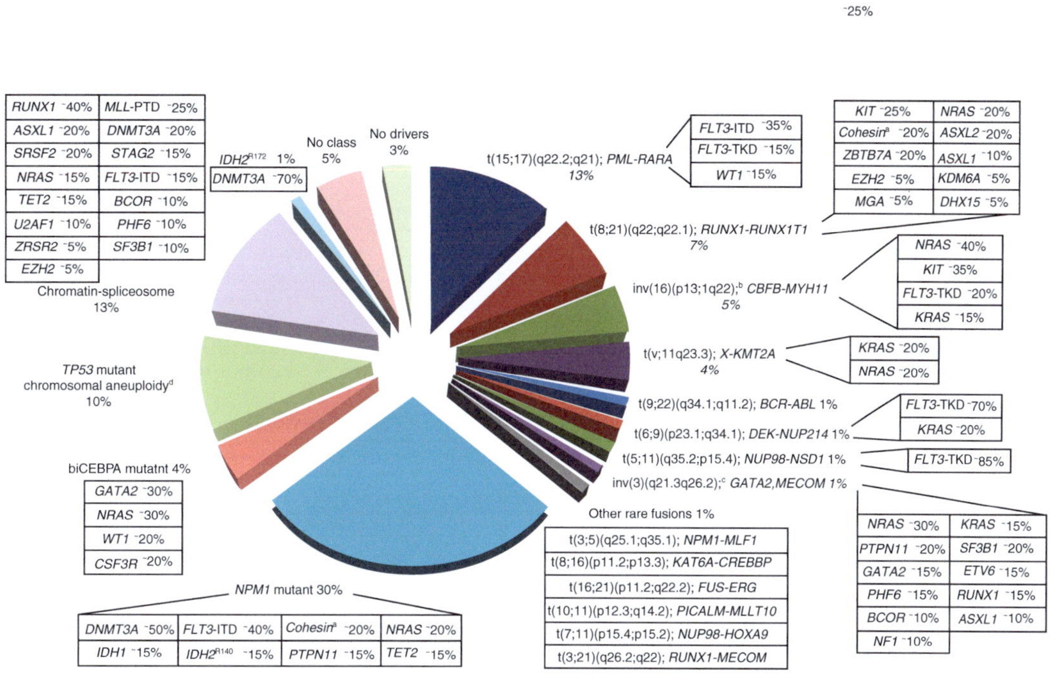


**Fig. 2.1** Molecular classes of AML and concurrent gene mutations in adult patients. (From Dohner et al. 2017)

level, undetectable by conventional approaches (Ottone et al. 2013; Angelini et al. 2015).

In this chapter, we will discuss recent guidelines for the diagnostic and prognostic stratification of AML. Diagnosis and monitoring of acute promyelocytic leukemia (APL) will be treated in a separate paragraph, due to the distinct clinical characteristics of this AML subtype, and the indications for prompt diagnosis and treatment start.

## 2.2 Diagnostic Procedures for AML Diagnosis

Figure 2.2 shows an algorithm for AML diagnosis.

### 2.2.1 Morphology

Morphology remains the basic diagnostic tool to assess the number and morphology of blasts in peripheral blood (PB) and bone marrow (BM). Starting from 2001, according to the WHO classification system, the diagnosis of AML requires ≥20% myeloblasts in the BM or PB, with some exceptions (Arber et al. 2016). Morphological evaluation of the BM aspirate or trephine biopsy, in cases with a dry tap (punctio sicca), represents the first indispensable tools for the routine diagnostic work-up for patients with a suspected AML. Marrow or PB smears are examined following May-Grünwald-Giemsa or Wright-Giemsa staining (Piaton et al. 2015). Myeloblasts, monoblasts, and megakaryoblasts must be included in the blast count. In AML with monocytic differentiation, monoblasts and promonocytes are counted as blast equivalents. The diagnosis of AML requires a BM blast count of 20% or more, except for AML with t(15;17), t(8;21), and inv(16), or t(16;16). In these AML subtypes, the genetic abnormality defines AML also in cases with BM blasts <20%. To identify lineage involvement, immunophenotyping is used with evaluation of myeloid differentiation markers, including myeloperoxidase (MPO). Cytochemistry with staining for nonspecific esterase (NSE), together with expression of lysozyme and monocytic markers, is required in cases with a mixed-phenotype AML (Grimwade 2001).

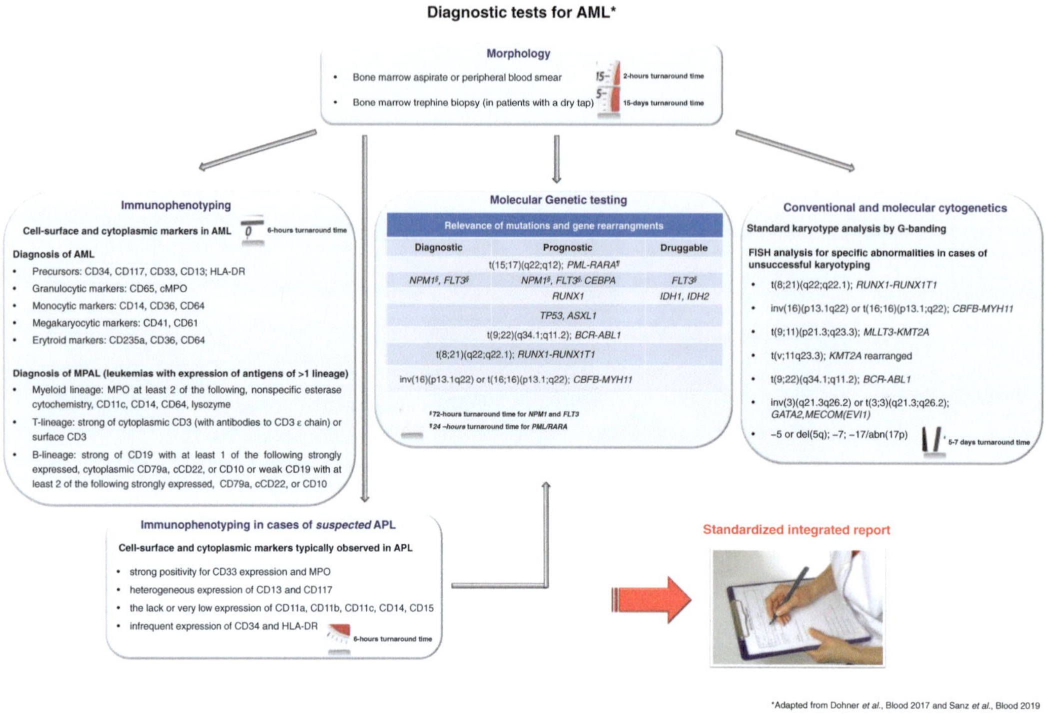


**Fig. 2.2** Diagnostic tests required for AML (Adapted from Dohner et al. 2017)

## 2.2.2 Immunophenotyping

Immunophenotyping using multiparameter flow cytometry (MFC) is a powerful tool to characterize cell surface and cytoplasmic markers, essential features for classification of AML subtypes. Common leucocyte antigen (CD45) and side scatter (SSC) gating are used to identify the blast population, (Borowitz et al. 1993) while expression of other lineage specific markers is useful for the phenotypic characterization of the blast population. The recommended panel includes the following antibodies: CD34, HLA-DR, TdT (stem cell/hematopoietic precursors), cMPO, CD13, CD33, CD117, CD15 (myeloid markers), monocytic markers (CD64, CD14, CD11b,CD11c), erythroid (CD71, CD235a), and megakaryocytic markers (CD41, CD61, CD36) (Venditti et al. 2019; Buccisano et al. 2018a; Maurillo et al. 2008). In addition, MFC is to identify monoblastic/monocytic AML (CD14+, CD64+, and CD36+), acute megakaryoblastic leukemia (CD41+ and CD61+), and pure erythroid leukemia (CD235a+ or CD36+ in the absence of CD64, MPO, or other myeloid-associated antigens) (Fig. 2.2) (Dohner et al. 2017; Del Principe et al. 2019).

## 2.2.3 Conventional and Molecular Cytogenetics

The WHO first added cytogenetic features to classify AML in 2001, while molecular subtypes were included in 2008 (Vardiman et al. 2009), in addition to morphologic and immunophenotypic features (Arber et al. 2016). The identification of recurrent cytogenetic abnormalities is mandatory for the diagnosis of AML, to define AML subtypes and prognostic groups, and to correctly address therapeutic strategies (Dohner et al. 2017; O'Donnell et al. 2013; Grimwade et al. 2010). Techniques used for cytogenetic analysis include karyotyping, analysis of G-banded chromosomes, and other cytogenetic banding techniques (Fig. 2.3a, b), such as fluorescent in situ

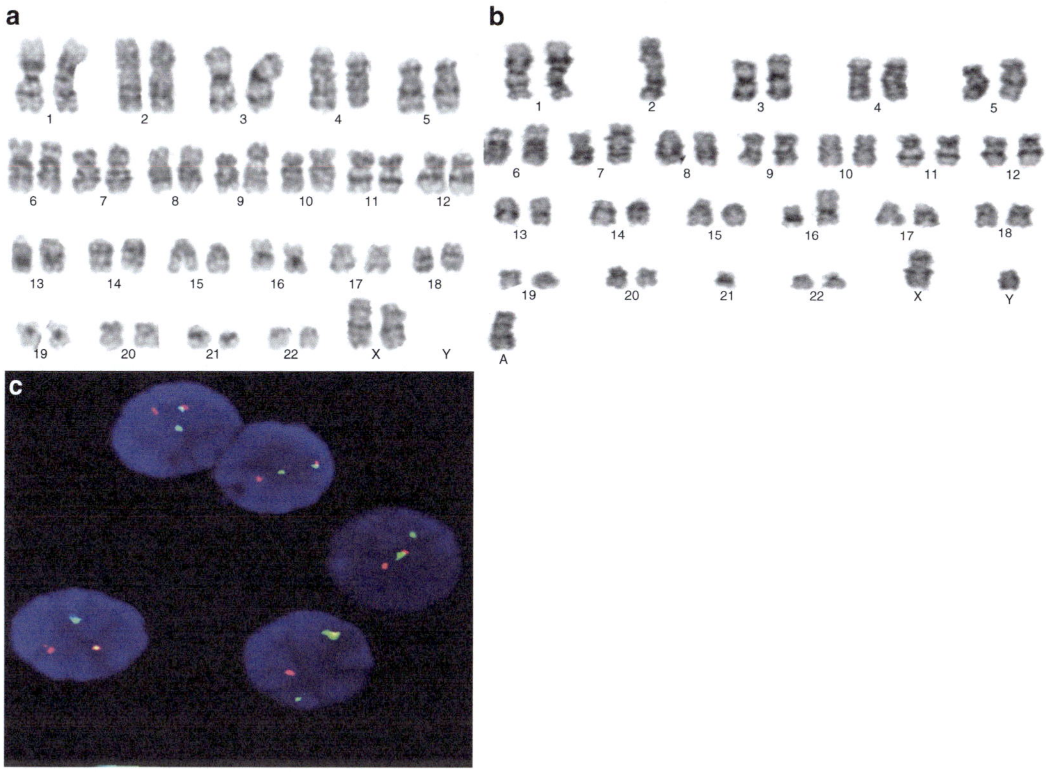


**Fig. 2.3** Cytogenetic analysis in AML. (**a**) G-banding of a cytogenetically *normal* male karyotype (46,XY). (**b**) G-banded analysis in a patient with complex karyotype (45,XY,-2,der(2)t(2;?),der(7)t(7;?),der(16)t(16;?),-21,+mar). (**c**) Interphase FISH showing a fusion signal between chromosome 15 and 17 in a patient with APL. The *PML* gene on chromosome 15 is labeled red, the *RARA* gene on chromosome 17 is labelled green and the *PML/RARA* fusion gene is yellow. Cells were counterstained with DAPI II

hybridization (FISH) (Fig. 2.3c). In AML, chromosome abnormalities are detected in approximately 55% of patients (Grimwade 2001; Mrozek et al. 2004) and eight recurrent balanced translocations and inversions are recognized in the WHO category "AML with recurrent genetic abnormalities" (Arber et al. 2016) (Table 2.1). A minimum of 20 metaphases are required to define normal or abnormal karyotype. If the cytogenetic analysis fails, FISH is an optional approach to detect translocations, *gene* rearrangements, and partial or complete chromosome losses (Fig. 2.2). AML with inv(3)(q21q26.2) or t(3;3)(q21;q26.2) has been recently included in the WHO classification as a distinct type of leukemia, associated with resistance to conventional chemotherapy (Weisser et al. 2007). A new provisional entity "AML with *BCR/ABL1*" has been introduced to recognize AML patients with this abnormality, candidates for tyrosine kinase inhibitors. Clinical and molecular factors useful to differentiate AML with *BCR/ABL1* from blast crisis of chronic myeloid leukemia (CML) are shown in Table 2.3.

### 2.2.4 Molecular Genetic Testing

In recent years, due to the availability of advanced technologies, in particular next-generation sequencing (NGS), several somatic mutations in myeloid genes have been identified in AML, some with diagnostic significance, others with prognostic or therapeutic relevance. The role of modern diagnostic in AML is to dissect these profiles, to accurately define individual entities, targetable by specific inhibitors, in the context of personalized medicine.

**Table 2.3** Biological features of AML with *BCR-ABL1* vs CML in blast crisis (BC)

| | AML with *BCR-ABL1* | CML-Blastic crisis | References |
|---|---|---|---|
| *NPM1*-mut | Present | Absent | Konoplev et al. (2013) |
| *ABL1*-mut | Absent | Present | |
| CD33/CD13/CD34+ | All 9 cases | | Cuneo et al. (1996) |
| Lymphoid-associated markers | 7 of 9 cases | | |
| IgH and/or TCR rearranged | 3 of 4 cases | | |
| Splenomegaly | Rare | Frequent | Soupir et al. (2007) |
| PB-basophilia | Rare | Frequent | |
| BM-cellularity | Low | High | |
| Additional cytogetical abnormalities | Rare | Frequent | |
| Mutations in Ig, TCR, IKZF1, CDKN2A genes | Frequent | Rare | Nacheva et al. (2013), Kang et al. (2016) |

The genetic algorithm of newly diagnosed AML patients according to ELN criteria (Dohner et al. 2017) should include screening by RT-PCR for core-binding factor (CBF) leukemias [AML with t(8;21)(q22;q22.1), with *RUNX1/RUNX1T1* rearrangement or inv(16)(p13.1q22)/t(16;16)(p13.1;q22), with *CBFB/MYH11* rearrangement]. This not only allows for the identification of patients with favorable outcome, but defines the specific rearrangement type, which can be used for measurable residual disease (MRD) monitoring. Indeed, positivity of molecular MRD currently represents a powerful marker to predict early relapse (Corbacioglu et al. 2010; Willekens et al. 2016). In acute promyelocytic leukemia, rapid genetic confirmation of the t(15;17)(q22;q12) translocation (detection of *PML/RARA* fusion transcripts) is mandatory in cases of suspected APL, to allow for a prompt initiation of tailored therapy and supportive care (Sanz et al. 2019). Fatal hemorrhage is the most common cause of early death in patients with APL. To prevent these deaths occurring prior to the start of treatment, individuals with suspected APL should be immediately hospitalized and managed as a medical emergency. The diagnosis must be confirmed at the genetic level by experienced reference laboratories (Sanz et al. 2019). Additional analyses mandatory in all patients, and in particular for those with a normal karyotype, include screening for mutations in *NPM1*, *CEBPA*, *ASLX1*, *TP53*, and *RUNX1* genes, which represent specific prognostic categories in the revised version of the ELN guidelines (Dohner et al. 2017). AML with *NPM1* and *CEBPA* biallelic (bi*CEBPA)* mutations have become full entities, while the new provisional entity "AML with mutated *RUNX1*" has been added.

*NPM1* mutations occur in approximately 30% of adult AML cases, and in 50–60% of AML cases with normal karyotype (NK-AML), which makes *NPM1* mutations the most frequent genetic lesions so far identified in de novo AML (Grisendi et al. 2006; Grimwade et al. 2016; Chang and Olson 1990). AML with *NPM1* mutations has distinctive genetic, immunophenotypic, and clinical features. Therefore, this type of leukemia was recognized as a distinct entity (Arber et al. 2016). Mutations in the *NPM1* gene predict favorable prognosis and represent a well-established marker for MRD-monitoring (Dohner et al. 2005). *NPM1* is a nucleolar phosphoprotein that belongs to the nucleoplasmin/nucleophosmin family of nuclear chaperones (Schmidt-Zachmann et al. 1987; Eirín-López et al. 2006) and maps on chromosome band 5q35 in humans (Chang and Olson 1990). *NPM1* mutations are mostly found in exon 12 of the *NPM1* gene, leading to cytoplasmic expression of the protein (normally found in the nucleolus), due to the generation of a novel nuclear export signal (Falini et al. 2009). Currently, more than 50 different mutations located within exon 12 of the *NPM1* gene have been described, and more than 95% of these involve an insertion of four nucleotides. The mutation types A, B, and D represent about 90% of *NPM1* mutations (Dohner et al. 2005) and the iden-

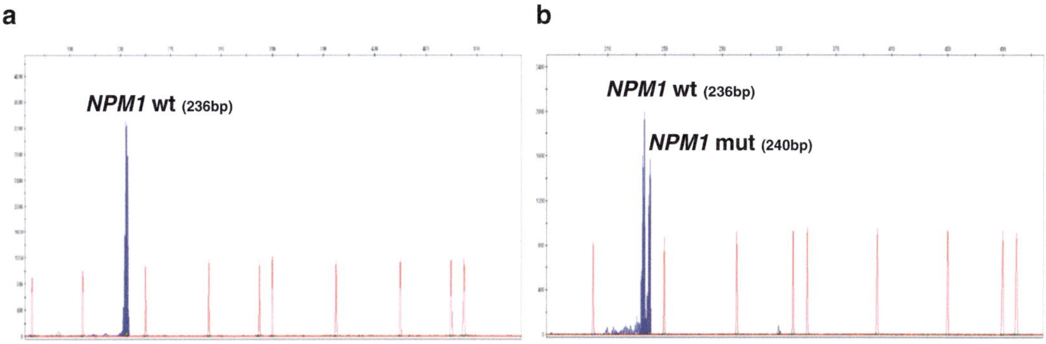


**Fig. 2.4** Genescan electropherograms of PCR reactions for *NPM1* mutations. (**a**) AML with *NPM1* wild-type gene. (**b**) AML mutated for *NPM1*. Normal amplicon sizes of *NPM1* wild-type allele correspond to 236 bp, while an additional PCR fragment amplification with an insertion of 4 bp corresponds to the *NPM1* mutated allele. PCR fragments are shown in blue (FAM) and GENESCAN-400HD (ROX) size markers in red

tification of the specific *NPM1* mutation by Sanger sequencing is particularly important for MRD monitoring. Figure 2.4 shows an example of PCR reaction for the detection of *NPM1* mutations, followed by capillary electrophoresis (Lin et al. 2006).

Other gene mutations are important clinicopathological features of AML. The *FLT3* gene is located on chromosome 13 at band q12 (Rosnet et al. 1991) and encodes for a receptor normally expressed on the surface of hematopoietic progenitor cells, and expression is lost upon cell maturation. *FLT3* is mutated in about 30% of adult AML (Stirewalt et al. 2001). Mutations in this gene result in constitutive activation of signaling through downstream pathways, leading to uncontrolled cell proliferation and survival. Two types of *FLT3* alterations have been reported: *FLT3*-ITD represents the most common mutation and corresponds to an internal tandem duplication (*FLT3*-ITD) in the cytoplasmic juxtamembrane (JM) region (exons 14 and 15) of the gene. The other *FLT3* mutation is located in the tyrosine kinase domain (*FLT3*-TKD), is located in the activation loop of FLT3, and includes the D835 point mutations or deletions of I836 (Gary Gilliland and Griffin 2002) (exon 20). Size of duplicated nucleotides in *FLT3*-ITD mutations vary from three to more than 400 base pairs, and are in-frame mutations caused by the duplication of various fragments from the JM *domain* of the FLT3 receptor. The FLT3-ITD receptor can homodimerize with mutant receptors or heterodimerize with wild-type receptors, independent of ligand stimulation, leading to distinct signaling responses to the ligand depending on the ratio of the wild-type to the mutant receptors (Gary Gilliland and Griffin 2002). Since the mutation is in-frame, the protein kinase domain remains functional (Kiyoi et al. 2002; Stirewalt and Radich 2003). Identification of the *FLT3*-ITD and TKD mutations requires a semi-quantitative assessment, using PCR followed by fragment length analysis are amplified by PCR (Thiede et al. 2002). Figure 2.5 shows representative electropherograms of *FLT3*-ITD, *FLT3*-TKD, and *FLT3* wild-type cases. Testing for FLT3-ITD and -TKD mutations is recommended by the ELN due to the unfavorable prognosis of these patients, who have increased risk of relapse and shorter overall survival (OS), as compared with patients without these mutations. Outcome in *FLT3*-ITD-positive patients is particularly unfavorable in cases with high allelic burden, who benefit from intensive consolidation treatments (Stone et al. 2017; Stirewalt and Radich 2003; Gale et al. 2008). For this reason, in addition to the presence of *FLT3*-ITD, which defines an adverse AML subtype in the 2010 edition of the ELN classification (Döhner et al. 2010), the revised ELN guidelines proposed that the *FLT3*-ITD allelic ratio (AR) is used for AML stratification, in particular in *NPM1*-mutated patients (Table 2.2). In these patients, a *low FLT3*-ITD AR (below 0.5) defines favorable risk AMLs,

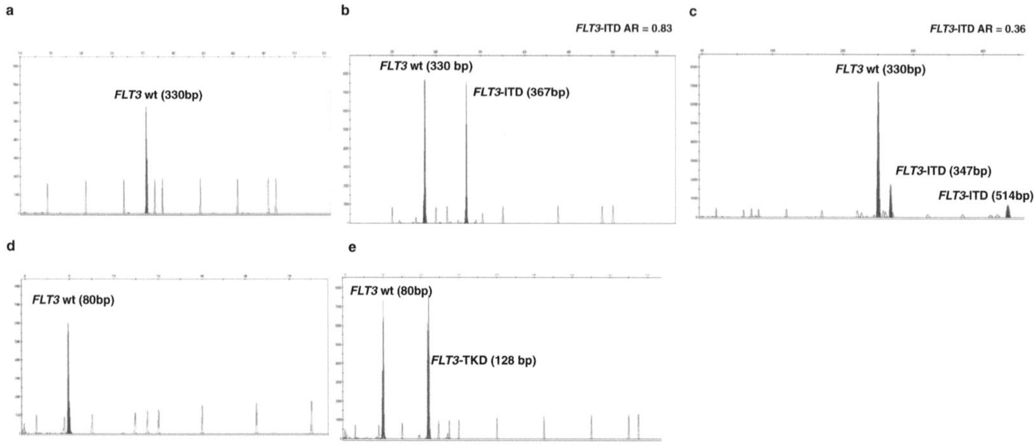


**Fig. 2.5** Genescan electropherograms of PCR reactions for *FLT3* mutations. (**a**) AML without the *FLT3*-ITD mutation. Normal amplicon sizes of *FLT3* wild-type allele correspond to 330 bp. (**b**) AML mutated for *FLT3*-ITD. An additional PCR fragment amplification of a mutated allele corresponding to 367 bp. The *FLT3*-ITD allelic ratio (AR) in this case is 0.83. (**c**) AML with two *FLT3*-ITD mutations. Additional PCR fragments amplification of two mutated alleles corresponding to 347 and 514 bp. The *FLT3*-ITD AR is 0.36 in this case. (**d**) AML without a *FLT3*-TKD mutation. Normal amplicon sizes of *FLT3* wild-type allele correspond to 80 bp. (**e**) AML mutated for *FLT3*-TKD. An additional PCR fragment amplification of a mutated allele corresponding to 128 bp

while a *high FLT3*-ITD AR (≥0.5) is associated with increasingly unfavorable prognosis, defining intermediate-risk AML if it is associated with *NPM1* mutations and high-risk AML if *NPM1* is wild-type. In addition to *FLT3*-ITD mutations, ELN also recommends that *FLT3*-TKD mutations at codons D835 and I836 should be assessed, although the prognostic impact of these mutations is less clear. Identification of *FLT3* mutations is not only of prognostic relevance, but these mutations may be targeted with the FLT3 tyrosine kinase inhibitor, as midostaurin and quizartinib (Stone et al. 2017; Perl 2019), which have significantly improved the outcome of these patients (Sutamtewagul and Vigil 2018).

*CEBPA* is a transcription factor upregulated during granulocytic differentiation (Koschmieder et al. 2009). Mutations in the *CEBPA* gene are reported in ~10–15% of NK-AML patients (Fasan et al. 2014) and may occur on the entire coding region. However, several studies showed an in-frame-shift mutation cluster in the N-terminal domain and in-frame insertions/deletions in the C-terminal region of the gene (Fasan et al. 2014). The mutated CEBPA protein inhibits the function of the full-length protein by a dominant negative mechanism and disrupt its DNA-binding ability. *CEPBA*-mutation may occur as single (single-mutated *CEPBA*sm) or as double (double-mutated *CEPBA, CEBPA*dm) events, in the N-terminal and C-terminal domains of the gene. When the mutations are biallelic, wild-type *CEBPA* is not expressed. Several reports showed a significantly improved outcome of patients with *CEPBA*dm as compared with *CEPBA*sm, and only biallelic *CEBPA* mutations define a distinct genetic entity (Fasan et al. 2014). Mutational analysis of *CEBPA* requires PCR sequencing of the entire *CEBPA* coding region, using four overlapping primer pairs. Technical details have been reported elsewhere (Frohling et al. 2004).

The *RUNX1* gene encodes for a myeloid transcription factor involved in the regulation differentiation of myeloid, megakaryocytic, and lymphocytic lineages (Ichikawa et al. 2004). *RUNX1* is mutated in 10% of de novo AML and is associated with unfavorable overall survival and rapid disease progression (Gaidzik et al. 2011). Missense and nonsense, or frameshift mutations in the *RUNX1* gene have been reported in AML; they are distributed throughout the entire gene and their identification requires a targeted next-generation sequencing (NGS) approach (Kohlmann et al. 2013).

Further gene mutations in combination with chromosome abnormalities are used for risk stratification and therapeutic decisions, and among these, *ASXL1* and *TP53* mutations have been included as adverse prognostic factors in the 2017 ELN recommendations. *ASXL1* is an epigenetic regulator, whose mutations represent early events in leukemogenesis. They have been described in 10% of AML patients (Devillier et al. 2015) and localize in exon 12, resulting in a truncated protein, with loss of the PHD domain (Pratcorona et al. 2012). These alterations are associated with marrow dysgranulopoiesis and have been frequently identified in intermediate-risk AML, where they predict inferior survival (Devillier et al. 2015). *ASLX1* mutations may be investigated by PCR amplification and Sanger sequencing or, more frequently, by NGS (Pratcorona et al. 2012). *TP53* is one of the most frequently mutated genes in human cancers, with a central role in aging, senescence, and DNA repair. In AML, *TP53* alterations are rare events, but are frequently associated with increased genomic instability, as observed in elderly and therapy-related AML/MDS. *TP53* mutations are mostly associated with complex karyotype and predict poor outcome (Devillier et al. 2015). The majority of TP53 mutations are localized in exons 5–8, and NGS analysis is commonly used to investigated the molecular status of the *TP53* gene (Leroy et al. 2013).

Following the discovery of the genomic landscape of AML (Papaemmanuil et al. 2016), other gene alterations have been shown to have prognostic relevance in AML, in particular epigenetic regulators such as *IDH1 and IDH2*. *IDH* mutations are mostly described in the intermediate-risk karyotype, are often associated with *NPM1* mutation, (Abbas et al. 2010) and are mutually exclusive with *TET2* alterations (Gaidzik et al. 2012). Some AML patients with *IDHs* mutations, mainly $IDH2^{R172}$, respond poorly to standard chemotherapy and have a higher relapse rate (Largeaud et al. 2019). *IDH1* and *IDH2* analysis may be performed by Sanger sequencing and Fig. 2.6 shows some electropherograms. Recently, the IDH inhibitors enasidenib and ivosidenib have shown activity in R/R AML with *IDH2* and *IDH1* mutations, respectively. Therefore, characterization of *IDHs'* molecular status represents an important step toward the use of individualized treatments.

In addition to the identification of novel driver mutations, NGS has highlighted the existence of multiple disease clones within a single AML case. Indeed, the genetic architecture of AML is extremely dynamic, and disease evolution/progression is mainly driven by the phenomenon of clonal evolution, characterized by the expansion/emergence of specific clones during the disease course (Ding et al. 2012; Genovese et al. 2014; Jaiswal et al. 2014). Interestingly, clonal evolution studies also indicate that mutations in genes involved in the regulation of DNA methylation and of chromatin state (i.e., *DNMT3A*, *TET2*, and *ASXL1*) may be present in pre-leukemic stem cells and may persist after therapy, leading to clonal expansion during remission, and eventually disease relapse. Large population-based cohorts have recently identified these pre-leukemic mutations in approximately 10% of elderly and healthy subjects; this phenomenon, termed "clonal hematopoiesis of indeterminate potential" (CHIP), has been associated with increased risks of hematologic neoplasms (Jongen-Lavrencic et al. 2018).

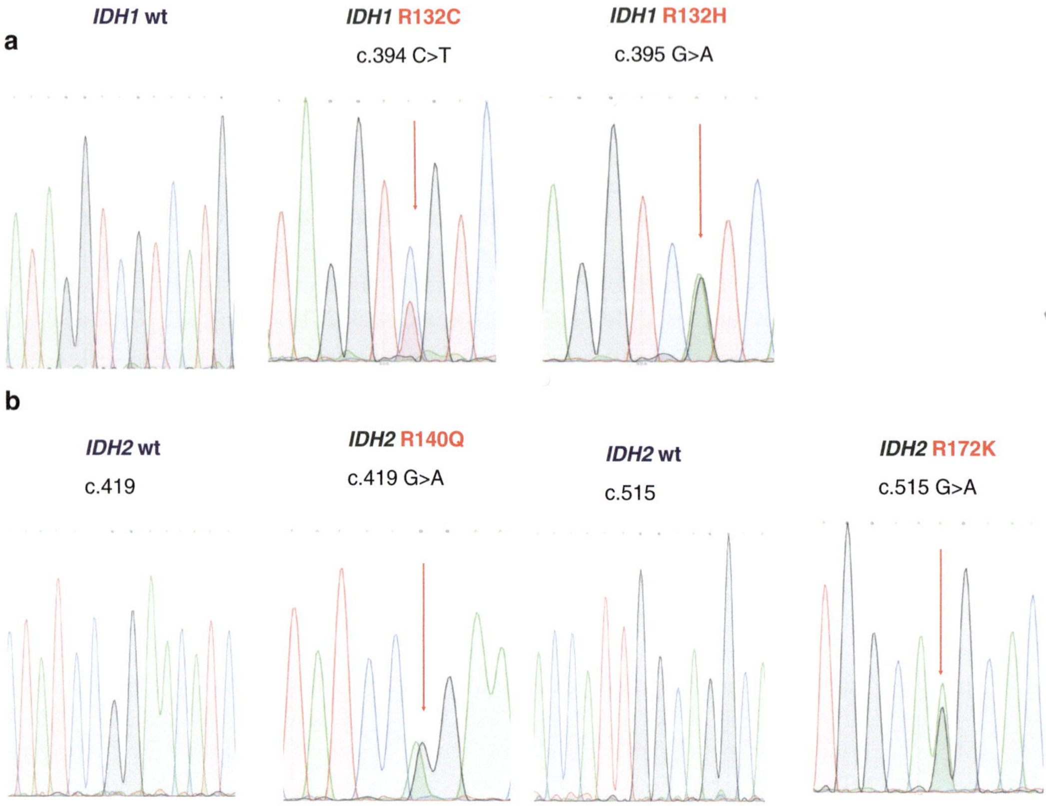


**Fig. 2.6** Sequence chromatograms for *IDH1* and *IDH2* mutations. (**a**) DNA sequence traces showing *IDH1* wild-type, *IDH1*$^{R132C}$ and *IDH1*$^{R132H}$ -mutated AML. The arrows indicate the nucleotide position (c.394 and c.395) of each missense mutations. (**b**) DNA sequence traces showing *IDH2* wild-type, *IDH2*$^{R140Q}$ and *IDH2*$^{R172K}$ mutated AML patients. The arrows indicate the nucleotide position (c.419 and c.515) of each missense mutations

## 2.3 Measurable Residual Disease (MRD) in AML and Available Technologies

MRD analysis represents a dynamic evaluation of disease course and has an independent prognostic value, important for risk stratification and treatment design, in combination with other well-established clinical, cytogenetic, and molecular data evaluated at AML diagnosis. Several techniques may be needed, but the results should be integrated in a final laboratory report that covers the different methodologies and maximizes clinically useful information, with the final goal of better addressing personalized treatment approaches.

In this chapter, we will focus on recent methodological advances in MRD assessment in AML, and their inclusion in the decision-making process for personalized treatment (Fig. 2.7) (Schuurhuis et al. 2018).

### 2.3.1 RT-qPCR

In AML, molecular MRD evaluation includes the quantification of *PML-RARA* (Cicconi and Lo-Coco 2016; Sanz et al. 2009), *RUNX1-RUNX1T1* (Jourdan et al. 2013), *CBFB-MYH11* (Corbacioglu et al. 2010), and mutated-*NPM1* (Ivey et al. 2016; Schnittger et al. 2005; Gorello et al. 2006). RT-qPCR methods for the above fusion genes have been standardized by the Europe Against Cancer (EAC) consortium (Gabert et al. 2003). Currently, clinical importance of MRD assessment has been best

| | Advantages | Disadvantages | Sensitivity | Applicability (% of AML) | Reference |
|---|---|---|---|---|---|
| Multiparametric Flow-cytometry (MFC) | Fast, less expensive | Less leukemia specific | $10^{-4}$ | Wide (>90%) | 61 |
| | Single cell analysis | Phenotypic shift | | | |
| | | Complex analysis | | | |
| PCR-based assays (QRT-PCR) | High DNA stability | Time consuming, expensive | $10^{-5}$ | NPM1 mutations (about 30%) | 67 |
| | Specific | False positive | | CBF-AML (about 12%) | 68 |
| | Very low background in normal cells | RNA instability | | PML-RARA (about 10%) | 69, 26 |
| ddPCR | Fast, sensitive, reduced false positive rate | Unique primers must be designed for each mutation type, not yet standardized | $10^{-6}$ | NPM1 | 84 |
| | | | $10^{-6}$ | PMLA216V (ATO-resistant APL) | 86 |

**Fig. 2.7** Methods for detection of minimal residual disease (MRD) in AML. (Adapted from 2018 ELN MRD Working Party documents (Schuurhuis et al. 2018))

established in APL, where achievement of molecular remission in BM after consolidation therapy is regarded as a treatment objective (Sanz et al. 2009) and a useful predictor of disease relapse (Grimwade et al. 2009). As of CBF fusion transcripts (*RUNX1-RUNX1T1* and *CBFB-MYH11*), several studies have reported the prognostic value of MRD assessment and quantification after induction therapy (Corbacioglu et al. 2010; Jourdan et al. 2013; Yin et al. 2012). *NPM1* mutations are a reliable marker of the disease course and represent an ideal leukemia-specific target for MRD monitoring (Ivey et al. 2016; Krönke et al. 2013; Ossenkoppele and Schuurhuis 2016). In particular, it has been shown that the positivity of *NPM1* transcripts after the second chemotherapy cycle has clinical relevance and is associated with a significantly higher relapse risk, independent of other known prognostic factors, when compared to persistent *NPM1*$^{mut}$ negativity, which is indeed associated with prolonged leukemia-free survival (Ivey et al. 2016).

Based on these findings, the ELN Working Party consensus document on MRD in AML (Dohner et al. 2017) indicates that molecular assessment for *NPM1* mutations, *RUNX1-RUNX1T1*, *CBFB-MYH11*, and *PML-RARA* fusion transcripts, should be performed at diagnosis, at least after two cycles of induction/consolidation therapy, and every 3 months, for 24 months after the end of treatment.

### 2.3.2 Next-Generation Sequencing (NGS)

NGS is an important approach to the molecular dissection of AML at the time of initial diagnosis, mainly in cytogenetically normal AML (Ley et al. 2008). Indeed, different clones, characterized by specific mutations or their combinations, may show variable sensitivity to therapy and distinct relapse tendency. The NGS-based MRD assessment can also identify potentially important changes occurring at the subclonal level during the disease course (Press et al. 2019; Thol et al. 2012; Ravandi 2018). Targeted NGS sequencing provides for profiling of genes of interest and is clinically relevant to dissect the impact of combined gene alterations as potential targets for MRD monitoring (Papaemmanuil et al. 2013, 2016). Indeed, MRD positivity at the time of complete remission (CR) represents an independent prognostic factor for survival (Schlenk 2016). This has been demonstrated by Jongen-Lavrencic and colleagues (Jongen-Lavrencic et al. 2018), who analyzed by targeted-NGS 482 AML patients, at diagnosis and in CR after induction therapy. Mutations persisted in about 50% of patients at the time of CR, and the presence of most mutations was associated with an increased risk of relapse. However, some of the persisting mutations such as *DNMT3A*, *ASXL1*, and *TET2* (Jongen-Lavrencic et al. 2018), collectively termed DTA, known to be associated with CHIP (Genovese et al. 2014; Zink et al. 2017), did not have a prognostic role. Novel molecular alterations are currently evaluated as targets for MRD assessment. Kohlmann and colleagues quantified *RUNX1* gene mutations in a large cohort of AML patients, using an amplicon-based NGS. *RUNX1*-mutated transcript levels correlated to clinical outcome (Kohlmann et al. 2013). *RUNX1*-MRD longitudinal assessment could be particularly useful in monitoring disease progression from a myelodysplastic syndrome to secondary AML (Kohlmann et al. 2013; Dicker et al. 2010).

### 2.3.3 Digital Droplet PCR (ddPCR)

Digital droplet PCR (ddPCR) is a molecular assay with great potential for MRD monitoring due to its high sensitivity and specificity. It is a high-throughput technology that, unlike conventional RT-qPCR, produces an absolute quantification, by amplifying the target genes without a reference standard curve (Coltoff et al. 2018; Ravandi et al. 2018). Indeed, although RT-qPCR assays are nowadays carefully standardized for accurate molecular quantifications (Gabert et al. 2003), since PCR amplification bias can influence reaction efficiency, leading to imprecise genetic quantification. *NPM1*-mutated monitoring is sometimes difficult due to the presence of several frameshift insertions and lack of information on the mutated sequence at diagnosis. A recent study showed that ddPCR can be used to monitor MRD using multiple *NPM1* mutation-specific primers (Mencia-Trinchant et al. 2017). The multiplex assay has an overall excellent concordance with single mutation-specific ddPCR assays, as well as with conventional RT-qPCR. In addition, although the prognostic value of conventional RT-qPCR in APL is well established (Brunetti et al. 2017), ddPCR may also be used to monitor patients at high risk of relapse. In particular, a ddPCR approach may detect mutations associated with arsenic trioxide (ATO) resistance such as the *PML*$^{A216V}$ mutation (Alfonso et al. 2019). The identification of the *PML*$^{A216V}$ mutation by ddPCR in APL cases at the time of molecular relapse may in the future help anticipate treatment decisions in ATO-resistant patients.

### 2.3.4 Multiparametric Flow-Cytometry (MFC)

Multiparameter flow cytometry (MFC) represents a great opportunity for MRD monitoring since it is applicable to virtually all patients (>90% of AML) (Buccisano et al. 2010). MFC can significantly contribute to risk assessment of patients with AML during and after treatment, and allows clinicians to consider alternative strategies. The harmonization of the analytical strategies has been recommended by the ELN group (Schuurhuis et al. 2018) and may overcome the concerns about the immunophenotypical shifts that make MRD by MFC a moving target in AML (Zeijlemaker et al. 2014). The application of panels including at least eight colors and the acquisition of a proper number of events minimize the possibility of missing minor populations present at diagnosis that may eventually generate relapse (Schuurhuis et al. 2018). The panel of the ELN MRD working party suggests that to achieve a reliable estimation with a threshold set at 0.1%, the amount of residual leukemic cells by MFC should be determined on a denominator of at least 0.5–1 × $10^6$ cells, excluding debris and CD45 negative cells (Schuurhuis et al. 2018; Buccisano et al. 2018b).

## 2.4 Classification of Acute Myeloid Leukemia

### 2.4.1 Background and History

In 1976, the French-American-British (FAB) Cooperative Group set up the first classification of AML that divided AML in seven categories, according to the morphologic and cytochemical features of blasts, coherently with their grade of maturation/differentiation. (Bennett et al. 1976)

With the improvement of diagnostic techniques, the description of the cytogenetic and genetic profiles of the disease was progressively included into the criteria for classifying AML. In 2001, the third edition of the WHO divided AML in four categories using for the first time a combination of clinical, morphologic, immunophenotypic, cytogenetic, and genetic features (Vardiman et al. 2002). The four categories were "AML with recurrent genetic abnormalities," "AML with multilineage dysplasia," "AML/MDS therapy-related (t-AML and t-MDS)," and "AML not otherwise categorized (NOC)." In the category of "AML with recurrent genetic abnormalities," four entities were included, three of them (AML with t(8;21)(q22;q22), with inv(16)(p13q22) or t(16;16)(p13;q22), and APL with t(15;17)(q22;q12)) characterized by a strict correlation between genetic and morphologic features, while abnormalities of 11q23 did not identify a particular morphologic subtype. The diagnosis of "AML with multilineage dysplasia" was based on a documented history of myelodysplastic syndrome (MDS) or a myelodysplastic/myeloproliferative disease (MDS/MPD), present for at least 6 months prior to the onset of AML, or on the presence of at least 50% of dysplastic cells in two or more myeloid lineages. The category of "therapy-related AML/MDS" also included MDS due to the aggressive clinical behavior of MDS in this setting. It was divided in two sub-groups according to the type of previous therapy received to treat the primary tumor or the autoimmune disease, including alkylating agents or radiation therapy, versus topoisomerase II inhibitors. The first type is usually preceded by MDS or may onset as AML with dysplastic features, and presents frequent abnormalities of chromosomes 5 or 7 and poor outcome. Therapy-related MDS/AML following treatment with topoisomerase II inhibitors is often associated with balanced translocations involving chromosome bands 11q23 or 21q22, or other translocations such as inv(16)(p13q22) or t(15;17)(q22;q12). Later editions of the WHO classification erased these subgroups, but we think that it is important to underline that the two subgroups are indeed characterized by distinct biologic features, despite the fact that modern oncologic treatments include combinations of different drugs and new agents. The remaining 2001 WHO category consisted of "AML not otherwise categorized (NOC)" and was divided into different subgroups, mostly following the FAB morphologic classification criteria.

A profound change introduced in 2001 was the reduction in the blast threshold necessary for AML diagnosis from 30 to 20% in the peripheral blood or bone marrow, as a result of a number of studies showing similar clinical behavior of 20–30%-blast MDS and AML. In addition, the recurrent cytogenetic abnormalities t(8;21)(q22;q22), inv(16)(p13q22) or t(16;16)(p13;q22), and t(15;17)(q22;q12) were defined as diagnostic of AML, regardless of the blast percentage.

The fourth edition of WHO Classification of Myeloid Neoplasms and Acute Leukemia published in 2008 added three new categories and brought important changes into the four preexisting ones (Vardiman et al. 2009). The threshold of 20% of blasts and the diagnostic role of one of the abovementioned balanced translocations regardless of the blast percentage were confirmed. In the category of "AML with recurrent genetic abnormalities," the group of AML with 11q23 abnormalities was better defined as AML with t(9;11)(p22;q23) (*MLLT3-MLL* rearrangement), while other rearrangements involving the *MLL* gene identified different biological entities. In APL with t(15;17)(q22;q12) (*PML-RARA*), variant *RARA* translocations with partner genes other than PML were recognized as different diseases, particularly for the resistance to all-*trans* retinoic acid (ATRA). Moreover, three new recurrent abnormalities, including AML with t(6;9)(p23;q34) (*DEK-NUP214*), AML with inv(3)(q21q26.2) or t(3;3)(q21;q26.2) (*RPN1-EVI1*), and AML (megakaryoblastic) with t(1;22)(p13;q13) (*RBM15-MKL1*), were recognized as full entities despite their low frequency. Two new provisional entities were added to this category, consistent with the multiple evidences of the prognostic significance of mutations in the *NPM1* gene, especially in combination with *FLT3*-ITD, and *CEBPA* mutations. The second 2008 category was renamed as "AML with myelodysplasia-related changes (AML-MRC)". AMLs were included in this group in case of (1) a previous history of MDS or MDS/MPN, and evolution to AML, (2) the presence of myelodysplasia-related cytogenetic abnormalities, or (3) the presence of 50% or more dysplastic cells in at least two myeloid lineages. Concerning the category of "therapy-related myeloid neoplasms," as previously mentioned, the division into subgroups according to the type of previous therapy was no longer recommended. In parallel, improvements in the diagnostic tools for AML diagnosis reduced the number of cases classifiable as "not otherwise specified (NOS)." Furthermore, three additional categories were included: "myeloid sarcoma," a tumor mass composed of myeloid blasts, occurring at an anatomical site different form bone marrow and that modifies the normal tissue architecture, "myeloid proliferations related to Down syndrome," and "blastic plasmacytoid dendritic cell neoplasm." Myeloid proliferations related to Down syndrome are characterized by specific clinical, morphologic, immunophenotypic, and molecular profiles, including mutation of the *GATA1 gene*. The inclusion of the "blastic plasmacytoid dendritic cell neoplasm" was due to the recognition of its derivation from precursors of a specialized subset of dendritic cells, the plasmacytoid dendritic cells. For this reason, they were re-classified as AML, as opposed to the third edition of WHO classification, in which they were classified as "blastic NK-cell lymphoma/leukemias."

### 2.4.2 The 2016 Revision of the WHO Classification of AML

The 2016 revision of WHO classification of myeloid neoplasms and acute leukemia was an update necessary to incorporate the advancements in the molecular characterization of AML, occurred from 2010 on (Arber et al. 2016). As shown in Table 2.1, the 2016 revision introduced major changes including (Arber et al. 2016) the acknowledgement of AML with mutated *NPM1* and AML with biallelic mutations of *CEBPA* as full entities; and (Papaemmanuil et al. 2013) the introduction of two provisional entities: AML with *BCR-ABL1*, which must be distinguished from a blastic transformation of CML, and may benefit from tyrosine-kinase inhibitors (TKI) treatment, and AML with mutated *RUNX1*, associated with poor prognosis. Criteria for defining "AML-MRC" were confirmed, but two points deserve our attention. First, AML with mutated *NPM1* or biallelic mutation of *CEBPA*, associated with multilineage dysplasia, must be classified according to the mutation, since the presence of dysplasia does not affect prognosis in these cases (Falini et al. 2010); second, the cytogenetic abnormality del(9q) has been removed from the AML-MRC category because of its frequent association with mutations of *NPM1* and *CEBPA*. However, in the presence of other MDS-related abnormalities, del(9q) is still included in the "AML-MRC" group (see Table 2.4).

Some changes have also been introduced in the "AML, NOS" category. The erythroleukemia, erythroid/myeloid subtype (previously defined by the presence of ≥50% erythroid precursors counted as proportion of bone marrow nucleated cells, and of ≥20% myeloblasts in non-erythroid cells) has been removed because of similar clinical and genetic features with cases of MDS or AML-MRC. In contrast, pure erythroid leukemia has been maintained as a subtype of "AML,

**Table 2.4** Cytogenetic abnormalities sufficient to diagnose AML with myelodisplasia-related changes in presence of ≥20% PB or BM blasts and excluded prior therapy (from the 2016 revision of WHO Classification (Arber et al. 2016))

| Unbalanced abnormalities | Balanced abnormalities |
|---|---|
| −7 or del(7q) | t(11;16)(q23.3;p13.3) |
| del(5q) or t(5q) | t(3;21)(q26.2;q22.1) |
| i(17q) or t(17p) | t(1;3)(p36.3;q21.2) |
| −13 or del(13q) | t(2;11)(p21;q23.3) |
| del(11q) | t(5;12)(q32;p13.2) |
| del(12p) or t(12p) | t(5;7)(q32;q11.2) |
| idic(X)(q13) | t(5;17)(q32;p13.2) |
| | t(5;10)(q32;q21.2) |
| | t(3;5)(q25.3;q35.1) |

Complex karyotype (three or more abnormalities)

NOS," defined by the presence of >80% (with ≥30% proerythroblasts) immature erythroid precursors, and myeloblasts <20% of bone marrow nucleated cells (Grossmann et al. 2013).

Minor nomenclature changes concern the definition of the category of "AML with recurrent genetic abnormalities": (1) APL with t(15;17)(q22;q12) was renamed APL with *PML-RARA* to emphasize the unique features of this gene fusion; (2) *MLL* was renamed *KMT2A*; and (3) inv(3)(q21.3q26.2) or t(3;3)(q21.3;q26.2), which does not appear to produce a fusion gene, but implies the repositioning of the *GATA2 enhancer*, driving to deregulation of *GATA2* and *MECOM* genes. The categories of "therapy-related myeloid neoplasms," "myeloid sarcoma," "myeloid proliferations related to Down syndrome," and "blastic plasmacytoid dendritic cell neoplasm" did not change in 2016.

The background and the recent criteria for classification of acute leukemia (AL) of ambiguous lineage will be dealt with in a distinct paragraph.

### 2.4.3 Rules for AML Classification According to WHO 2016

Sometimes, different entities may overlap in the same patient: the heart of the matter is to prioritize a criterion (clinical, morphologic, immunophenotypic, cytogenetic, or genetic) in order to assign the disease to the right category (Arber 2019).

The first criterion to be taken into consideration to correctly classify AML is patient history. A prior chemotherapy or radiotherapy supersedes every other feature, leading to classification of the disease as a "therapy-related myeloid neoplasm." In fact, regardless of the genetic/cytogenetic profile, these patients appear to generally have a worse prognosis than those with a corresponding de novo AML (Rowley and Olney 2002), with the exception of CBF-AML (Kayser et al. 2011), and t-APL, whose clinical course is similar to that of de novo APL (Kayser et al. 2017). The same applies to a prior history of MDS or MPN, defining "AML-MRC," except for AML with inv(3)(q21.3q26.2)/t(3;3)(q21.3;q26.2) or t(6;9)(p23;q34.1), which are classified as AML with recurrent genetic abnormalities.

The second important parameter is the presence of a balanced translocation or gene mutation, characterizing the nine full entities belonging to the category of "AML with recurrent genetic abnormalities."

In the absence of a history of cytotoxic therapy, or of a recurrent cytogenetic abnormality, detection of balanced or unbalanced aberrations considered associated with MDS defines the disease as "AML-MRC," which is the third criterion (Table 2.4).

At this point, the role of morphology becomes significant, both for its capability of forewarning of the presence of particular genetic/cytogenetic abnormalities, and the detection of multilineage dysplasia, which, even in the absence of prior MDS or an MDS-related cytogenetic abnormality, leads to the diagnosis of "AML-MRC" (Rozman et al. 2014). Last, when the disease cannot be classified in another category, the morphologic exam of bone marrow and peripheral blood is the only parameter useful in the subcategorization of "AML, NOS" (Walter et al. 2013).

### 2.4.4 Acute Myeloid Leukemia with Recurrent Genetic Abnormalities

#### 2.4.4.1 AML with t(8;21)(q22;q22.1);RUNX1-RUNX1T1

AML with t(8;21)(q22;q22.1) accounts for 4–8% of cases. This balanced translocation is commonly found in younger patients and in cases with granulocytic maturation, and is associated with a good outcome when treated with intensive consolidation therapy (Al-Harbi et al. 2020).

Usually, the percentage of bone marrow blasts is ≥20%; rarely it could be inferior, but the presence of this translocation is diagnostic for AML, independent of blast percentage. The typical morphologic features are those of the M2 subtype of FAB classification, with large size blasts, and abundant basophilic cytoplasm with the presence of numerous azurophilic granules and perinuclear clearing (hofs). In some cases, blasts show very large granules (pseudo-Chediak-Higashi granules) and Auer rods (Fig. 2.7). Dysplasia is a common finding, but usually it does not affect erythroblasts or megakaryocytes. The percentage of eosinophils, basophils, and mast cells could be increased. The immunophenotype follows the granulocytic differentiation: blasts usually express CD15 and/or CD65, together with immaturity markers such as CD34, MPO, HLA-DR, and CD13. Maturation asynchrony may be observed in the same blast population. Expression of lymphoid-aberrant antigens such as CD19, PAX5, and CD79a is frequent and expression of CD56 has been reported, correlating with worse prognosis (Baer et al. 1997). A cytogenetic analysis may demonstrate co-existing abnormalities, including loss of chromosome X (Chen et al. 2020) or Y (Zhou et al. 2020), del(9q), and trisomy 8.

The t(8;21)(q22;q22.1) generates a chimeric fusion gene, involving the *RUNX1* gene on chromosome 21 and the *RUNX1T1* gene on chromosome 8. *RUNX1*, the alpha subunit of the core-binding factor, is a key transcriptional factor crucial for hematopoietic differentiation and myeloid development, while *RUNX1T1* is a transcriptional corepressor. In this way, *RUNX1-RUNX1T1* works as a repressor for all *RUNX1*-regulated hematopoietic genes to disrupt normal hematopoietic differentiation and promote a preleukemic state (Goyama and Mulloy 2011). The t(8;21)(q22;q22.1);*RUNX1-RUNX1T1* seems to be an early event, and secondary genetic events are needed to develop leukemia. Many other genes are involved in the process of leukemogenesis: 96% of t(8;21) AML cases carry additional cytogenetic or genetic abnormalities (Duployez et al. 2016). The most frequent association is with *c-KIT* mutations: reported in up to 46% of patients with t(8;21) AML, and associated with unfavorable outcome (Cairoli et al. 2006). *FLT3* mutations have been reported in up to 16% of t(8;21) patients, although evidence for their impact on prognosis appears controversial: while *FLT3-ITD* mutations with a high allelic burden have been associated with poor prognosis, *FLT3-TKD* mutations seem associated with improved outcome (Christen et al. 2019). Other possible additional mutations concern *NRAS/KRAS*, *CBL*, *JAK2*, and *PTPN11 genes, and also epigenetic regulators such as TET2*, *ASXL1*, and *ASXL2* (Al-Harbi et al. 2020).

#### 2.4.4.2 AML with inv(16)(p13.1q22) or t(16;16)(p13.1;q22);CBFB-MYH11

The inv(16)(p13.1q22) or t(16;16)(p13,1;q22) are found in 5–8% of younger patients with AML, with decreasing prevalence in elderly adults. This AML subtype is characterized by granulocytic and monocytic differentiation, good response to intensive chemotherapy, and low incidence of relapse. Also in these cases, detection of ˂20% bone marrow blasts is infrequent, but similar to t(8;21), the presence of *CBFB-MYH11* defines AML per se, independent of blast proportion.

The bone marrow morphologic examination shows typical features of the M4Eo subtype of the FAB classification. Blasts are characterized by myelomonocytic features, in addition to a relevant infiltration of eosinophils at all stages of maturation, without maturation arrest. The immature eosinophilic granules are larger and thicker than normal, and have a typical intense purple-violet color (Swerdlow et al. 2017).

The immunophenotypic evaluation often shows the presence of multiple blast populations, one characterized by immaturity markers such as CD34 and CD117, and others with features belonging to the granulocytic (CD13, CD33, CD15, CD65, and MPO) and/or the monocytic differentiation (CD14, CD4, CD11b, CD11c, CD64, CD36, and lysozyme). Maturation asynchrony may be observed in the same blast population. One antigen aberration frequently detected in this type of AML is the co-expression of CD2 with myeloid markers.

Additional cytogenetic abnormalities have been documented in approximately 40% of cases, including trisomy of chromosomes 22 and 8 (each occurring in 10–15% of cases), and less frequently del(7q) and trisomy of chromosome 21 (Marcucci et al. 2005). Co-existing trisomy 22 seems to be associated with improved outcome, while trisomy 8 has been associated with a worse prognosis.

The translocation or, most frequently, the pericentric inversion of chromosome 16 generates the chimeric fusion gene *CBFB-MYH11*. The gene *MYH11* encodes for the myosin heavy chain, while *CBFB* encodes for the beta subunit of core-binding factor. The fusion gene encodes for a protein called CBFβ–SMMHC, acting as a dominant negative regulator of transcription, increasing the viability of pre-leukemic myeloid cells, and enhancing their resistance to genotoxic stress (Kuo et al. 2006). As in AML with t(8;21)(q22;q22.1), secondary gene mutations are present in >90% of cases. Mutations of *c-KIT* are the most frequent, being observed in 30–40% of cases of this AML subtype; other mutations include *NRAS* (in 45% of cases), *KRAS* (in 13%), and *FLT3* (in 14%), the last one associated with decreased prognosis (Paschka et al. 2013).

#### 2.4.4.3 Acute Promyelocytic Leukemia (APL) with PML/RARA

APL is a distinct subtype of AML, representing 5–8% of AML cases. The median age of APL onset is 35–40 years, but it can occur at any age. The genetic hallmark of APL is the balanced reciprocal t(15;17) translocation, which results in the fusion between the promyelocytic leukemia *(PML)* and the retinoic acid receptor α (*RAR*A) genes. The disease presentation is frequently associated with a life-threatening coagulopathy that can cause fatal hemorrhages and thrombosis. APL is stratified according to the risk of relapse, based on initial white blood (WBC) and platelet counts at diagnosis. Low/intermediate-risk categories include patients with WBC count $\leq 10 \times 10^9$/L and platelet count $<40 \times 10^9$/L or $> 40 \times 10^9$/L in low and intermediate risk, respectively; in the high-risk group, patients present with WBC $>10 \times 10^9$/L (Sanz et al. 2000).

A rapid diagnosis of APL and the institution of adequate anti-leukemic and supportive care are of relevant importance in preventing early death, which is currently considered the most important issue in the final cure of this disease (Cicconi and Lo-Coco 2016). Morphologically, it is identified as AML-M3 by the French-American-British (FAB) classification (Bennett et al. 1976) and is characterized by a differentiation block resulting in accumulation in the BM of immature, hypergranular promyelocytes with abundant cytoplasm, irregular nuclei with fine azurophilic granules, and Auer rods, often piled up (Faggott cells) in 90% of cases. Morphologically, there are three possible presentations: the classical hypergranular variant, the microgranular variant (hypogranular), and the hyperbasophilic variant. Classical APL promyelocytes are hypergranular, with the possible observation of giant granules that tend to invade all the cytoplasm; the nucleus is bilobed, but sometimes not easily visible due to the high prevalence of granules. Auer rods are frequent (Fig. 2.8). The microgranular variant of APL also presents a bilobed nucleus, while cytoplasm is hypogranular, with a nude perinuclear zone representing the Golgi zone. However, although not frequent, some hypergranular promyelocytes containing Auer rods may be present. The third type of APL, the hyperbasophilic variant, presents with a poor and basophilic cytoplasm, characterized by the presence of blebs (Bain and Bene 2019). In the majority of cases, the diagnosis of APL is suggested by the characteristic morphology of leukemic blasts (Cicconi and Lo-Coco 2016; Sanz et al. 2009). Immunophenotypic

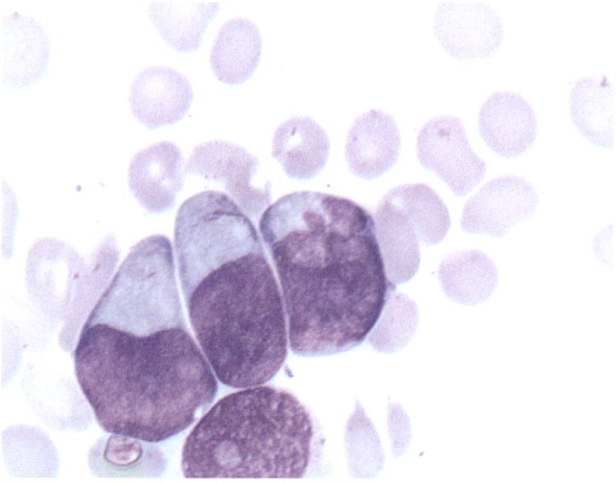

**Fig. 2.8** AML with t(8;21)(q22;q22.1);*RUNX1-RUNX1T1*. Typical large size myeloblasts with abundant basophilic cytoplasm with the presence of numerous azurophilic granules and single Auer rods

evaluation often shows a typical image called "flame-like" in the SSC/CD45 plot: this reflects the morphologic/immunophenotypic features of abnormal promyelocytes that are characterized by hypergranular cytoplasm, and express intermediate levels of CD45. Usually CD34 and HLA-DR antigens are absent or low, while CD13, CD33, CD117, and MPO are strongly expressed (Rahman et al. 2018). Approximately 10% of APL cases express CD56, which has been associated with a decreased outcome. Cytogenetics detects the t(15;17)(q22;q12) translocation in most of cases, leading to *PML-RARA* fusion gene, between the *RARA* and *PML* gene. In some cases, a submicroscopic insertion of *RARA* into *PML* has been described: the result is a *PML-RARA* transcript detectable by molecular studies, but not by cytogenetics. These cases are considered to have cryptic or masked t(15;17)(q22;q12), and are included in the category of APL with *PML-RARA* (Swerdlow et al. 2017), different from other variant translocations described below. Coexisting cytogenetical abnormalities are frequent and present in almost 40% of cases, with trisomy 8 as the most frequent.

Some rare cytogenetic variant involving the *RARA* gene has been observed. The variant fusion partners may include *PLZF* at 11q23.2, *NPM1* at 5q35.1, *NUMA1* at 11q13.4, and *STATSB* at 17q21.2. Cases with these variant translocations are not true APL and should be classified as "AML with a variant *RARA* translocation," since they have different treatment indications and worse prognosis compared to APL.

Confirmation of genetic diagnosis with a rapid *PML/RARA* genetic test is crucial for patient management. Current methods for genetic confirmation of APL diagnosis include RT-PCR, RT-qPCR, RT-QLAMP, and FISH approaches (Sanz et al. 2019). However, a rapid diagnosis of APL could be confirmed by analyzing the immunocytochemical pattern of the *PML* protein, using the anti-PML PG-M3 monoclonal antibody (Falini et al. 1997). This assay analyses the nuclear distribution of the PML protein, differentiating the typical "microspeckled pattern" associated with *PML/RARA*-positivity from the "nuclear body pattern," characteristic of other

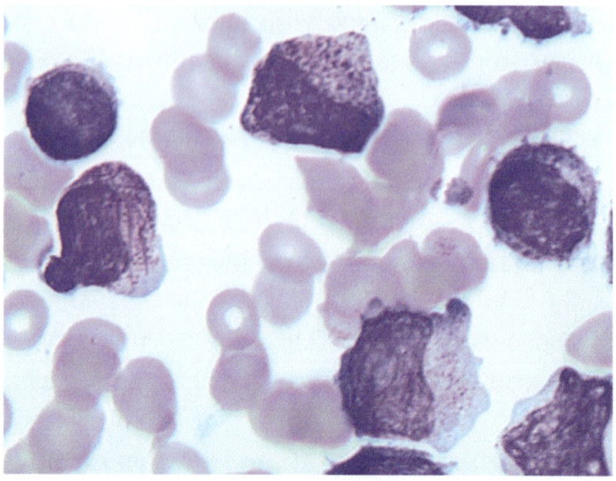

**Fig. 2.9** AML with *PML/RARA*: classic variant. Promyelocytes are characterized by a hypergranular cytoplasm, with the presence of giant granules that tend to invade all the cytoplasm, and multiple Auer rods

leukemias and normal hematopoietic cells (Fig. 2.9). This assay is cheap and useful for rapid diagnosis, available within 2 h (Dimov et al. 2010). However, as reported by ELN guidelines for APL diagnosis (Sanz et al. 2019), RT-PCR represents the "gold standard" for genetic confirmation of APL, as it allows for the identification of the specific *PML/RARA* isoform (Van Dongen et al. 1999). This information is important for subsequent molecular monitoring of minimal residual disease. Depending on *PML* breakpoint, usually located in intron 6, exon 6, or intron 3, different *PML/RARA* transcript isoforms may be generated, that is, long (bcr1), variant (bcr2), and short (bcr3), respectively (Pandolfi et al. 1992). The long and short isoforms are detectable in 95% of APL cases, whereas only 5% harbor the variant form. In contrast, *RARA* breakpoints are always located within intron 2 (Borrow et al. 1990). The FISH methodology is highly specific and sensitive, and less expensive and time-consuming than karyotyping on G-banded metaphases; thus, it is preferred at diagnosis (Sanz et al. 2009). Once the correct *PML/RARA* fusion transcript has been identified, RT-qPCR allows for a sensitive assessment of the response to therapy through MRD monitoring during follow-up and early identification of molecular relapse (Gabert et al. 2003; Grimwade et al. 2009). In this setting, APL represents a model for MRD-driven therapy, since molecular relapse is an indication for salvage treatment. Currently, the use of all-trans retinoic acid (ATRA), combined with arsenic trioxide (ATO) or with chemotherapy, induces long-term remissions in at least 85%–90% of patients. However, some patients relapse after ATRA-ATO-based treatments and the mechanisms associated with resistance to these agents are still poorly understood. The A216V mutation in the *PML* gene has been shown to prevent ATO binding, inhibiting degradation of the oncoprotein, thus hindering oligomerization into nuclear bodies (Zhu et al. 2014). The $PML^{A216V}$ mutation may be efficiently identified by ddPCR, and $PML^{A216V}$ is associated with ATO resistance. Additional genetic aberrations such as *FLT3* mutations are frequently found in APL: *FLT3*-ITD occurs in 40% of patients, while *FLT3*-TKD has been observed in 8% of cases (Breccia et al. 2013). In both cases, a correlation with hyperleukocytosis has been described, and the presence of *FLT3*-ITD mutations results in the context of ATRA/chemotherapy is associated to reduced response rates and shorter overall survival (Breccia et al. 2013; Picharski et al. 2019). In contrast, the ATRA-ATO combination abrogates the adverse prognostic role of *FLT3*-ITD mutations in standard-risk APL (Cicconi et al. 2016).

#### 2.4.4.4 AML with t(9;11)(p21.3;q23.3);MLLT3-KMT2A

This recurrent genetic abnormality accounts for 9–12% of pediatric and 2% of adult AML cases. Morphologic and immunophenotypic features often follow monoblastic/monocytic differentiation, with overexpression of CD33, CD65, CD4, and HLA-DR, whereas the expression of CD13, CD34, and CD14 is usually low.

The (9;11)(p21.3;q23.3) (*MLLT3-KMT2A)* translocation involves the *KMT2A* gene, which encodes for a histone methyltransferase that regulates gene transcription via chromatin remodeling, and the *MLLT3* gene, which encodes for AF9, a protein involved in cell growth and maintenance. Secondary additional cytogenetic abnormalities are common, and the most frequent is trisomy of chromosome 8, without clear prognostic significance (Mrozek et al. 1997).

#### 2.4.4.5 AML with t(6;9)(p23;q34.1);DEK-NUP214

AML with t(6;9)(p23;q34.1) (*DEK-NUP214*) is a rare disease, more frequent in children and younger adults, accounting for 0.7–1.8% of AML cases. It is characterized by poor outcome. Morphologically, this entity may present as an AML with maturation, or sometimes as acute myelomonocytic leukemia. Both peripheral blood and bone marrow are often (44–62% of cases) characterized by an increase in the basophil proportion (≥2%), and signs of multilineage dysplasia can be observed.

The immunophenotypic profile is characterized by high expression of MPO, CD9, CD13, CD33, CD38, CD123, and HLA-DR. The basophil population can be detected and separated for its positivity for CD123, CD33, and CD38, and negativity for HLA-DR (Swerdlow et al. 2017).

The t(6;9) translocation involves the *DEK* gene at 6p22, and the *NUP214* gene (formerly known as *CAN*), located at 9q34, creating the *DEK-NUP214* fusion gene, which acts as an aberrant transcription factor and alters nuclear transport by binding soluble transportins. Moreover, *DEK-NUP214* has been reported to enhance protein synthesis in myeloid cells. In most of cases, there are no other cytogenetic abnormalities, but a minor percentage of patients present a complex karyotype. *FLT3*-ITD has been observed in 42–69% of pediatric and 73–90% of adult AML patients (Kayser et al. 2020).

#### 2.4.4.6 AML with inv(3)(q21.3q26.2) or t(3;3)(q21.3;q26.2);GATA2, MECOM

AML with inv(3)(q21,3q26.2) or t(3;3)(q21.3;q26.2) accounts for 1–2% of all AML and is more common in the adult population. It may often present with normal or even increased platelet counts, and it must be considered a poor prognosis disease.

The morphologic features of bone marrow blasts reflect those of AML without maturation, acute myelomonocytic leukemia or acute megakaryoblastic leukemia. A frequent finding is multilineage dysplasia of non-blast bone marrow cells, especially in megakaryocytes, which are often small non-lobated or bilobated. Megakaryocytic differentiation, when present, may be confirmed by the expression of CD41, CD42, and/or CD61 on blasts. In other cases, markers of immaturity like CD34, CD117, CD13, and CD33 are expressed by the blast population, together with CD7, CD11c, CD11b, and CD123 (Bain and Bene 2019).

The inv(3)(q21.3q26.2) and t(3;3)(q21.3;q26.2) involve the *MECOM* oncogene at 3q26.2, and a distal *GATA2 enhancer,* located at 3q21.3. These abnormalities result in the activation of *MECOM* expression and in *GATA2* haploinsufficiency at the same time.

Frequently, these cytogenetic abnormalities are associated with other adverse-risk anomalies, as monosomy of chromosome 7, del(5q), or complex karyotype. The association with *BCR-ABL1* positive CML has been described, and it must be considered a marker of accelerated phase or blastic transformation of the disease. Secondary gene mutations are found in almost all cases of AML with inv(3) or t(3;3), with high frequency of *NRAS* mutations (45.0%), followed by *SF3B1* (15.0%), *GATA2* (15.0%), *FLT3*-ITD (10.0%), *c-KIT/D816* (5.0%), and *CEBPA* (5.0%) (Gong et al. 2019).

#### 2.4.4.7 AML (Megakaryoblastic) with t(1;22) (p13.3;q13.3);RBM15-MKL1

AML with t(1;22)(p13,3;q13.1) accounts for <1% of all cases of AML and is typical of infants and young children, with the highest incidence in the first 6 months of life. It is characterized by megakaryoblastic differentiation and hepatosplenomegaly at onset, and it must be considered an aggressive disease.

Morphological examination of bone marrow aspirate usually shows megakaryoblasts with a basophilic agranular cytoplasm and numerous blebs; signs of dysplasia of the other cell lines are infrequent. Fibrosis is a common finding, so that a bone marrow biopsy results helpful or even mandatory for diagnosis.

Immunophenotyping may confirm the megakaryoblastic differentiation through expression of CD41, CD42, and/or CD61. The myeloid-associated markers CD33 and CD13 may also be positive, while CD45, CD34, and HLA-DR are often negative.

In most cases, t(1;22)(p13.3;q13.1) is the sole karyotypic abnormality. Rarely, trisomy of chromosome 21, 19, or 8, may be present, without clear prognostic significance (Inaba et al. 2015).

#### 2.4.4.8 AML with Mutated NPM1

Mutations of the *NPM1* gene occur in 2–8% of childhood, and 27%–35% of adult AML, as well as in 45–64% of adult cases with normal karyotype (Swerdlow et al. 2017). Initially described as a favorable-risk entity, in the last few years, AML with mutated *NPM1* showed heterogeneous outcome, primarily depending on the presence of co-mutations, and on the MRD status post-consolidation treatment (Ivey et al. 2016).

Most cases of AML with mutated *NPM1* present morphologic features of acute myelomonocytic leukemia or acute monocytic leukemia, but characteristics of AML with or without maturation have also been described. The bone marrow is often hypercellular with signs of multilineage dysplasia that, as mentioned above, does not affect prognosis. The immunophenotypic profiling identifies two subgroups: one expressing antigens of monocytic differentiation (CD36, CD64, CD11b, and CD14), and the other with a pattern of myeloblastic differentiation (CD33, CD117, and MPO). CD34 is usually negative and, in a minor percentage, HLA-DR may also be absent (Bain and Bene 2019). Presence of CD34+/CD25+/CD123+/CD99+ blasts is predictive for the presence of *FLT3*-ITD mutations (Angelini et al. 2015).

AML with mutated *NPM1* is usually de novo and has a normal karyotype. However, 5–15% of cases show additional chromosomal abnormalities, including gain of chromosome 8 and del(9q), and adverse-risk karyotypes, which impact prognosis (Angenendt et al. 2019).

Secondary mutations are common in AML with mutated *NPM1* and most frequently involve the *FLT3* gene (ITD or TKD mutations) and, in 70% of cases, genes regulating DNA methylation, such as *DNMT3A* (50% of cases), *TET2*, *IDH1*, and *IDH2* (each occurring in 15% of cases) (Mason et al. 2019). The combination of *NPM1* and *FLT3*-ITD mutations, quantified in terms of ITD allelic ratios >0.5 or <0.5, identifies patients with significantly different outcome, and has been included in the 2017 ELN genetic/cytogenetic risk stratification (Dohner et al. 2017).

#### 2.4.4.9 AML with Biallelic Mutations of CEBPA

Mutations in the *CEBPA* gene occur in 5–10% cases of AML, mostly in children and younger adults. Biallelic mutations are typically associated with de novo AML, normal karyotype, and favorable outcome.

AML with biallelic mutation of *CEBPA* does not have typical morphologic features. Similar to AML with mutated *NPM1*, a possible finding is multilineage dysplasia, without adverse prognostic significance. Cytological features are not specific, but the immunophenotypic profile may be suggestive of this AML subtype. Recently, Mannelli et al. identified a pattern of antigens predictive of *CEBPA* biallelic mutation, with overexpression of CD34, CD117, HLA-DR, and MPO in blasts, and asynchronous CD15 and CD65 expression. CD64 has also been found overexpressed, not only by blasts but also by granulocytes, and patterns of erythroblast dysplasia with CD117 and CD105 expression associated with low levels of CD36 and CD71 have been described (Mannelli et al. 2017). This immunophenotypic profile suggests further investigation of *CEBPA* mutations.

Most cases of AML with biallelic mutation of *CEBPA* have a normal karyotype, but in some patients, other cytogenetic abnormalities may be found, usually del(9q), which has no prognostic impact. Co-mutations of *GATA2* and *FLT3*-ITD occur in 39% and 5–9% cases of AML with biallelic *CEBPA* mutations, respectively (Swerdlow et al. 2017).

#### 2.4.4.10 AML with t(9; 22)(q34.1;q11.2);BCR-ABL1

AML with *BCR-ABL1* is a provisional entity, firstly introduced in 2016 WHO Classification revision but not yet recognized as a full entity. This new group includes de novo AML cases with *BCR-ABL1* rearrangements without evidence of a previous CML. The incidence of *BCR-ABL1* de novo AML ranges from 0.5 to 3% (Konoplev et al. 2013).

There are no specific morphologic features of myeloblasts, while the presence of peripheral blood basophilia is usually lower than those observed in cases of blastic transformation of CML. Immunophenotypic features include positivity for myeloid antigens of immaturity and lineage aberrations, like CD7, CD19, or TdT. In these cases, it is recommended to exclude the diagnosis of MPAL with *BCR-ABL1* (Bain and Bene 2019).

The cytogenetic/genetic profile shows the presence of the translocation t(9;22)(q34.1;q11.2) and/or the *BCR-ABL1* fusion gene, in both p210 and p190 types. Other secondary abnormalities include gain or loss of chromosomes or the presence of a complex karyotype. Moreover, cases of AML with *BCR-ABL1* and *NPM1* or *FLT3*-ITD mutations have been described. Being a provisional entity, the eventual presence of another recurrent abnormality supersedes in the classification the detection of *BCR-ABL1*. Treatment strategies in these cases of AML should include the use of tyrosine kinase inhibitors (TKI) (Swerdlow et al. 2017; Neuendorff et al. 2016).

#### 2.4.4.11 AML with Mutated RUNX1

This is the second de novo provisional entity introduced with the 2016 revision of the WHO Classification of AML and is associated with poor prognosis.

*RUNX1* gene mutations occur in 6–18% of AML cases. They are also found in about 28% of AML secondary to MDS, and they are often associated with prior radiotherapy or chemotherapy. These latter must be classified, as "AML-MRC" and "therapy-related myeloid neoplasms," respectively (Yokota et al. 2020). The cytological features often follow those of AML with minimal differentiation, but not exclusively. Immunophenotypic evaluation usually shows expression of markers of immaturity, as CD34, CD13, and HLA-DR, while markers of differentiation, such as CD33 and CD15, are less common (Bain and Bene 2019). The cytogenetic profile is often characterized by alterations of karyotype, including trisomy 8 and trisomy 13 in most cases; additional mutations have been described in 41–95% of AML with *RUNX1* mutations, mostly involving *FLT3, NRAS, MLL, ASXL1, IDH1/IDH2, TET2, BCOR, DNMT3A, SRSF2, SF3B1,* and *WT1* genes (Yokota et al. 2020).

### 2.4.5 AML with Myelodysplasia-Related Changes (AML-MRC)

"AML-MRC" is a WHO category that includes cases with a documented history of MDS or MDS/MPN, or with MDS-related cytogenetic abnormalities, and/or cases with multilineage dysplasia. It accounts for 24–35% of AML with a higher incidence in elderly patients, and is considered a category with poor outcome for its frequent resistance to therapy.

Multilineage dysplasia is defined by the observation of over 50% of dysplastic non-blast cells in two or more hematopoietic cell lineages in bone marrow and/or peripheral blood smears. Features of dysgranulopoiesis include the presence of hyposegmented nuclei and hypogranular cytoplasm, while features of dysmegakaryopoiesis include the presence of normal/large megakaryocytes with non-lobated or multiple nuclei, or micromegakaryocites. Cytological features defining dyserythropoiesis are fragmentation/

**a** **b**

**Microspeckled pattern in *PML/RARA*-positive APL** **Nuclear body pattern *PML/RARA*-negative AML**

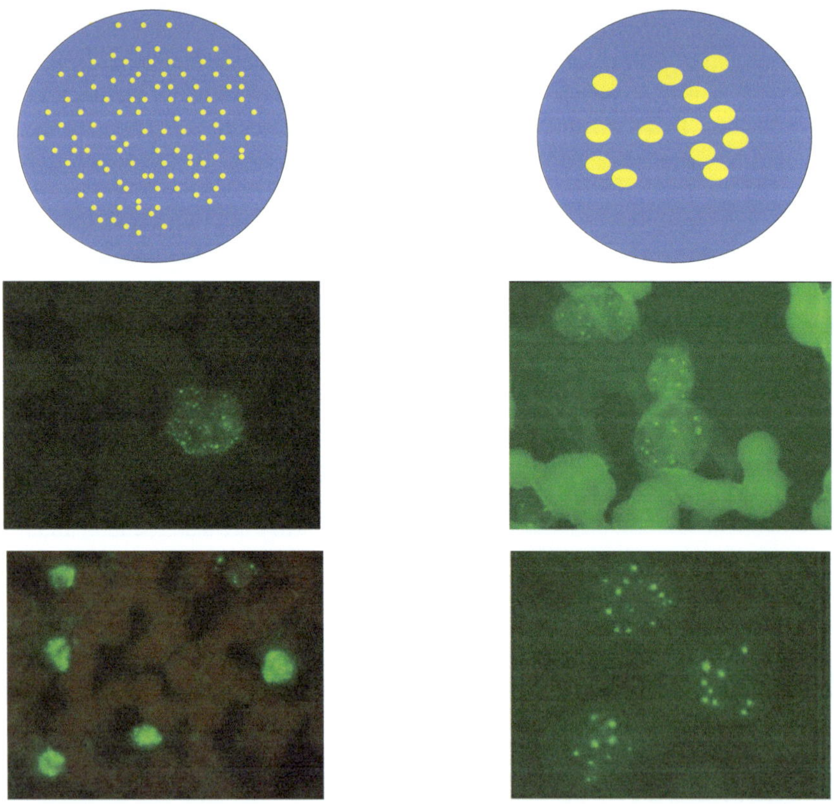

**Fig. 2.10** Patterns of PML nuclear staining. (**a**) Typical "microspeckled pattern" of two *PML/RARA*-positive APL samples. (**b**) "Nuclear bodies pattern" of two *PML/RARA*-negative samples

irregularity of nuclei, megaloblastosis, karyorrhexis, and the presence of ring sideroblasts (Fig. 2.10) (Swerdlow et al. 2017). Hypogranularity of neutrophils, studied with MFC-SSC, is one of the immunophenotypic features considered suggestive of the diagnosis of MDS and "AML-MRC." Other immunophenotypic characteristics suggesting dysplasia are aberrant differentiation patterns with expression of antigens belonging to different maturative stages, reduction of hematogones, and aberrant expression of lineage-infidelity markers (LIM), such as CD7 and CD56 (Porwit et al. 2014). However, immunophenotype characteristics are not formally included in the diagnostic criteria of AML-MRC.

Multilineage dysplasia is a sufficient criterion for defining AML-MRC, unless mutations of *NPM1* or *CEBPA* are detected. These cases are then classified as "AML with recurrent genetic abnormalities." Conversely, detection of an MDS-related karyotype (see Table 2.4) is sufficient to define "AML-MRC," even in the presence of these mutations. However, *NPM1* and *CEBPA* mutations are very uncommon in this category of AML, while other mutations, such as *ASXL1* and *TP53*, are often observed. Mutations of *TP53* occur in up to 70% of cases with complex-karyotype AML, explaining why *TP53*-mutated cases are included in the AML-MRC category. *TP53* mutations typically lead to chemo-resistance and are one of the most important unfavorable prognostic factors in AML (Vardiman and Reichard 2015).

### 2.4.6 Therapy-Related Myeloid Neoplasms (t-MN)

This category includes both MDS and AML developing after radiation therapy, chemotherapy, or immunomodulating treatment for a previous tumor or autoimmune disease. The definition does not include any criterion of time-to-exposure. It accounts for 10–20% of all AML cases, median age at diagnosis is 64 years, and it generally has a poor outcome, with the exception of CBF-AML and APL (McNerney et al. 2017).

Morphologic, immunophenotypic, and cytogenetic features are often similar to those observed in "AML-MRC," especially in cases following radiation therapy and/or alkylating agents. These characteristics include multilineage dysplasia, expression of LIM, and aberrations of differentiation antigens, and cytogenetic alterations, mostly affecting chromosomes 5 and 7, or complex karyotype. Other cases, usually preceded by therapy with topoisomerase II inhibitors, are characterized by various morphologic features, including monoblastic or myelomonocytic presentation, with heterogeneous immunophenotypes. Balanced translocations have also been reported in t-MN, mostly involving 11q23 or 21q22.1 rearrangements, but also cases with inv(16) or t(16;16) and t(15;17) have been described. This latter defines APL with *PML/RARA,* although the correct classification is t-AML with *PML/RARA* (Swerdlow et al. 2017). As for the genetic profile, mutations of the *TP53* gene are very common and have been detected in 80% of cases with del(5q); instead, alterations affecting the *RAS* pathway are frequently associated with −7/del(7q) cases (Side et al. 2004). *TP53* mutations are strongly associated with chemo-resistance and a very poor outcome; other genes frequently mutated are *TET2*, *PTPN11*, *IDH1/2*, *NRAS*, and *FLT3*.

### 2.4.7 AML, Not Otherwise Specified (NOS)

To define the diagnosis of "AML NOS," it is necessary to rule out other WHO categories according to medical history, and morphology, immunophenotype, and genetics: "AML NOS" includes cases that do not fulfill the criteria for any of the other categories. Morphology and immunophenotyping are crucial for the diagnosis and subclassification, since these features are different for each entity belonging to this category, and indicate the major lineages involved and their degree of maturation/differentiation.

AML with minimal differentiation coincides with FAB classification M0: most commonly, blasts are medium size with agranular cytoplasm and round or indented nuclei, with dispersed chromatin and presence of nucleoli. Cytochemical staining demonstrates the negativity for MPO and Sudan Black B; immunophenotypic features include the expression of markers of immaturity as CD34 and HLA-DR, while antigens of monocytic maturation are absent. Immunophenotypic evaluation is helpful in identifying those cases that are morphologically indistinguishable from acute lymphoblastic leukemias or acute leukemias of ambiguous lineage. About 16–22% *FLT3* mutations have been described.

AML without maturation coincides with FAB classification M1 and requires <10% maturing cells of the granulocytic lineage counted as proportion of all the nucleated bone marrow cells. Blasts may have azurophilic granules or may be agranular, looking like lymphoblasts, but MPO and Sudan Black B are positive in about 3% of blasts. Immunophenotypic features include expression of myeloblastic differentiation markers (CD33, CD13, and CD117) and markers of immaturity (CD34 and HLA-DR), while antigens of granulocytic and monocytic maturation are absent; it is possible to find lineage aberration antigens, as CD7, CD2, CD19, or CD56.

AML with maturation coincides with FAB classification M2: for diagnosis, ≥10% maturing cells of the granulocytic lineage and <20% cells with monocytic differentiation counted as proportion of bone marrow cells are required. Morphologic features of blasts are the same described for AML with t(8;21)(q22;q22.1), and this balanced translocation must be excluded. Immunophenotypic characteristics include the expression of myeloid-associated markers with granulocytic differentiation antigens (CD13, CD33, CD65, CD11b, and CD15 positivity); some cases have shown aberrant expression of CD7.

Acute myelomonocytic leukemia coincides with FAB classification M4, and ≥20% cells with granulocytic differentiation and ≥20% with monocytic differentiation are necessary for diagnosis. Morphologic examination shows the same features described for AML with inv(16)(p13.1q22) or t(16;16)(p13.1;q22), and this recurrent abnormality has to be excluded by genetic/cytogenetic evaluation for a correct classification. Cytochemical staining with MPO and NSE may be helpful in the diagnosis since these reactions are positive in most of the cases. Immunophenotyping typically shows more than one blast population: one expressing granulocytic differentiation antigens and another expressing monocytic differentiation markers, while in some cases it is possible to identify a third group of blasts expressing immaturity antigens; positivity for CD7 may be revealed.

Acute monoblastic/monocytic leukemia coincides with FAB M5 classification, with >80% of blasts belonging to monocytic lineage, including monoblasts, promonocytes, and monocytes. Monoblasts are typically large, with abundant basophilic cytoplasm and round nuclei with lacy chromatin, and one or more large prominent nucleoli; pseudopods may be observed. Promonocytes have a less basophilic, more granulated cytoplasm, and irregular and delicately convoluted nuclear configuration, sometimes hypersegmented. NSE reaction is positive in 80–90% of cases. Immunophenotyping usually shows expression of myeloid antigens and monocytic differentiation markers, while aberrant presence of CD7 and/or CD56 may be observed. The t(8;16)(p11.2;p13.3) translocation has been associated with acute monocytic leukemia (but also with acute myelomonocytic leukemia), and in most cases, the clinical presentation includes hemophagocytosis by leukemic cells and coagulopathy. Acute monoblastic/monocytic leukemia, in general, may present with bleeding disorders and extramedullary infiltration, especially in the central nervous system (CNS), cutis, and gingiva (Swerdlow et al. 2017).

Pure erythroid leukemia coincides with FAB classification M6 and is characterized by the presence of >80% (with ≥30% proerythroblasts) immature erythroid precursors, and myeloblasts <20% of bone marrow nucleated cells. Pathological erythroblasts have basophilic agranular cytoplasm, round nuclei with fine chromatin, and frequently cytoplasmatic elongated vacuoles that are often positive for periodic acid-Schiff (PAS) reaction. Immunophenotypic features include the expression of CD235a (glycophorin A), CD36, and strong CD71, while

CD34 and HLA-DR are usually negative. The prognosis of this entity is particularly poor.

Acute megakaryoblastic leukemia coincides with FAB classification M7 and, for diagnosis, >50% of bone marrow blasts must belong to the megakaryocyte lineage. Morphologic aspects include the presence of megakaryoblasts with blebs and moderately basophilic, agranular cytoplasm; also micromegakaryocytes may be observed, but they must not be included in the leukemic cell count. Since aspiration often results in a dry tap, bone marrow biopsy may be necessary for diagnosis. Immunophenotyping typically shows expression of CD41, CD42b, and/or CD61, and in some cases, aberrant expression of CD7 has been described. For diagnosis, the t(1;22) balanced translocation must be excluded.

Acute basophilic leukemia is a very rare AML in which the primary differentiation of blasts is toward basophils. This entity can be easily recognized by cytological features: the blast cytoplasm results basophilic since it contains a variable number of coarse basophilic granules that are positive for metachromatic staining with toluidine blue. The immunophenotypic profile shows expression of CD123, CD203c, and CD11b in addition to other myeloid antigens, while CD117 is not expressed.

Acute panmyelosis with myelofibrosis (APMF) is a very rare form of de novo AML, associated by definition with the presence of medullary fibrosis: for this reason, bone marrow biopsy with immunohistochemistry is required for diagnosis. The term panmyelosis indicates the presence of a hypercellular bone marrow with an increase in multiple cell lines (erythroid precursors, granulocytic precursors, and megakaryocytes): the multilineage nature of the proliferation may be confirmed by immunohistochemistry, using a panel of antibodies including MPO, lysozyme, megakaryocytic, and erythroid markers (Bain and Bene 2019).

### 2.4.8 Myeloid Sarcoma

Myeloid sarcoma is a rare AML manifestation. It is defined as a tumor mass composed of myeloid blasts, occurring at an anatomical site different from bone marrow and that modifies the normal tissue architecture, which distinguishes myeloid sarcoma from other types of AML with infiltration by myeloid blasts. Myeloid sarcoma may present without an underlying AML or other myeloid neoplasms in about 25% of cases; more commonly, it may precede or coincide with AML onset or with acute blastic transformation of MDS, MDS/MPN, or MPN. It may also represent the first manifestation of relapse in a patient with previously diagnosed AML, as well as one of the possible complications of allogenic hematopoietic stem cell transplantation (allo-HSCT) (Almond et al. 2017).

About 90% of myeloid sarcoma cases involve a unique site, commonly skin, lymph nodes, gastrointestinal tract, bone, soft tissue, peritoneum, and testes. The diagnosis is based on histological and immunohistochemical evaluation: the absence of a significant blast population assessed by morphologic and immunohistochemical studies, brings to the diagnosis of extramedullary hematopoiesis (myeloid metaplasia), and excludes a myeloid sarcoma. Morphology usually presents blasts with myeloblastic, myelomonocytic, or monoblastic/monocytic features. Frequently, the blastic population mimics a metastatic carcinoma by forming cohesive nests, and/or a linear stretch, surrounded by fibrotic septa. Immunohistochemistry is helpful in distinguishing myeloid sarcoma from solid tumors or lymphomas: CD68-KP1 is the most commonly expressed marker, followed by MPO, CD117, CD99, CD68/PG-M1, lysozyme, CD34, TdT, CD56, CD61, CD30, glycophorin A, and CD4 (Magdy et al. 2019). Cytogenetic alterations have been reported in more than 50% of cases, balanced or unbalanced, including 11q23 rearrangements, t(8;21), monosomy of chromosomes 7 or 16, trisomy of chromosomes 8, 11, or 4, inv(16), and the deletion of (16q), (5q), or (20q). About 16% of cases of myeloid sarcoma stains for NPM1 at the nuclear and cytoplasmic level, reflecting the presence of *NPM1* gene mutations; these mutations seem more frequent when studied by NGS, reaching more than 50% of cases (Swerdlow et al. 2017).

### 2.4.9 Myeloid Proliferations Related to Down Syndrome

In general, individuals affected by Down syndrome have an increased risk of leukemia at all ages. However, in these patients, the probability of developing an AML is high during childhood, and 1–2% of children affected by Down syndrome develop AML before the age of 5 years. Most cases (70%) of Down syndrome associated myeloid leukemia (ML-DS) correspond to a specific subtype of acute megakaryoblastic leukemia, characterized by distinct clinical, morphological, immunophenotypic, and genetic features, including transcription factor *GATA1* mutations (absent in the other forms of acute megakaryoblastic leukemia) (Swerdlow et al. 2017).

The other disorder included in this category is transient abnormal myelopoiesis (TAM); it is a pre-leukemic condition that onsets in 10–15% of neonates affected by Down syndrome, spontaneously resolving in most cases within some months. Further 10–20% of patients will develop an ML-DS within the first 5 years of life. Few patients go through life-threatening or fatal complications. *GATA1* mutations acquired during fetal life lead to the development of TAM in Down syndrome newborns; in a second phase, GATA1 mutated cells tend to acquire additional transforming mutations in other oncogenes, resulting in ML-DS onset (Labuhn et al. 2019). Both entities are characterized by morphologic and immunophenotypic features belonging to megakaryoblastic differentiation leukemia. In patients affected by ML-DS, additional cytogenetic abnormalities have been described, such as trisomy 8, trisomy 11, del(6q), del(7p), del(16q), and dup(1p) (Bhatnagar et al. 2016).

### 2.4.10 Blastic Plasmacytoid Dendritic Cell Neoplasm

Blastic plasmacytoid dendritic cell neoplasm (BPDCN) is a rare type of AML, particularly aggressive, derived from precursors of plasmacytoid dendritic cells; the median age of incidence is 60–70 years old, but it may present at any age, with a prevalence in males. The clinical presentation includes the involvement of cutis, with single or disseminated nodular/popular lesions, and bone marrow in almost all cases; other sites that may be infiltrated are lymph nodes, soft tissue, and SNC (Pagano et al. 2013).

Morphologic features of blasts are very heterogeneous and both myeloid-like and lymphoid-like characteristics are possible findings. In most of cases, blasts are medium sized with basophilic agranular cytoplasm, characterized by the presence of gray zones, with a "granite" or "cloudy sky" coloration; nucleus may be rounded or irregular, peripheral, and containing small nucleoli. A circumferential nuclear rimming by vacuoles (pearl neck appearance), and the presence of pseudopod cytoplasmic extensions may be evident. Immunophenotyping is mandatory to confirm the diagnosis of BPDCN. Blasts usually express CD4 and CD56, but their negativity (infrequent) does not rule out the diagnosis if other PDC-associated antigens (such as CD123, IL3 alpha-chain receptor), CD303, TCL1A, CD2AP, and SPIB) are expressed. Expression of isolated myeloid markers (CD33, CD117, or CD13) and aberrant expression of isolated lymphoid antigens (CD7, CD2, CD22, or CD79a) have been described; in contrast, MPO, CD14, CD64, cCD3, and CD19 are typically negative. As mentioned above, almost all cases of BPDCN present with cutaneous manifestations: histopathological evaluation of cutaneous lesions is an important complementary tool, using PDC-associated markers, such as TCL1, CD2AP, SPIB, TCF4, and MX1 (Garnache-Ottou et al. 2019). More than 50% patients have an altered cytogenetic profile, and in most of cases, it is characterized by abnormalities of chromosomes 5, 6, 9, 11, 12, 13, 15, or complex karyotype. *TET2* is the most commonly mutated gene in BPDCN; other mutations affect *NPM1, ASXL1, NRAS, ATM, KRAS, IDH2, KIT, ARC, RB1, VHL, BRAE, MLH1, TP53,* and *RET* genes (Swerdlow et al. 2017).

## 2.5 Classification of Acute Leukemias (AL) of Ambiguous Lineage

AL of ambiguous lineage is a heterogenous group of diseases, including two possible scenarios: (Arber et al. 2016) the absence of lineage-specific (myeloid, B-lymphoid, and T-lymphoid) antigens on blasts, or (Papaemmanuil et al. 2013) the expression of markers of more than one lineage on leukemic cells, resulting in the impossibility to assign the AL to a specific lineage-related category.

The 2008 edition of the WHO classification placed AL of ambiguous lineage in a chapter distinct from AML and ALL, and introduced new criteria to defining the largest subset of cases expressing antigens related to more than one lineage. Cases without lineage-specific markers are named "acute undifferentiated leukemia" (AUL), while the term "mixed-phenotype acute leukemia" (MPAL) has been introduced to collectively include entities previously defined "bi-phenotypic AL" (BAL) and "acute bilineal leukemia" (ABL) (Vardiman et al. 2009).

In the 2016 revision of the WHO classification, the category of AL of ambiguous lineage includes seven subgroups, according to the presence of specific-lineage antigens and genetic abnormalities: AL undifferentiated (AUL); MPAL with t(9;22)(q34.1;q11.2) (*BCR-ABL1*); MPAL with t(v;11q23.3) (*KMT2A* rearranged); MPAL, B/myeloid, NOS; MPAL, T/myeloid, NOS; MPAL, NOS, rare types; and AL of ambiguous lineage, NOS (Arber et al. 2016).

This category accounts for only <4% of all AL cases and it is considered an aggressive group of leukemias, with worse prognosis than AML or acute lymphoid leukemia (ALL). MFC is the method of choice to diagnose AUL and MPAL, and a recommended *minimum* panel of antibodies to is: (1) anti-CD3; (2) anti-CD19 and three other B-specific markers (CD22, CD79a, CD10); (3) anti-MPO and two to three markers associated with the monocytic lineage (CD14, CD11c, CD64, CD36, or anti-lysozyme) (Matutes et al. 2011).

The immunophenotypic criteria for lineage assignment are:

1. myeloid lineage: MPO (by flow cytometry, immunohistochemistry, or cytochemistry) *OR* monocytic differentiation (>2 of the following: NSE, CD11c, CD14, CD64, lysozyme);
2. T-cell lineage: cytoplasmic CD3 (by flow cytometry with antibodies to CDS epsilon chain; immunohistochemistry using polyclonal anti-CD3 antibody may detect the CD3 zeta chain, which is not T-cell-specific) *OR* surface CD3 (rare in mixed-phenotype acute leukemias);
3. B-cell lineage (multiple antigens required): strong CD19 expression, with >1 of the following strongly expressed: CD79a, cytoplasmic CD22, CD10 *OR* weak CD19 with >2 of the following strongly expressed: CD79a, cytoplasmic CD22, CD10.

Immunophenotypic criteria for lineage assignment are used to identify the subgroup of MPAL, B/myeloid, NOS and MPAL, T/myeloid, NOS. Conversely, AUL blasts often express HLA-DR, CD34, and/or CD38, and may be positive for TdT, but by definition, they lack the T-cell and myeloid markers cCD3 and MPO, and also lack B-cell markers such as cCD22, cCD79a, or CD19. Moreover, they do not express the specific antigens of other lineages, such as megakaryocytes or plasmacytoid dendritic cells (Swerdlow et al. 2017).

Genetic and cytogenetic analyses assume an important role in identifying two separated entities: MPAL with t(9;22)(q34.1;q11.2) (*BCR-ABL1*) and MPAL with t(v;11q23.3) (*KMT2A* rearranged), with the first one benefiting from TKI-based treatments. In the presence of a recurrent genetic abnormality different from t(9;22)(q34.1;q11.2) and t(v;11q23.3), the AML must be classified following the balanced translocation or mutation (Khan et al. 2018) (Fig. 2.11).

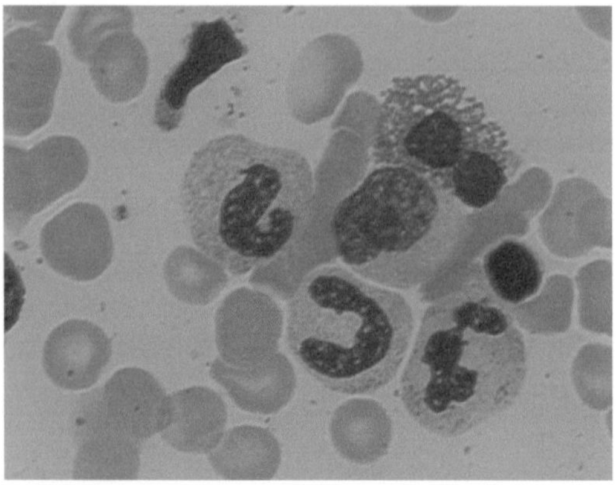

**Fig. 2.11** AML with myelodysplasia-related changes (AML-MRC). One myeloblast surrounded by three granulocytes with evident signs of digranulopyesis (hyposegmented nuclei and hypogranular cytoplasm)

## References


Abbas S et al (2010) Acquired mutations in the genes encoding IDH1 and IDH2 both are recurrent aberrations in acute myeloid leukemia: prevalence and prognostic value. Blood 116:2122–2126

Alfonso V et al (2019) Early and sensitive detection of PML-A216V mutation by droplet digital PCR in ATO-resistant acute promyelocytic leukemia. Leukemia 33(6):1527–1530. https://doi.org/10.1038/s41375-018-0298-3

Al-Harbi S et al (2020) An update on the molecular pathogenesis and potential therapeutic targeting of AML with t(8;21)(q22;q22.1);RUNX1-RUNX1T1. Blood Adv 4:229–238

Almond LM et al (2017) Myeloid sarcoma: presentation, diagnosis, and treatment. Clin Lymphoma Myeloma Leuk 17:263–267

Angelini DF et al (2015) A leukemia-associated CD34/CD123/CD25/CD99+immunophenotype identifies FLT3-mutated clones in acute myeloid leukemia. Clin Cancer Res 21:3977–3985

Angenendt L et al (2019) Chromosomal abnormalities and prognosis in NPM1-mutated acute myeloid leukemia: a pooled analysis of individual patient data from nine international cohorts. J Clin Oncol 37:2632–2642

Arber DA (2019) The 2016 WHO classification of acute myeloid leukemia: what the practicing clinician needs to know. Semin Hematol 56:90–95

Arber DA et al (2016) The 2016 revision to the World Health Organization (WHO) classification of myeloid neoplasms and acute leukemia. Blood 127:2391–2405

Baer MR et al (1997) Expression of the neural cell adhesion molecule CD56 is associated with short remission duration and survival in acute myeloid leukemia with t(8;21)(q22;q22). Blood 90:1643–1648

Bain BJ, Bene MC (2019) Morphological and immunophenotypic clues to the WHO categories of acute myeloid leukaemia. Acta Haematol 141:232–244

Bennett J et al (1976) Proposals for the classification of the acute Leukaemias. Br J Haematol 33:451–458

Bhatnagar N et al (2016) Transient abnormal myelopoiesis and AML in Down syndrome: an update. Curr Hematol Malig Rep 11:333–341

Borowitz MJ et al (1993) Immunophenotyping of acute leukemia by flow cytometric analysis. Use of CD45 and right-angle light scatter to gate on leukemic blasts in three-color analysis. Am J Clin Pathol 100:534–540

Borrow J et al (1990) Molecular analysis of acute promyelocytic leukemia breakpoint cluster region on chromosome 17. Science 249:1577–1580

Breccia M et al (2013) FLT3-ITD confers poor prognosis in patients with acute promyelocytic leukemia treated with AIDA protocols: long-term follow-up analysis. Haematologica 98:e161–e163

Brunetti C et al (2017) Droplet digital PCR is a reliable tool for monitoring minimal residual disease in acute promyelocytic leukemia. J Mol Diagn 19:437–444

Buccisano F et al (2010) Cytogenetic and molecular diagnostic characterization combined to postconsolidation minimal residual disease assessment by flow cytometry improves risk stratification in adult acute myeloid leukemia. Blood 116(13):2295–2303

Buccisano F et al (2018a) Role of minimal (measurable) residual disease assessment in older patients with acute myeloid leukemia. Cancers (Basel) 10

Buccisano F et al (2018b) Minimal residual disease as a biomarker for outcome prediction and therapy optimization in acute myeloid leukemia. Expert Rev Hematol 11:307–313

Cairoli R et al (2006) Prognostic impact of c-KIT mutations in core binding factor leukemias: an Italian retrospective study. Blood 107:3463–3468

Chang JH, Olson MO (1990) Structure of the gene for rat nucleolar protein B23. J Biol Chem 265:18227–18233

Chen G et al (2020) Loss of X chromosome predicts favorable prognosis in female patients with t(8;21) acute myeloid leukemia. Leuk Lymphoma 61(5):1168–1177. https://doi.org/10.1080/10428194.2019.1709836

Christen F et al (2019) Genomic landscape and clonal evolution of acute myeloid leukemia with t(8;21): an international study on 331 patients. Blood 133:1140–1151

Cicconi L, Lo-Coco F (2016) Current management of newly diagnosed acute promyelocytic leukemia. Ann Oncol 27:1474–1481

Cicconi L et al (2016) PML-RAR? Kinetics and impact of FLT3-ITD mutations in newly diagnosed acute promyelocytic leukaemia treated with ATRA and ATO or ATRA and chemotherapy. Leukemia 30:1987–1992

Coltoff A et al (2018) Role of minimal residual disease in the management of acute myeloid leukemia-a case-based discussion. Ann Hematol 97:1155–1167

Corbacioglu A et al (2010) Prognostic impact of minimal residual disease in CBFB-MYH11-positive acute myeloid leukemia. J Clin Oncol 28:3724–3729

Cuneo A et al (1996) Philadelphia chromosome-positive acute myeloid leukemia: cytoimmunologic and cytogenetic features. Haematologica 81:423–427

Del Principe MI et al (2019) Applications and efficiency of flow cytometry for leukemia diagnostics. Expert Rev Mol Diagn 19:1089–1097

Devillier R et al (2015) Role of ASXL1 and TP53 mutations in the molecular classification and prognosis of acute myeloid leukemias with myelodysplasia-related changes. Oncotarget 6:8388–8396

Dicker F et al (2010) Mutation analysis for RUNX1, MLL-PTD, FLT3-ITD, NPM1 and NRAS in 269 patients with MDS or secondary AML. Leukemia 24:1528–1532

Dimov ND et al (2010) Rapid and reliable confirmation of acute promyelocytic leukemia by immunofluorescence staining with an antipromyelocytic leukemia antibody: The M. D. Anderson cancer center experience of 349 patients. Cancer 116:369–376

Ding L et al (2012) Clonal evolution in relapsed acute myeloid leukaemia revealed by whole-genome sequencing. Nature 481:506–510

Dohner K et al (2005) Mutant nucleophosmin (NPM1) predicts favorable prognosis in younger adults with acute myeloid leukemia and normal cytogenetics: interaction with other gene mutations. Blood 106:3740–3746

Döhner H et al (2010) Diagnosis and management of acute myeloid leukemia in adults: recommendations from an international expert panel, on behalf of the European LeukemiaNet. Blood 115:453–474

Dohner H et al (2017) Diagnosis and management of AML in adults: 2017 ELN recommendations from an international expert panel. Blood 129:424–447

Duployez N et al (2016) Comprehensive mutational profiling of core binding factor acute myeloid leukemia. Blood 127:2451–2459

Eirín-López JM et al (2006) Long-term evolution and functional diversification in the members of the nucleophosmin/nucleoplasmin family of nuclear chaperones. Genetics 173:1835–1850

Falini B et al (1997) Immunocytochemical diagnosis of acute promyelocytic leukemia (M3) with the monoclonal antibody PG-M3 (anti-PML). Blood 90:4046–4053

Falini B et al (2009) Altered nucleophosmin transport in acute myeloid leukaemia with mutated NPM1: molecular basis and clinical implications. Leukemia 23:1731–1743

Falini B et al (2010) Multilineage dysplasia has no impact on biologic, clinicopathologic, and prognostic features of AML with mutated nucleophosmin (NPM1). Blood 115:3776–3786

Fasan A et al (2014) The role of different genetic subtypes of CEBPA mutated AML. Leukemia 28:794–803

Frohling S et al (2004) CEBPA mutations in younger adults with acute myeloid leukemia and normal cytogenetics: prognostic relevance and analysis of cooperating mutations. J Clin Oncol 22:624–633

Gabert J et al (2003) Standardization and quality control studies of 'real-time' quantitative reverse transcriptase polymerase chain reaction of fusion gene transcripts for residual disease detection in leukemia—a Europe against cancer program. Leukemia 17:2318–2357

Gaidzik VI et al (2011) RUNX1 mutations in acute myeloid leukemia: results from a comprehensive genetic and clinical analysis from the AML study group. J Clin Oncol 29:1364–1372

Gaidzik VI et al (2012) TET2 mutations in acute myeloid leukemia (AML): results from a comprehensive genetic and clinical analysis of the AML study group. J Clin Oncol 30:1350–1357

Gale RE et al (2008) The impact of FLT3 internal tandem duplication mutant level, number, size, and interaction with NPM1 mutations in a large cohort of young adult patients with acute myeloid leukemia. Blood 111:2776–2784

Garnache-Ottou F et al (2019) How should we diagnose and treat blastic plasmacytoid dendritic cell neoplasm patients? Blood Adv 3:4238–4251

Gary Gilliland D, Griffin JD (2002) The roles of FLT3 in hematopoiesis and leukemia. Blood 100:1532–1542

Genovese G et al (2014) Clonal hematopoiesis and blood-Cancer risk inferred from blood DNA sequence. N Engl J Med 371:2477–2487

Gong X et al (2019) Unusual findings of acute myeloid leukemia with inv(3)(q21q26.2) or t(3;3)(q21;q26.2): a multicenter study. Int J Lab Hematol 41:380–386

Gorello P et al (2006) Quantitative assessment of minimal residual disease in acute myeloid leukemia carrying nucleophosmin (NPM1) gene mutations. Leukemia 20:1103–1108

Goyama S, Mulloy JC (2011) Molecular pathogenesis of core binding factor leukemia: current knowledge and future prospects. Int J Hematol 94:126–133

Grimwade D (2001) The clinical significance of cytogenetic abnormalities in acute myeloid leukaemia. Best Pract Res Clin Haematol 14:497–529

Grimwade D et al (2009) Prospective minimal residual disease monitoring to predict relapse of acute promyelocytic leukemia and to direct pre emptive arsenic trioxide therapy. J Clin Oncol 27:3650–3658

Grimwade D et al (2010) Refinement of cytogenetic classification in acute myeloid leukemia: determination of prognostic significance of rare recurring chromosomal abnormalities among 5876 younger adult patients treated in the United Kingdom Medical Research Council trials. Blood 116:354–365

Grimwade D et al (2016) Molecular landscape of acute myeloid leukemia in younger adults and its clinical relevance. Blood 127:29–41

Grisendi S et al (2006) Nucleophosmin and cancer. Nat Rev Cancer 6:493–505

Grossmann V et al (2013) Acute erythroid leukemia (AEL) can be separated into distinct prognostic subsets based on cytogenetic and molecular genetic characteristics. Leukemia 27:1940–1943

Heuser M et al (2019) How precision medicine is changing acute myeloid leukemia therapy. Am Soc Clin Oncol Educ book 39:411–420

Ichikawa M et al (2004) AML-1 is required for megakaryocytic maturation and lymphocytic differentiation, but not for maintenance of hematopoietic stem cells in adult hematopoiesis. Nat Med 10:299–304

Inaba H et al (2015) Heterogeneous cytogenetic subgroups and outcomes in childhood acute megakaryoblastic leukemia: a retrospective international study. Blood 126:1575–1584

Ivey A et al (2016) Assessment of minimal residual disease in standard-risk AML. N Engl J Med 374:422–433

Jaiswal S et al (2014) Age-related clonal hematopoiesis associated with adverse outcomes. N Engl J Med 371:2488–2498

Jongen-Lavrencic M et al (2018) Molecular Minimal Residual Disease in Acute Myeloid Leukemia. N Engl J Med 378:1189–1199

Jourdan E et al (2013) Prospective evaluation of gene mutations and minimal residual disease in patients with core binding factor acute myeloid leukemia. Blood 121:2213–2223

Kang Z-J et al (2016) The Philadelphia chromosome in leukemogenesis. Chin J Cancer 35:48

Kayser S et al (2011) The impact of therapy-related acute myeloid leukemia (AML) on outcome in 2853 adult patients with newly diagnosed AML. Blood 117:2137–2145

Kayser S et al (2017) Characteristics and outcome of patients with therapy-related acute promyelocytic leukemia front-line treated with or without arsenic trioxide. Leukemia 31:2347–2354

Kayser S et al (2020) Allogeneic hematopoietic cell transplantation improves outcome of adults with t(6;9) acute myeloid leukemia: results from an international collaborative study. Haematologica 105:161–169

Khan M et al (2018) An update on classification, genetics, and clinical approach to mixed phenotype acute leukemia (MPAL). Ann Hematol 97:945–953

Kiyoi H et al (2002) Mechanism of constitutive activation of FLT3 with internal tandem duplication in the juxtamembrane domain. Oncogene 21:2555–2563

Kohlmann A et al (2013) Monitoring of residual disease by next-generation deep-sequencing of RUNX1 mutations can identify acute myeloid leukemia patients with resistant disease. Leukemia 28:129

Konoplev S et al (2013) Molecular characterization of de novo Philadelphia chromosome-positive acute myeloid leukemia. Leuk Lymphoma 54:138–144

Koschmieder S et al (2009) Dysregulation of the C/EBPalpha differentiation pathway in human cancer. J Clin Oncol 27:619–628

Krönke J et al (2013) Clonal evolution in relapsed NPM1-mutated acute myeloid leukemia. Blood 122:100–108

Kuo Y-H et al (2006) Cbf beta-SMMHC induces distinct abnormal myeloid progenitors able to develop acute myeloid leukemia. Cancer Cell 9:57–68

Labuhn M et al (2019) Mechanisms of progression of myeloid preleukemia to transformed myeloid leukemia in children with Down syndrome. Cancer Cell 36:123–138.e10

Largeaud L et al (2019) Outcome of AML patients with IDH2 mutations in real world before the era of IDH2 inhibitors. Leuk Res 81:82–87

Leroy B et al (2013) The TP53 website: an integrative resource centre for the TP53 mutation database and TP53 mutant analysis. Nucleic Acids Res 41:D962–D969

Ley TJ et al (2008) DNA sequencing of a cytogenetically normal acute myeloid leukaemia genome. Nature 456:66–72

Lin L-I et al (2006) A novel fluorescence-based multiplex PCR assay for rapid simultaneous detection of CEBPA mutations and NPM mutations in patients with acute myeloid leukemias. Leukemia 20:1899–1903

Magdy M et al (2019) Myeloid sarcoma. Oncol Res Treat 42:224–229

Mannelli F et al (2017) CEBPA-double-mutated acute myeloid leukemia displays a unique phenotypic profile: a reliable screening method and insight into biological features. Haematologica 102:529–540

Marcucci G et al (2005) Prognostic factors and outcome of core binding factor acute myeloid leukemia patients with t(8;21) differ from those of patients with inv(16): a cancer and leukemia group B study. J Clin Oncol 23:5705–5717

Mason EF, Hasserjian RP, Aggarwal N, Seegmiller AC, Pozdnyakova O (2019) Blast phenotype and comutations in acute myeloid leukemia with mutated NPM1 influence disease biology and outcome. Blood Adv 3:3322–3332

Matutes E et al (2011) Mixed-phenotype acute leukemia: clinical and laboratory features and outcome in 100 patients defined according to the WHO 2008 classification. Blood 117:3163–3171

Maurillo L et al (2008) Toward optimization of postremission therapy for residual disease-positive patients with acute myeloid leukemia. J Clin Oncol 26:4944–4951

McNerney ME et al (2017) Therapy-related myeloid neoplasms: when genetics and environment collide. Nat Rev Cancer 17:513–527

Mencia-Trinchant N et al (2017) Minimal residual disease monitoring of acute myeloid leukemia by massively multiplex digital PCR in patients with NPM1 mutations. J Mol Diagn 19:537–548

Mrozek K et al (1997) Adult patients with de novo acute myeloid leukemia and t(9; 11)(p22; q23) have a superior outcome to patients with other translocations involving band 11q23: a cancer and leukemia group B study. Blood 90:4532–4538

Mrozek K et al (2004) Cytogenetics in acute leukemia. Blood Rev 18:115–136

Nacheva EP et al (2013) Does BCR/ABL1 positive acute myeloid leukaemia exist? Br J Haematol 161:541–550

Neuendorff NR et al (2016) BCR-ABL-positive acute myeloid leukemia: a new entity? Analysis of clinical and molecular features. Ann Hematol 95:1211–1221

O'Donnell MR et al (2013) Acute myeloid leukemia, version 2.2013. J Natl Compr Canc Netw 11:1047–1055

Ossenkoppele G, Schuurhuis GJ (2016) MRD in AML: does it already guide therapy decision-making? Hematology Am Soc Hematol Educ Program 2016:356–365
Ottone T et al (2013) Identification of emerging FLT3 ITD-positive clones during clinical remission and kinetics of disease relapse in acute myeloid leukaemia with mutated nucleophosmin. Br J Haematol 161:533–540
Pagano L et al (2013) Blastic plasmacytoid dendritic cell neoplasm with leukemic presentation: an Italian multicenter study. Haematologica 98:239–246
Pandolfi PP et al (1992) Genomic variability and alternative splicing generate multiple PML/RAR alpha transcripts that encode aberrant PML proteins and PML/RAR alpha isoforms in acute promyelocytic leukaemia. EMBO J 11:1397–1407
Papaemmanuil E et al (2013) Genomic and epigenomic landscapes of adult de novo acute myeloid leukemia. N Engl J Med 368:2209–2221
Papaemmanuil E et al (2016) Genomic classification and prognosis in acute myeloid leukemia. N Engl J Med 374:2209–2221
Paschka P et al (2013) Secondary genetic lesions in acute myeloid leukemia with inv(16) or t(16;16): a study of the German-Austrian AML study group (AMLSG). Blood 121:170–177
Perl AE (2019) Availability of FLT3 inhibitors: how do we use them? Blood 134:741–745
Piaton E, et al (2015) [Technical recommendations and best practice guidelines for May-Grunwald-Giemsa staining: literature review and insights from the quality assurance]. Ann Pathol 35:294–305
Picharski GL et al (2019) The impact of Flt3 gene mutations in acute promyelocytic leukemia: a meta-analysis. Cancers (Basel) 11:1311
Porwit A et al (2014) Revisiting guidelines for integration of flow cytometry results in the WHO classification of myelodysplastic syndromes-proposal from the International/European LeukemiaNet Working Group for flow cytometry in MDS. Leukemia 28:1793–1798
Pratcorona M et al (2012) Acquired mutations in ASXL1 in acute myeloid leukemia: prevalence and prognostic value. Haematologica 97:388–392
Press RD et al (2019) Next-generation sequencing-defined minimal residual disease before stem cell transplantation predicts acute myeloid leukemia relapse. Am J Hematol 94:902–912
Rahman K et al (2018) The triple-negative (CD34-/HLA-DR-/CD11b-) profile rapidly and specifically identifies an acute promyelocytic leukemia. Int J Lab Hematol 40:144–151
Ravandi F (2018) Is it time to routinely incorporate MRD into practice? Best Pract Res Clin Haematol 31:396–400
Ravandi F et al (2018) Evaluating measurable residual disease in acute myeloid leukemia. Blood Adv 2:1356–1366
Rosnet O et al (1991) Isolation and chromosomal localization of a novel FMS-like tyrosine kinase gene. Genomics 9:380–385
Rowley JD, Olney HJ (2002) International workshop on the relationship of prior therapy to balanced chromosome aberrations in therapy-related myelodysplastic syndromes and acute leukemia: overview report. Genes Chromosomes Cancer 33:331–345
Rozman M et al (2014) Multilineage dysplasia is associated with a poorer prognosis in patients with de novo acute myeloid leukemia with intermediate-risk cytogenetics and wild-type NPM1. Ann Hematol 93:1695–1703
Sanz MA et al (2000) Definition of relapse risk and role of nonanthracycline drugs for consolidation in patients with acute promyelocytic leukemia: a joint study of the PETHEMA and GIMEMA cooperative groups. Blood 96:1247–1253
Sanz MA et al (2009) Management of acute promyelocytic leukemia: recommendations from an expert panel on behalf of the European LeukemiaNet. Blood 113:1875–1891
Sanz MA et al (2019) Management of acute promyelocytic leukemia: updated recommendations from an expert panel of the European LeukemiaNet. Blood 133:1630–1643
Schlenk RF (2016) Is there justification for 4 cycles of consolidation therapy in AML? Best Pract Res Clin Haematol 29:341–344
Schmidt-Zachmann MS et al (1987) A constitutive nucleolar protein identified as a member of the nucleoplasmin family. EMBO J 6:1881–1890
Schnittger S et al (2005) Nucleophosmin gene mutations are predictors of favorable prognosis in acute myelogenous leukemia with a normal karyotype. Blood 106:3733–3739
Schuurhuis GJ et al (2018) Minimal/measurable residual disease in AML: a consensus document from the European LeukemiaNet MRD working party. Blood 131:1275–1291
Side LE et al (2004) RAS, FLT3, and TP53 mutations in therapy-related myeloid malignancies with abnormal ities of chromosomes 5 and 7. Genes Chromosomes Cancer 39:217–223
Soupir CP et al (2007) Philadelphia chromosome-positive acute myeloid leukemia: a rare aggressive leukemia with clinicopathologic features distinct from chronic myeloid leukemia in myeloid blast crisis. Am J Clin Pathol 127:642–650
Stirewalt DL, Radich JP (2003) The role of FLT3 in haematopoietic malignancies. Nat Rev Cancer 3:650–665
Stirewalt DL et al (2001) FLT3, RAS, and TP53 mutations in elderly patients with acute myeloid leukemia. Blood 97:3589–3595
Stone RM et al (2017) Midostaurin plus chemotherapy for acute myeloid leukemia with a *FLT3* mutation. N Engl J Med 377:454–464
Sutamtewagul G, Vigil CE (2018) Clinical use of FLT3 inhibitors in acute myeloid leukemia. Onco Targets Ther 11:7041–7052

Swerdlow SH et al (2017) WHO classification of tumors of hematopoietic and lymphoid tissues. IARC

Thiede C et al (2002) Analysis of FLT3-activating mutations in 979 patients with acute myelogenous leukemia: association with FAB subtypes and identification of subgroups with poor prognosis. Blood 99:4326–4335

Thol F et al (2012) Next-generation sequencing for minimal residual disease monitoring in acute myeloid leukemia patients with FLT3-ITD or NPM1 mutations. Genes Chromosomes Cancer 51:689–695

Van Dongen JJ et al (1999) Standardized RT-PCR analysis of fusion gene transcripts from chromosome aberrations in acute leukemia for detection of minimal residual disease. Report of the BIOMED-1 concerted action: investigation of minimal residual disease in acute leukemia. Leukemia 13:1901–1928

Vardiman J, Reichard K (2015) Acute myeloid leukemia with myelodysplasia-related changes. Am J Clin Pathol 144:29–43

Vardiman JW et al (2002) The World Health Organization (WHO) classification of the myeloid neoplasms. Blood 100:2292–2302

Vardiman JW et al (2009) The 2008 revision of the World Health Organization (WHO) classification of myeloid neoplasms and acute leukemia: rationale and important changes. Blood 114:937–951

Venditti A et al (2019) GIMEMA AML1310 trial of risk-adapted, MRD-directed therapy for young adults with newly diagnosed acute myeloid leukemia. *Blood* 134:935–945

Walter RB et al (2013) Significance of FAB subclassification of 'acute myeloid leukemia, NOS' in the 2008 WHO classification: analysis of 5848 newly diagnosed patients. Blood 121:2424–2431

Weisser M et al (2007) Advanced age and high initial WBC influence the outcome of inv(3) (q21q26)/t(3;3) (q21;q26) positive AML. Leuk Lymphoma 48:2145–2151

Willekens C et al (2016) Prospective long-term minimal residual disease monitoring using RQ-PCR in RUNX1-RUNX1T1-positive acute myeloid leukemia: results of the French CBF-2006 trial. Haematologica 101:328–335

Yin JAL et al (2012) Minimal residual disease monitoring by quantitative RT-PCR in core binding factor AML allows risk stratification and predicts relapse: results of the United Kingdom MRC AML-15 trial. Blood 120:2826–2835

Yokota A et al (2020) The clinical, molecular, and mechanistic basis of RUNX1 mutations identified in hematological malignancies. Mol Cells 43(2):145–152

Zeijlemaker W et al (2014) Tumor heterogeneity makes AML a 'moving target' for detection of residual disease. Cytometry B Clin Cytom 86:3–14

Zhou W et al (2020) Loss of the Y chromosome predicts a high relapse risk in younger adult male patients with t(8;21) acute myeloid leukemia on high-dose cytarabine consolidation therapy: a retrospective multicenter study. Leuk Lymphoma 61(4):820–830. https://doi.org/10.1080/10428194.2019.1683734

Zhu H-H et al (2014) Resistance to arsenic therapy in acute promyelocytic leukemia. N Engl J Med 370:1864–1866

Zink F et al (2017) Clonal hematopoiesis, with and without candidate driver mutations, is common in the elderly. Blood 130:742–752

# Germline Predisposition in AML

# 3

M. P. T. Ernst and M. H. G. P. Raaijmakers

## 3.1 Genetic Predisposition to Myeloid Neoplasms: Definition and Epidemiology

Genetic predisposition to MN is defined by the presence of a constitutional mutation, or variant, that occurred in a germline cell (and is thus present in every cell in a person's body), associated with an increased risk of developing MN. This is in contrast to somatic mutations, which are acquired in specific somatic (hematopoietic) cells and may drive or precede malignant transformation. Table 3.1 provides an overview of the genes that are implicated in germline predisposition to MN, or underlie syndromes that predispose to MN.

The exact incidence of germline predisposition to MN is unknown. It is estimated that ~5 to 9% of adult AML patients harbor germline mutations that predispose them to MN (Lu et al. 2015; Huang et al. 2018; Wartiovaara-Kautto et al. 2018; Akpan et al. 2018). However, it is reasonable to assume that the discovery of new predisposition genes in the gene sequencing era will lead to higher estimations on the prevalence of germline predisposition. This is exemplified by the recent finding of the high frequency of germline *DDX41* variants in MDS/AML patients. In a large cohort of unselected adult patients, 2.4% harbored a germline *DDX41* variant (Sebert et al. 2019), making this gene the most common cause of germline predisposition to MDS/AML in the adult patient population (Obrochta and Godley 2018). In spite of the recent discovery of founder mutations that predispose to MN in specific populations (Douglas et al. 2019; Sarasin et al. 2019), it is not known whether the prevalence of germline predisposition to MN differs between ethnicities.

The frequency of germline mutations might be substantially increased in certain subgroups of patients. In cohorts of patients that are clinically suspected of harboring germline predisposition to MN, the diagnosis was molecularly verified in 11–21% of patients (Dinardo et al. 2016; Guidugli et al. 2017). Also, in therapy-related AML (t-AML), germline mutations seem to be more frequent than primary AML (Mcnerney et al. 2017). Of note, germline *TP53* mutations were found in 5.6% of t-AML patients, most of whom had previously received radiotherapy (Zebisch et al. 2016). Additionally, in a cohort of 47 breast cancer patients who developed t-AML, over 20% were found to have a mutation in breast cancer and/or ovarian cancer predisposition genes (*BRCA1*, *BRCA2*, *TP53*, *CHEK2,* or *PALB2*) (Churpek et al. 2016).

It has also become evident that the penetrance of MN, that is, the proportion of patients with a certain variant that will develop MN, depends on

M. P. T. Ernst · M. H. G. P. Raaijmakers (✉)
Department of Hematology, Erasmus MC Cancer Institute, Rotterdam, The Netherlands
e-mail: m.h.g.raaijmakers@erasmusmc.nl



C. Röllig, G. J. Ossenkoppele (eds.), *Acute Myeloid Leukemia*, Hematologic Malignancies,
https://doi.org/10.1007/978-3-030-72676-8_3

**Table 3.1** Genes currently implicated in germline predisposition to MN or in syndromes that predispose to MN

| Not syndromal | Syndromal | |
|---|---|---|
| *ATG2B* in 14q32 duplication | *ATM* (AT) | *GATA2* (Emberger/MonoMAC) |
| *CEBPA* | *BLM* (Bloom syndrome) | *LIG4* (LIG4 syndrome) |
| *GSKIP* in 14q32 duplication | Diamond-Blackfan anemia<br>*GATA1, RPL5, RPL11*<br>*RPL15, RPL23, RPL26, RPL27, RPL31, RPL35A, RPL36, RPS7, RPS10, RPS15, RPS17,RPS19, RPS24, RPS26, RPS27, RPS27A, RPS28, RPS29* | *MECOM* |
| *RBBP6* | | *NBN/NBS* (NBS) |
| *SH2B3* | | *RASopathies*<br>*BRAF1, CBL, KRAS, NF1, MAP2K1/MEK1, MAP2K2/MEK2, NRAS, PTPN11, RAF1, RASA1, SHOC2, SOS1, SPRED1* |
| **Congenital thrombocytopenia** | | |
| *ANKRD26* (thrombocytopenia 2) | | |
| *ETV6* (thrombocytopenia 5) | | *RBM8A* (TAR) |
| *RUNX1* (FPD/AML) | *DDX41* | *SAMD9* (MIRAGE syndrome) |
| *MPL* (CAMT) | *ERCLL2* (BMFS2) | *SAMD9L* (Ataxia Pancytopenia syndrome) |
| **Congenital neutropenia** | Fanconi anemia<br>*BRCA1/FANCS, BRCA2/FANCD1, BRIP1/FANCJ, ERCC4/FANCQ, FANCA, FANCB, FANCC, FANCD2, FANCE, FANCF, FANCG, FANCI, FANCL, FANCM, PALB2/FANCN, RAD51/FANCR, RAD51C/FANCO, UBE2T/FANCT, SLX4F/FANCP* | Schwachman-Diamond (like) syndrome<br>*DNAJC21, EFL1, SBDS, SRP54* |
| *CXCR4* (WHIM syndrome) | | *SRP72* (BMFS1) |
| Severe congenital neutropenia<br>*CSF3R, ELANE, HAX1, G6PC3, GFI1, JAGN1, LAMTOR2, LYST2, TAZ1, TCIRG1, VPS45 VPSB13, WAS* | | Telomere biology disorders<br>*ACD, CTC1, DKC1, NAF1, NHP2, NOP10, PARN, POT1, RTEL1, STN1, TERC, TERT, TINF2, USB1, WRAP53* |
| | | *WRN* (Werner syndrome) |
| **Cancer predisposition** | | |
| CMMRD<br>*EPCAM, MLH1, MSH2, MSH6, PMS2* | | |
| Li-Fraumeni syndrome<br>*CHEK2, TP53* | | |
| *MBD4* | | |

These genes are mentioned in recommendations, guidelines, or reviews on germline predisposition to MN, or reviews of specific syndromes (Baliakas et al. 2019; Bezzerri and Cipolli 2019; Crysandt et al. 2018; Dinardo et al. 2018; Furutani and Shimamura 2017; Raaijmakers et al. 2018; Rauen 2013; Skokowa et al. 2017; University of Chicago Hematopoietic Malignancies Cancer Risk Team 2016; Obrochta and Godley 2018; Rafei and Dinardo 2019; Akpan et al. 2018; Jameson-Lee et al. 2018). Genes are categorized by associated clinical features (although these are not uniformly present). Multiple genes causing the same syndrome are grouped with the name of the syndrome. Otherwise, the syndrome is provided between brackets. This table does not provide a definitive list of predisposition genes, as germline predisposition to MN is a swiftly evolving field. Over the last decade, multiple new predisposition genes have been identified, and it is reasonable to expect that more will be identified in the near future. In contrast, future research might show that a few of these genes confer minimal or no germline predisposition to MN.

*FPD/AML* familial platelet disorder with propensity to AML, *CAMT* congenital amegakaryocytic thrombocytopenia, *WHIM* warts, hypogammaglobulinemia, infections and myelokathexis, *CMMRD* constitutional mismatch repair deficiency, *AT* ataxia telangiectasia, *BMFS2/1* bone marrow failure syndrome 2/1, *MonoMAC* monocytopenia and mycobacterial infection, *NBS* Nijmegen breakage syndrome, *TAR* thrombocytopenia with absent radii the specific gene that is mutated. Penetrance can be nearly complete, as is the case for AML associated with germline *CEBPA* mutations (Owen et al. 2008a; Tawana et al. 2015), but also lower, such as MDS/AML development in patients carrying pathogenic germline mutations in *RUNX1* (~45%) (Godley 2014) and *GATA2* (~75%) (Wlodarski et al. 2017). For some genes, current data is insufficient to determine to what extent a variant predisposes to MN. An example is *RBM8A*, which causes the rare thrombocytopenia with absent radii (TAR) syndrome. Only a couple of cases are reported in which AML occurred (Jameson-Lee et al. 2018). Future research should further elucidate the association between predisposition genes and MN development.

This chapter aims to provide a general overview of genetic predisposition to MN, in which specific predisposition genes will serve to exemplify the broader relevance.

## 3.2 Biological Mechanisms in Genetic Predisposition to Myeloid Neoplasms

Genes currently implicated in MN predisposition are involved in a variety of biological pathways and molecular processes. Some of the molecular mechanisms in which multiple predisposition genes are involved are shown in Figs. 3.1 and 3.2.

First, (loss-of-function) mutations in transcription factors that are important for hematopoietic stem/progenitor cell maintenance and differentiation, such as *RUNX1*, *GATA2*, *CEBPA*, and *ETV6* (Churpek and Bresnick 2019), may be implicated. Additionally, pathogenic germline variants in genes involved in the maintenance of DNA integrity and response to DNA damage can result in a propensity to develop MN (Quinn and Nichols 2017; Rafei and Dinardo 2019). These variants result, for example, in Fanconi anemia,

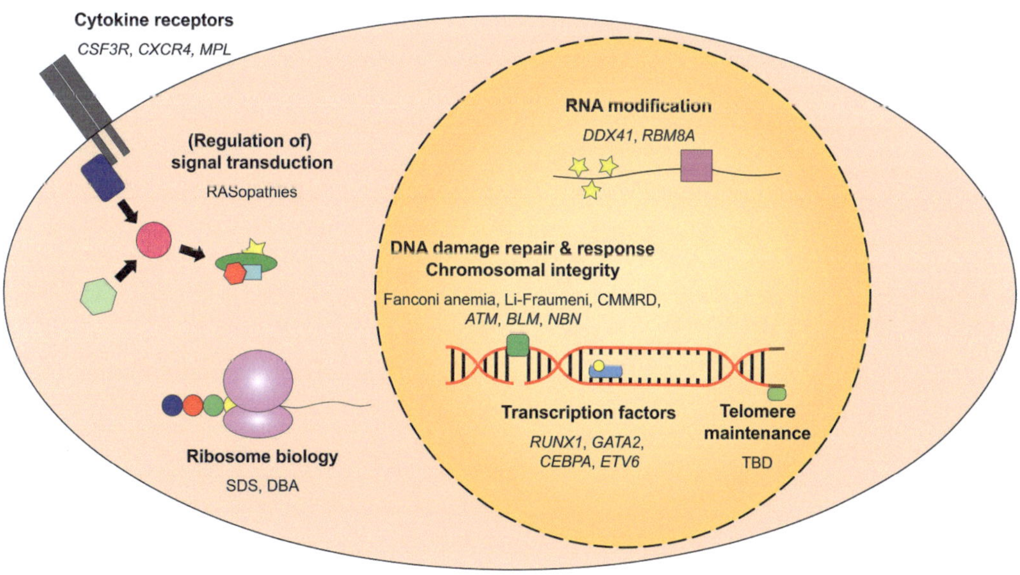


**Fig. 3.1** Recurrent molecular processes and functions of genes implicated in myeloid neoplasms predisposition. Genes implicated in myeloid neoplasms (MN) predisposition cover a variety of cellular functions. Some biological processes in which multiple of these genes are involved are depicted in bold, together with a selection of applicable genes (in italics) or syndromes. This illustration does not cover all genes implicated in MN predisposition. *SDS* Shwachman-Diamond syndrome, *DBA* Diamond-Blackfan anemia, *CMMRD* constitutional mismatch repair deficiency, *TBD* telomere biology disorder. (Adapted from University of Chicago Hematopoietic Malignancies Cancer Risk Team 2016)

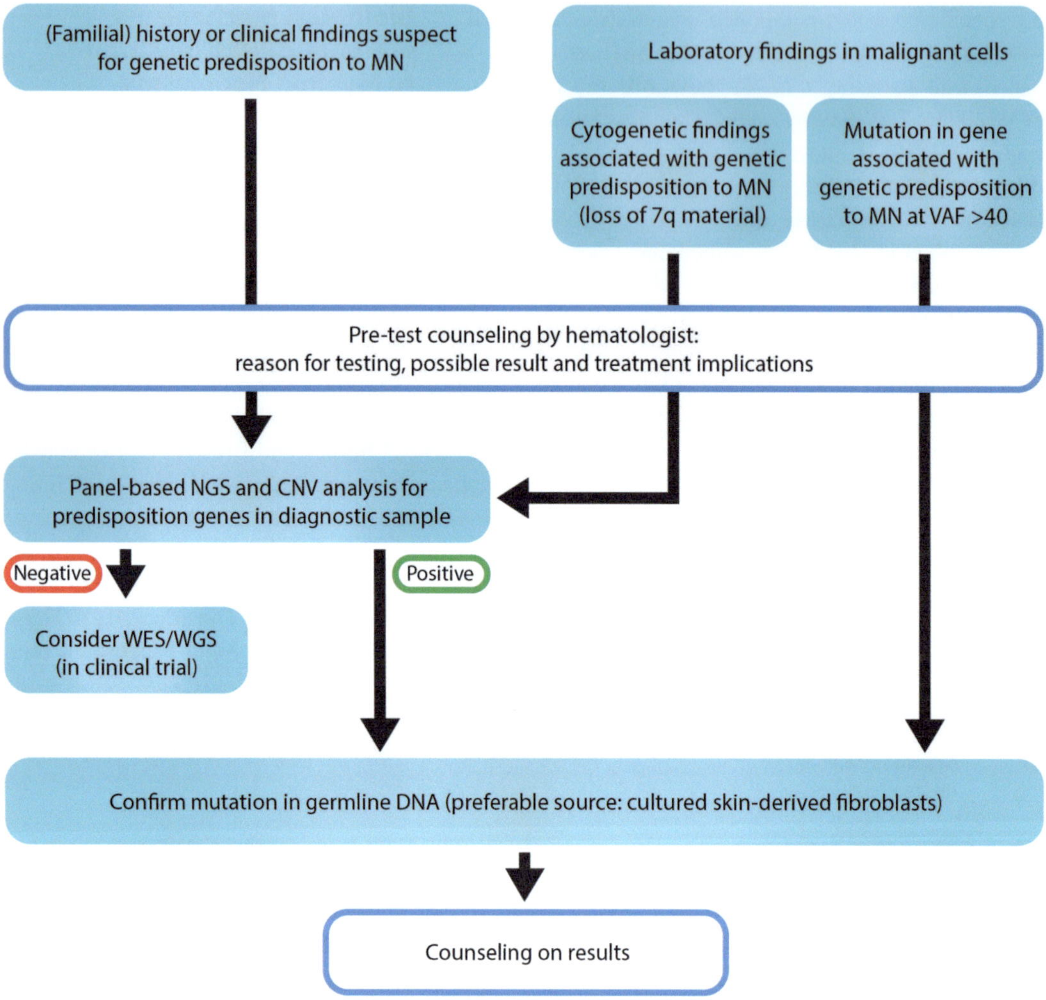


**Fig. 3.2** Decision tree indicating the general diagnostic algorithm for genetic predisposition to myeloid neoplasms. Either clinical suspicion or laboratory findings may warrant testing for germline predisposition. In all cases, patients should be counseled before testing commences. In case of clinical suspicion, or if loss of 7q material was detected in malignant cells from (young) patients, diagnostic material may serve as initial source of DNA for (panel-based) next generation sequencing (NGS) and copy number variant (CNV) analysis (for candidate genes). Mutations detected in this work-up, or mutations in a gene implicated in genetic predisposition with a variant allele frequency (VAF) > 40% in diagnostic samples, should be confirmed in germline DNA. In case of negative results despite a strong suspicion of predisposition, whole exome sequencing (WES) or whole genome sequencing (WGS) in the context of a clinical trial should be considered. In any case, patients should be counseled on the results of germline testing. (Adapted from Raaijmakers et al. 2018)

Li-Fraumeni syndrome, constitutional mismatch repair deficiency (CMMRD) syndrome, ataxia telangiectasia (AT), Bloom syndrome, and Nijmegen breakage syndrome (NBS). As might be expected, these syndromes predispose to more types of cancer besides MN (see "Clinical and genetic principles of familial predisposition to myeloid neoplasms"). Another DNA-related mechanism in which some MN predisposition genes are involved is telomere maintenance. Pathogenic variants in these genes result in telomere biology disorders (TBD), of which dyskeratosis congenita is the prototype example (Mason and Bessler 2011).

Other MN predisposition genes have functions in the processing and translation of RNA and RNA modification, in which *DDX41* and *RBM8A* are involved (Jameson-Lee et al. 2018; Rafei and Dinardo 2019). Germline deficiencies in genes governing ribosome biogenesis and/or encoding ribosomal components can lead to bone marrow failure and leukemia predisposition. These disorders are collectively known as "ribosomopathies," including Shwachman-Diamond syndrome (SDS) and Diamond-Blackfan anemia (DBA) (Aspesi and Ellis 2019).

Specific deficiencies in signal reception and transduction may cause predisposition to MN. Germline mutations in cytokine receptors *CSF3R*, *CXCR4,* and *MPL* may result in Severe Congenital Neutropenia (SCN), warts, hypogammaglobulinemia, infections, and myelokathexis (WHIM) syndrome, and congenital amegakaryocytic thrombocytopenia, respectively (Skokowa et al. 2017; Geddis 2011). Additionally, variants in genes involved in (regulating) the RAS pathway cause a plethora of syndromes, collectively known as "RASopathies" (Rauen 2013). In these patients, multiple hematological malignancies have been reported.

These biologic pathways do not represent all processes in which MN predisposition genes are involved. The functions of some genes associated with MN predisposition have not yet been elucidated and genes that might be discovered in the future could be involved in different processes. Future research should also elucidate the exact role of these genes in the pathophysiology of malignant transformation, as this is largely unknown for many genes.

## 3.3 Clinical and Genetic Principles of Familial Predisposition to Myeloid Neoplasms

### 3.3.1 Genetic Predisposition to MN May Be Inherited (Familial) or May Occur De Novo

Germline variants can originate in the germ cells of a parent, possibly leading to passing this variant on to progeny. This can result in familial clustering of MN. Initial reports from expertise centers for hereditary hematological malignancies state that in 18–30% of families with two or more (biological) relatives that develop MDS and/or AML, a pathological germline variant was identified (Churpek et al. 2015; Dinardo et al. 2016; Holme et al. 2012).

However, the absence of familial MN does not rule out the presence of germline predisposition. Mutations can occur "de novo" in a (parental) gamete or in a developing fertilized oocyte. In this case, the presenting patient will be the first family member in whom the germline mutation occurred. De novo mutations seem to be especially abundant in the case of *SAMD9* germline mutations (Veitia 2019). Noteworthy in the context of familial predisposition is also the concept of "anticipation," meaning that the phenotype (e.g., MDS/AML development) occurs at a younger age in subsequent generations (Desai et al. 2017; Tegg et al. 2011). In such cases, a patient might develop a hematological malignancy at a younger age than an affected parent, possibly even before the parent.

### 3.3.2 Genetic Predisposition to MN May or May Not Be Accompanied by Syndromic Organ Pathology

Some germline variants that predispose to MN can also cause dysfunction in (multiple) other organ systems and symptoms resulting from these pathologies. Examples of diseases that are classically accompanied by such syndromic pathologies include, but are not limited to, SDS (Bezzerri and Cipolli 2019), TBD (Mason and Bessler 2011; Opresko and Shay 2017), and Fanconi anemia (Nalepa and Clapp 2018) (see Table 3.1). Additionally, *GATA2* insufficiency can cause the Emberger/MonoMAC-syndrome (Wlodarski et al. 2017) and patients rarely remain symptom free (Donadieu et al. 2018). However, it should be noted that the penetrance of these syndromic pathologies can vary widely and syndrome-associated germline variants can even be present asymptomatically. Also, differences in expressivity (severity of symptoms) can result in a wide variety of clinical presentations that may become manifest only at an (advanced) adult age. Due to these differences in penetrance and expressivity, variants in predisposition genes that are classically accompanied by syndromic pathologies can be coincidental diagnostic findings, even in adults, as is described for germline *FANCA* variants (Guidugli et al. 2017) and biallelic *SBDS* variants (Lindsley et al. 2017).

### 3.3.3 Genetic Predisposition to MN May or May Not Be Accompanied by Cytopenia

In some cases of genetic predisposition to MN, (isolated) cytopenia is a characteristic finding. Some syndromic pathologies can include cytopenia, such as anemia in DBA (Bartels and Bierings 2019), neutropenia in SDS (Bezzerri and Cipolli 2019), or cytopenia in case of TBD (Mason and Bessler 2011, Opresko and Shay 2017), and Fanconi anemia (Nalepa and Clapp 2018). However, cytopenia can also be an isolated finding in germline predisposition to MN. Examples include thrombocytopenia in the context of germline variants in *RUNX1* (Bellissimo and Speck 2017), *ETV6* (Hock and Shimamura 2017), or *ANKRD26* (Noris et al. 2013), or neutropenia in the case of SCN (see Table 3.1) (Skokowa et al. 2017). In cytopenia related to germline predisposition to MDS/AML, penetrance and expressivity can differ, even between family members (who share the same mutation, as is exemplified by families carrying *RUNX1* mutations) (Latger-Cannard et al. 2016).

On the other hand, germline predisposition may present without any clinical manifestation other than the development of MN. Germline mutations in *CEBPA* form one prime example (Tawana et al. 2017). Pathogenic germline variants in *DDX41* also frequently present without clinical manifestation (Cheah et al. 2017), although recent data indicates that AML caused by these variants may be preceded by cytopenia (Sebert et al. 2019) or syndromic pathology in childhood (Diness et al. 2018).

### 3.3.4 Genetic Predisposition to MN May or May Not Be Associated with Predisposition to Other Forms of Cancer

Predisposition to MN can occur in the context of a generally increased risk of malignant transformation and cancer (in other organs) (Quinn and Nichols 2017). This is, for example, the case in loss-of-function mutations in tumor suppressor genes such as *TP53* (in Li-Fraumeni syndrome) (Valdez et al. 2017), in DNA-repair pathway genes such as those involved in the Fanconi anemia pathway (in Fanconi anemia) (Nalepa and Clapp 2018), and in genes involved in telomere biology (in TBD) (Mason and Bessler 2011; Opresko and Shay 2017). In other cases, the increased risk of malignant transformation seems to be largely confined to the hematopoietic system. Examples of this include mutations in transcription factors that are involved in the regulation of hematopoiesis, such as *CEBPA*, *ETV6,* and *RUNX1*. Malignant transformation in these cases may be confined to a propensity for the development of MDS/AML (*CEBPA*), or for both myeloid and lymphoid malignancies (albeit to a different degree, in *RUNX1* and *ETV6* mutations) (Churpek and Bresnick 2019; Rafei and Dinardo 2019).

### 3.3.5 Genetic Predisposition to MN May Cause AML/MDS at an Advanced Age

The traditional notion that genetic predisposition will always lead to hematological malignancy at a young age is incorrect. Hematological malignancies may develop in adulthood or even at an advanced age, the latter even being characteristic for *DDX41* germline mutations (Polprasert et al. 2015). As another example, multiple cases have been described in which germline *GATA2* mutations underlie MN development between the ages of 50 and 80 years (Wlodarski et al. 2017).

## 3.4 Relevance of Diagnosing Genetic Predisposition

A molecular diagnosis that confirms germline predisposition as the underlying cause of familial cancer, including hematological malignancy, can be of great support to patients and their family members. In these families, the occurrence of multiple (rare) tumors can be a psychological burden and a cause of distress, anxiety, and insecurity. A diagnosis explaining this "fate of the family" can be of comfort.

Furthermore, the recognition and subsequent diagnosis of germline predisposition may be of important clinical consequence to the management of a patient (and family members).

### 3.4.1 Making a Correct Diagnosis and Avoiding Ineffective Treatment

The identification of germline predisposition to MN as the cause of bone marrow failure and other associated pathologies can be vital to effectively treat patients. For example, misdiagnosing thrombocytopenia in the context of genetic variants such as *ANKRD26* or *RUNX1* for immune thrombocytopenia can result in the ineffective administration of immunosuppressive therapy or even splenectomy (Noris et al. 2011). Similarly, a missed diagnosis of Fanconi anemia or TBD in the context of aplastic anemia may lead to the ineffective administration of immunosuppressive therapy (Al-Rahawan et al. 2006). Making a correct diagnosis opens up the possibility of administering effective therapy, such as androgens (especially danazol) in TBD (Townsley et al. 2016).

In the treatment of MN, the presence of germline predisposition mainly influences decisions concerning stem cell transplantation (SCT), as will be discussed in the following subparagraph.

### 3.4.2 Determining the Indication for Allogeneic Stem Cell Transplantation and Considerations in Making Treatment Strategy Decisions

A critical reason not to miss genetic predisposition concerns its impact on clinical decision-making. The diagnosis of genetic predisposition to MN has implications for the indication, eligibility, choice of donor, and conditioning regimen for allogeneic SCT.

First, allogeneic SCT should be considered for MDS/AML patients with molecularly defined germline predisposition, regardless of risk classification and prognostic factors. At least in theory, it seems reasonable to assume that the germline propensity for malignant transformation needs to be removed to reduce the risk for relapse and secondary MN in these patients. It seems counterintuitive to consolidate a patient with germline predisposition for myeloid transformation with chemotherapeutic regimens and/or autologous transplantation. On the other hand, evidence of better clinical outcomes with allogeneic transplant vs. other consolidation regimens, for example, in the context of patients with *DDX41* germline mutations, is currently lacking. Moreover, patients with germline, biallelic *CEBPA* mutations have a high likelihood of long-lasting remission after chemotherapeutic consolidation and relapsed disease is typically chemosensitive, allowing remission induction and allogeneic transplant in the relapsed setting (Tawana et al. 2015). Future clinical trialing, testing the value of allogeneic transplant regardless of disease risk classification in these settings, should instruct optimal treatment.

Gene therapy might enable autologous SCT with engineered hematopoietic stem and progenitor cells (HSPCs) in the future. Recently, it was found that engineered autologous HSPCs were able to engraft in non-conditioned Fanconi anemia patients (Rio et al. 2019), paving the way for exciting advances in this area that might drastically reduce treatment-related toxicity.

Second, the diagnosis of germline predisposition with syndromic features might be of consequence to the eligibility of a patient toward allogeneic SCT. This is exemplified by TBD, which may be accompanied by, previously unrecognized, liver cirrhosis and/or lung fibrosis upon clinical testing, possibly resulting in ineligibility for allogeneic stem cell transplantation. Therefore, if a germline variant that predisposes to MN is diagnosed, testing for syndrome-associated comorbidity should be included in the work-up prior to determining the eligibility of a patient for allogeneic SCT. This includes additional diagnostic tests to identify (asymptomatic) solid tumors in case of cancer-predisposition syndromes.

Importantly, the presence of a predisposing germline variant strongly impacts donor choice in allogeneic SCT. Unfortunately, multiple cases have been described in which patients received stem cells from a sibling carrying the same germline variant and subsequently developed donor-derived leukemia (Galera et al. 2018; Kobayashi et al. 2017; Owen et al. 2008b; Xiao et al. 2011). Therefore, family members should be precluded from serving as a donor for patients with documented germline predisposition, unless the genetic variant can be ruled out in the potential donor. Naturally, this requires genetic-molecular testing of the potential donor, which is accompanied by ethical and emotional considerations (see "How to incorporate testing for germline predisposition into daily practice").

Additionally, the diagnosis of germline predisposition to MN might be of influence in determining the conditioning regiment preceding allogeneic SCT. It is important to realize that cancer predisposition syndromes confer an increased risk to malignant transformation (Mcnerney et al. 2017). Thus, genotoxicity of conditioning modalities should be taken into account in these cases, particularly when regiments include full-body irradiation and/or certain cytotoxic drugs (such as busulfan and cyclophosphamide). This should be weighed on a case-by-case basis against the importance of the particular modality in the treatment of AML. In absence of suitable alternatives for the individual patient (for example, in case of poor-risk AML), the standard conditioning regiment might still be the best option but should be discussed with the patient.

Lastly, germline variants may further instruct the choice of prophylactic antimicrobial therapy around allogeneic SCT. For example, patients with MonoMAC syndrome (in the context of *GATA2* insufficiency) should receive adapted prophylaxis including agents against atypical mycobacteria, as they are extremely susceptible to such infections (Spinner et al. 2014).

### 3.4.3 Enabling Adequate Surveillance and Genetic Counseling

If MDS/AML predisposition is part of a general cancer predisposition, surveillance is generally indicated. This is particularly important after allogeneic SCT, as the treatment is genotoxic. Recently, specific guidelines for Fanconi anemia, Li-Fraumeni, and TBD have been published (Hays et al. 2014; Kratz et al. 2017; Savage and Cook 2015). No general recommendations have been published on follow-up after HSCT in patients with germline predisposition to MN, besides specific cancer predisposing syndromes and bone marrow failure syndromes. However, it is stressed that HSCT does not cure non-hematologic manifestations of disease, for which long-term follow-up might be indicated for adequate monitoring and treatment (Godley and Shimamura 2017; Baliakas et al. 2019).

In all cases, there is an indication to refer patients to a genetic counselor. Pre-test counseling offers patients insight into the potential consequences of identifying germline predisposition, and post-test counseling is required to instruct patients how to interpret their disease and the treatment decisions in the context of the test results. Hereditary predisposition to MN has implications for family members as well, which are discussed in "Incorporating germline predisposition testing in daily practice."

## 3.5 Incorporating Germline Predisposition Testing into Daily Practice

### 3.5.1 In Which Patients Should Molecular-Genetic Testing to Identify Germline Predisposition to MDS/AML Be Considered?

It is not straightforward to determine when to speak of familial predisposition and which patients to test. The (emotional) burden of testing for hereditary predisposition should be weighed against the significance of the diagnosis and the clinical consequences for the patient. The matter of which patients to test for germline variants has been addressed in several expert recommendations, based on reviews and/or experiences of single institutions, either by generally outlining when to suspect genetic predisposition (Akpan et al. 2018; Baptista et al. 2017; Crysandt et al. 2018; Furutani and Shimamura 2017; Niemeyer and Mecucci 2017; Obrochta and Godley 2018) or by providing defined criteria for whom to refer (Churpek et al. 2013) or whom to test (Bochtler et al. 2018; Desai et al. 2017; Dinardo et al. 2018; Duployez et al. 2016; Raaijmakers et al. 2018; University of Chicago Hematopoietic Malignancies Cancer Risk Team 2016). Recently, the first guideline proposed by an international working group has been published (Baliakas et al. 2019). Four scenarios warranting the consideration of germline testing can be discerned, which are discussed below and summarized in Table 3.2. Based on previous recommendations and guidelines, we include a general decision tree indicating the diagnostic algorithm for genetic predisposition to MN in Fig. 3.2. Diagnostic checklists have been published to guide the clinical implementation of screening for genetic predisposition (Duployez et al. 2016; University of Chicago Hematopoietic Malignancies Cancer Risk Team 2016).

**Table 3.2** Indications to test for genetic predisposition to myeloid malignancies

| |
|---|
| **1. Family history**<br>– Hematological (myeloid) malignancies<br>– Solid tumors<br>– Persistent cytopenia/aplastic anemia<br>– Any other organ manifestation/specific finding that can be related to germline predisposition to MN (see Table 3.3) |
| **2. Organ manifestations/specific findings** See Table 3.3 |
| **3. Molecular/cytogenetic aberrations**<br>Mutation in gene represented on a somatic panel at diagnosis that is known to be potentially related to genetic predisposition (VAF > 40%) or loss of chromosome 7 material at diagnosis (in young patients) |
| **4. Age**<br>– Young patients with MDS<br>– Young MN patients with loss of chromosome 7 material |

This table contains findings that should raise awareness of a possible underlying genetic predisposition for myeloid neoplasms (MN). Current recommendations and guidelines have not reached consensus on specified criteria for testing

*VAF* variant allele frequencies

#### 3.5.1.1 Family History of (Hematological) Malignancy and Other Signs

First, as germline predisposition can result in familial clustering of MN, a detailed family history is vital for the diagnostic work-up of any MN patient. In case of cancer predisposition syndromes, familial occurrence of solid malignancies is potentially another indicator of germline predisposition, as can other hematological malignancies be in case of pathological variants in certain predisposition genes.

It should be noted that the number of affected relatives, the genetic distance of affected relatives (degree), and the nature of (hematological) disorders and/or malignancies these relatives suffer from, which are used as indication to perform germline testing, are somewhat arbitrary. Institutions differ in their specific recommendations on this aspect. In general, applying less strict criteria will lead to a larger

**Table 3.3** Findings in genetic predisposition to myeloid malignancies

| | |
|---|---|
| **Hematological** | |
| – (Persistent) Cytopenia of any or multiple lineages | *ANKRD26, ETV6, RUNX1*, CAMT, SCN, DBA, Fanconi, TBD, *SAMD9, SAMD9L* |
| – Bleeding tendency | *ANKRD26, ETV6, RUNX1* |
| **Oral mucosa & dentition** | |
| – Leukoplakia | TBD |
| – Abnormal dentition/dental caries | TBD |
| **Skin and adnexa** | |
| – Café-au-lait spots | Fanconi, RASopathy, CMMRD |
| – Pigmentation abnormalities/freckling | Fanconi, RASopathy, CMMRD |
| – Warts (genital, hands, feet) | *GATA2, CXCR4* |
| – Lymphedema | *GATA2* |
| – Nail dystrophy | TBD |
| – Early greying | TBD |
| **Skeletal system** | |
| – Osteoporosis | TBD, SDS, *WRN* |
| – Skeletal abnormalities | SDS, TAR, Fanconi |
| – Short stature | Fanconi, DBA, SDS, *NBN, BLM* |
| **Lungs** | |
| – Fibrosis | TBD |
| – Early onset emphysema | TBD |
| – Organizing pneumonia | TBD |
| – Pulmonary alveolar proteinosis | *GATA2* |
| **Liver & pancreas** | |
| – Cirrhosis | TBD |
| – Exocrine pancreatic insufficiency | SDS |
| **Nervous system & sensory organs** | |
| – Intellectual disability | Fanconi |
| – Neurologic disorders | *SAMD9, SAMD9L, ELANE*, Fanconi, AT, TBD |
| – Deafness (sensorineural) | *SRP72, GATA2* |
| – Ophthalmic abnormalities | TBD |
| **Endocrine system** | |
| – Hypergonadotrophic hypogonadism | Fanconi |
| **Other** | |
| – Congenital anatomical abnormalities and dysmorphic features | TAR, RASopathies, Fanconi, DBA, *NBN* |
| – Immunodeficiency, repetitive (opportunistic) infections (atypical mycobacteria) | SCN, SDS, GATA2, *CXCR4* |
| – (Multiple) other forms of cancer (at young age) | Li-Fraumeni, CMMRD, TBD, AT, *BLM, WRN, MBD4* |
| – Severe toxicity with cytotoxic exposures | AT |

In the left column, a summarized overview of signs and symptoms that may be present in germline predisposition to MN is listed. In the right column, some of the genes or syndromes that are associated with these findings are listed (per sign). Note that per sign, only some important examples are provided, and that this list is not exhaustive
*CAMT* congenital amegakaryocytic thrombocytopenia, *SCN* severe congenital neutropenia, *DBA* Diamond-Blackfan anemia, *Fanconi* Fanconi anemia, *TBD* telomere biology disorders, *CMMRD constitutional mismatch repair deficiency, SDS* Shwachman-Diamond syndrome, *AT* ataxia telangiectasia, *TAR* thrombocytopenia with absent radii

number of patients to test, resulting in higher costs and a decrease in diagnostic yield.

#### 3.5.1.2 Specific Findings in Personal Medical History, Physical Examination, or Diagnostic Tests

As discussed before, germline predisposition to MN might be accompanied by syndromic pathologies or cytopenia (preceding the diagnosis of AML). A thorough medical history and physical examination are key to identifying these signs. Some of the previously mentioned recommendations provide a comprehensive list of predisposition genes with associated signs (Baliakas et al. 2019; Crysandt et al. 2018; Dinardo et al. 2018; Furutani and Shimamura 2017; University of Chicago Hematopoietic Malignancies Cancer Risk Team 2016; Godley and Shimamura 2017), and these are also discussed in other reviews (Rafei and Dinardo 2019).

Table 3.3 provides a summary of findings that have been reported to associate with pathologic variants in predisposition genes and are potentially indicative of genetic predisposition to

MN. It should be noted that this table is not exhaustive. Also, future research might result in other findings that correlate with pathogenic variants in currently known or newly discovered predisposition genes. Although most recommendations do not specifically state how many and which signs in particular should be present in MN patients to justify germline testing, most include these as one of the criteria for testing. In general, these signs increase the likelihood of genetic predisposition to MN and should affect the differential diagnoses of the malignancy and lower the threshold for germline testing. This should be considered on a case-by-case basis and weighed against the differential diagnosis for the specific clinical finding(s).

#### 3.5.1.3 Specific Molecular and Cytogenetic Aberrations in AML Diagnostics

In the diagnostic work-up of AML, molecular testing of tissues containing malignant cells (peripheral blood, bone marrow) is routinely performed to identify mutations that affect risk classification and choice of treatment regimen. Some of these mutations can be associated with germline predisposition.

The genes included in the ELN 2017 risk classification, which can also cause predisposition to MN when mutated in the germline, are *CEBPA, RUNX1,* and *TP53* (Dohner et al. 2017). Monoallelic germline variants in these genes may underlie predisposition, and MN might develop by acquiring a second (somatic) mutation in the other allele of the same gene (or other genes) in hematopoietic (stem and progenitor) cells. If a *CEBPA* mutation is found in AML, 7–11% of these mutations are in fact of germline origin (Pabst et al. 2008; Taskesen et al. 2011). This percentage might be higher in biallelic *CEBPA*-mutated AML (Tawana et al. 2017), although a recent study found lower percentages of germline mutations in these cases (Zhang et al. 2020). Although small series mostly show a percentage of 8–10% of germline *RUNX1* variants in *RUNX1*-mutated AML (Drazer et al. 2018; Gaidzik et al. 2016; Mendler et al. 2012), frequencies as low as 0% (Schnittger et al. 2011) and, most recently, as high as 30% have been reported (Simon et al. 2020), with secondary acquired mutations in the other *RUNX1* allele in some cases. Recent data suggests that secondary acquired mutations in *RUNX1* represent the most frequent somatic event in AML related to germline *RUNX1* mutations (Brown et al. 2020).

One study confirmed a germline origin for 11.5% of pathogenic mutations that were identified in genes associated with MN predisposition on a prognostic, tumor-based sequencing panel (Drazer et al. 2018). In this study, all germline variants had a variant allele frequency (VAF) above 40% on the prognostic sequencing panel. Based on this study, most recent recommendations advice to use a VAF of 40% as a threshold for germline testing, in case mutations in genes associated with predisposition to MN are found in diagnostic tumor samples. However, as data is still limited, this threshold should be used with some caution. The number of patients in whom germline testing was performed in this study was small, and the panel contained more potentially predisposing genes than the ELN 2017 risk classification panel. Moreover, interpretation may be complicated by somatic cytogenetic abnormalities leading to loss of the gene in question. However, the results indicate that it might be of interest to expand somatic panels and include, besides risk-associated genes, predisposition genes that are relatively frequently causative of hereditary MN and might present without clinical signs (such as *DDX41*).

Certain cytogenetic anomalies can be related to genetic predisposition to MN. Aberrations in chromosome 7 (monosomy 7/del7q or other aberrations with loss of 7q material) seem to be particularly common in hematopoietic cells of young patients harboring *GATA2*, *SAMD9,* and *SAMD9L* variants (Davidsson et al. 2018; Wlodarski et al. 2017). Monosomy 7 is also a recurrent cytogenetic event in syndromes such as Fanconi anemia, TBD, SDS, and SCN (Babushok et al. 2016). Therefore, some recommend to perform germline testing if loss of chromosome 7 material is found in malignant cells from (young) patients (Baliakas et al. 2019; Bochtler et al. 2018; Duployez et al. 2016).

#### 3.5.1.4 Myeloid Malignancy at a Young Age

In general, myeloid malignancies are associated with ageing and thus atypically present at a young age (Babushok et al. 2016). Data in MDS suggests that prevalence of germline predisposition is 13% in patients diagnosed at a younger age (arbitrarily defined as <40 years) (Lindsley et al. 2017). These may include clinically unrecognized cases of SDS that have a particularly dismal outcome (Lindsley et al. 2017). Additionally, in a select cohort of pediatric patients suspected of having germline predisposition, this diagnosis was molecularly confirmed in 15% of cases (Guidugli et al. 2017).

There is, however, no international consensus on whether an age limit for germline testing should be applied to MN, and to what patients in particular. Some recommend to test MDS patients under a certain age (Raaijmakers et al. 2018), specifically in the case of loss of chromosome 7 material (Baliakas et al. 2019; Bochtler et al. 2018). Others recommend germline testing for young patients with familial malignancy only (Crysandt et al. 2018) or do not seem to apply any age limit in their criteria for germline testing (Churpek et al. 2013; Niemeyer and Mecucci 2017; Obrochta and Godley 2018; University of Chicago Hematopoietic Malignancies Cancer Risk Team 2016). Moreover, the age limit under which patients are considered "young patients" is variable and arbitrary.

### 3.5.2 How Should Molecular-Genetic Testing to Identify Germline Predisposition to Hematological Malignancies Be Performed?

It is important to note that the assessment whether germline testing is indicated in a certain patient or not should be made early in the diagnostic trajectory (shortly after first presentation) to allow timely diagnostic germline testing and incorporation of clinical consequences (such as the indication for allogeneic SCT and donor search).

Genetic-molecular testing to identify germline variants that are associated with genetic predisposition is performed by whole exome sequencing or by a select gene panel that covers known predisposition genes. Most published data is based on panel-based sequencing, in combination with micro-array techniques to detect large deletions and/or rearrangements. In limited datasets of select patients, this method yields positive results in 12–21% (Dinardo et al. 2016; Guidugli et al. 2017). It should be noted that these results were limited by the panel that was being applied.

Although initial screening can be performed on DNA isolated from bone marrow samples, it is essential to verify the results in germline DNA. Blood and bone marrow samples do not suffice, as these are contaminated with malignant cells that have acquired somatic mutations. Possible sources of germline DNA include saliva, buccal swabs, nails, hair follicles, or cultured fibroblasts. In general, cultured fibroblasts are considered the golden standard as source of DNA for germline testing, mainly based on expert opinion (Akpan et al. 2018; Baptista et al. 2017; University of Chicago Hematopoietic Malignancies Cancer Risk Team 2016). To acquire fibroblasts, a skin biopsy can be performed simultaneously with bone marrow aspiration/biopsy on locally anesthetized skin at the time of diagnosis or response evaluation. However, depending on the growth rate of the fibroblasts, results can take up to 6 weeks to become available. Recent data suggests that buccal swabs and hair follicles are good alternatives (Padron et al. 2018), but recommendations advice that results obtained from these materials should be interpreted with caution and should preferably be validated on cultured fibroblasts as contamination with blood is possible (Akpan et al. 2018, Baptista et al. 2017, University of Chicago Hematopoietic Malignancies Cancer Risk Team 2016). Germline DNA can also be isolated from nails or urine, but these methods often yield low amounts of DNA (Padron et al. 2018).

Interpretation of DNA-sequencing results can be difficult or ambiguous, as the pathogenicity of variants is not always clear. Variants may not have been reported earlier and/or be unique to a family. Multiple guidelines exist for variant classification (i.e., determining the probability that a variant leads to a dysfunctional protein that contributes to genetic predisposition), such as the guidelines published by the American College of Medical Genetics and Genomics (Richards et al. 2015). For *RUNX1* germline variation specifically, guidelines have been recently published by ClinGen (Luo et al. 2019). Additionally, segregation analysis (relating occurrence of the variant to clinical phenotypes within a family) and functional experiments (testing the in vitro and/or in vivo consequences of a genetic variant on protein function) may shed light on the pathogenicity of variants of unknown significance. Furthermore, next-generation sequencing panels might miss deletions or gene rearrangements if the analyzing software is not designed to detect such aberrations (Obrochta and Godley 2018). Examples have been reported for *RUNX1* germline deletions (Duployez et al. 2019; Obrochta and Godley 2018). Based on this notion, copy number variant testing should complement mutational analysis, at least in case of negative results on a sequencing panel alongside a suspicion of predisposition to MN. In case of clear familial clustering of MDS/AML with negative germline results in panel-based sequencing and copy number variant testing, whole exome sequencing or whole genome sequencing (on a clinical research basis) can be considered.

### 3.5.3 How to Proceed when Genetic Predisposition Is Diagnosed?

If a germline variant is identified, it is important to distinguish the management of the patient from the management of the family members.

The testing results and consequences for treatment should be discussed with the patient. Besides direct consequences for treatment (for example, concerning allogeneic SCT or additional testing for organ pathologies), this should also include the possible indication for entering a screening program for other forms of cancer (see paragraph "3.4.3. Enabling Adequate Surveillance and Genetic Counseling"). Additionally, the consequences for family members should be discussed.

Patients and family members should also be offered the opportunity for counseling on inheritability of the variant, including considerations on family planning and screening. Hematologists should closely cooperate with clinical geneticists in these consultations. Family members that harbor a pathogenic variant should be counseled on subsequent follow-up and implications of results.

As previously discussed, guidelines for the surveillance of certain cancer predisposition syndromes and bone marrow failure syndromes are available. For other germline variants predisposing to MN, specific guidelines are lacking and general recommendations are mainly based on expert opinion (Akpan et al. 2018; Baliakas et al. 2019; Churpek et al. 2013; Crysandt et al. 2018; Desai et al. 2017; Duployez et al. 2016; Furutani and Shimamura 2017; Godley and Shimamura 2017; Niemeyer and Mecucci 2017; Raaijmakers et al. 2018; University of Chicago Hematopoietic Malignancies Cancer Risk Team 2016). In summary, recommendations state that follow-up of relatives with genetic predisposition may consist of periodic blood counts every 3–12 months (depending on the estimated risk of developing MN) with persistent changes warranting bone marrow analysis.

The benefit of both germline testing and surveillance should be weighed against the (emotional) burden that it causes. Of note, biomarkers that predict leukemic evolution in genetic predisposition are currently lacking. Findings such as clonal hematopoiesis and/or (mild) dysplastic features do not always herald imminent leukemic transformation; cytopenia might not develop until overt malignancy is present. This knowledge gap has precluded evidence-based recommendations for preemptive SCT, which should be considered on an individual basis.

The complexity of the results and the considerations that follow demand an interdisciplinary approach to the management of patients and family members with genetic predisposition to hematological malignancies. Referral of patients that are suspected of genetic predisposition to expert centers for counseling, treatment, and/or follow-up should be considered.

## 3.6 Conclusion

Since it was recognized that genetic predisposition to myeloid neoplasms is not restricted to some rare childhood syndromes, the field is rapidly evolving. Many genes, with myriad functions, have been implicated in predisposition to MN, and more can be expected to be identified in the near future. This also extends to other hematological malignancies, such as lymphoid leukemia, lymphomas, and multiple myeloma. Although it can be challenging to make the diagnosis, it is of vital importance for direct treatment of patients with MN. Also, it enables tailored genetic counseling and surveillance. Although current recommendations depend heavily on expert opinion, increasing clinical and translational research efforts are being made to increase our knowledge of these diseases with the goal of improving diagnosis and treatment, and ultimately prevent cancer.

## References


Akpan IJ, Osman AEG, Drazer MW et al (2018) Hereditary myelodysplastic syndrome and acute myeloid leukemia: diagnosis, questions, and controversies. Curr Hematol Malig Rep 13:426–434

Al-Rahawan MM, Giri N, Alter BP (2006) Intensive immunosuppression therapy for aplastic anemia associated with dyskeratosis congenita. Int J Hematol 83:275–276

Aspesi A, Ellis SR (2019) Rare ribosomopathies: insights into mechanisms of cancer. Nat Rev Cancer 19:228–238

Babushok DV, Bessler M, Olson TS (2016) Genetic predisposition to myelodysplastic syndrome and acute myeloid leukemia in children and young adults. Leuk Lymphoma 57:520–536

Baliakas P, Tesi B, Wartiovaara-Kautto U et al (2019) Nordic guidelines for germline predisposition to myeloid neoplasms in adults: recommendations for genetic diagnosis, clinical management and follow-up. Hema 3:e321

Baptista RLR, Dos Santos ACE, Gutiyama LM et al (2017) Familial myelodysplastic/acute leukemia syndromes-myeloid neoplasms with germline predisposition. Front Oncol 7:206

Bartels M, Bierings M (2019) How I manage children with Diamond-Blackfan anaemia. Br J Haematol 184:123–133

Bellissimo DC, Speck NA (2017) RUNX1 mutations in inherited and sporadic leukemia. Front Cell Dev Biol 5:111

Bezzerri V, Cipolli M (2019) Shwachman-Diamond syndrome: molecular mechanisms and current perspectives. Mol Diagn Ther 23:281–290

Bochtler T, Haag GM, Schott S et al (2018) Hematological malignancies in adults with a family predisposition. Dtsch Arztebl Int 115:848–854

Brown AL, Arts P, Carmichael CL et al (2020) RUNX1-mutated families show phenotype heterogeneity and a somatic mutation profile unique to germline predisposed AML. Blood Adv 4:1131–1144

Cheah JJC, Hahn CN, Hiwase DK et al (2017) Myeloid neoplasms with germline DDX41 mutation. Int J Hematol 106:163–174

Churpek JE, Bresnick EH (2019) Transcription factor mutations as a cause of familial myeloid neoplasms. J Clin Invest 129:476–488

Churpek JE, Lorenz R, Nedumgottil S et al (2013) Proposal for the clinical detection and management of patients and their family members with familial myelodysplastic syndrome/acute leukemia predisposition syndromes. Leuk Lymphoma 54:28–35

Churpek JE, Pyrtel K, Kanchi KL et al (2015) Genomic analysis of germ line and somatic variants in familial myelodysplasia/acute myeloid leukemia. Blood 126:2484–2490

Churpek JE, Marquez R, Neistadt B et al (2016) Inherited mutations in cancer susceptibility genes are common among survivors of breast cancer who develop therapy-related leukemia. Cancer 122:304–311

Crysandt M, Brings K, Beier F et al (2018) Germ line predisposition to myeloid malignancies appearing in adulthood. Expert Rev Hematol 11:625–636

Davidsson J, Puschmann A, Tedgard U et al (2018) SAMD9 and SAMD9L in inherited predisposition to ataxia, pancytopenia, and myeloid malignancies. Leukemia 32:1106–1115

Desai AV, Perpich M, Godley LA (2017) Clinical assessment and diagnosis of germline predisposition to hematopoietic malignancies: the University of Chicago experience. Front Pediatr 5:252

Dinardo CD, Bannon SA, Routbort M et al (2016) Evaluation of patients and families with concern for predispositions to hematologic malignancies within the hereditary hematologic malignancy clinic (HHMC). Clin Lymphoma Myeloma Leuk 16:417–428.e2

Dinardo CD, Routbort MJ, Bannon SA et al (2018) Improving the detection of patients with inherited predispositions to hematologic malignancies using next-generation sequencing-based leukemia prognostication panels. Cancer 124:2704–2713

Diness BR, Risom L, Frandsen TL et al (2018) Putative new childhood leukemia cancer predisposition syndrome caused by germline bi-allelic missense mutations in DDX41. Genes Chromosomes Cancer 57:670–674

Dohner H, Estey E, Grimwade D et al (2017) Diagnosis and management of AML in adults: 2017 ELN recommendations from an international expert panel. Blood 129:424–447

Donadieu J, Lamant M, Fieschi C et al (2018) Natural history of GATA2 deficiency in a survey of 79 French and Belgian patients. Haematologica 103:1278–1287

Douglas SPM, Siipola P, Kovanen PE et al (2019) ERCC6L2 defines a novel entity within inherited acute myeloid leukemia. Blood 133:2724–2728

Drazer MW, Kadri S, Sukhanova M et al (2018) Prognostic tumor sequencing panels frequently identify germ line variants associated with hereditary hematopoietic malignancies. Blood Adv 2:146–150

Duployez N, Lejeune S, Renneville A et al (2016) Myelodysplastic syndromes and acute leukemia with genetic predispositions: a new challenge for hematologists. Expert Rev Hematol 9:1189–1202

Duployez N, Martin JE, Khalife-Hachem S et al (2019) Germline RUNX1 intragenic deletion: implications for accurate diagnosis of FPD/AML. Hema 3:e203

Furutani E, Shimamura A (2017) Germline genetic predisposition to hematologic malignancy. J Clin Oncol 35:1018–1028

Gaidzik VI, Teleanu V, Papaemmanuil E et al (2016) RUNX1 mutations in acute myeloid leukemia are associated with distinct clinico-pathologic and genetic features. Leukemia 30:2160–2168

Galera P, Hsu AP, Wang W et al (2018) Donor-derived MDS/AML in families with germline GATA2 mutation. Blood 132:1994–1998

Geddis AE (2011) Congenital amegakaryocytic thrombocytopenia. Pediatr Blood Cancer 57:199–203

Godley LA (2014) Inherited predisposition to acute myeloid leukemia. Semin Hematol 51:306–321

Godley LA, Shimamura A (2017) Genetic predisposition to hematologic malignancies: management and surveillance. Blood 130:424–432

Guidugli L, Johnson AK, Alkorta-Aranburu G et al (2017) Clinical utility of gene panel-based testing for hereditary myelodysplastic syndrome/acute leukemia predisposition syndromes. Leukemia 31:1226–1229

Hays L, Frohnmayer D, Frohnmayer L, et al 2014 Fanconi anemia: guidelines for diagnosis and management. 4th edn [Online]. Fanconi Anemia Research Fund. https://www.fanconi.org/images/uploads/other/Guidelines_4th_Edition.pdf. Accessed 2 Apr 2020

Hock H, Shimamura A (2017) ETV6 in hematopoiesis and leukemia predisposition. Semin Hematol 54:98–104

Holme H, Hossain U, Kirwan M et al (2012) Marked genetic heterogeneity in familial myelodysplasia/acute myeloid leukaemia. Br J Haematol 158:242–248

Huang KL, Mashl RJ, Wu Y et al (2018) Pathogenic germline variants in 10,389 adult cancers. Cell 173:355–370.e14

Jameson-Lee M, Chen K, Ritchie E et al (2018) Acute myeloid leukemia in a patient with thrombocytopenia with absent radii: a case report and review of the literature. Hematol Oncol Stem Cell Ther 11:245–247

Kobayashi S, Kobayashi A, Osawa Y et al (2017) Donor cell leukemia arising from preleukemic clones with a novel germline DDX41 mutation after allogenic hematopoietic stem cell transplantation. Leukemia 31:1020–1022

Kratz CP, Achatz MI, Brugieres L et al (2017) Cancer screening recommendations for individuals with Li-Fraumeni syndrome. Clin Cancer Res 23:e38–e45

Latger-Cannard V, Philippe C, Bouquet A et al (2016) Haematological spectrum and genotype-phenotype correlations in nine unrelated families with RUNX1 mutations from the French network on inherited platelet disorders. Orphanet J Rare Dis 11:49

Lindsley RC, Saber W, Mar BG et al (2017) Prognostic mutations in myelodysplastic syndrome after stem-cell transplantation. N Engl J Med 376:536–547

Lu C, Xie M, Wendl MC et al (2015) Patterns and functional implications of rare germline variants across 12 cancer types. Nat Commun 6:10086

Luo X, Feurstein S, Mohan S et al (2019) ClinGen myeloid malignancy variant curation expert panel recommendations for germline RUNX1 variants. Blood Adv 3:2962–2979

Mason PJ, Bessler M (2011) The genetics of dyskeratosis congenita. Cancer Genet 204:635–645

Mcnerney ME, Godley LA, Le Beau MM (2017) Therapy-related myeloid neoplasms: when genetics and environment collide. Nat Rev Cancer 17:513–527

Mendler JH, Maharry K, Radmacher MD et al (2012) RUNX1 mutations are associated with poor outcome in younger and older patients with cytogenetically normal acute myeloid leukemia and with distinct gene and microRNA expression signatures. J Clin Oncol 30:3109–3118

Nalepa G, Clapp DW (2018) Fanconi anaemia and cancer: an intricate relationship. Nat Rev Cancer 18:168–185

Niemeyer CM, Mecucci C (2017) Practical considerations for diagnosis and management of patients and carriers. Semin Hematol 54:69–74

Noris P, Perrotta S, Seri M et al (2011) Mutations in ANKRD26 are responsible for a frequent form of inherited thrombocytopenia: analysis of 78 patients from 21 families. Blood 117:6673–6680

Noris P, Favier R, Alessi MC et al (2013) ANKRD26-related thrombocytopenia and myeloid malignancies. Blood 122:1987–1989

Obrochta E, Godley LA (2018) Identifying patients with genetic predisposition to acute myeloid leukemia. Best Pract Res Clin Haematol 31:373–378

Opresko PL, Shay JW (2017) Telomere-associated aging disorders. Ageing Res Rev 33:52–66

Owen C, Barnett M, Fitzgibbon J (2008a) Familial myelodysplasia and acute myeloid leukaemia—a review. Br J Haematol 140:123–132

Owen CJ, Toze CL, Koochin A et al (2008b) Five new pedigrees with inherited RUNX1 mutations causing familial platelet disorder with propensity to myeloid malignancy. Blood 112:4639–4645

Pabst T, Eyholzer M, Haefliger S et al (2008) Somatic CEBPA mutations are a frequent second event in families with germline CEBPA mutations and familial acute myeloid leukemia. J Clin Oncol 26:5088–5093
Padron E, Ball MC, Teer JK et al (2018) Germ line tissues for optimal detection of somatic variants in myelodysplastic syndromes. Blood 131:2402–2405
Polprasert C, Schulze I, Sekeres MA et al (2015) Inherited and somatic defects in DDX41 in myeloid neoplasms. Cancer Cell 27:658–670
Quinn E, Nichols KE (2017) Cancer predisposition syndromes associated with myeloid malignancy. Semin Hematol 54:115–122
Raaijmakers MHGP, Joosten M, Wouters BJ et al (2018) Genetic predisposition for myeloid malignancies: diagnosis and management. Ned Tijdschr Hematol 15:208–2017
Rafei H, Dinardo CD (2019) Hereditary myeloid malignancies. Best Pract Res Clin Haematol 32:163–176
Rauen KA (2013) The RASopathies. Annu Rev Genomics Hum Genet 14:355–369
Richards S, Aziz N, Bale S et al (2015) Standards and guidelines for the interpretation of sequence variants: a joint consensus recommendation of the American College of Medical Genetics and Genomics and the Association for Molecular Pathology. Genet Med 17:405–424
Rio P, Navarro S, Wang W et al (2019) Successful engraftment of gene-corrected hematopoietic stem cells in non-conditioned patients with Fanconi anemia. Nat Med 25:1396–1401
Sarasin A, Quentin S, Droin N et al (2019) Familial predisposition to TP53/complex karyotype MDS and leukemia in DNA repair-deficient xeroderma pigmentosum. Blood 133:2718–2724
Savage SA, Cook EF 2015 Dyskeratosis congenita and telomere biology disorders: diagnosis and management guidelines. 1st edn. [Online]. Dyskeratosis Congenital Outreach. https://teamtelomere.org/wp-content/uploads/2018/07/DC-TBD-Diagnosis-And-Management-Guidelines.pdf. Accessed 2 Apr 2020
Schnittger S, Dicker F, Kern W et al (2011) RUNX1 mutations are frequent in de novo AML with noncomplex karyotype and confer an unfavorable prognosis. Blood 117:2348–2357
Sebert M, Passet M, Raimbault A et al (2019) Germline DDX41 mutations define a significant entity within adult MDS/AML patients. Blood 134:1441–1444
Simon L, Spinella JF, Yao CY et al (2020) High frequency of germline RUNX1 mutations in AML patients. Blood 135(21):1882–1886
Skokowa J, Dale DC, Touw IP et al (2017) Severe congenital neutropenias. Nat Rev Dis Primers 3:17032
Spinner MA, Sanchez LA, Hsu AP et al (2014) GATA2 deficiency: a protean disorder of hematopoiesis, lymphatics, and immunity. Blood 123:809–821
Swerdlow SH, Campo E, Harris NL, et al (eds) (2017) WHO classification of tumours of haematopoietic and lymphoid tissues. WHO classification of tumours, revised 4th edn. vol. 2. International Agency for Research on Cancer: Lyon
Taskesen E, Bullinger L, Corbacioglu A et al (2011) Prognostic impact, concurrent genetic mutations, and gene expression features of AML with CEBPA mutations in a cohort of 1182 cytogenetically normal AML patients: further evidence for CEBPA double mutant AML as a distinctive disease entity. Blood 117:2469–2475
Tawana K, Wang J, Renneville A et al (2015) Disease evolution and outcomes in familial AML with germline CEBPA mutations. Blood 126:1214–1223
Tawana K, Rio-Machin A, Preudhomme C et al (2017) Familial CEBPA-mutated acute myeloid leukemia. Semin Hematol 54:87–93
Tegg EM, Thomson RJ, Stankovich JM et al (2011) Anticipation in familial hematologic malignancies. Blood 117:1308–1310
Townsley DM, Dumitriu B, Liu D et al (2016) Danazol treatment for telomere diseases. N Engl J Med 374:1922–1931
University of Chicago Hematopoietic Malignancies Cancer Risk Team (2016) How I diagnose and manage individuals at risk for inherited myeloid malignancies. Blood 128:1800–1813
Valdez JM, Nichols KE, Kesserwan C (2017) Li-Fraumeni syndrome: a paradigm for the understanding of hereditary cancer predisposition. Br J Haematol 176:539–552
Veitia RA (2019) MIRAGE syndrome: phenotypic rescue by somatic mutation and selection. Trends Mol Med 25:937–940
Wartiovaara-Kautto U, Hirvonen EM, Pitkanen E et al (2018) Germline alterations in a consecutive series of acute myeloid leukemia. Leukemia 32:2282–2285
Wlodarski MW, Collin M, Horwitz MS (2017) GATA2 deficiency and related myeloid neoplasms. Semin Hematol 54:81–86
Xiao H, Shi J, Luo Y et al (2011) First report of multiple CEBPA mutations contributing to donor origin of leukemia relapse after allogeneic hematopoietic stem cell transplantation. Blood 117:5257–5260
Zebisch A, Lal R, Muller M et al (2016) Acute myeloid leukemia with TP53 germ line mutations. Blood 128:2270–2272
Zhang Y, Wang F, Chen X et al (2020) Companion gene mutations and their clinical significance in AML with double mutant CEBPA. Cancer Gene Ther 27:599–606

# Secondary AML

**4**

Pau Montesinos and David Martínez-Cuadrón

## 4.1 Introduction

Secondary acute myeloid leukemia (sAML) comprises all AML cases diagnosed after receiving cytotoxic agents, radiation therapy, immunosuppressive treatments, and those arising from prior hematologic disorders, such as myelodysplastic syndromes (MDS) or myeloproliferative neoplasms (MPN) (Hulegårdh et al. 2015; Østgård et al. 2010; Godley and Larson 2008; Larson 2007). According to the 2016 World Health Organization (WHO) classification, the majority of sAML are included in two different entities, therapy-related myeloid neoplasms (t-MN) and AML with myelodysplasia-related changes (AML-MRC). However, AML-MRC not only contains sAML, but also de novo AML with certain criteria (see below) (Arber et al. 2016; Döhner et al. 2017). Although it is generally believed that a higher risk to develop a t-MN exists after a primary neoplasia, there is no consensus on whether it is due to an individual predisposition for developing tumors or a consequence of prior exposure to leukemogenic agents. The term AML with antecedent hematological disorders (AHD-AML) can be used for AML derived from MDS or MPN, but also for those cases in which a prior diagnosis of MDS or MPN was suspected on the basis of documented blood count abnormalities. The term AHD-AML has been abandoned by the WHO, and has been replaced by MRC-AML, which is more inclusive and accurate. As sAML patients achieve lower complete remission (CR) rates and shorter overall survival (OS) compared with de novo AML, the diagnosis of sAML has been considered an independent prognostic factor per se (Larson 2007; Stölzel et al. 2011; Pulsoni and Pagano 2005; Rizzieri et al. 2009). However, its independent prognostic value has been questioned because sAML is associated with other well-established adverse prognostic features such as older age, worse performance status (PS), and unfavorable cytogenetic or molecular profile (Østgård et al. 2010; Stölzel et al. 2011; Pulsoni and Pagano 2005; Rizzieri et al. 2009).

Secondary acute promyelocytic leukemia (sAPL) cases are almost exclusively diagnosed after a primary neoplasia treated with chemotherapy, radiotherapy, or immunosuppressive agents for a previous non-malignant disease, and the term therapy-related APL (t-APL) is recommended (Lo-Coco et al. 2013). In contrast to sAML, only anecdotal cases of sAPL evolving from MDS or MPN have been reported. The available evidence shows a relationship between developing t-APL and prior exposure to alkylating agents and topoisomer-

P. Montesinos (✉) · D. Martínez-Cuadrón
Hematology Department, Hospital Universitari i Politècnic La Fe, Avinguda Fernando Abril Martorell, València, Spain
e-mail: montesinos_pau@gva.es



C. Röllig, G. J. Ossenkoppele (eds.), *Acute Myeloid Leukemia*, Hematologic Malignancies,
https://doi.org/10.1007/978-3-030-72676-8_4

ase II inhibitors (Beaumont et al. 2003; Mays et al. 2010; Mistry et al. 2005; Cowell and Austin 2012). Unlike sAML, main characteristics and clinical outcomes of t-APL seem similar to de novo APL, and prognosis of t-APL patients is significantly better than in patients with other t-MN (Lo-Coco et al. 2013; Pulsoni et al. 2002).

## 4.2 Epidemiology

The reported incidence of sAML ranges between 20 and 30% of all AML cases (Juliusson et al. 2009; Bertoli et al. 2017; Medeiros et al. 2015; Hulegårdh et al. 2015; Østgård et al. 2010, 2015; Gangatharan et al. 2013; Szotkowski et al. 2010). Nevertheless, the real frequency could be higher as sAML patients are usually excluded from clinical trials and protocols. Furthermore, it is difficult to calculate how many patients diagnosed with de novo AML had previously an undiagnosed MDS or MPN (Sengsayadeth et al. 2018). It is estimated that in two-thirds of patients, the sAML was preceded by MDS or MPN, whereas one-third of them are considered t-MN (86% related to cytotoxic agents or radiation therapy and 13% after immunosuppressive treatments) (Hulegårdh et al. 2015; Østgård et al. 2010). In patients younger than 40 years, t-AML occurs in about 5% of cases, and its prevalence increases up to 10% in patients above 40 years. Likewise, AHD-AML is uncommon before the age of 40 years, increasing up to 30% between 70 and 79 years (Hulegårdh et al. 2015). Table 4.1 shows the main studies reporting the frequency of sAML.

Regarding secondary APL, few studies have reported the frequency of t-APL, ranging from 15 to 21% of all APL cases (Braun et al. 2015; Beaumont et al. 2003; Elliott et al. 2012). Although overall t-APL incidence appears to be constant throughout the time, some authors suggest that evolving treatment strategies for breast cancer (with less frequent use of alkylating agents, topoisomerase II inhibitors, and anthracyclines) could have decreased its occurrence in this setting (Braun et al. 2015).

**Table 4.1** Frequency of sAML

| Author (Year) [Reference] | Age, years | sAML, % | AHD-AML, % | t-AML, % |
|---|---|---|---|---|
| Hulegårdh et al. (2015) | ≥17 | 26.4 | 18.7<br>MDS-AML: 12.1<br>MPN-AML: 5.6 | 7.7 |
| Østgård et al. (2010) | ≥15 | 25 | 19<br>MDS-AML: 12<br>MPN-AML: 7 | 6 (24% of sAML) |
| Juliusson et al. (2009) | ≥16 | 28 | 24 | 4 |
| | 70–74 | 38 | 32 | 6 |
| Bertoli et al. (2017) | ≥15 | 18 | – | – |
| Medeiros et al. (2015) | >65 | – | 17.3 | – |
| Østgård et al. (2015) | ≥15 | 26.4 | 19.8 | 6.6<br>CHT:50.7<br>RT: 22.6<br>Both: 26.7 |
| Gangatharan et al. (2013) | ≥16 | 26 | – | – |
| | >60 | 53 | MDS-AML: 34<br>MPN-AML: 10 | – |
| Nagel et al. (2017) | ≥18 | 18 | MDS-AML: 13.6 | 4.3 |
| Wheatley et al. (2009) | ≥60 | 22 | – | – |
| Szotkowski et al. (2010) | ≥18 | 25 | MDS-AML: 15 | 10 |

*sAML* secondary acute myeloid leukemia, *AHD-AML* AML with an antecedent hematological disease, *t-AML* therapy-related AML, *MDS* myelodysplastic syndrome, *MPN* myeloproliferative neoplasm, *CHT* intensive chemotherapy, *RT* radiotherapy

## 4.3 Etiology and Pathogenesis

Prior exposure to cytotoxic drugs, radiation therapy, or immunosuppressive agents for treating neoplastic or non-neoplastic diseases are considered etiopathogenetic factors for the development of t-AML. Several cytostatic drugs, such as alkylating agents or topoisomerase II inhibitors, have clearly been related to the development of sAML, and thus were defining pathological entities according to 2001 WHO classification (Mistry et al. 2005; Kayser et al. 2017; Schoch et al. 2004; Felix 1998). However, since the WHO 2008 version, these subgroups were no more independent entities (Vardiman 2008), and the t-AML definition included other types of therapy, as no practical advantages were expected from further subcategorizations. Although t-AML seems to increase with age (median age at diagnosis is around 69 years) (Østgård et al. 2010), it can be found in younger patients, too. It has been proposed that some younger patients may have inheritable predisposition to the development of t-AML (Godley and Larson 2008).

The pathogenesis of t-AML may occur by direct induction of a fusion oncogene through chromosomal translocation, induction of genome instability, or selection of pre-existing treatment-resistant hematopoietic cell clones (Heuser 2016). The latter mechanism can explain the high frequency of *TP53* mutations in patients with t-AML. Longitudinal assessments performed in some t-AML patients showed that these mutations were detected at low-variant allele frequency before AML diagnosis and even before exposure to any cytotoxic therapy. Thus, it has been suggested that chemotherapy or radiotherapy may not directly induce *TP53* mutations but more probably select *TP53* mutated clones of hematopoietic progenitor cells, which may expand after treatment for primary neoplasia. Moreover, de novo AML and t-AML show a similar percentage of therapy-related transversions and number of somatic nucleotide variants, suggesting that prior treatment may not inflict genome-wide DNA damage (Wong et al. 2015; Takahashi et al. 2017; Ok et al. 2015a).

The genetic evolution from MDS to sAML is not well known. Studies based on whole genome sequencing have shown that bone marrow cells from patients diagnosed with MDS progressing to sAML are clonally derived throughout a dynamic process based on numerous cycles of mutation acquisition and clonal selection (Walter et al. 2012). During this progression, acquired mutations often interfere with normal hematopoietic differentiation (e.g., mutations in *RUNX1*, *GATA2*, and *CEBPA*) and/or activate signaling pathways that upregulate proliferation (e.g., mutations in *FLT3* or *RAS* family members) (Sperling et al. 2017).

Although the mechanisms and pathways that contribute to transformation from MPN to AML have not been well established, two distinct routes for leukemic transformation have been described: (1) *JAK2/MPL*-positive MPN progress to *JAK2/MPL*-positive AML—this pathway is associated with the acquisition of additional genetic alterations, and (2) *JAK2/MPL*-positive MPN progress to *JAK2/MPL*-negative AML, which are clonally related on account of a pre-*JAK2/MPL*-mutant clone (Zhang et al. 2012; Abdel-Wahab et al. 2010; Harutyunyan et al. 2011; Green and Beer 2010; Theocharides et al. 2007; Campbell et al. 2006). Some studies have shown that post-MPN-AML has a somatic mutational spectrum different from that observed in de novo AML (e.g., *JAK2*V617F mutations are rare in de novo AML, and AML patients with *JAK2*V617F mutations normally have a history of previous MPN; moreover common mutations in de novo AML, such as *NPM1* and *FLT3*, are usually absent in MPN-AML) (Fröhling et al. 2006a). In addition, MPN-AML is frequently characterized by mutations in *TP53*, *IDH2*, and *ASXL1*, and the acquisition of these somatic mutations may contribute to the progression from MPN to AML (e.g., loss of *TP53* in combination with expression of *JAK2V617F* results in the development of post-MPN-AML) (Rampal et al. 2014).

The latency period between diagnosis of the primary disease or previous cytostatic therapy and sAML can range from few months to several years. While the median latency was 1.1 years in MDS-AML (Hulegårdh et al. 2015), leukemic transformation occurs over a 10-year period in essential thrombocythemia (7.6 years), polycythemia vera (7.3 years), and primary myelofibrosis (Cervantes et al. 1991). Median latency time in t-AML can vary between 4.0 and 6.2 years, being shorter after malignancies (5.8 years) and longer after non-malignant disorders (14.3 years) (Hulegårdh et al. 2015; Kayser et al. 2011). The latency period could depend on the cumulative dose, dose intensity, and type of preceding chemotherapy and/or radiation therapy (Godley and Larson 2008; Borthakur and Estey 2007). For instance, after receiving alkylating agents and/or radiation, patients can develop a t-AML in 5–10 years. However, patients who receive agents targeting topoisomerase II have often shorter latency period, approximately 1–5 years. In any case, such discrimination according to type of preceding therapy is not realistic, as patients often receive various types of agents. However, controversial data arise from some studies, which showed similar latency periods in patients with solid cancer who had not been exposed to previous therapy compared with those exposed to chemotherapy (Østgård et al. 2015). These findings suggest that, beyond clonal hematopoiesis selection or direct damage by leukemogenic agents, there might be a potential role of immune escape mechanisms in the pathogenesis of sAML in patients with a primary malignancy or autoimmune disease.

Regarding APL patients, those diagnosed with t-APL are older than those with de novo APL (mean age, 60.2 vs 48.7 years, respectively) (Braun et al. 2015). There is more prevalence of female gender, which may be related to the higher incidence of breast cancer and autoimmune diseases among primary disorders in female patients (Lo-Coco et al. 2013; Pulsoni et al. 2002; Kayser et al. 2017). The knowledge of the molecular pathogenesis of t-APL gained insights after identification of the role of DNA topoisomerase II (TOP2), a dimeric enzyme that plays an essential role in replication, transcription, chromosome condensation, and segregation. TOP2 facilitates one double-stranded DNA segment to pass through another, thus altering DNA topology. Before the re-ligation step, each monomer of TOP2 remains linked to DNA, forming double-strand breaks (DSB). Topoisomerase II inhibitors interfere in this re-ligation step, resulting in accumulation of DSB, which are cytotoxic and lead to apoptosis thought activation of the DNA damage response. Thus, chemotherapy-induced lesions are poorly repaired and generate a wide variety of genetic alterations like novel fusion genes, including t(15,17)(*PML-RARA*) (Mistry et al. 2005; Cowell and Austin 2012). Uneven distribution of DNA breakpoints at both *PML* and *RARA* loci suggest the existence of specific pathogenetic mechanisms in t-APL as compared with de novo APL (Hasan et al. 2010).

Latency between primary disorder and t-APL diagnosis ranges from few months to several years, with a median interval lower than 3.5 years (Kayser et al. 2017). Treatment with topoisomerase II-targeted drugs has commonly been related to shorter latency period, but recent studies suggested that only younger age at diagnosis of primary disorder was correlated with a shorter latency time (Beaumont et al. 2003; Kayser et al. 2011, 2017).

## 4.4 Clinical Features

Clinical presentation of sAML is variable and, similar to de novo AML, depending on three main factors: (1) bone marrow insufficiency, (2) presence of extramedullary disease, and (3) number of white blood cell (WBC) counts and presence of thrombogenic factors.

- Clinical features related to medullar insufficiency:
  - Anemia: weakness, fatigue, tachycardia, dyspnea, headache, etc.
  - Neutropenia: fever and infections
  - Thrombocytopenia: hemorrhage symptoms (coagulopathy, gingival bleeding, epistaxis, menorrhagia, etc.)
- Clinical features related to extramedullary disease:
  - Central nervous system (neurological disorders)
  - Hepatomegaly, splenomegaly, and lymphatic nodes
  - Skin (leukemia cutis)
  - Gingival hyperplasia
  - Granulocytic sarcoma

- Clinical features related to number of WBC and release of intracellular substances:
  - Leukostasis (frequently related to hyperleukocytosis): lungs (respiratory failure, infiltrates), central nervous system (neurological disorders without blast cells in cerebrospinal fluid)
  - Thrombogenic substances delivery (coagulopathy, disseminated vascular coagulopathy with fibrinogen decreased, and thrombosis)
  - Tumor lysis syndrome: hyperuricemia, creatinine increase, hypocalcemia, hyperkalemia, hyperphosphatemia

In relation with the aforementioned characteristics, some patients can present at diagnosis some specific features according to the type of sAML. MPNs are hematopoietic disorders characterized by clonal proliferation of mature myeloid elements that manifest clinically as an excess of red blood cells, platelets, or WBC (Campbell et al. 2006). In these instances, sAML may present clinical symptoms related to the previous MPN, such as hepatomegaly and splenomegaly, or other manifestations related to the increased number of peripheral blood cells. AML from MDS is usually less proliferative and t-AML patients can show signs and symptoms of hematopoietic insufficiency due to prior antineoplastic therapies, in addition to damage in different organs because of therapy-related sequalae (Appelbaum et al. 2006). Moreover, concomitant activity or relapse of previous tumors can complicate the clinical course of t-AML.

Characteristics of t-APL seem to be similar to de novo APL, with no differences reported for baseline hemoglobin, WBC, or platelets counts (Lo-Coco et al. 2013; Beaumont et al. 2003; Yin et al. 2005). However, like non-APL sAML, t-APL patients are older than de novo APL and have worse PS at diagnosis, which may determine the treatment choice and the outcomes (Lo-Coco et al. 2013; Pulsoni et al. 2002).

## 4.5 Diagnosis

Diagnosis of AML is based on morphological findings, so the detection of ≥20% blast cells in peripheral blood or bone marrow is a requisite, except for t(8;21), t(16:16)/inv(16), or t(15;17). Although dysplasia is frequent in sAML, its presence is not a diagnostic criteria (Arber et al. 2016; Döhner et al. 2017).

sAML diagnosis requires a documented clinical history of previous diagnosis of MDS, MPN, or MDS/MPN (AHD-AML); or prior treatment with chemotherapy, radiotherapy, or immunosuppressive therapy for an unrelated malignancy or immune disorder (t-AML).

Immunophenotypic characterization by multiparameter flow cytometry (MFC) can be helpful to support the diagnosis of sAML, distinguishing myeloid lineage from ambiguous, mixed, or lymphoid leukemias, which might be classified as different entities. Another utility of MFC is to detect the minimal residual disease (MRD) after initial therapy, allowing to establish relapse risk in order to adapt the intensity of post-remission strategies.

Cytogenetics and molecular tests remain mandatory in the assessment of AML, in order to complete diagnosis and to identify those sAML patients with favorable recurrent genetic abnormalities (RGAs) who may benefit from intensive approaches not including allogeneic stem cell transplant. In addition to conventional karyotyping, fluorescent in situ hybridization (FISH) and reverse transcription polymerase chain reaction (RT-PCR) are useful tools to classify sAML patients. According to the 2017 panel of European Leukemia Net experts, genetic risk can be stratified in favorable, intermediate, and adverse, in both de novo AML and sAML.

The relevance of chromosomal alterations and gene variants for diagnosis, risk stratification, and choice of targeted therapies (i.e., FLT3 and IDH1/2 inhibitors) has remarkably increased the complexity of routine molecular diagnostic strategies. Next-generation sequencing (NGS) has been established as a new molecular diagnostic tool rapidly adopted by clinical laboratories, being able to simultaneously assess different genetic alterations such as rearrangements, single nucleotide variants, insertions-deletions, and copy number variations in a wide variety of genes. NGS gene panels have been preferentially adopted rather than whole genome or exome sequencing due to an easier interpretation of results, lower cost, and less time. As compared to NGS, conventional single-gene approaches by PCR are laborious and less efficient to detect minor clones, but they are still needed as rapid-screening tests for druggable variants. In addition, NGS has some limitations, which are often restricting its use to the context of research programs.

As compared to de novo AML, some gene mutations could be more frequent in t-AML patients (*TP53* [36%], *PTPN11* [12%], *NRAS* [10%], *KRAS* [5%]), equally frequent (*IDH1* [10%], *IDH2* [10%]), or less frequent (*FLT3* [7%], *DNMT3A* [7%]) (Ok et al. 2015a).

No differences have been reported regarding morphological and immunophenotypic characterization between t-APL and de novo APL (Duffield et al. 2012). To diagnose t-APL, demonstration of the t(15;17) or *PML/RARA* rearrangement is also mandatory. Some studies suggested that patients developing t-APL after mitoxantrone show a higher prevalence of long-type (bcr 1) *PML/RARA* isoform due to a specific DNA-break hotspot in the *PML* gene (Hasan et al. 2008). However, this has not been confirmed later (Kayser et al. 2017). It is expected that NGS studies will help to elucidate the genetic features of t-APL and the potential differences with de novo APL (Lo-Coco et al. 2013).

## 4.6 Classification

According to the WHO 2016 classification, patients diagnosed with AML diagnosed after receiving cytotoxic drugs, radiation therapy, or immunosuppressive agents for neoplastic and non-neoplastic diseases should be classified in the t-MN group (Arber et al. 2016; Döhner et al. 2017). However, this designation includes also patients diagnosed with MDS or MDS/MPN after mutagenic therapy, so t-AML seems to be a better term to differentiate AML from other t-MN diseases (Kayser et al. 2017). According to the WHO 2016, if a recurrent genetic abnormality is diagnosed, this should be added to the nomenclature (see Table 4.2). It remains controversial whether well-defined entities with particular treatment approaches and prognosis, such as APL or core-binding-factor (CBF) AML, should be included in the t-MN cluster, as recommended by WHO, or could preferably remain in their respective groups of recurrent genetic abnormalities.

The 2016 WHO AML with myelodysplasia-related changes (MRC-AML) is a wide entity that encompasses both sAML and de novo AML. The WHO 2001 defined AML with multilineage dysplasia (AML-MLD) as a new category, which was only defined by the presence of ≥50% dysplastic abnormalities in ≥2 hematopoietic cell lines. The AML-MLD was replaced by the MRC-AML in the WHO 2008 revision since several studies showed that MLD was not an independent factor when cytogenetics was incorporated into the prognostic models (Vardiman et al. 2009). With hindsight, more authors have insinuated the lack of prognostic significance of MLD (Miesner et al. 2010).

The WHO 2008 AML-MRC is defined as AML (≥20% blasts of bone marrow [BM] or peripheral blood [PB]) with at least one of the following criteria: (1) ≥50% dysplastic abnormalities in ≥2 hematopoietic cell lines (MLD); (2) prior history of MDS or MDS/MPN; and (3) MDS-related cytogenetic abnormalities and absence of recurrent genetic abnormalities.

Regarding MLD assessment, these are the current recommendations by WHO:

**Table 4.2** sAML classification according to antecedents, RGA, and WHO 2016

| Antecedents | RGA | WHO 2016 classification | sAML |
|---|---|---|---|
| Previous therapy (unrelated disease) | No | t-MN | Yes |
| | Yes | t-MN with RGA | Yes |
| Previous history of MDS or MDS/MPN[a] | No | MRC-AML | Yes |
| | Yes | AML with RGA | Yes |
| Myelodysplasia-related cytogenetic abnormality[a] | No | MRC-AML | No |
| • Complex karyotype: $\geq$3 unrelated abnormalities (not including the recurrent genetic abnormalities encountered in AML)<br>• Unbalanced abnormalities:<br>– −7/del(7q)<br>– del(5q)/t(5q)<br>– i(17q)/t(17p)<br>– −13/del(13q)<br>– del(11q)<br>– del(12p)/t(12p)<br>– Idic(X)(q13)<br>• Balanced abnormalities:<br>– t(11;16)(q23.3;p13.3)<br>– t(3;21)(q26.2;q22.1)<br>– t(1;3)(p36.3;q21.2)<br>– t(2;11)(p21;q23.3)<br>– t(5;12)(q32;p13.2)<br>– t(5;7)(q32;q11.2)<br>– t(5;17)(q32;p13.2)<br>– t(5;10)(q32;q21.2)<br>– t(3;5)(q25.3;q35.1) | Yes | AML with RGA | No |
| Multilineage dysplasia[a] | No | MRC-AML | No |
| • Dysgranulopoiesis, dyserythropoiesis, and/or dysmegakaryopoiesis (>50% in $\geq$2 cell lineages) | Yes | AML with RGA | No |

*AML* acute myeloid leukemia, *MDS* myelodysplastic syndrome, *MDS/MPN* myelodysplastic syndrome/myeloproliferative neoplasm, *MRC-AML* acute myeloid leukemia with myelodysplasia-related changes, *RGA* recurrent genetic abnormalities, *sAML* secondary acute myeloid leukemia, *t-MN* therapy-related myeloid neoplasms, *WHO* World Health Organization

[a]Absence of prior mutagenic therapy for unrelated disease. Recurrent genetic abnormalities (RGA): t(8;21)(q22;q22.1); *RUNX1-RUNX1T1;* inv.(16)(p13.1q22) or t(16;16)(p13.1;q22); *CBFB-MYH11; PML-RARA;* t(9;11)(p21.3;q23.3); *MLLT3-KMT2A;* t(6;9)(p23;q34.1); *DEK-NUP214;* inv(3)(q21.3q26.2) or t(3;3)(q21.3;q26.2); *GATA2, MECOM;*t(1;22)(p13.3;q13.3); *RBM15-MKL1*; Mutated *NPM1;* Biallelic mutations of *CEBPA*

- Dysgranulopoiesis: 25–100 neutrophils—hypogranular cytoplasm, hyposegmented nuclei or bizarrely segmented nuclei, cytoplasmic vacuoles—myeloperoxidase deficiency (50%, 20 cells)
- Dyserythropoiesis: at least 25 mature erythroblasts—megaloblastosis, karyorrhexis and nuclear irregularity, fragmentation or multinucleation—ring sideroblasts, PAS positivity
- Dysmegakaryopoiesis: at least six megakaryocytes—micromegakaryocytes, normal sized, or large megakaryocytes with non-lobulated or multiple nuclei

According to the WHO 2016 update, patients diagnosed with MRC-AML must meet at least one of the following criteria (along with the absence of both prior cytotoxic therapy for unrelated disease and recurrent genetic abnormalities [RGA]):

- Previous history of MDS or MDS/MPN
- Myelodysplasia-related cytogenetic abnormality (see Table 4.2)
- Multilineage dysplasia (see Table 4.2)

Thus, AML patients with a medical history of hematologic disorder who have received therapy for any unrelated disease or show any RGA should not be classified as MRC-AML. Table 4.2 shows detailed information regarding sAML classification according to antecedent disorders, presence of RGA, and WHO 2016 terminology.

Although the WHO pathological classification attempts to define biologically homogeneous entities with similar prognosis, the WHO definitions should be used together with age, performance status (PS), cytogenetics, and molecular profile in order to decide the best available regimen for each entity and patient (Hulegårdh et al. 2015; Juliusson et al. 2009; Nilsson et al. 2019).

## 4.7 Prognosis

Similar to de novo AML patients, the prognosis of sAML patients is related to several factors as age, PS, cytogenetics, and molecular profile (Fig. 4.1) (Wheatley et al. 2009). However, sAML patients are often older, with worse PS and genetic features, so they tend to be more frequently considered unfit for intensive chemotherapy. Other baseline characteristics, such as WBC counts, previous comorbidities, or response to induction treatment, have been also associated with worse prognosis in AML (Wheatley et al. 2009; Schoch et al. 2004). It is expected that sAML patients could present with more comorbidities, since prior treatments or malignant dis-

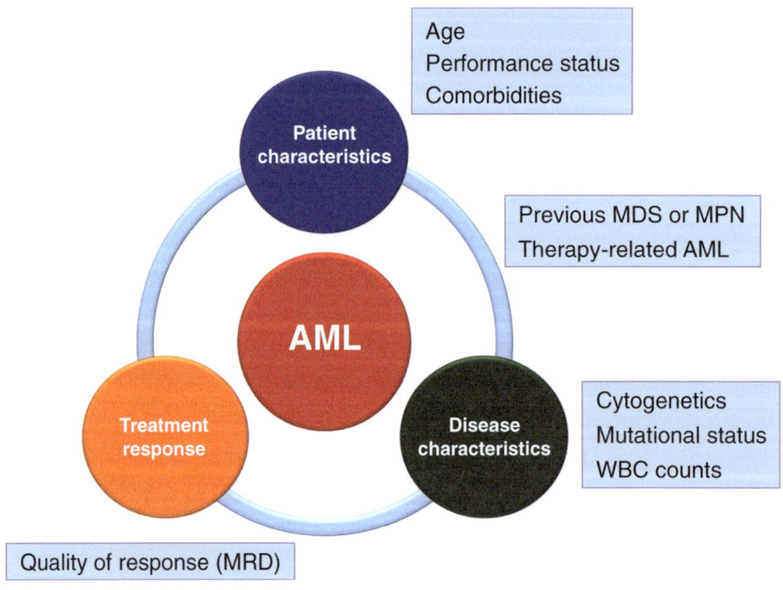


**Fig. 4.1** Main prognostic factors in AML: the place of sAML (MDS-MPN-AML and t-AML), between patient factors and disease-related factors

orders could have caused sequelae (e.g., other organ damage, low hematopoietic stem cell reserve, persistence of malignant disease). In addition, the prognostic impact of some well-established gene mutations in sAML is unclear (e.g., *FLT3*, *NPM1*), as available data mainly derive from studies performed in de novo AML patients with normal karyotype.

The dilemma about considering sAML as an independent prognostic factor remains unsolved as published manuscripts revealed discrepant results (Juliusson et al. 2009; Wheatley et al. 2009; Fröhling et al. 2006b; Szotkowski et al. 2010). Some studies have shown a different prognosis depending on the type of sAML: MPN patients who develop a leukemic transformation show the worst clinical outcomes, with a median survival between 6–11 months and 1-year OS of 10%, which is worse than 20% in t-AML, 41% in de novo AML, and 43% in AML from MDS (Østgård et al. 2015; Mesa et al. 2005; Thepot et al. 2010). As in de novo AML, molecular and cytogenetic changes play a relevant role in establishing the prognosis of sAML. t-AML patients with CBF have a longer OS than those with intermediate and adverse genetic risk, but prognosis seems to be worse than in de novo CBF AML patients (Borthakur et al. 2009). Mutations and loss of heterozygosity of *TP53*, which have been identified as independent negative prognostic factors for OS, are common in sAML (reported in 17–37% of t-MN patients) (Christiansen et al. 2001; Ok et al. 2015b). Similarly, shorter OS has also been observed in t-MN patients with amplification of the *MLL* gene, compared with patients without these mutations (Andersen et al. 2001). Table 4.3 shows the main studies analyzing the prognostic factors in sAML.

Unlike t-MN, the prognosis of t-APL is favorable with anthracycline-based chemotherapy plus all-trans-retinoic acid (ATRA) or ATRA plus arsenic trioxide (ATO). Several studies showed a similar prognosis as compared to de novo APL, particularly after adjusting by age and PS (Ammatuna et al. 2011; Dayyani et al. 2011; Lo-Coco et al. 2013).

**Table 4.3** Prognostic factors in studies performed in sAML patients

| Author (Year) [Reference] | Characteristics | Prognostic factors: findings |
|---|---|---|
| Juliusson et al. (2009) | Registry<br>All AML<br>*N* = 2767<br>Intensive treatment: 62% | PS III-IV. Higher ED in all ages |
| | | Intensive treatment: Improves ED rates and OS |
| | | sAML: No differences between de novo and sAML in ED at the same age |
| Østgård et al. (2010) | Registry<br>All AML<br>*N* = 630 (sAML: 157 [25%]; de novo: 473 [75%])<br>Intensive treatment: 58% | Age ≥ 60 (CR, OS, and DFS): More sAML patients ≥60 yo did not receive curative treatment |
| | | PS (OS) |
| | | Unfavorable cytogenetics (CR, OS, and DFS): MDS-AML (34%) > t-AML plus MPN-AML (20%) |
| | | To achieve CR:<br>• Age<br>• Treatment protocol<br>• Cytogenetics |
| | | sAML patients in CR: Similar DFS than de novo |
| | | CR, OS, and DFS: When correcting for age, cytogenetics, PS, and WBC, sAML lost prognostic significance |

(continued)

**Table 4.3** (continued)

| Author (Year) [Reference] | Characteristics | Prognostic factors: findings |
|---|---|---|
| Schoch et al. (2004) | Retrospective<br>*N* = 1184 (t-AML: 93 [8%]; de novo: 1091 [92%])<br>Intensive treatment: 100% | Favorable cytogenetics: Better OS (independent of age and WBC) |
| | | Unfavorable cytogenetics:<br>• Worse OS (independent of age and WBC)<br>• More adverse cytogenetics in t-AML (46%) than in de novo AML (20%), but the same abnormalities |
| | | Age:<br>• For OS (t-AML + de novo)<br>• No impact for OS in t-AML group |
| | | WBC:<br>• For OS (t-AML + de novo)<br>• No impact for OS in t-AML group |
| Kayser et al. (2011) | Prospective<br>*N* = 2853 (t-AML: 200 [7%]; de novo: 2653 [93%])<br>Intensive treatment: 100% | t-AML:<br>• An adverse prognostic factor for death in CR in young intensive pts. (not for relapse) → cumulative toxicity of treatments<br>• An adverse prognostic factor for relapse old pts (not for death in CR) → lower dose in elderly<br>• An adverse prognostic factor for OS in young intensive pts<br>• Similar rates of CR in both groups (sAML and de novo), refractory disease and ED (differences by age) |
| Hulegårdh et al. (2015) | Registry<br>*N* = 3363 (AHD-AML: 630 [18.7%]; t-AML: 259 [7.7%]; de novo: 2474 [73.6%])<br>Intensive treatment: 58% | De novo vs sAML: Different age, gender, and cytogenetics<br>• sAML: Impact in OS in young patients (no impact on elderly)<br>• sAML: Worse OS than de novo in all cytogenetic groups (sAML independent of karyotype)<br>• AHD-AML and t-AML independently associated to poor OS<br>• AHD-AML: Worse PS than t-AML<br>• AHD-AML: Low-risk cytogenetics is uncommon<br>• High-risk cytogenetics: t-AML (46%) >AHD-AML (40%) > de novo (26%)<br>• Worse CR and OS in t-AML and MRC-AML vs de novo, regardless of PS |
| Østgård et al. (2015) | Registry | Response to therapy (prognostic factor for OS)<br>Prognostic factor for OS: Cytogenetic group and type of sAML<br>• MDS-AML no impact on OS (dismal outcomes)<br>• t-AML: Higher frequency of adverse risk<br>• OS in intermediate risk: t-AML similar to MPN-AML < de novo AML<br>• 1-year OS in adverse risk: MPN-AML (10%), t-AML (20%), de novo AML (41%), MDS-AML (43%)<br>• MDS-AML and t-AML impact on OS:<br>– <60 yo: Worse OS<br>– (≥60 yo: Longer OS<br>• MPN-AML: Worse OS than MDS-AML (age- and ctyogenetics-independent)<br>• Less HSCT in MPN-AML and t-AML due to lower CR rate, higher induction death, older age, more comorbidities, and worse PS) |
| Szotkowski et al. (2010) | Retrospective<br>*N* = 574<br>Intensive treatment: 66% | sAML: Unfavorable for younger and older than 60 years<br>Intensive treatment according to type of AML:<br>• sAML: 69 (48% of sAML)<br>• De novo: 307 (71% of de novo AML) |

**Table 4.3** (continued)

| Author (Year) [Reference] | Characteristics | Prognostic factors: findings |
|---|---|---|
| Zeichner and Arellano (2015) | Retrospective<br>De novo AML<br>sAML | ECOG >2 is unfavorable in AML (including sAML)<br>Higher risk of induction death → require less intensive therapy |
| Armand et al. (2007) | Retrospective<br>*N* = 556 (t-MN: 80 [14%]; AML or MDS: 476 [16%])<br>Previous HSCT | Cytogenetics<br>• OS and DFS in t-MN: Favorable > unfavorable<br>• After stratifying by cytogenetics: No differences between de novo and t-MN |
| Christiansen et al. (2001) | Retrospective<br>*N* = 77 (t-MN/t-MDS: 52 [68%]; t-AML: 25 [32%])<br>Treatment: NA | Mutations of *p53* were significantly associated with:<br>• Deletion or loss of 5q<br>• Complex karyotype<br>• Old patients<br>• Extremely poor prognosis |
| Ok et al. (2015b) | Retrospective<br>*N* = 108 (t-MN/t-MDS: 53 [49%]; t-AML: 55 [51%])<br>Treatment: NA | Loss of heterozygosity of *TP53*: Worse OS |
| Andersen et al. (2001) | Retrospective<br>*N* = 70<br>t-MN<br>Treatment: NA | Amplification of the *MLL* gene significantly associated with:<br>• Deletion or loss of 5q<br>• Complex karyotype<br>• Old patients<br>• Alkylating agents<br>• Worse OS |
| Borthakur et al. (2009) | Retrospective<br>*N* = 188 CBF-AML (sAML: 17 [9%]; de novo: 171 [91%])<br>Intensive treatment: 100% | CBF sAML: Worse OS and EFS than CBF de novo AML (but only after matched-analysis by age, ECOG, and the presence of additional chromosomal abnormalities) |
| Fröhling et al. (2006b) | Retrospective<br>*N* = 361 (sAML: 119 [33%]; de novo: 242 [67%])<br>Age ≥ 60 yo<br>Intensive treatment: 100% | sAML no impact<br>Independent impact on OS:<br>• Age<br>• Cytogenetics |
| Wheatley et al. (2009) | Retrospective<br>*N* = 2483 (sAML: 544 [22%]; de novo: 1939 [78%])<br>Age ≥ 60 yo<br>Intensive treatment: 100% | Independent impact on OS:<br>• Age<br>• sAML<br>• WBC<br>• PS<br>• Cytogenetics |
| Stölzel et al. (2011) | Retrospective<br>sAML<br>*N* = 305 (MDS-AML: 233 [76%]; t-AML: 72 [24%])<br>Intensive treatment: 100% | Age (OS and EFS)<br>Cytogenetic risk (OS)<br>Platelets count (OS and EFS)<br>NPM1 positivity (OS and EFS)<br>Type of sAML was not a prognostic factor |
| Thepot et al. (2010) | Retrospective<br>*N* = 54 (MPN-AML: 26 [48%]; MPN-MDS: 28 [52%])<br>Azacitidine | For CR:<br>• Underlying MPN: 14% CR for PV vs 43% for ET<br>• WHO classification at diagnosis: 36% CR in MDS vs 12% in AML |

*AHD-AML* acute myeloid leukemia with an antecedent hematological disease, *AML* acute myeloid leukemia, *CBF* core binding factor, *CR* complete remission, *DFS* disease-free survival, *ECOG* Eastern Cooperative Oncology Group score, *ED* early death, *EFS* event-free survival, *ET* essential thrombocythemia, *HSCT* hematopoietic stem cell transplantation, *MDS-AML* AML after myelodysplastic syndrome, *MPN-AML* AML after myeloproliferative neoplasm, *MRC-AML* AML with myelodysplasia-related changes, *NA* not available, *OS* overall survival, *PV* polycythemia vera, *PS* performance status, *pts* patients, *sAML* secondary AML, *t-AML* therapy-related AML, *t-MDS* therapy-related myeloproliferative neoplasm, *t-MN* therapy-related myeloid neoplasm, *WBC* white blood cell, *yo* years old

## 4.8 Treatment

The optimal treatment options for sAML patients are not yet established. This therapeutic dilemma comes from the lack of well-designed studies in this subset of patients, as they are commonly excluded from trials and protocols (Juliusson et al. 2009; Mengis et al. 2003).

Despite new advances, front-line therapy remains a challenge in sAML. In addition to older age and worse PS of these patients, deteriorated baseline characteristics because of the preceding treatments or concomitant malignant disease activity must be taken into account to judge the best approach for each patient. As in de novo AML, genetic and molecular characterization is mandatory for the initial risk-assessment of sAML patients, which can be categorized in favorable, intermediate, and adverse groups. Although, in general, we can recommend that sAML patients should receive similar treatment as de novo AML, specific characteristics of sAML patients may justify a distinct approach in some instances. Table 4.4 shows detailed information on studies who analyzed treatment outcomes in sAML.

### 4.8.1 Younger Patients

As in young patients with de novo AML, induction therapy in sAML is based on intensive 3 + 7 chemotherapy, with a combination of cytarabine for 7 days plus an anthracycline for 3 days, usually idarubicin or daunorubicin. Nevertheless, other schedules have also been explored (Döhner et al. 2017; Fey and Buske 2013; Tallman et al. 2019; De Kouchkovsky and Abdul-Hay 2016; Lee et al. 2011; Burnett et al. 2013; Zeidner et al. 2015; Stone et al. 2015; Lee et al. 2017; Holowiecki et al. 2012; Burnett et al. 2015). Due to the high risk of relapse, the majority of sAML fit patients achieving a first complete remission (CR) will be candidates to receive an allogeneic hematopoietic stem cell transplantation (HSCT). In consequence, an early search for a suitable donor should be started at diagnosis. After achieving CR, consolidation cycles with high-dose cytarabine-based schedules are recommended for patients with optimal PS and favorable cytogenetic risk. In contrast, the preferred strategy to achieve long-term survival in patients with intermediate-risk genetics is to perform an allogeneic HSCT (De Kouchkovsky and Abdul-Hay 2016; Li et al. 2018; Sengsayadeth et al. 2018; Litzow et al. 2010; Yakoub-Agha et al. 2000). Unfortunately, the prognosis in patients with poor-risk cytogenetics is dismal, regardless of the treatment administered. Despite this, allogeneic HSCT remains the most appropriate post-remission modality for patients with high-risk cytogenetics sAML, especially in younger patients with good PS (Sengsayadeth et al. 2018; Kennedy et al. 2013). Few data have been published comparing patients with or without HSCT after induction therapy in sAML patients. Although treatment-related mortality and toxicity after allogeneic HSCT is suspected to be higher in sAML patients than in de novo AML, allogeneic HSCT improves survival and is considered the only realistic curative option in patients with sAML (Nilsson et al. 2019).

In younger patients who are considered unfit for intensive schedules (e.g., because of another active malignancy or end-organ failure), front-line approaches using hypomethylating agents (HMAs) could prolong OS (Zeichner and Arellano 2015).

As a general recommendation, participating in clinical trials should be the preferred option for all sAML patients (Fey and Buske 2013; Tallman et al. 2019).

### 4.8.2 Older Patients

Older patients (especially those aged more than 70–75 years) are usually considered unfit and often receive non-curative schemes or supportive care exclusively. Intensive therapies in older patients are limited to those with optimal PS, and considered able to withstand very toxic schedules (Löwenberg et al. 1998; Anderson et al. 2002). In the last decades, through a more accurate risk stratification of patients and improvements in supportive therapy, intensive schedules have also

**Table 4.4** Studies of induction therapy in secondary AML patients

| Author (Year) [Reference] | Design | Treatment schedule | *N* | Age, median (range) | Induction outcome (*n* [%]) | Median OS | Other survival outcomes |
|---|---|---|---|---|---|---|---|
| *Registries and observational studies* | | | | | | | |
| Schoch et al. (2004) | Registry<br>AML<br>t-AML | Intensive chemotherapy | 93 t-AML<br>1091 de novo | 57 (16–82)<br>58 (16–84) | No differences in the CR rate | t-AML:10 m<br>De novo: 15 m<br>($p = 0.0007$) | See Table 4.3 |
| Hulegårdh et al. (2015) | Registry<br>Age ≥ 17 yo<br>AML<br>APL | AML: IDA + Ara-C (3 + 7)<br>APL: ATRA + IDA/DNR<br>BSC<br>Intensive: 1967 (58%)<br>Non-intensive: 1396 (42%) | 3363<br>De novo AML: 2474 (74%)<br>AHD-AML: 630 (19%)<br>t-AML: 259 (8%)<br><65 yo: 1165 (35%)<br>≥65 yo: 2198 (65%) | De novo: 70 (17–98)<br>AHD-AML: 73<br>t-AML: 70 | IDA + Ara-C (3 + 7): <65 yo<br>• De novo: CR 82%<br>• AHD-AML: CR 43%<br>• t-AML: CR 56%<br>IDA + Ara-C (3 + 7): ≥65 yo<br>• De novo: CR 59%<br>• AHD-AML: CR 37%<br>• t-AML: CR 53%<br>Non-intensive <65 yo<br>• De novo: CR 11%<br>• AHD-AML: CR 7%<br>• t-AML: CR 0%<br>Non-intensive ≥65 yo<br>• De novo: CR 3%<br>• AHD-AML: CR 1%<br>• t-AML: CR 3% | IDA + Ara-C (3 + 7): <65 yo<br>• De novo: ~3 y<br>• AHD-AML: < 1 y<br>• t-AML: ~1 y<br>Patients <65 yo + sAML: Similar mOS to elderly patients with sAML | • De novo: Higher CR in younger<br>• sAML: Similar CR rates in younger and older |

(continued)

**Table 4.4** (continued)

| Author (Year) [Reference] | Design | Treatment schedule | *N* | Age, median (range) | Induction outcome (*n* [%]) | Median OS | Other survival outcomes |
|---|---|---|---|---|---|---|---|
| Østgård et al. (2015) | Registry<br>Age ≥ 15 yo<br>Non-APL | Intensive CHT: 1567 (51%)<br>• DNR + Ara-C (3 + 7): 41%<br>• IDA + Ara-C (3 + 7): 35%<br>• MIT + Ara-C (3 + 7): 18% | 3205<br>De novo AML: 2249 (74%)<br>MDS-AML: 350 (11%)<br>MPN-AML: 253 (8%)<br>t-AML: 203 (7%) | Intensive CHT:<br>De novo: 58 (15–86)<br>MDS-AML: 64 (18–82)<br>MPN-AML: 62 (38–87)<br>t-AML: 58 (22–76) | Intensive CHT:<br>De novo: CR 75%<br>MDS-AML: CR 59%<br>MPN-AML: CR 54%<br>t-AML: CR 61% | OS 1- and 3y (intensive CHT):<br>• De novo: 65%, 39%<br>• t-AML: 45%, 24%<br>• Non-MDS-sAML: 31%, 11% | See Table 4.3 |
| Østgård et al. (2010) | RETROSP<br>Age ≥ 15 yo<br>AML (includes APL) | Anthracycline + Ara-C (intensive): 364 (58%) | 630 AML<br>157 sAML (25%) | Intensive: 58<br>sAML: 69<br>De novo: 66 | sAML: CR 56%<br>De novo: CR 73% | Intensive: 13 m<br>sAML: 5.7 m<br>De novo: 16 m | See Table 4.3 |
| Szotkowski et al. (2010) | RETROSP<br>Age ≥ 18 yo<br>AML<br>APL | Intensive treatment:<br>De novo: 305 (71%)<br>sAML: 69 (48%) | 574<br>De novo AML: 430 (75%)<br>MDS-AML: 86 (15%)<br>t-AML: 58 (10%) | De novo: 58 (18–80)<br>sAML: 64 (20–87)<br>Intensive CHT:<br>De novo: 53 (18–80)<br>sAML: 55 (20–76) | Intensive CHT:<br>De novo: CR 73%<br>sAML: CR 46% | Intensive CHT:<br>Shorter OS in sAML than de novo ($p < 0001$) | See Table 4.3 |
| Mesa et al. (2005) | RETROSP<br>MPN-AML | AML-like CHT: 24 (26%)<br>Non-intensive: 19 (21%)<br>BSC: 48 (53%) | 91 | 66 (41–82) | AML-like: CR 0% (41% reverted into chronic-phase, TRM 33%) | 2.6 m (all patients)<br>AML-like OS: 3.9 m<br>Non-intensive CHT: 2.9 m<br>BSC: 2.1 m | 2 patients alive after 41 and 57 m with either cytarabine-based induction CHT or HSCT |

| Author (Year) [Reference] | Design | Treatment schedule | *N* | Age, median (range) | Induction outcome (*n* [%]) | Median OS | Other survival outcomes |
|---|---|---|---|---|---|---|---|
| Nilsson et al. (2019) | RETROSP<br>AML<br>sAML | Intensive treatment (100%) | 3337<br>De novo: 2613 (78%)<br>AHD-AML: 442 (13%)<br>t-AML: 282 (8%)<br>HSCT:<br>• De novo: 576 (17%)<br>• AHD-AML: 74 (17%)<br>• t-AML: 57 (20%) | HSCT:<br>• De novo: 48 (17–72)<br>• AHD-AML: 58 (28–77)<br>• t-AML: 51 (18–68)<br>No HSCT:<br>• De novo: 64 (17–86)<br>• AHD–AML: 68 (24–83)<br>• t-AML: 66 (34–83) | De novo: CR 72%<br>AHD-AML: CR 45%<br>t-AML: CR 60% | HSCT OS 3 y, 5 y:<br>• De novo: 55%, 40%<br>• MDS-AML: 31%, 18%<br>• MPN-AML: 37%, 32%<br>• t-AML: 42%, 25%<br>No HSCT OS 3 y, 5 y:<br>• De novo: 24%, 16%<br>• MDS-AML: 5%, 2%<br>• MPN-AML: 3%, 0%<br>• t-AML: 21%, 10% | NA |
| Li et al. (2018) | RETROSP<br>sAML | Haplo-HSCT:<br>Myeloablative conditioning: 57 (38%)<br>RIC: 97 (62%) | 154<br>At HSCT: CR 69; active sAML 85 | 60 (at HSCT) | Not applicable | OS 2 y: 43% | LFS 2 y: 37% |
| Yakoub-Agha et al. (2000) | RETROSP<br>t-MDS<br>t-AML | Allo-HSCT | 70<br>t-MDS: 31<br>t-AML: 39<br>At HSCT: CR 24; active 46 | 37 (16–55) | Not applicable | OS 2 y: 30% | EFS 2 y: 28%<br>TRM 2 y: 49%<br>Relapse 2 y: 42% |
| Litzow et al. (2010) | RETROSP<br>t-MDS<br>t-AML | Allo-HSCT<br>Myeloablative conditioning: 670 (77%)<br>RIC: 198 (23%) | 868<br>t-MDS: 323 (37%)<br>t-AML: 545 (63%)<br>At HSCT: CR 317 (37%);<br>Active 551 (63%)<br>(t-AML: 228, t-MDS: 323) | 40 (4–72) | Not applicable | OS 1 y, 5 y: 37%, 22% | DFS 1 y, 5 y: 32%, 21%<br>TRM 1 y, 5 y: 41%, 48%<br>Relapse 1 y, 5 y: 27%, 31% |

(continued)

**Table 4.4** (continued)

| Author (Year) [Reference] | Design | Treatment schedule | *N* | Age, median (range) | Induction outcome (*n* [%]) | Median OS | Other survival outcomes |
|---|---|---|---|---|---|---|---|
| Sengsayadeth et al. (2018) | RETROSP<br>sAML | Allo-HSCT | 4997 | 58 (at HSCT) | Not applicable | OS 2 y: 45% | DFS 2 y: 39%<br>NRM 2 y: 28%<br>Inferior OS and DFS:<br>• Active disease<br>• Poor-risk cytogenetics<br>• Older age<br>• Lower ECOG<br>• Hematologic malignancies |
| Kennedy et al. (2013) | MPN-AML | Curative intent:<br>CHT ± Allo-HSCT<br>BSC<br>(CHT = 3 + 7 or MIT + ETOP+HiDAC) | 75<br>CHT ± Allo-HSCT: 39 (52%)<br>BSC: 36 (48%) | 65 (36–89)<br>CHT ± Allo-HSCT: 57 (36–88)<br>BSC: 72 (54–89) | CHT ± Allo-HSCT: CR: 18 (46%) → Allo-HSCT in 17 | 6.6 m<br>CHT ± Allo-HSCT: 9.4 m<br>BSC: 2.3 m | All: OS 2 y: 15%<br>CHT ± Allo-HSCT: OS 2 y: 26%<br>CHT + Allo-HSCT: OS 2 y: 47%<br>CHT: OS 2 y: 15%<br>BSC: OS 2 y: 3% |
| Thepot et al. (2010) | MPN-AML<br>MPN-MDS | Azacitidine | 54<br>MPN-AML: 26 (48%)<br>MPN-MDS: 28 (52%) | 69.5 (37–89) | MPN-AML CR: 12%<br>MPN-MDS CR: 36% | 11 m (all patients)<br>MPN-AML OS: 8 m<br>MPN-MDS OS: 14 m | NA |
| Borthakur et al. (2009) | CBF-AML | Intermediate-dose to high-dose cytarabine-based CHT | *N* = 188 CBF-AML (sAML: 17 [9%]; De novo: 171 [91%]) | sAML: 62 (31–75)<br>De novo: 61 (31–73) | CR + CRp: 92% | CBF-AML OS: 62 m<br>sAML OS: 23 m<br>De novo OS: 143 m | See Table 4.3 |
| Dumas et al. (2017) | RETROSP<br>sAML (MDS-AML: 69 [37.5%]; MPN-AML: 32 [17.4%]; t-AML: 83 [45%]) | Intensive CHT<br>Azacitidine | 199<br>Intensive CHT: 92 (46%)<br>Azacitidine: 107 (54%) | Intensive CHT: 66 (IQR: 63–71)<br>Azacitidine: 76 (IQR: 71–80) | CR + CRi:<br>Intensive: 58 (63%)<br>Azacitidine: 21 (20%) | Intensive mOS: 9.6 m<br>Azacitidine mOS: 10.8 m<br>($p = 0.899$) | Azacitidine versus intensive CHT: OS was not significantly different according to AML subtypes |

| Author (Year) [Reference] | Design | Treatment schedule | *N* | Age, median (range) | Induction outcome (*n* [%]) | Median OS | Other survival outcomes |
|---|---|---|---|---|---|---|---|
| *Acute promyelocytic leukemia* | | | | | | | |
| Kayser et al. (2017) | RETROSP t-APL | ATRA+CHT (intensive)<br>ATO + ATRA (intensive)<br>ATO + ATRA + CHT (intensive)<br>ATRA alone | 103<br>ATRA + CHT: 53 (51.5%)<br>ATO + ATRA: 24 (23.3%)<br>ATO + ATRA + CHT: 19 (18.4%)<br>ATRA: 7 (6.3%) | 59 (18–80) | ATRA + CHT: ED 12%, CR 78%<br>ATO + ATRA: ED 0%, CR 100%<br>ATO + ATRA + CHT: ED 5%, CR 95%<br>ATRA alone:<br>ED 43%, CR 57% | 3.7 y<br>OS 2 y (intensive): 88%<br>ATRA + CHT: OS 2 y 84%<br>ATO + ATRA: OS 2 y 89%<br>ATO + ATRA + CHT: OS 2 y 95% | EFS 2 y (intensive): 84%<br>RFS 2 y (intensive): 84%<br>ATRA+CHT: EFS 2 y 78%, RFS 2 y 78%<br>ATO + ATRA: 2 y EFS 89%, RFS 2 y 90%<br>ATO + ATRA + CHT: 2 y EFS 95%, RFS 2 y 95%<br>EFS 2 y (censoring died patients due to primary malignancy): ATO-based 95%, ATRA + CHT 78% ($p = 0.042$) |
| Elliott et al. (2012) | | ATRA+CHT | 64 (1[illegible] t-APL) | 56 (18–80) | sAPL: CR 64% (RES 0%)<br>De novo APL: CR 92% (RES 0%) | sAPL: OS 51%<br>De novo APL: 84% | NA |
| Beaumont et al. (2003) | RETROSP t-APL | Anthracycline + Ara-C<br>ATRA + CHT | 106 | 55 (12–82) | Anthracycline + Ara-C CR: 87% (ED: 13%) ATRA + CHT: CR 80%<br>(ED: 20%) | OS 5 y: 59% | OS 8y:<br>• After CHT alone: 68%<br>• After RT alone: 59%<br>• Both: 52% |
| Pulsoni et al. (2002) | RETROSP sAPL (secondary) | AIDA (31 sAPL; 641 de novo) | 692 (51 sAPL) | sAPL: 57 (27–76)<br>De novo: 39 (1–74) | sAPL CR: 97%<br>De novo CR: 68% | sAPL OS 4 y: 65%<br>De novo OS 4 y: 78% | sAPL EFS 4 y: 93%<br>De novo EFS 4 y: 85% |

(continued)

**Table 4.4** (continued)

| Author (Year) [Reference] | Design | Treatment schedule | *N* | Age, median (range) | Induction outcome (*n* [%]) | Median OS | Other survival outcomes |
|---|---|---|---|---|---|---|---|
| Dayyani et al. (2011) | RETROSP t-APL | ATRA+CHT<br>ATO + ATRA | 29 both arms<br>ATRA + CHT: 10<br>ATO + ATRA: 19 | ATRA+CHT: 54 (35–75)<br>ATO + ATRA: 53 (36–81) | ATRA+CHT: CR 70<br>ATO + ATRA: CR 89<br>($p = 0.35$) | ATRA+CHT: mOS 171 w;<br>ATO + ATRA: mOS not achieved<br>($p = 0.79$) | NA |
| *Clinical trials* | | | | | | | |
| Löwenberg et al. (1998) | RCT, PROSP, phase-III | Ara-C (100 mg/m$^2$ d: 1–7) + DNR (30 mg/m$^2$ d: 1–3)<br>or<br>Ara-C (100 mg/m$^2$ d: 1–7) + MIT (8 mg/m$^2$ d: 1–3) | 63<br>61<br>124 both arms | 68 (60–88) in both arms | Mixing 2 arms:<br>CR: 46 (37)<br>vs AML de novo<br>CR: 207 (44);<br>$p = 0.21$ | Mixing 2 arms:<br>OS sAML vs AML 1st<br>$\mathbf{p = 0.02}$ | NA |
| Anderson et al. (2002) | RCT, PROSP, Phase-III | Ara-C (200 mg/m$^2$ d: 1–7) + DNR (45 mg/m$^2$ d: 1–3)<br>or<br>MIT (10 mg/m$^2$ d: 1–5) + ETOP (100 mg/m$^2$ d: 1–5) | 36<br>38<br>Both: 74 | 68 (56–84)<br>67 (56–86) | Mixing 2 arms:<br>CR: 19 (26)<br>vs<br>AML de novo<br>CR: 107 (42);<br>$p = 0.011$ | Mixing 2 arms:<br>OS 2 y: 7 (10)<br>vs AML de novo<br>OS 2 y: 41 (16); $p = 0.11$ | Mixing 2 arms:<br>RFS 2 y: 8 (11)<br>vs AML de novo<br>RFS 2 y: 46 (18)<br>$P = 0.89$ |
| Löwenberg et al. (2009) | RCT, PROSP | Ara-C (200 mg/m$^2$ d: 1–7) + DNR (45 mg/m$^2$ d: 1–3)<br>or<br>Ara-C (200 mg/m$^2$ d: 1–7) + DNR (90 mg/m$^2$ d: 1–3)<br>Both arms 2° cycle: Ara-C (1000 mg/m$^2$ d: 1–6) | 75<br>MDS-AML: 52<br>t-AML: 23<br>94<br>MDS-AML: 67<br>t-AML: 27<br>169 both arms<br>MDS-AML: 119<br>t-AML: 50 | 68 (60–79)<br>68 (60–83) | Mixing 2 arms:<br>CR: 80 (47)<br>MDS-AML: CR: 54 (45)<br>t-AML: CR: 26 (52)<br>vs AML de novo<br>CR: 399 (62);<br>$p < 0.001$ | OS 2 y: 37 (22)<br>MDS-AML: CR: 54 (45)<br>t-AML: CR: 26 (52)<br>vs AML de novo<br>OS 2 y: 193 (30);<br>$p = 0.01$ | EFS 2 y: 19 (11)<br>MDS-AML: EFS 2 y: 11 (9)<br>t-AML: EFS 2 y: 8 (16)<br>vs AML de novo<br>EFS 2 y: 129 (20);<br>$p = 0.003$<br>DFS 2 y: 36 (21)<br>MDS-AML: DFS 2 y: 21 (18)<br>t-AML: DFS 2 y: 15 (30)<br>vs AML de novo<br>DFS 2 y: 200 (31);<br>$p = 0.27$ |

| Author (Year) [Reference] | Design | Treatment schedule | $N$ | Age, median (range) | Induction outcome ($n$ [%]) | Median OS | Other survival outcomes |
|---|---|---|---|---|---|---|---|
| Chauncey et al. (2010) | RCT, PROSP, Phase-II, 2-Arms | Ara-C (200 mg/m² d: 1–7) + DNR (45 mg/m² d: 1–3)<br>or<br>Ara-C (200 mg/m² d: 1–7) + DNR (45 mg/m² d: 1–3) + CSA (loading dose of 6 mg/kg over 2 h and 16 mg/kg CI d: 1–3) | 16<br>MDS-AML: 14<br>t-AML: 2<br>7<br>MDS-AML: 7<br>t-AML: 0 | 68 (56–85)<br>65 (56–81) | CR: 1 (6)<br>MDS-AML: CR: 0 (0)<br>t-AML: CR: 1 (50)<br>CR: 2 (29)<br>MDS-AML: CR: 2 (29)<br>t-AML: Not applicable | NA | NA |
| Röllig et al. (2010) | RCT, PROSP, 1-Arm | Ara-C (100 mg/m² d: 1–7) + DNR (45 mg/m² d: 1–3) | 236 | 67 (61–87) | CR: 100 (42)<br>vs<br>AML de novo<br>CR: 354 (53);<br>***p* = 0.007** | mOS 8.4 m<br>OS 3 y: 27 (11.4)<br>OS 5 y: 12 (5.2)<br>vs AML 1st L, ***p* = 0.016** | mDFS 8.5 m<br>DFS 3 y: 21 (8.8)<br>DFS 5 y: 16 (6.6) |
| Lee et al. (2011) | RCT, PROSP, Phase-III MDS-AML | Ara-C (200 mg/m² d: 1–7) + DNR (45 mg/m² d: 1–3)<br>or<br>Ara-C (200 mg/m² d: 1–7) + DNR (90 mg/m² d: 1–3) | 6<br>11<br>17 both arms | 43 (15–60) in both arms | Mixing 2 arms:<br>CR: 10 (59)<br>vs AML de novo<br>CR: 286 (78);<br>$p = 0.063$ | Mixing 2 arms:<br>OS at 5 y: 2 (14.1)<br>vs AML de novo<br>OS at 5 y: 153 (41.8);<br>***p* = 0.009** | Mixing 2 arms:<br>EFS 5 y: 4 (23.5)<br>RFS 5 y: 7 (40)<br>vs AML de novo<br>EFS 5 y: (40.8)<br>RFS 5 y: 129 (35)<br>$p = 0.056; 0.307$ |
| Holowiecki et al. (2012) | RCT, PROSP, Phase-III MDS-AML | Ara-C (200 mg/m² d: 1–7) + DNR (60 mg/m² d: 1–3)<br>or<br>2-CdA (5 mg/m² d: 1–5) + DNR (60 mg/m² d: 1–3)<br>or<br>FLU (25 mg/m² d: 1–5) + DNR (60 mg/m² d: 1–3) | 22<br>20<br>27 | 48 (18–60)<br>47 (17–60)<br>47 (18–60) | NA | OS at 3 y: 3 (12)<br>OS at 3 y: 4 (20)<br>OS at 3 y: 6 (22)<br>$p = 0.94$ | NA |

(continued)

**Table 4.4** (continued)

| Author (Year) [Reference] | Design | Treatment schedule | *N* | Age, median (range) | Induction outcome (*n* [%]) | Median OS | Other survival outcomes |
|---|---|---|---|---|---|---|---|
| Burnett et al. (2013) | RCT, PROSP, 2-Arms | Ara-C (100 mg/m² d: 1–7) + DNR (50 mg/m² d: 1–3)<br>or<br>Ara-C (100 mg/m² d: 1–7) + DNR (50 mg/m² d: 1–3) + ETOP (100 mg/m² d: 1–5) | 88<br>84 | 53 (16–72)<br>53 (16–72) | NA | OS 5 y: 22 (25)<br>OS 5 y: 17 (20.2) | NA |
| Lancet et al. (2014) | RCT, PROSP, Phase-II, 2-Arms | Ara-C (100 mg/m² d: 1–7) + DNR (60 mg/m² d: 1–3)<br>or<br>CPX-351 (100 units/m² d: 1, 3, 5) | 19<br>33 | 68 (61–77)<br>68 (60–77) | CR: 6 (32)<br>CR: 12 (58)<br>$p = 0.06$ | 6.1 m<br>12.1 m<br>$\mathbf{p = 0.01}$ | mEFS, 1.3 m<br>mEFS, 4.5 m<br>$p = 0.08$ |
| Burnett et al. (2015) | RCT, PROSP, 2-Arms | Ara-C (100 mg/m² d: 1–7) + DNR (60 mg/m² d: 1–3)<br>or<br>Ara-C (100 mg/m² d: 1–7) + DNR (90 mg/m² d: 1–3) | 58<br>59 | 53 (16–72)<br>53 (16–72) | NA | OS 2 y: 34 (58.6)<br>OS 2 y: 29 (49.2) | NA |
| Müller-Tidow et al. (2016) | RCT, PROSP, 2-Arms | Ara-C (100 mg/m² d: 1–7) + DNR (60 mg/m² d: 1–3)<br>or<br>Ara-C (100 mg/m² d: 1–7) + DNR (60 mg/m² d: 1–3) + Azacitidine (75 mg/m² d: −5 to 1) | 32<br>30 | 69 (all ≥61)<br>70 (all ≥61) | NA | OS 2 y: 16 (50)<br>OS 2 y: 10 (33.3)<br>$\mathbf{p = 0.048}$ | EFS: 7 (21.9)<br>EFS: 5 (16.7)<br>$p = 0.627$ |

| Author (Year) [Reference] | Design | Treatment schedule | $N$ | Age, median (range) | Induction outcome ($n$ [%]) | Median OS | Other survival outcomes |
|---|---|---|---|---|---|---|---|
| Zeidner et al. (2015) | RCT, PROSP, Phase-II, 2-Arms | Ara-C (100 mg/m² d: 1–7) + DNR (90 mg/m² d: 1–3)<br>or<br>FLAM: Flavopiridol (50 mg/m² d: 1–3) + Ara-C (667 mg/m² CI d: 6–8) + MIT (40 mg/m² d: 9) | 26<br>52 | 60 (22–69)<br>59 (19–70) | CR: 9 (35)<br>CR: 31 (60) | NA | NA |
| Stone et al. (2015) | RCT, PROSP, Phase-III | Ara-C (200 mg/m² d: 1–7) + DNR (45 mg/m² d: 1–3)<br>or<br>Ara-C (200 mg/m² d: 1–7) + Amonafide (60 mg/m² d: 1–5) | 217<br>MDS-AML: 104<br>t-AML: 88<br>t-AML-MDS: 24<br>216<br>MDS-AML: 111<br>t-AML: 85<br>t-AML-MDS: 20 | 63 (27–83)<br>65 (19–84) | CR: 97 (45)<br>MDS-AML: CR: 43 (41)<br>t-AML: CR: 49 (56)<br>t-AML-MDS: CR: 7 (29)<br>CR: 99 (46)<br>MDS-AML: CR: 44 (40)<br>t-AML: CR: 49 (58)<br>t-AML-MDS: CR: 4 (20)<br>All $p > 0.05$ | 7 m<br>7 m<br>$p > 0.05$ | NA |
| Lee et al. (2017) | RCT, PROSP, Phase-III | Ara-C (200 mg/m² d: 1–7) + DNR (90 mg/m² d: 1–3)<br>or<br>Ara-C (200 mg/m² d: 1–7) + IDA (12 mg/m² d: 1–3) | 17<br>7 | 49 (15–65)<br>49 (15–65) | CR: 2 (12)<br>CR: 2 (29)<br>$P = 0.32$ | OS 4 y: 0 (0)<br>OS 4 y: 0 (0)<br>$p = 0.18$ | EFS 4 y: 0 (0)<br>EFS 4 y: 2 (33.3)<br>$p = 0.083$ |

(continued)

**Table 4.4** (continued)

| Author (Year) [Reference] | Design | Treatment schedule | *N* | Age, median (range) | Induction outcome (*n* [%]) | Median OS | Other survival outcomes |
|---|---|---|---|---|---|---|---|
| Lancet et al. (2018) | RCT, PROSP, Phase-III | Ara-C (100 mg/$m^2$ d: 1–7) + DNR (60 mg/$m^2$ d: 1–3)<br>or<br>CPX-351 (100 units/$m^2$ d: 1, 3, 5) | 119<br>MDS-AML: 74<br>CMML-AML: 12<br>t-AML: 33<br>112<br>MDS-AML: 71<br>CMML-AML: 11<br>t-AML: 30 | 67.7 (60–75)<br>67.8 (60–75) | CR: 40 (34)<br>MDS-AML, CR: 25 (34)<br>CMML-AML, CR: 3 (25)<br>t-AML, CR: 12 (36)<br>CR: 50 (45)<br>MDS-AML, CR: 32 (45)<br>CMML-AML, CR: 4 (36)<br>t-AML, CR: 14 (47) | 6.0 m<br>MDS-AML: 6.0 m<br>CMML-AML: 2.3 m<br>t-AML: 6 m<br>NA<br>MDS-AML: 7.4 m<br>CMML-AML: 9.3 m<br>t-AML: 12.2 m | NA |

*AHD-AML* AML with an antecedent hematological disease, *AIDA* ATRA+IDA, *AML* acute myeloid leukemia, *APL* acute promyelocytic leukemia, *Ara-C* cytarabine, *ATO* arsenic trioxide, *ATRA* all-trans-retinoic acid, *BSC* best supportive care, *CBF* core binding factor, *CHT* intensive chemotherapy, *CI* continuous infusion, *CMML-AML* AML with chronic myelomonocytic leukemia, *CR* complete remission, *CRi* complete response with incomplete blood recovery, *CRp* CR with incomplete platelet recovery, *CSA* ciclosporin, *d* days, *DNR* daunorubicin, *ECOG* Eastern Cooperative Oncology Group score, *ED* early death, *EFS* event-free survival, *ETOP* etoposide, *FLU* fludarabine, *HiDAC* high-dose cytarabine, *HSCT* hematopoietic stem cell transplantation, *IDA* idarubicin, *IQR* interquartile range, *LFS* leukemia-free survival, *m* months, *mDFS* median disease-free survival, *mEFS* median event-free survival, *MDS* myelodysplastic syndrome, *MDS-AML*: AML with MDS antecedent, *MPN* myeloproliferative neoplasm, *MIT* mitoxantrone, *mOS* median overall survival, *MPN-AML* AML with MPM antecedent, *N* population of the cohort, *NA* not available, *NRM* non-relapse mortality, *OS* overall survival, *PROSP* prospective study, *RCT* randomized clinical trial, *RES* resistance, *RETROSP* retrospective study, *RFS* relapse-free mortality, *RIC* reduced intensity conditioning, *RT* radiotherapy, *sAML* secondary AML, *sAPL* secondary APL, *t-AML* therapy-related AML, *t-AML-MDS* t-AML and MDS antecedent, *TRM* treatment-related mortality, *w* weeks, *y* year, *yo* years old, *2-CdA* cladribine been a more accessible option for some older patients, mainly in those with favorable genetic risk (Zeidner et al. 2015; Stone et al. 2015; Löwenberg et al. 2009; Chauncey et al. 2010; Röllig et al. 2010; Müller-Tidow et al. 2016; Lancet et al. 2014). On the contrary, patients with poor PS, poor cytogenetics, high age (>75 years old), active malignant disease, or serious comorbidities should be considered for non-intensive approaches (e.g., HMAs, low-dose cytarabine [LDAC]) (Dumas et al. 2017).

Due to the poor prognosis, enrolment in clinical trials also remains the first option in this population (Fey and Buske 2013; Tallman et al. 2019). This strategy could allow some patients to benefit from innovative treatments and targeted therapies.

### 4.8.3 APL

Patients diagnosed with t-APL must receive therapeutic approaches comprising differentiating agents, such as anthracycline-based chemotherapy plus all-trans-retinoic acid (ATRA) or ATRA plus arsenic trioxide (ATO). Several studies have reported comparable results in t-APL as comparted to de novo APL in patients treated with ATRA plus chemotherapy regimens, while there is scarce information for t-APL patients treated with ATO-based regimens (Beaumont et al. 2003; Pulsoni et al. 2002; Elliott et al. 2012; Kayser et al. 2017; Dayyani et al. 2011). ATO plus ATRA regimens are now considered standard front-line for low- and intermediate-risk de novo APL, and are under investigation for high-risk patients (>10 × $10^9$/L WBC counts). As t-APL patients are systematically excluded from clinical trials, clinical outcomes under chemotherapy-free approaches must be extrapolated from studies performed in de novo cases. Although upfront approaches with ATRA plus anthracycline can be suitable for t-APL, chemotherapy-free schedules are more appealing for t-APL patients to avoid additive toxicity of chemotherapy (Kayser et al. 2017; Dayyani et al. 2011). As suggested by some authors, the cumulative dose of chemotherapy may be related to higher rates of death during induction, higher incidence of toxic death, and development of t-MN after APL (Kayser et al. 2017).

### 4.8.4 New Approaches

Novel therapies have recently been approved for the treatment of AML. Although the majority of studies have focused on de novo AML patients, some of the following agents have been properly evaluated in sAML.

#### 4.8.4.1 CPX-351

CPX-351 (Vyxeos®, Jazz Pharmaceuticals) is a liposomal formulation of cytarabine and daunorubicin at a 5:1 molar ratio, which is delivered into leukemic cells (Kim et al. 2011; Lim et al. 2010). CPX-351 liposomes could deliver daunorubicin and cytarabine in optimal ratio to maintain a synergistic effect. In addition, the liposomal formulation could lead to selective accumulation of both drugs in the bone marrow.

In a randomized phase 3 trial, CPX-351 showed longer OS and higher CR plus CR with incomplete recovery (CRi) rate in comparison with 7 + 3 schedule (median OS: 9.6 vs 5.6 months, $p = 0.005$; and CR + CRi: 47.7% vs 33.3%, $p = 0.016$, respectively) in fit patients aged between 60 and 75 years with untreated AML and the following characteristics: t-AML, MDS-AML with and without prior HMA, AML with a history of chronic myelomonocytic leukemia (CMML), and de novo AML with MDS-related cytogenetic abnormalities (Lancet et al. 2018).Toxicity was similar in both groups.

Currently, CPX-351 is the only therapy specifically approved for adults with newly diagnosed t-AML and MRC-AML by the US Food and Drug Administration (FDA) since 2017 and by the European Medicines Agency (EMA) since 2018 (Talati and Lancet 2018; Vyxeos n.d.).

#### 4.8.4.2 Venetoclax

Venetoclax (Venclyxto/Venclexta®, AbbVie) is a small-molecule inhibitor of Bcl-2 that targets

AML cells whose survival could depend on anti-apoptotic proteins of the Bcl-2 family (Mihalyova et al. 2018).

Two studies contributed to the approval of venetoclax by the FDA in 2018, in combination with azacitidine or decitabine or LDAC, for the treatment of adult newly diagnosed AML patients aged 75 years or older, or who have comorbidities that preclude use of intensive induction chemotherapy (VENCLEXTA 2018). One of them was a phase 1/2 trial in which venetoclax plus LDAC was tested in 82 older patients with untreated AML, showing a CR + CRi rate of 35% in the group of patients with sAML (which represented 49% of the study cohort) (Wei et al. 2019). A phase 1b study explored venetoclax combined with HMA therapy (decitabine or azacitidine) in a similar cohort, but enrolled subjects could not have received HMAs for prior MDS or MDS/MPN. The CR + CRi rate in the subset of patients with sAML was 67% (DiNardo et al. 2019). Continued FDA approval for this indication is contingent upon verification of clinical benefit in confirmatory trials. Recently, the phase 3 trial VIALE-C comparing venetoclax plus LDAC versus placebo plus LDAC failed its primary endpoint of OS, although this was almost doubled in the experimental arm.

#### 4.8.4.3 Gemtuzumab Ozogamicin (GO)

Gemtuzumab ozogamicin (GO; Mylotarg™, Pfizer) is a conjugate of an anti-CD33 antibody and the toxin calicheamicin. Its mechanism of action is based on the advantage of selective expression of CD33 by leukemic cells, but not in normal hematopoietic stem cells (Appelbaum and Bernstein 2017; Jen et al. 2018).

GO was approved by the FDA in 2017 and the EMA in 2018 for the treatment of adult patients with newly diagnosed CD33-positive AML, in combination with standard cytarabine and daunorubicin. Moreover, GO was also approved by the FDA as monotherapy for the treatment of patients ≥2 years of age with relapsed/refractory CD33-positive AML.

Although recent clinical trials have evaluated the possibility of adding GO to traditional schedules for the treatment of sAML patients, their results have not supported further development in this setting (de Witte et al. 2015; Burnett et al. 2011).

#### 4.8.4.4 Glasdegib

The hedgehog signaling pathway is an attractive novel therapeutic target because of its biologic role in the maintenance and expansion of leukemic stem cells and the acquisition of a drug-resistant phenotype in AML (Aberger et al. 2017; Campbell and Copland 2015). Glasdegib (Daurismo™, Pfizer) blocks hedgehog signaling by inhibiting Smoothened, a transmembrane receptor with an integral function in the canonical hedgehog pathway (DAURISMO 2018).

In a randomized phase 2 study performed in unfit patients with newly diagnosed AML or high-risk MDS, glasdegib in combination with LDAC showed longer OS and achieved a higher CR rate than LDAC alone (Cortes et al. 2019). Afterward, glasdegib plus LDAC was approved by the FDA in 2018 for the treatment of newly diagnosed adult AML patients aged ≥75 years or who have comorbidities that preclude use of intensive induction chemotherapy (DAURISMO 2018). However, analysis of sAML patient group included in this study has not yet been published.

#### 4.8.4.5 *IDH* Inhibitors

Leukemic IDH1 and IDH2 mutations confer a neomorphic enzymatic activity, impairing hematopoietic differentiation and promoting leukemogenesis (Figueroa et al. 2010). Mutations in IDH1 occur in approximately 6–10% of patients with AML and IDH2 mutations occur in 9–13% (DiNardo et al. 2018). Similar incidence has been reported in sAML (Ok et al. 2015a).

Ivosidenib (Tibsovo®, Agios) and enasidenib (Idhifa®, Celgene) induce myeloid differentiation and reduce blast counts by inhibiting mutant IDH1 and mutant IDH2, respectively (IDHIFA 2017; TIBSOVO 2018). The approval of ivosidenib by the FDA in 2018 was based on results of a phase 1 study, performed in adult patients with relapsed/refractory IDH1-mutated AML (35% were sAML). With ivosidenib monotherapy, a CR + CRi rate of 30% was achieved

(DiNardo et al. 2018). Enasidenib was approved by the FDA in 2017 for the treatment of adult patients with relapsed or refractory IDH2-mutated AML. The results of a phase 1/2 trial with a CR + CRi rate of 26% and median OS of 9.3 months led to its approval (Stein et al. 2017).

#### 4.8.4.6 *FLT3* Inhibitors

FMS-like tyrosine kinase 3 (FLT3) is a transmembrane receptor tyrosine kinase specially expressed on hematopoietic progenitor cells and is involved in differentiation and proliferation (Lyman and Jacobsen 1998; McKenna et al. 2000). *FLT3-ITD* mutation occurs less frequently in patients with sAML than in de novo (9% vs 26%, respectively) and predicts a poor prognosis (Fröhling et al. 2002; Stone et al. 2018). Midostaurin (Rydapt®, Novartis), a small-molecule inhibitor of FLT3, was approved by the FDA and EMA in 2017 for the treatment of adult patients with newly diagnosed FLT3-mutated AML, in combination with cytarabine and daunorubicin chemotherapy (Stone et al. 2018). In a randomized phase 3 RATIFY study, midostaurin plus conventional chemotherapy showed longer OS and EFS compared with chemotherapy alone in *FLT3* mutated patients aged ≤60 years with newly diagnosed AML (Stone et al. 2017). Of note, sAML patients were excluded from the RATIFY trial. Gilteritinib (Xospata®, Astellas Pharma) is other FLT3 kinase inhibitor, recently approved by FDA in 2018 for the treatment of adult patients with relapsed/refractory AML (XOSPATA 2018). Unfortunately, t-AML patients were excluded in all phase 3 trials with FLT3 inhibitors, and no data for second-generation inhibitors (gilteritinib or quizartinib) have yet been published with regard to MDS-AML.

## 4.9 Future Directions

Currently, patients diagnosed with sAML have a dismal prognosis, either because of the adverse biological features of the disease or the patient's clinical characteristics. Scientific groups are continuously updating their treatment protocols to design tailored therapies according to prognostic factors, including sAML as a relevant decision factor. Nevertheless, there is an increasing need to improve treatment strategies for sAML patients, which may represent one of the most challenging AML subsets. In particular, older patients with sAML may represent a very frequent subgroup where no specific approaches have been designed. There is room for advances in this challenging population, but these will be obtained only through well-designed specific protocols. In this regard, the clinical development of CPX-351, from phase 2 to phase 3, is a good example of success within this therapeutic area.

The better understanding of molecular mechanisms of leukemogenesis has led to the development of new targeted molecules focusing on actionable mutations and pathways. Unfortunately, patients with sAML are often excluded from clinical trials and only some new agents have been tested in this subset of patients with promising results. CPX-351 was approved for adults with newly diagnosed t-AML or MRC-AML, venetoclax in combination with LDAC or HMAs has remarkable activity in unfit subjects, glasdegib was shown to be able to benefit unfit sAML patients, and *IDH1/IDH2* inhibitors may be an option at least for relapsed/refractory sAML.

Based on new scientific evidence, the treatment landscape in sAML may change toward: (1) replacement of conventional 7 + 3 chemotherapy by CPX-351 as a backbone for fit patients; (2) combination of CPX-351 with a *FLT3* or *IDH* inhibitor in sAML fit patients with *FLT3* or *IDH* mutations; and (3) combination of venetoclax with HMAs or LDAC for patients considered unfit to receive intensive chemotherapy. The role of targeted- vs venetoclax- vs triple combinations-based approaches for unfit sAML harboring actionable mutations must be elucidated in the future.

We should highlight two groups of sAML patients in whom therapeutic improvements have not been achieved yet. The first group constitutes MRC-AML following HMA therapy. These patients are systematically excluded from phase 3 clinical trials in which an HMA is the control arm, so no evidence-based advances will be available for these patients from the majority of ongoing phase 3 trials. Only the combinations of glasdegib plus LDAC or venetoclax plus LDAC regimens could be applied in these patients with some background evidence, but unfortunately those regimens do not represent a therapeutic breakthrough for this population. On the other hand, younger fit patients developing sAML after HMA therapy have been classically treated with 3 + 7 or similar regimens and more recently with CPX-351, showing poor clinical outcomes in both scenarios. The second group of very difficult-to-treat sAML is composed by MRC-AML evolving from MPN. These patients are usually excluded from clinical trials, including the recently sAML-focused CPX-351 phase 3 trial.

Additionally, some early development stage therapies for AML may become promising treatment approaches for sAML patients. Some examples are chimeric antigen receptor T cells or agents targeting the *TP53* pathway, which should be evaluated in patients with sAML in forthcoming studies.

## 4.10 Conclusions

According to the 2016 WHO classification, sAML is included in two diagnostic groups: t-MN, along with therapy-related MDS/MPN; and MRC-AML, along with non-secondary AML subtypes (Arber et al. 2016; Döhner et al. 2017). The incidence of sAML is estimated between 20 and 30% of all AML (Juliusson et al. 2009; Bertoli et al. 2017; Medeiros et al. 2015; Hulegårdh et al. 2015; Østgård et al. 2010, 2015; Gangatharan et al. 2013; Szotkowski et al. 2010), with most of them having a prior history of MDS or MPN (Hulegårdh et al. 2015; Østgård et al. 2010). Although sAML has commonly been considered an independent adverse prognostic condition, this might be questionable as sAML is closely related to older age, comorbidities, worse PS, and unfavorable genetic features (Larson 2007; Stölzel et al. 2011; Pulsoni and Pagano 2005; Rizzieri et al. 2009). These baseline characteristics also lead physicians to frequently consider sAML patients unfit to receive curative therapies or be included in clinical trials.

The frequency of adverse features, such as older age, worse PS, and adverse karyotype and molecular profile, is by far higher in sAML than in de novo AML. However, the most relevant prognostic factor in AML is the therapeutic approach itself, which is probably intended as curative option in the minority sAML patients. Enrolling sAML patients in clinical trials should be a priority, and whenever possible, they should be referred to an appropriate research center where experimental options are available. Only patients with hopeless prognosis who do not meet criteria to participate in these studies should be approached in a palliative way. Given the challenging condition that they represent, obtaining improvements in sAML should be a priority, warranting that this field is becoming an active area of basic and clinical research in the forthcoming years.

## References

Abdel-Wahab O, Manshouri T, Patel J et al (2010) Genetic analysis of transforming events that convert chronic myeloproliferative neoplasms to leukemias. Cancer Res 70(2):447–452. https://doi.org/10.1158/0008-5472.CAN-09-3783

Aberger F, Hutterer E, Sternberg C, Del Burgo PJ, Hartmann TN (2017) Acute myeloid leukemia—strategies and challenges for targeting oncogenic hedgehog/GLI signaling. Cell Commun Signal 15(1):8. https://doi.org/10.1186/s12964-017-0163-4

Ammatuna E, Montesinos P, Hasan SK et al (2011) Presenting features and treatment outcome of acute promyelocytic leukemia arising after multiple sclerosis. Haematologica 96(4):621–625. https://doi.org/10.3324/haematol.2010.036657

Andersen MK, Christiansen DH, Kirchhoff M, Pedersen-Bjergaard J (2001) Duplication or amplification of chromosome band 11q23, including the unrearranged MLL gene, is a recurrent abnormality in therapy-related MDS and AML, and is closely related to mutation of the TP53 gene and to previous therapy with alkylating agents. Genes Chromosom Cancer 31(1):33–41. https://doi.org/10.1002/gcc.1115

Anderson JE, Kopecky KJ, Willman CL et al (2002) Outcome after induction chemotherapy for older patients with acute myeloid leukemia is not improved with mitoxantrone and etoposide compared to cyta-

rabine and daunorubicin: a southwest oncology group study. Blood 100(12):3869–3876. https://doi.org/10.1182/blood-2001-12-0354
Appelbaum FR, Bernstein ID (2017) Gemtuzumab ozogamicin for acute myeloid leukemia. Blood 130(22):2373–2376. https://doi.org/10.1182/blood-2017-09-797712
Appelbaum FR, Gundacker H, Head DR et al (2006) Age and acute myeloid leukemia. Blood 107(9):3481–3485. https://doi.org/10.1182/blood-2005-09-3724
Arber DA, Orazi A, Hasserjian R et al (2016) The 2016 revision to the World Health Organization classification of myeloid neoplasms and acute leukemia. Blood 127(20):2391–2405. https://doi.org/10.1182/blood-2016-03-643544
Armand P, Kim HT, DeAngelo DJ et al (2007) Impact of cytogenetics on outcome of de novo and therapy-related AML and MDS after allogeneic transplantation. Biol Blood Marrow Transplant 13(6):655–664. https://doi.org/10.1016/j.bbmt.2007.01.079
Beaumont M, Sanz M, Carli PM et al (2003) Therapy-related acute promyelocytic leukemia. J Clin Oncol 21(11):2123–2137. https://doi.org/10.1200/JCO.2003.09.072
Bertoli S, Tavitian S, Huynh A et al (2017) Improved outcome for AML patients over the years 2000-2014. Blood Cancer J 7(12):1–8. https://doi.org/10.1038/s41408-017-0011-1
Borthakur G, Estey EE (2007) Therapy-related acute myelogenous leukemia and myelodysplastic syndrome. Curr Oncol Rep 9(5):373–377. https://doi.org/10.1007/s11912-007-0050-z
Borthakur G, Lin E, Jain N et al (2009) Survival is poorer in patients with secondary core-binding factor acute myelogenous leukemia compared with de novo core-binding factor leukemia. Cancer 115(14):3217–3221. https://doi.org/10.1002/cncr.24367
Braun T, Cereja S, Chevret S et al (2015) Evolving characteristics and outcome of secondary acute promyelocytic leukemia (APL): a prospective analysis by the French-Belgian-Swiss APL group. Cancer 121(14):2393–2399. https://doi.org/10.1002/cncr.29389
Burnett AK, Hills RK, Milligan D et al (2011) Identification of patients with acute myeloblastic leukemia who benefit from the addition of Gemtuzumab Ozogamicin: results of the MRC AML15 trial. J Clin Oncol 29(4):369–377. https://doi.org/10.1200/JCO.2010.31.4310
Burnett AK, Russell NH, Hills RK et al (2013) Optimization of chemotherapy for younger patients with acute myeloid leukemia: results of the medical research council AML15 trial. J Clin Oncol 31(27):3360–3368. https://doi.org/10.1200/JCO.2012.47.4874
Burnett AK, Russell NH, Hills RK et al (2015) A randomized comparison of daunorubicin 90 mg/m2 vs 60 mg/m2in AML induction: results from the UK NCRI AML17 trial in 1206 patients. Blood 125(25):3878–3885. https://doi.org/10.1182/blood-2015-01-623447
Campbell V, Copland M (2015) Hedgehog signaling in cancer stem cells: a focus on hematological cancers. Stem Cells Cloning Adv Appl 8:27–38. https://doi.org/10.2147/SCCAA.S58613
Campbell PJ, Baxter EJ, Beer PA et al (2006) Mutation of JAK2 in the myeloproliferative disorders: timing, clonality studies, cytogenetic associations, and role in leukemic transformation. Blood 108(10):3548–3555. https://doi.org/10.1182/blood-2005-12-013748
Cervantes F, Tassies D, Salgado C, Rovira M, Pereira A, Rozman C (1991) Acute transformation in nonleukemic chronic myeloproliferative disorders: actuarial probability and main characteristics in a series of 218 patients. Acta Haematol 85(3):124–127. https://doi.org/10.1159/000204873
Chauncey TR, Gundacker H, Shadman M et al (2010) Sequential phase II southwest oncology group studies (S0112 and S0301) of daunorubicin and cytarabine by continuous infusion, without and with ciclosporin, in older patients with previously untreated acute myeloid leukaemia. Br J Haematol 148(1):48–58. https://doi.org/10.1111/j.1365-2141.2009.07919.x
Christiansen DH, Andersen MK, Pedersen-Bjergaard J (2001) Mutations with loss of heterozygosity of p53 are common in therapy-related myelodysplasia and acute myeloid leukemia after exposure to alkylating agents and significantly associated with deletion or loss of 5q, a complex karyotype, and a poor prognosis. J Clin Oncol 19(5):1405–1413. https://doi.org/10.1200/JCO.2001.19.5.1405
Cortes JE, Heidel FH, Hellmann A et al (2019) Randomized comparison of low dose cytarabine with or without glasdegib in patients with newly diagnosed acute myeloid leukemia or high-risk myelodysplastic syndrome. Leukemia 33(2):379–389. https://doi.org/10.1038/s41375-018-0312-9
Cowell IG, Austin CA (2012) Mechanism of generation of therapy related leukemia in response to anti-topoisomerase II agents. Int J Environ Res Public Health 9(6):2075–2091. https://doi.org/10.3390/ijerph9062075
DAURISMO™ (glasdegib) tablets [packet insert]. New York: Pfizer Labs; 2018
Dayyani F, Kantarjian H, O'Brien S et al (2011) Outcome of therapy-related acute promyelocytic leukemia with or without arsenic trioxide as a component of front-line therapy. Cancer 117(1):110–115. https://doi.org/10.1002/cncr.25585
De Kouchkovsky I, Abdul-Hay M (2016) Acute myeloid leukemia: a comprehensive review and 2016 update. Blood Cancer J. 6(7):e441. https://doi.org/10.1038/bcj.2016.50
de Witte T, Suciu S, Meert L et al (2015) Idarubicin and cytarabine in combination with gemtuzumab ozogamicin (IAGO) for untreated patients with high-risk MDS or AML evolved from MDS: a phase II study from the EORTC and GIMEMA leukemia groups (protocol 06013). Ann Hematol 94(12):1981–1989. https://doi.org/10.1007/s00277-015-2486-9

DiNardo CD, Stein EM, De Botton S et al (2018) Durable remissions with ivosidenib in IDH1-mutated relapsed or refractory AML. N Engl J Med 378(25):2386–2398. https://doi.org/10.1056/NEJMoa1716984
DiNardo CD, Pratz K, Pullarkat V et al (2019) Venetoclax combined with decitabine or azacitidine in treatment-naive, elderly patients with acute myeloid leukemia. Blood 133(1):7–17. https://doi.org/10.1182/blood-2018-08-868752
Döhner H, Estey E, Grimwade D et al (2017) Diagnosis and management of AML in adults: 2017 ELN recommendations from an international expert panel. Blood 129(4):424–447. https://doi.org/10.1182/blood-2016-08-733196
Duffield AS, Aoki J, Levis M et al (2012) Clinical and pathologic features of secondary acute promyelocytic leukemia. Am J Clin Pathol 137(3):395–402. https://doi.org/10.1309/AJCPE0MV0YTWLUUE
Dumas PY, Bertoli S, Bérard E et al (2017) Azacitidine or intensive chemotherapy for older patients with secondary or therapy-related acute myeloid leukemia. Oncotarget 8(45):79126–79136. https://doi.org/10.18632/oncotarget.15988
Elliott MA, Letendre L, Tefferi A et al (2012) Therapy-related acute promyelocytic leukemia: observations relating to APL pathogenesis and therapy. Eur J Haematol 88(3):237–243. https://doi.org/10.1111/j.1600-0609.2011.01727.x
Felix CA (1998) Secondary leukemias induced by topoisomerase-targeted drugs. Biochim Biophys Acta 1400(1-3):233–255. https://doi.org/10.1016/S0167-4781(98)00139-0
Fey MF, Buske C (2013) Acute myeloblastic leukaemias in adult patients: ESMO clinical practice guidelines for diagnosis, treatment and follow-up. Ann Oncol 24 Suppl 6:vi138–vi143. https://doi.org/10.1093/annonc/mdt320
Figueroa ME, Abdel-Wahab O, Lu C et al (2010) Leukemic IDH1 and IDH2 mutations result in a hypermethylation phenotype, disrupt TET2 function, and impair hematopoietic differentiation. Cancer Cell 18(6):553–567. https://doi.org/10.1016/j.ccr.2010.11.015
Fröhling S, Schlenk RF, Breitruck J et al (2002) Prognostic significance of activating FLT3 mutations in younger adults (16 to 60 years) with acute myeloid leukemia and normal cytogenetics: a study of the AML study group Ulm. Blood 100(13):4372–4380. https://doi.org/10.1182/blood-2002-05-1440
Fröhling S, Lipka DB, Kayser S et al (2006a) Rare occurrence of the JAK2 V617F mutation in AML subtypes M5, M6, and M7. Blood 107(3):1242–1243. https://doi.org/10.1182/blood-2005-09-3644
Fröhling S, Schlenk RF, Kayser S et al (2006b) Cytogenetics and age are major determinants of outcome in intensively treated acute myeloid leukemia patients older than 60 years: results from AMLSG trial AML HD98-B. Blood 108(10):3280–3288. https://doi.org/10.1182/blood-2006-04-014324
Gangatharan S, Grove CS, P'ng S et al (2013) Acute myeloid leukaemia in Western Australia 1991-2005: a retrospective population-based study of 898 patients regarding epidemiology, cytogenetics, treatment and outcome. Intern Med J 43(8):903–911. https://doi.org/10.1111/imj.12169
Godley LA, Larson RA (2008) Therapy-related myeloid leukemia. Semin Oncol 35(4):418–429. https://doi.org/10.1053/j.seminoncol.2008.04.012
Green A, Beer P (2010) Somatic mutations of IDH1 and IDH2 in the leukemic transformation of myeloproliferative neoplasms. N Engl J Med 362(4):369–370. https://doi.org/10.1056/NEJMc0910063
Harutyunyan A, Klampfl T, Cazzola M, Kralovics R (2011) p53 lesions in leukemic transformation. N Engl J Med 364(5):488–490. https://doi.org/10.1056/NEJMc1012718
Hasan SK, Mays AN, Ottone T et al (2008) Molecular analysis of t(15;17) genomic breakpoints in secondary acute promyelocytic leukemia arising after treatment of multiple sclerosis. Blood 112(8):3383–3390. https://doi.org/10.1182/blood-2007-10-115600
Hasan SK, Ottone T, Schlenk RF et al (2010) Analysis of t(15;17) chromosomal breakpoint sequences in therapy-related versus de novo acute promyelocytic leukemia: association of DNA breaks with specific DNA motifs at PML and RARA loci. Genes Chromosom Cancer 49(8):726–732. https://doi.org/10.1002/gcc.20783
Heuser M (2016) Therapy-related myeloid neoplasms: does knowing the origin help to guide treatment? Hematology 2016(1):24–32. https://doi.org/10.1182/asheducation-2016.1.24
Holowiecki J, Grosicki S, Giebel S et al (2012) Cladribine, but not fludarabine, added to daunorubicin and cytarabine during induction prolongs survival of patients with acute myeloid leukemia: a multicenter, randomized phase III study. J Clin Oncol 30(20):2441–2448. https://doi.org/10.1200/JCO.2011.37.1286
Hulegårdh E, Nilsson C, Lazarevic V et al (2015) Characterization and prognostic features of secondary acute myeloid leukemia in a population-based setting: a report from the Swedish acute leukemia registry. Am J Hematol 90(3):208–214. https://doi.org/10.1002/ajh.23908
IDHIFA® (enasidenib) tablets [packet insert]. Summit: Celgene Corporation; 2017
Jen EY, Ko CW, Eun Lee J et al (2018) FDA approval: Gemtuzumab ozogamicin for the treatment of adults with newly diagnosed CD33-positive acute myeloid leukemia. Clin Cancer Res 24(14):3242–3246. https://doi.org/10.1158/1078-0432.CCR-17-3179
Juliusson G, Antunovic P, Derolf A et al (2009) Age and acute myeloid leukemia: real world data on decision to treat and outcomes from the Swedish acute leukemia registry. Blood 113(18):4179–4187. https://doi.org/10.1182/blood-2008-07-172007.An
Kayser S, Döhner K, Krauter J et al (2011) The impact of therapy-related acute myeloid leukemia (AML) on outcome in 2853 adult patients with newly diagnosed AML. Blood 117(7):2137–2145. https://doi.org/10.1182/blood-2010-08-301713

Kayser S, Krzykalla J, Elliott MA et al (2017) Characteristics and outcome of patients with therapy-related acute promyelocytic leukemia front-line treated with or without arsenic trioxide. Leukemia 31(11):2347–2354. https://doi.org/10.1038/leu.2017.92

Kennedy JA, Atenafu EG, Messner HA et al (2013) Treatment outcomes following leukemic transformation in Philadelphia-negative myeloproliferative neoplasms. Blood 121(14):2725–2733. https://doi.org/10.1182/blood-2012-10-464248

Kim HP, Gerhard B, Harasym TO, Mayer LD, Hogge DE (2011) Liposomal encapsulation of a synergistic molar ratio of cytarabine and daunorubicin enhances selective toxicity for acute myeloid leukemia progenitors as compared to analogous normal hematopoietic cells. Exp Hematol 39(7):741–750. https://doi.org/10.1016/j.exphem.2011.04.001

Lancet JE, Cortes JE, Hogge DE et al (2014) Phase 2 trial of CPX-351, a fixed 5:1 molar ratio of cytarabine/daunorubicin, vs cytarabine/daunorubicin in older adults with untreated AML. Blood 123(21):3239–3246. https://doi.org/10.1182/blood-2013-12-540971

Lancet JE, Uy GL, Cortes JE et al (2018) Cpx-351 (cytarabine and daunorubicin) liposome for injection versus conventional cytarabine plus daunorubicin in older patients with newly diagnosed secondary acute myeloid leukemia. J Clin Oncol 36(26):2684–2692. https://doi.org/10.1200/JCO.2017.77.6112

Larson RA (2007) Is secondary leukemia an independent poor prognostic factor in acute myeloid leukemia? Best Pract Res Clin Haematol 20(1):29–37. https://doi.org/10.1016/j.beha.2006.10.006

Lee JH, Joo YD, Kim H et al (2011) A randomized trial comparing standard versus high-dose daunorubicin induction in patients with acute myeloid leukemia. Blood. 118(14):3832–3841. https://doi.org/10.1182/blood-2011-06-361410

Lee JH, Kim H, Joo YD et al (2017) Prospective randomized comparison of idarubicin and high-dose daunorubicin in induction chemotherapy for newly diagnosed acute myeloid leukemia. J Clin Oncol 35(24):2754–2763. https://doi.org/10.1200/JCO.2017.72.8618

Li Z, Labopin M, Ciceri F et al (2018) Haploidentical transplantation outcomes for secondary acute myeloid leukemia: acute leukemia working party (ALWP) of the European Society for Blood and Marrow Transplantation (EBMT) study. Am J Hematol 93(6):769–777. https://doi.org/10.1002/ajh.25087

Lim WS, Tardi PG, Dos Santos N et al (2010) Leukemia-selective uptake and cytotoxicity of CPX-351, a synergistic fixed-ratio cytarabine: Daunorubicin formulation, in bone marrow xenografts. Leuk Res 34(9):1214–1223. https://doi.org/10.1016/j.leukres.2010.01.015

Litzow MR, Tarima S, Pérez WS et al (2010) Allogeneic transplantation for therapy-related myelodysplastic syndrome and acute myeloid leukemia. Blood 115(9):1850–1857. https://doi.org/10.1182/blood-2009-10-249128

Lo-Coco F, Hasan SK, Montesinos P, Sanz MA (2013) Biology and management of therapy-related acute promyelocytic leukemia. Curr Opin Oncol 25(6):695–700. https://doi.org/10.1097/CCO.0000000000000013

Löwenberg B, Suciu S, Archimbaud E et al (1998) Mitoxantrone versus daunorubicin in induction-consolidation chemotherapy—the value of low-dose cytarabine for maintenance of remission, and an assessment of prognostic factors in acute myeloid leukemia in the elderly. J Clin Oncol 16(3):872–881. https://doi.org/10.1200/JCO.1998.16.3.872

Löwenberg B, Ossenkoppele GJ, Van Putten W et al (2009) High-dose daunorubicin in older patients with acute myeloid leukemia. N Engl J Med 361(13):1235–1248. https://doi.org/10.1056/NEJMoa0901409

Lyman SD, Jacobsen SEW (1998) C-kit ligand and flt3 ligand: stem/progenitor cell factors with overlapping yet distinct activities. Blood 91(4):1101–1134. https://doi.org/10.1182/blood.V91.4.1101

Mays AN, Osheroff N, Xiao Y et al (2010) Evidence for direct involvement of epirubicin in the formation of chromosomal translocations in t(15;17) therapy-related acute promyelocytic leukemia. Blood 115(2):326–330. https://doi.org/10.1182/blood-2009-07-235051

McKenna HJ, Stocking KL, Miller RE et al (2000) Mice lacking flt3 ligand have deficient hematopoiesis affecting hematopoietic progenitor cells, dendritic cells, and natural killer cells. Blood 95(11):3489–3497. https://doi.org/10.1182/blood.v95.11.3489.011k45_3489_3497

Medeiros BC, Satram-Hoang S, Hurst D, Hoang KQ, Momin F, Reyes C (2015) Big data analysis of treatment patterns and outcomes among elderly acute myeloid leukemia patients in the United States. Ann Hematol 94(7):1127–1138. https://doi.org/10.1007/s00277-015-2351-x

Mengis C, Aebi S, Tobler A, Dähler W, Fey MF (2003) Assessment of differences in patient populations selected for or excluded from participation in clinical phase III acute myelogenous leukemia trials. J Clin Oncol 21(21):3933–3939. https://doi.org/10.1200/JCO.2003.03.186

Mesa RA, Li CY, Ketterling RP, Schroeder GS, Knudson RA, Tefferi A (2005) Leukemic transformation in myelofibrosis with myeloid metaplasia: a single-institution experience with 91 cases. Blood 105(3):973–977. https://doi.org/10.1182/blood-2004-07-2864

Miesner M, Haferlach C, Bacher U et al (2010) Multilineage dysplasia (MLD) in acute myeloid leukemia (AML) correlates with MDS-related cytogenetic abnormalities and a prior history of MDS or MDS/MPN but has no independent prognostic relevance: a comparison of 408 cases classified as "AML not otherwise specified" (AML-NOS) or "AML with myelodysplasia-related changes" (AML-MRC). Blood 116(15):2742–2751. https://doi.org/10.1182/blood-2010-04-279794

Mihalyova J, Jelinek T, Growkova K, Hrdinka M, Simicek M, Hajek R (2018) Venetoclax: a new wave in hema-

tooncology. Exp Hematol 61:10–25. https://doi.org/10.1016/j.exphem.2018.02.002
Mistry AR, Felix CA, Whitmarsh RJ et al (2005) DNA topoisomerase II in therapy-related acute promyelocytic leukemia. N Engl J Med 352(15):1529–1538. https://doi.org/10.1056/NEJMoa042715
Müller-Tidow C, Tschanter P, Röllig C et al (2016) Azacitidine in combination with intensive induction chemotherapy in older patients with acute myeloid leukemia: the AML-AZA trial of the study alliance leukemia. Leukemia 30(3):555–561. https://doi.org/10.1038/leu.2015.306
Nagel G, Weber D, Fromm E et al (2017) Epidemiological, genetic, and clinical characterization by age of newly diagnosed acute myeloid leukemia based on an academic population-based registry study (AMLSG BiO). Ann Hematol 96(12):1993–2003. https://doi.org/10.1007/s00277-017-3150-3
Nilsson C, Hulegårdh E, Garelius H et al (2019) Secondary acute myeloid leukemia and the role of allogeneic stem cell transplantation in a population-based setting. Biol Blood Marrow Transplant 25(9):1770–1778. https://doi.org/10.1016/j.bbmt.2019.05.038
Ok CY, Patel KP, Garcia-Manero G et al (2015a) Mutational profiling of therapy-related myelodysplastic syndromes and acute myeloid leukemia by next generation sequencing, a comparison with de novo diseases. Leuk Res 39(3):348–354. https://doi.org/10.1016/j.leukres.2014.12.006
Ok CY, Patel KP, Garcia-Manero G et al (2015b) TP53 mutation characteristics in therapy-related myelodysplastic syndromes and acute myeloid leukemia is similar to de novo diseases. J Hematol Oncol 8:45. https://doi.org/10.1186/s13045-015-0139-z
Østgård LSG, Kjeldsen E, Holm MS et al (2010) Reasons for treating secondary AML as de novo AML. Eur J Haematol 85(3):217–226. https://doi.org/10.1111/j.1600-0609.2010.01464.x
Østgård LSG, Medeiros BC, Sengeløv H et al (2015) Epidemiology and clinical significance of secondary and therapy-related acute myeloid leukemia: a national population-based cohort study. J Clin Oncol 33(31):3641–3649. https://doi.org/10.1200/JCO.2014.60.0890
Pulsoni A, Pagano L (2005) Treatment of secondary acute myeloid leukemia. J Clin Oncol 23(4):926–927. https://doi.org/10.1200/JCO.2005.05.202
Pulsoni A, Pagano L, Lo Coco F et al (2002) Clinicobiological features and outcome of acute promyelocytic leukemia occurring as a second tumor: the GIMEMA experience. Blood 100(6):1972–1976. https://doi.org/10.1182/blood-2001-12-0312
Rampal R, Ahn J, Abdel-Wahaba O et al (2014) Genomic and functional analysis of leukemic transformation of myeloproliferative neoplasms. Proc Natl Acad Sci U S A 111(50):E5401–E5410. https://doi.org/10.1073/pnas.1407792111
Rizzieri DA, O'Brien JA, Broadwater G et al (2009) Outcomes of patients who undergo aggressive induction therapy for secondary acute myeloid leukemia. Cancer 115(13):2922–2929. https://doi.org/10.1002/cncr.24379
Röllig C, Thiede C, Gramatzki M et al (2010) A novel prognostic model in elderly patients with acute myeloid leukemia: results of 909 patients entered into the prospective AML96 trial. Blood 116(6):971–978. https://doi.org/10.1182/blood-2010-01-267302
Schoch C, Kern W, Schnittger S, Hiddemann W, Haferlach T (2004) Karyotype is an independent prognostic parameter in therapy-related acute myeloid leukemia (t-AML): an analysis of 93 patients with t-AML in comparison to 1091 patients with de novo AML. Leukemia 18(1):120–125. https://doi.org/10.1038/sj.leu.2403187
Sengsayadeth S, Labopin M, Boumendil A et al (2018) Transplant outcomes for secondary acute myeloid leukemia: acute leukemia working party of the European Society for blood and bone marrow transplantation study. Biol Blood Marrow Transplant 24(7):1406–1414. https://doi.org/10.1016/j.bbmt.2018.04.008
Sperling AS, Gibson CJ, Ebert BL (2017) The genetics of myelodysplastic syndrome: from clonal haematopoiesis to secondary leukaemia. Nat Rev Cancer 17(1):5–19. https://doi.org/10.1038/nrc.2016.112
Stein EM, DiNardo CD, Pollyea DA et al (2017) Enasidenib in mutant IDH2 relapsed or refractory acute myeloid leukemia. Blood 130(6):722–731. https://doi.org/10.1182/blood-2017-04-779405
Stölzel F, Pfirrmann M, Aulitzky WE et al (2011) Risk stratification using a new prognostic score for patients with secondary acute myeloid leukemia: results of the prospective AML96 trial. Leukemia 25(3):420–428. https://doi.org/10.1038/leu.2010.279
Stone RM, Mazzola E, Neuberg D et al (2015) Phase III open-label randomized study of cytarabine in combination with amonafide L-malate or daunorubicin as induction therapy for patients with secondary acute myeloid leukemia. J Clin Oncol 33(11):1252–1257. https://doi.org/10.1200/JCO.2014.57.0952
Stone RM, Mandrekar SJ, Sanford BL et al (2017) Midostaurin plus chemotherapy for acute myeloid leukemia with a FLT3 mutation. N Engl J Med 377(5):454–464. https://doi.org/10.1056/NEJMoa1614359
Stone RM, Manley PW, Larson RA, Capdeville R (2018) Midostaurin: its odyssey from discovery to approval for treating acute myeloid leukemia and advanced systemic mastocytosis. Blood Adv 2(4):444–453. https://doi.org/10.1182/bloodadvances.2017011080
Szotkowski T, Rohon P, Zapletalova J, Sicova K, Hubacek J, Indrak K (2010) Secondary acute myeloid leukemia—a single center experience. Neoplasma 57(2):170–178. https://doi.org/10.4149/neo_2010_02_170
Takahashi K, Wang F, Kantarjian H et al (2017) Preleukaemic clonal haemopoiesis and risk of therapy-related myeloid neoplasms: a case-control study. Lancet Oncol 18(1):100–111. https://doi.org/10.1016/S1470-2045(16)30626-X
Talati C, Lancet JE (2018) CPX-351: changing the landscape of treatment for patients with secondary acute

myeloid leukemia. Future Oncol 14(12):1147–1154. https://doi.org/10.2217/fon-2017-0603
Tallman MS, Wang ES, Altman JK et al (2019) Acute myeloid leukemia, version 3.2019, NCCN clinical practice guidelines in oncology. J Natl Compr Cancer Netw 17(6):721–749. https://doi.org/10.6004/jnccn.2019.0028
Theocharides A, Boissinot M, Girodon F et al (2007) Leukemic blasts in transformed JAK2-V617F-positive myeloproliferative disorders are frequently negative for the JAK2-V617F mutation. Blood 110(1):375–379. https://doi.org/10.1182/blood-2006-12-062125
Thepot S, Itzykson R, Seegers V et al (2010) Treatment of progression of Philadelphia-negative myeloproliferative neoplasms to myelodysplastic syndrome or acute myeloid leukemia by azacitidine: a report on 54 cases on the behalf of the Groupe francophone des Myelodysplasies (GFM). Blood 116(19):3735–3742. https://doi.org/10.1182/blood-2010-03-274811
TIBSOVO® (ivosidenib tablets) [packet insert]. Cambridge: Agios Pharmaceuticals, Inc.; 2018
Vardiman J, SSHCEHNLJESPSASHTJ, Swerdlow SH, Campo E, et al (2008) WHO classification of tumours of haematopoietic and lymphoid tissues. Lyon
Vardiman JW, Thiele J, Arber DA et al (2009) The 2008 revision of the World Health Organization (WHO) classification of myeloid neoplasms and acute leukemia: rationale and important changes. Blood 114(5):937–951. https://doi.org/10.1182/blood-2009-03-209262
VENCLEXTA® (venetoclax tablets) [packet insert]. North Chicago: AbbVie Inc. 2018
Vyxeos (n.d.) Summary of product characteristics. https://www.ema.europa.eu/en/documents/product-information/vyxeos-liposomal-epar-product-information_es.pdf. Accessed 17 May 2020
Walter MJ, Shen D, Ding L et al (2012) Clonal architecture of secondary acute myeloid leukemia. N Engl J Med 366(12):1090–1098. https://doi.org/10.1056/NEJMoa1106968
Wei A, Strickland SA, Hou J-Z, et al (2019) Venetoclax with low-dose Cytarabine induces rapid, deep, and durable responses in previously untreated older adults with AML ineligible for intensive chemotherapy. Blood. https://doi.org/10.1182/blood-2018-99-118729
Wheatley K, Brookes CL, Howman AJ et al (2009) Prognostic factor analysis of the survival of elderly patients with AML in the MRC AML11 and LRF AML14 trials. Br J Haematol 145(5):598–605. https://doi.org/10.1111/j.1365-2141.2009.07663.x
Wong TN, Ramsingh G, Young AL et al (2015) Role of TP53 mutations in the origin and evolution of therapy-related acute myeloid leukaemia. Nature 518(7540):552–555. https://doi.org/10.1038/nature13968
XOSPATA® (gilteritinib)[packet insert]. Northbrook: Astellas Pharma US, Inc.; 2018.
Yakoub-Agha I, De La Salmonière P, Ribaud P et al (2000) Allogeneic bone marrow transplantation for therapy-related myelodysplastic syndrome and acute myeloid leukemia: a long-term study of 70 patients—report of the French society of bone marrow transplantation. J Clin Oncol 18(5):963–971. https://doi.org/10.1200/JCO.2000.18.5.963
Yin CC, Glassman AB, Lin P et al (2005) Morphologic, cytogenetic, and molecular abnormalities in therapy-related acute promyelocytic leukemia. Am J Clin Pathol 123(6):840–848. https://doi.org/10.1309/TJFFK819RPCLFKJ0
Zeichner SB, Arellano ML (2015) Secondary adult acute myeloid leukemia: a review of our evolving understanding of a complex disease process. Curr Treat Options Oncol 16(8):37. https://doi.org/10.1007/s11864-015-0355-3
Zeidner JF, Foster MC, Blackford AL et al (2015) Randomized multicenter phase II study of flavopiridol (alvocidib), cytarabine, and mitoxantrone (FLAM) versus cytarabine/daunorubicin (7+3) in newly diagnosed acute myeloid leukemia. Haematologica 100(9):1172–1179. https://doi.org/10.3324/haematol.2015.125849
Zhang SJ, Rampal R, Manshouri T et al (2012) Genetic analysis of patients with leukemic transformation of myeloproliferative neoplasms shows recurrent SRSF2 mutations that are associated with adverse outcome. Blood 119(19):4480–4485. https://doi.org/10.1182/blood-2011-11-390252

# 5 Genomic Landscape and Clonal Evolution of AML

Daniel Noerenberg, Frederik Damm, and Lars Bullinger

## 5.1 Introduction

Acute myeloid leukemia (AML) develops as a clonal expansion of undifferentiated myeloid precursors. It remains challenging to treat due to patient factors such as age and coexisting disease and its intrinsic heterogeneous biology. The majority of patients will respond to induction therapy. However, refractory disease is common and many patients relapse during the course of disease. Recurrent cytogenetic abnormalities have been widely used to study the genetic pathogenesis of AML and provided the backbone for stratifying patients into different risk groups and predicting response for decades (Mrozek et al. 2004; Dohner et al. 2015). Approximately 50% of AML patients have a normal karyotype and their outcome is heterogeneous. After completion of the human genome project, recurrent somatic mutations such as *FLT3*, *NPM1*, *CEBPA*, *DNMT3A*, *IDH1/2*, *KIT*, and *TET2* have been identified and further shaped the molecular landscape in AML (Cancer Genome Atlas Research Network 2013; Stirewalt and Radich 2003; Patel et al. 2012; Ley et al. 2010; Delhommeau et al. 2009; Mardis et al. 2009). Identifying these mutations has not only deepened our understanding of AML pathophysiology, but also opened the door for the development of novel targeted therapies in a disease, in which the cytarabine + anthracycline (7 + 3) induction regimen remained standard of care for the last four decades. Recently, next-generation sequencing (NGS) has led to the discovery of numerous other recurrent molecular mutations, which can currently be identified in >95% of AML patients (Papaemmanuil et al. 2016a; Metzeler et al. 2016; Bullinger et al. 2017). Mechanisms of clonal leukemia evolution and disease dynamics are on the verge of being understood, especially as novel technologies allow us to capture multiple competing clones coexisting at any disease time point (Welch et al. 2012; Wong et al. 2015; Pellegrino et al. 2018). However, despite advances in sequencing techniques and bioinformatics, the translation of this knowledge into clinical practice has been cumbersome in the past. Later, midostaurin was added to the induction regimen for the treatment of adult patients with newly diagnosed *FLT3*-mutated AML. After all-trans retinoic acid (ATRA) in acute promyelocytic leukemia (APL), midostaurin became the first targeted therapy that significantly improved overall survival and changed the standard of care for AML patients (Stone et al. 2017). In addition, ivosidenib and enasidenib, targeting small-molecule inhibitors of mutant *IDH1* and *IDH2*, have been approved by the US Food and Drug Administration (FDA) in *IDH*$^{mut}$ disease (DiNardo et al. 2018; Richard-Carpentier and

D. Noerenberg · F. Damm · L. Bullinger (✉)
Charité Universitätsmedizin Berlin, Berlin, Germany
e-mail: lars.bullinger@charite.de



C. Röllig, G. J. Ossenkoppele (eds.), *Acute Myeloid Leukemia*, Hematologic Malignancies,
https://doi.org/10.1007/978-3-030-72676-8_5

DiNardo 2019), and recently the hedgehog inhibitor glasdegib was approved for the treatment of AML (Cortes et al. 2019). Targeting other common mutations such as *NPM1*, *DNMT3A*, and *TET2* remains challenging due to disease- and patient-specific factors, but numbers of clinical trials using other small-molecule inhibitors for targeted therapy have been launched. In this article, we will give an overview of the genomic landscape in AML and its impact on molecular diagnostics. We will further summarize the use of molecular aberrations for monitoring measurable residual disease (MRD) and their prognostic value in AML.

## 5.2 Classification of De Novo AML

The recognition of the biological and clinical heterogeneity of AML was historically based largely on morphology prompting the French-American-British (FAB) Cooperative Group to develop a classification system based on conventional morphologic and cytochemical characteristics several decades ago (Bennett et al. 1976, 1985a, b). Since the late 1990s, leukemia-associated chromosomal structural variations have become one of the pillars of risk stratification of de novo AML and opened the door toward its genetic classification (Mrozek et al. 2004; Grimwade et al. 1998, 2001). Despite the prognostic information available from cytogenetics (e.g., t(15;17) for M3 or inv(16) for M4Eo), AML has been categorized according to the FAB classification for a long time. More importantly, almost half of AML genomes lack structural abnormalities, even when analyzed with high-density comparative genomic hybridization (array-CGH) or single-nucleotide polymorphism (SNP) arrays (Suela et al. 2007). Since the turn of the century, advances in targeted sequencing, microarray, and next-generation sequencing (NGS)-based "omics" technologies have identified several somatic mutations that play an integral part in AML pathogenesis and prognosis (Cancer Genome Atlas Research Network 2013; Papaemmanuil et al. 2016b; Ley et al. 2008). This exponential knowledge growth, the biological insights into causative genetic lesions, and their clinical utility has been cumulated in a revised World Health Organization (WHO) classification that integrated genetic, immunophenotypic, biological, and clinical features to define specific disease entities (Vardiman et al. 2002, 2009). The WHO classification scheme essentially replaced the outdated FAB classification. A molecular-diagnostics-based novel genomic classification scheme has considerable advantages over one based on only clinical and morphological features with the main reason being that a genomic classification is more robust and reproducible.

In AML, molecular disease classification has already begun to translate into improved disease classification with direct impact on clinical decision-making. The revised WHO classification of 2016 incorporates this knew knowledge (Vardiman et al. 2009; Arber et al. 2016). Disease categories are mostly defined by non-overlapping genetic features with 25 subtypes in total such as t(8;21), t(15;17), inv(16)/t(16;16), t(6;9), inv(3)/t(3;3), AML with 11q23/*MLL*-abnormalities, or AML (megakaryoblastic) with t(1;22). Major changes in comparison to the previous version from 2008 were the change of "AML with *NPM1* mutation" and "AML with biallelic *CEBPA*" from provisional to full entities. Additionally, the presence of mutated *NPM1* or biallelic mutation of *CEBPA* does now supersede the presence of multilineage dysplasia (MLD) in patients without myelodysplastic syndrome (MDS)-related cytogenetic findings. Likewise, in *RUNX1*$^{mut}$ AML, the detection of MLD did not show independent influence on survival in multivariate analysis (Haferlach et al. 2016). With the recognition that biallelic mutation of *CEBPA* is necessary to translate into improved prognosis (Wouters et al. 2009; Green et al. 2010; Taskesen et al. 2011; Dufour et al. 2010), and the addition of AML with *RUNX1* mutation as well as AML with *BCR-ABL1* as new provisional entities, new genetic entities emerged. Importantly, a new category "myeloid neoplasms with germ line predisposition" was added. Since the 2016 WHO classification, a number of sequencing studies have extended the number of somatic, clonal, and pathogenetically relevant driver mutations; and, in accordance, next to the well-established molecular markers *NPM1*, *CEBPA*, and *FLT3*, an update of the European LeukemiaNet (ELN) guidelines does now also recommend the screening for *RUNX1*, *TP53*, and *ASXL1* mutations as novel poor prognostic markers (Table 5.1) (Dohner et al. 2017).

**Table 5.1** 2017 European LeukemiaNet (ELN) risk stratification by genetics[a]

| Risk category[b] | Genetic lesion |
|---|---|
| Favorable | t(8;21)(q22;q22.1); *RUNX1-RUNX1T1*<br>inv(16)(p13.1q22) or t(16;16)(p13.1;q22); *CBFB-MYH11*<br>Mutated *NPM1* without *FLT3*-ITD or with *FLT3*-ITD$^{low(h)}$<br>Biallelic mutated *CEBPA* |
| Intermediate | Mutated *NPM1* and *FLT3*-ITD$^{high(c)}$<br>Wildtype *NPM1* without *FLT3*-ITD or with *FLT3*-ITD$^{low(h)}$ (w/o adverse-risk gene mutations)<br>t(9;11)(p21.3;q23.3); *MLLT3-KMT2A*[c]<br>Cytogenetic abnormalities not classified as favorable or adverse |
| Adverse | t(6;9)(p23;q34.1); *DEK-NUP214*<br>t(v;11q23.3); *KMT2A* rearranged<br>t(9;22)(q34.1;q11.2); *BCR-ABL1*<br>inv(3)(q21.3q26.2) or t(3;3)(q21.3;q26.2); *GATA2*, *MECOM(EVI1)*<br>−5 or del(5q); −7; −17/abn(17p)<br>Complex karyotype[d], monosomal karyotype[e]<br>Wildtype *NPM1* and *FLT3*-ITD$^{high(h)}$<br>Mutated *RUNX1*[f]<br>Mutated *ASXL1*[f]<br>Mutated *TP53*[g] |

Adapted from reference (Dohner et al. 2017)

[a]Frequencies, response rates, and outcome measures should be reported by risk category, and, if sufficient numbers are available, by specific genetic lesions indicated

[b]Prognostic impact of a marker is treatment-dependent and may change with new therapies

[c]The presence of t(9;11)(p21.3;q23.3) takes precedence over rare, concurrent adverse-risk gene mutations

[d]Three or more unrelated chromosome abnormalities in the absence of one of the WHO-designated recurring translocations or inversions, that is, t(8;21), inv(16) or t(16;16), t(9;11), t(v;11)(v;q23.3), t(6;9), inv(3) or t(3;3); AML with *BCR-ABL1*

[e]Defined by the presence of one single monosomy (excluding loss of X or Y) in association with at least one additional monosomy or structural chromosome abnormality (excluding core-binding factor AML)

[f]These markers should not be used as an adverse prognostic marker if they co-occur with favorable-risk AML subtypes

[g]*TP53* mutations are significantly associated with AML with complex and monosomal karyotype

[h]Low, low-allelic ratio (<0.5); high, high-allelic ratio (≥0.5); semi-quantitative assessment of *FLT3*-ITD allelic ratio (using DNA fragment analysis) is determined as ratio of the area under the curve (AUC) "*FLT3*-ITD" divided by AUC "*FLT3*-wildtype"; recent studies indicate that AML with *NPM1* mutation and *FLT3*-ITD low-allelic ratio may also have a more favorable prognosis and patients should not routinely be assigned to allogeneic hematopoietic-cell transplantation

## 5.3 Genomic Landscape

Since the identification of the t(8;21)(q22;q22) translocation and the AML1/ETO Fusion in 1973 by Janet Rowley (Rowley 1973), AML has a long history of "being first" (Fig. 5.1). Based on cloning of the breakpoint of the t(15;17) fusion in APL, all-trans retinoic acid (ATRA) became the first targeted therapy in cancer (Wang and Chen 2008). Following the proof of the cancer stem cell model in AML by John Dick's group (Bonnet and Dick 1997), there has been a growing knowledge on the pathogenic relevance of genomic aberrations in AML. Cytogenetic aberrations have been extensively studied and deepened our knowledge about AML as a genetically driven disease. Following first comprehensive studies using high-throughput microarray technologies (Golub et al. 1999), AML was also the first tumor genome to be completely sequenced using novel NGS technologies in 2008 (Ley et al. 2008) (Fig. 5.1). Subsequent studies led to the identification of novel recurrent somatic mutations of biologic, prognostic, and therapeutic relevance, and they identified AML as complex and dynamic disease characterized by a high inter- and intra-individual heterogeneity. Genome-wide profiling of 200 de novo AML cases within the "The Cancer Genome Atlas (TCGA)" project revealed an average of 13 coding mutations

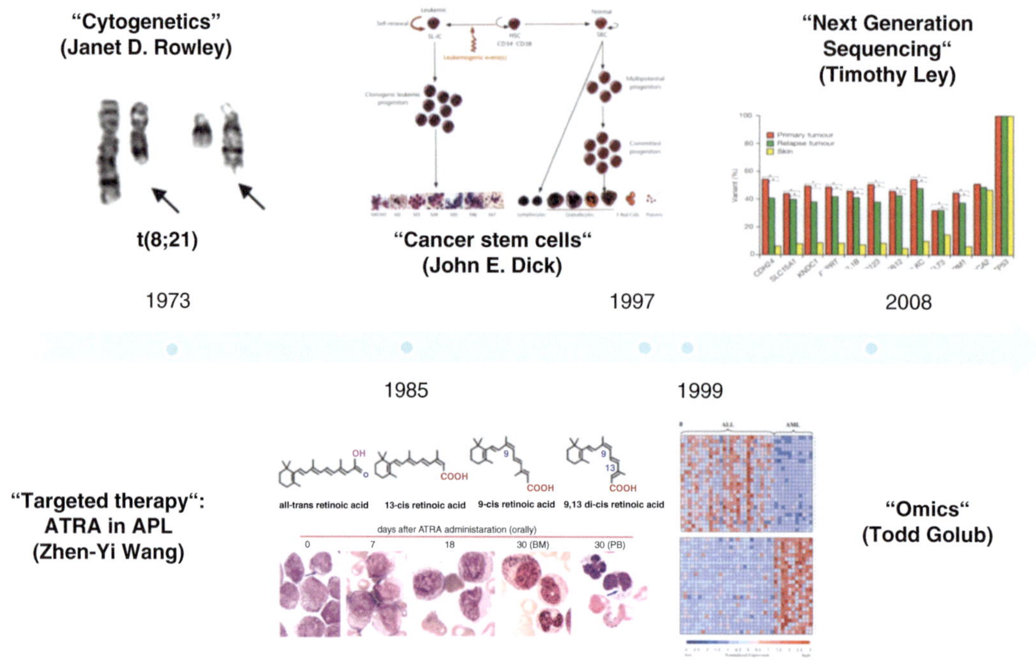


**Fig. 5.1** Acute myeloid leukemia (AML): "a long tradition of being first"

(single-nucleotide variations [SNVs], and insertions/deletions [indels]) per adult AML as well as a median of one somatic copy-number variant (e.g., trisomies or monosomies) and an average of less than one gene-fusion event (Cancer Genome Atlas Research Network 2013). Based on the TCGA study findings as well as other comprehensive genomic studies, the mutations found in AML can be subgrouped into eight functionally and pathogenetically relevant gene categories (Dohner et al. 2015): mutations/structural aberrations in (1) signaling genes, such as *FLT3*; (2) myeloid transcription factors (TFs), such as *RUNX1*; (3) nucleophosmin (*NPM1*) gene; (4) spliceosome complex genes, such as *SRSF2, SF3B1, U2AF1*, and *ZRSR2*; (5) cohesion complex genes, such as *RAD21* and *STAG2*; (6) chromatin modifiers, such as *ASXL1, EZH2*, and *KMT2A*; (7) DNA methylation regulators, such as *DNMT3A, IDH1, IDH2*, and *TET2*; and (8) tumor-suppressor genes, such as *TP53* (Fig. 5.2).

A recent NGS-based landmark study of Papaemmanuil and colleagues led to a revised leukemia classification based on refined molecular genetics (Papaemmanuil et al. 2016a). By using comprehensive cytogenetic analysis and targeted deep-sequencing of 111 pre-defined genes, they identified at least 1 driver mutation in 96%, and 2 drivers in 86% of the 1540 AML patients analyzed. The most frequently mutated loci included known drivers such as *FLT3, NPM1, DNMT3A, NRAS, CEBPA*, and *TET2* and complex cytogenetics all of which being mutated in >10% of the patients and contributing for approximately 40% of all driver mutations observed. Interestingly, point mutations accounted for 73% of all drivers. The recurrently mutated genes also included other known and potentially druggable candidates such as *IDH1* and *IDH2* as well as genes just recently implicated in leukemogenesis (including *EZH2, U2AF1, SMC1A*, and *SMC3*) or a novel hotspot mutation cluster in the *MYC* gene. The mutational patterns in this study compartmentalized the cohort into 11 non-overlapping classes, each with distinct diagnostic features and clinical outcomes (Table 5.2). Beyond currently defined classes such as inv(16), t(15;17), t(8;21), inv(3), t(6;9), and *MLL* fusions as relatively small subgroups (<5% prevalence), AML with mutated

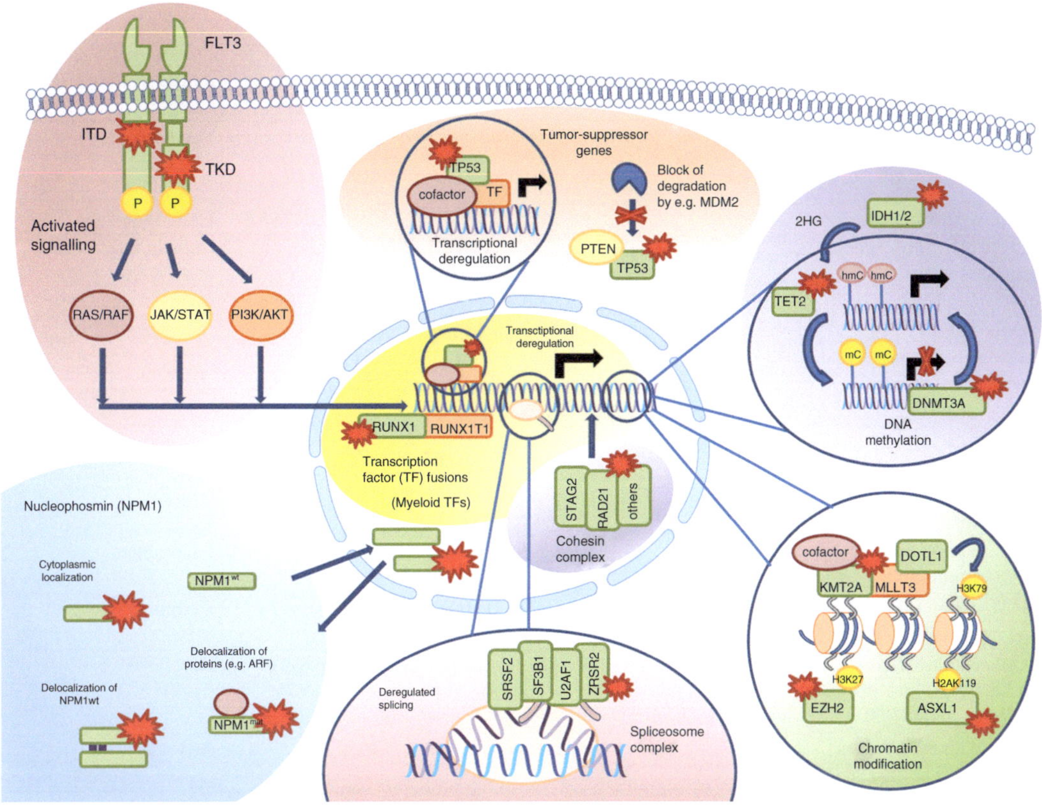


**Fig. 5.2** Mutational landscape in acute myeloid leukemia (AML): illustration of eight functional categories of genes commonly mutated in AML. (Adapted from reference (Papaemmanuil et al. 2016b)). (1) Mutations in signaling genes, such as the class III tyrosine kinase receptor gene *FLT3* (ITD, internal tandem duplications; TKD, tyrosine kinase domain mutations), confer proliferative advantage through activated signaling (upper left panel in lilac); (2) mutations in myeloid transcription factors (TFs), such as RUNX1, and/or transcription factor (TF) fusions by chromosomal rearrangements, such as t(8;21)(q22;q22) [RUNX1-RUNX1T1], lead to transcriptional deregulation and impaired hematopoietic differentiation (center panel in yellow); (3) mutations in the nucleophosmin (*NPM1*) gene, encoding a multifunctional nucleocytoplasmic shuttling protein, result in the aberrant cytoplasmic localization of NPM1 and NPM1-interacting proteins (lower left panel in blue); (4) mutations of spliceosome complex genes, such as *SRSF2, SF3B1, U2AF1*, and *ZRSR2*, are involved in deregulated RNA processing (lower middle panel in lilac); (5) cohesion complex gene mutations, such *RAD21* and *STAG2*, might impair accurate chromosome segregation and transcriptional regulation (center panel in purple); mutations of genes involved in the epigenetic homeostasis of cells lead to either (6) deregulation of chromatin modification, such as *ASXL1, EZH2*, and *KMT2A* mutations (lower right panel in green) or (7) deregulation of DNA methylation, such as *DNMT3A, IDH1, IDH2,* and *TET2* mutations (upper right panel in purple); and (8) mutations of tumor-suppressor genes, such as *TP53*, can, for example, lead to transcriptional deregulation (upper middle panel in orange)

*NPM1*, or biallelic mutated *CEBPA*, three more heterogeneous classes emerged, that is, "*AML with mutated chromatin, RNA-splicing genes, or both*," "*AML with TP53 mutations, chromosomal aneuploidy, or both*," and "*AML with IDH2*$^{R172}$ *mutation*" (Table 5.2). *NPM1*$^{mut}$ AML was the largest class in the cohort, comprising 27% of patients. The chromatin-spliceosome group, accounting for 18% of the cohort, was defined by mutations in RNA-splicing genes (*SRSF2, SF3B1, U2AF1*, and *ZRSR2*), chromatin modifiers (*ASXL1, BCOR, MLL*$^{PTD}$, and *EZH2*), or transcription factors (*RUNX1 and PHF6*). A group with particular dismal outcome accounted for 13% of the patients, and included mutations in *TP53*, complex karyotype alterations, cytogenetically visible copy-number alterations (aneuploidies), or a combination. Last, the authors

**Table 5.2** Proposed genomic classification of AML into 11 distinct genetic subgroups

| Genomic subgroup | Frequency in reference (Papaemmanuil et al. 2016b) (%) | Most frequently mutated genes (%)[a] | Predominant corresponding risk category (ELN 2017)[b] |
|---|---|---|---|
| AML with *NPM1* mutation | 27 | ***NPM1*** (100), *DNMT3A* (54), *FLT3*$^{ITD}$ (39), *NRAS* (19), *TET2* (16), *PTPN11* (15) | Favorable (intermediate) |
| AML with mutated chromatin, RNA-splicing genes, or both[c] | 18 | ***RUNX1*** (39), ***MLL***$^{\mathbf{PTD}}$ (25), ***SRSF2*** (22), *DNMT3A* (20), ***ASXL1*** (17), ***STAG2*** (16), *NRAS* (16), *TET2* (15), *FLT3*$^{ITD}$ (15) | Heterogeneous (mostly intermediate or adverse) |
| AML with *TP53* mutations, chromosomal aneuploidy, or both[d] | 13 | **Complex karyotype** (68), **−5/5q** (47), **−7/7q** (44), ***TP53*** (44), **−17/17p** (31), **−12/12p** (17), +8/8q (16) | Adverse |
| AML with inv(16)(p13.1q22) or t(16;16)(p13.1;q22); *CBFB–MYH11* | 5 | **inv(16)** (100), *NRAS* (53), +8/8q (16), +22 (16), *KIT* (15), *FLT3*$^{TKD}$ (15) | Favorable |
| AML with biallelic *CEBPA* mutations | 4 | ***CEBPA***$^{\mathbf{biallelic}}$ (100), *NRAS* (30), *WT1* (21), *GATA2* (20) | Favorable |
| AML with t(15;17)(q22;q12); *PML–RARA* | 4 | **t(15;17)** (100), *FLT3*$^{ITD}$ (35), *WT1* (17) | Favorable |
| AML with t(8;21)(q22;q22); *RUNX1–RUNX1T1* | 4 | **t(8;21)** (100), *KIT* (38), −Y (33), −9q (18) | Favorable |
| AML with *MLL* fusion genes; t(x;11)(x;q23)[e] | 3 | **t(x;11q23)** (100), *NRAS* (23) | Adverse |
| AML with inv(3)(q21q26.2) or t(3;3)(q21;q26.2); *GATA2, MECOM(EVI1)* | 1 | **inv(3)** (100), −7 (85), *KRAS* (30), *NRAS* (30), *PTPN11* (30), *ETV6* (15), *PHF6* (15), *SF3B1* (15) | Adverse |
| AML with *IDH2*R$^{172}$ mutations and no other class-defining lesions | 1 | ***IDH2***$^{\mathbf{R172}}$ (100), *DNMT3A* (67), +8/8q (17) | Intermediate |
| AML with t(6;9)(p23;q34); *DEK–NUP214* | 1 | **t(6;9)** (100), *FLT3*$^{ITD}$ (80), *KRAS* (20) | Adverse |
| AML with driver mutations but no detected class-defining lesions | 11 | *FLT3*$^{ITD}$ (39), *DNMT3A* (16) | Heterogeneous (mostly intermediate) |
| AML with no detected driver mutations | 4 | – | Intermediate |
| AML meeting criteria for ≥2 genomic subgroups | 4 | – | NA |

*AML* acute myeloid leukemia, *ELN* European LeukemiaNet, *NA* not available, *RNA* ribonucleic acid
Adapted from reference (Papaemmanuil et al. 2016b)

[a]Genes with a frequency of 15% or higher are shown in descending order of frequency. Key contributing genes in each class are shown in boldface type

[b]Only the most predominant risk-groups are mentioned according to the 2017 ELN guidelines (Dohner et al. 2017), cp. Table 5.1

[c]Classification in this subgroup requires one or more driver mutations in *RUNX1*, *ASXL1*, *BCOR*, *STAG2*, *EZH2*, *SRSF2*, *SF3B1*, *U2AF1*, *ZRSR2*, or *MLL*$^{PTD}$. In the presence of other class-defining lesions—namely, inv(16), t(15;17), t(8;21), t(6;9), *MLL* fusion genes, or complex karyo- type or driver mutations in *TP53*, *NPM1*, or *CEBPA*$^{biallelic}$—two or more chromatin–spliceosome mutations are required

[d]Classification in this subgroup requires TP53 mutation, complex karyotype, or in the absence of other class-defining lesions, one or more of the following: −7/7q, −5/5q, −4/4q, −9q, −12/12p, −17/−17p, −18/18q, −20/20q, +11/11q, +13, +21, or +22

[e]Multiple fusion partners for *MLL* were found, with the clinical implications depending on the specific fusion partner

identified a new minor group with *IDH2*$^{R172}$ mutations, accounting for 1% of the cohort. Interestingly, *IDH2*$^{R172}$-mutated AML (in contrast to *IDH2*$^{R140}$) was mutually exclusive with *NPM1*$^{mut}$ AML. Using this classification scheme, at least 80% of AML could unambiguously be categorized in a single group based upon the underlying genetic abnormalities (Papaemmanuil et al. 2016a; Gerstung et al. 2017). However, considering that 20% of AML patients can still not be unambiguously categorized in a distinct genetic subgroup and given the "long tail" of low-frequency mutations that is still to be characterized for its genomic associations and clinical impact, an updated and even more comprehensive molecular classification scheme is currently being developed and will indubitably be clinically relevant in the future.

The overall mutational spectrum in AML is non-random with distinct patterns of co-occurrences and mutual exclusivities reflecting underlying biological interactions among driver mutations. For instance, *DNMT3A* mutations are predominantly observed in *NPM1*$^{mut}$ AML and less frequently in patients with mutations in chromatin or splicing (Papaemmanuil et al. 2016a; Thol et al. 2011). The chromatin/spliceosome group as well as *NPM1*$^{mut}$ AML (which was the largest class in the Papaemmanuil cohort, 27% respectively) showed enrichment in the other hydroxymethylation genes *TET2*, *IDH1*, and *IDH2*. Interestingly, the epigenetic regulators *DNMT3A* and *ASXL1* were mutually exclusive. When analyzing gene-gene correlations, *NPM1* preferentially associates with *NRAS*$^{G12/13}$, whereas there is no significant co-occurrence with the *NRAS*$^{Q61}$ hotspot mutation. Distinct patterns are also observed for *FLT3*: *FLT3*$^{ITD}$ associates with *DNMT3A* and *NPM1*, whereas *FLT3*$^{TKD}$ occurred more often with inv(16) and +22. Differences in co-mutations are also observed for *IDH2*$^{R140}$ and *IDH2*$^{R172}$. These findings suggest that functional consequences of distinct hotspot mutations in the same gene may significantly differ (Green et al. 2011). With the assumption that clinical associations with mutation hotspots/clusters could be altered by differences in co-mutated genes, this is of high-translational importance for the development of targeted therapies such as FLT3 or IDH1/2 inhibitors. Likewise, it emphasizes a thorough description of the mutational spectrum also in entities other than AML and favors even larger-scale genomic studies when aiming to identify (even minor) clinically relevant genetic subgroups (Mead et al. 2007; Ward et al. 2013).

At the same time, large-scale studies as the one from Papaemmanuil and colleagues also allow studying mutational patterns of low-frequency oncogenic drivers with a prevalence below 2–5%. In AML, these rare drivers, such as *RAD21* and *MYC*, seem to be enriched in particular molecular subgroups; for example, mutations in *RAD21* with an overall prevalence of 3% are significantly enriched in *NPM1*$^{mut}$ and t(8;21) AML, 8% and 11%, respectively. Rare drivers may thus be more oncogenic in a particular genomic context and play a role in the relapse setting after targeting the major clone.

## 5.4 Clonal Evolution: Clonal and Subclonal Driver

Cancer evolves by a complex and reiterative process of sequential acquisition, genetic diversification, and clonal selection of vertically transmittable genetic/epigenetic elements (Shlush and Hershkovitz 2015; Greaves and Maley 2012). An initial genetic or epigenetic hit in hematopoietic stem cells (HSCs) leads to the formation of a premalignant clone that further gains selective survival advantages in a changing environment over time. The acquisition of additional molecular events in a highly adaptive and Darwinian fashion with subsequent reprogramming of intracellular programs, and clonal expansion under internal and external pressures over time will lead to the acquisition of additional hallmarks of cancer in later stages (Hanahan and Weinberg 2000, 2011). The dynamics in cancer evolution are highly complex with variable patterns of genetic diversity and resulting clonal architecture. Understanding these processes and the dynamics of cancer evolvement and clonal expansion, that define and shape the molecular landscape of individual cancers, is of key importance not only for effective disease monitoring, but also to improve therapeutic strategies for initial diagnosis and relapse.

Mutant or variant allele fractions (VAFs) of mutations can be used to determine whether a mutation is clonal or subclonal and provide first insights into the phylogenetic tree leading to the development of overt leukemia. Mutations occurring in the founding clone as initiators of disease have a high VAF, whereas mutations in minor clones with lower VAF typically drive disease. The mutational landscape in AML has been well documented in a number of whole exome, whole genome, and targeted sequencing studies with varying reliability to infer clonal evolution due to varying sample size (Cancer Genome Atlas Research Network 2013; Papaemmanuil et al. 2016a; Hughes et al. 2014; Walter et al. 2011, 2012; Damm et al. 2013, 2014a). Analysis of the variant allele frequency (VAF) in the TCGA cohort demonstrated that over half of the cases exhibited at least one subclone in addition to a founding leukemia clone (the clone showing the highest VAF values). Hematopoietic stem cells that bear a *DNMT3A* mutation have a significant fitness advantage in repopulation assays when compared to wildtype HSCs in xenograft models, leading to a clonally expanded pool of pre-leukemic HSCs (Shlush et al. 2014; Kronke et al. 2013). Reliable data in AML support a clonal evolution concept in which mutations affecting epigenetic regulators of transcription (e.g., *DNMT3A, TET2*, and *ASXL1* mutations) or splicing factor gene mutations (e.g., *SF3B1* and *SRSF2* mutations), each with preferred co-operating lesions, occur as early founder events in pre-leukemic stem or progenitor cells that precede transforming leukemogenic events (e.g., *NPM1, FLT3*, or other signaling molecule mutations). In addition, *IDH1/2* mutations appear to be early events as well (Paschka et al. 2010). These data are further supported by single-cell sequencing studies and patient-derived xenograft models (Shlush et al. 2014; Kronke et al. 2013; Jan et al. 2012; Wang et al. 2017; Quek et al. 2018).

In accordance, the occurrence of somatic mutations in genes primarily associated with myeloid neoplasms that can be found in the blood of elderly individuals without clinical signs of overt disease has been commonly termed "clonal hematopoiesis of indeterminate potential" (CHIP) (Jaiswal et al. 2014; Genovese et al. 2014; Steensma et al. 2015; Xie et al. 2014). Patients with CHIP bear a significantly increased risk of developing hematopoietic neoplasms. However, a single alteration in one of these founder mutations in the pre-leukemic niche is probably not sufficient to lead to overt leukemia. *DNMT3A* mutations, as initiators of AML, when present at diagnosis, appear to occur exclusively in the major AML clone, often persist during remission, and increase again at relapse (Ploen et al. 2014; Gaidzik et al. 2018; Jongen-Lavrencic et al. 2018). In turn, *FLT3* mutations, as driver of the disease, are present at diagnosis and frequently disappear at relapse, and are thus unlikely to represent initiators of disease in AML (Miller et al. 2013). In the study by Papaemmanuil and colleagues, *CEPBA* and *RUNX1* mutations were mutually exclusive of transcription factor fusions, thereby indicating that these aberrations might be leukemia-initiating or at least "early" events similar to the fusion genes. These mutually exclusive patterns suggest that "early" molecular hits pre-configure the disease to a distinct subsequent molecular evolution (Cancer Genome Atlas Research Network 2013).

The nucleophosmin (*NPM1*) gene encodes for a multifunctional phosphoprotein involved in ribogenesis, DNA repair, centrosome duplication during cell cycle, and the ARF-p53 pathway (Falini et al. 2007; Lindstrom 2011). *NPM1* mutations that alter the C-terminal DNA-binding domain lead to aberrant cytoplasmatic localization of the protein and concurrent impaired function of the nucleolar wildtype protein (Dohner et al. 2015; Tarlock and Meshinchi 2015; Federici and Falini 2013). Given the importance of founder mutations, it may seem counter-intuitive that *NPM1* mutations as intermediate/late driver-events appear as class-defining lesions. However, whereas early mutations such as the DNA methylation/hydroxymethylation genes *DNMT3A*, *TET2*, and *IDH1/2* are present in a number of hematologic neoplasms and also appear in healthy individuals with CHIP, *NPM1* mutations are considerably more specific to AML and shape the leukemic phenotype. Accordingly, as the second-most recurrent mutation in de novo AML (Falini et al. 2005), *NPM1* emerged as a separate entity with its clinical course depending on co-operating mutations. For example, in *NPM1/DNMT3A* double-mutated AML, *NPM1* was subclonal to *DNMT3A* in 78% of cases, whereas in 21% of the cases, both mutations co-occurred in the same clone, and in less than 1%, *NPM1* mutation was an earlier event than *DNMT3A*. These data are consistent with longitudinal studies in *NPM1*$^{mut}$AML, showing loss of the *NMP1* mutation during relapse, suggesting an early branching of an *NPM1* negative clone that gets dominant in the relapse setting (Kronke et al. 2013). The authors hypothesize that *NPM1* may have transformative effects in the context of an epigenetic landscape shaped by above-mentioned initiating mutations such as *DNMT3A*, *TET2*, or *IDH1/2*. Additional whole exome studies in this cohort finally revealed that in *NPM1* negative relapse cases, a second independent transforming event based on persistent clonal hematopoiesis has caused a second leukemia, which is besides the clonal hematopoiesis lesion on the genomic level independent from the primary disease (Fig. 5.3) (Cocciardi et al. 2019).

In contrast to epigenetic regulators, mutations in transcription factors (*WT1*, *GATA2*), RNA splicing genes (*SF3B1*, *SRSF2*, *U2AF1*), and chromatin modifiers (*EZH2*, *BCOR*) appear to occur at intermediate time points (Papaemmanuil et al. 2016a). Lesions in receptor tyrosine kinase (RTK) and RAS signaling genes (*NRAS*, *KRAS*, *PTPN11*, *KIT*, *FLT3*$^{TKD}$, *NF1*) are distributed among many subgroups with a high overall frequency of 55%, often affected my multiple mutations in the same sample and appearing late in AML evolution. When comparing the mutational landscape of primary and corresponding relapsed samples, two major evolution patterns in AML emerge: (1) evolvement of the founding clone by acquisition of additional mutations, and (2) survival of a subclone(s) with acquisition of mutations and expansion at relapse (Ding et al. 2012). In all cases analyzed, conventional chemotherapy failed to eradicate the founding clone.

Delineating the dynamic intratumoral heterogeneity, with identification of AML-initiating molecular events and the temporal acquisition of mutations over time, is not only important for our understanding of AML biology, but also central to the development of targeted therapies and combination strategies tailored to the genomic landscape and clonal evolution in AML. Founding clones with mutations in ancestral cells capable of multilineage engraftment may survive (or are not even targeted) by therapy, can lead to clonal expansion during remission, and cause recurrent disease with acquisition of new/other driver mutations. Minor clones may also coexist with the major founding clone, become dominant under selective pressure, and lead to relapsed disease with a different mutational pattern and change of disease biology (Fig. 5.3). Based on novel single-cell sequencing strategies, capturing not only the heterogeneity of stem cells but also allowing us to dissect the tumor microenvironment (Baccin et al. 2020), we will better understand clonal evolution, and this will allow us to better target individual resistant subclones in the future.

## 5.5 Clonal Hematopoiesis of Indeterminate Potential (CHIP)

Recurrent somatic mutations in epigenetic regulators and splicing factor genes (e.g., *ASXL1*, *DNMT3A*, and *TET2*) can be found in the blood of at least 10% of people older than 60 years of age. The term CHIP was proposed to describe the presence of these hematologic cancer-associated mutations with a VAF of at least 2% and in the absence of conventional diagnostic criteria for a

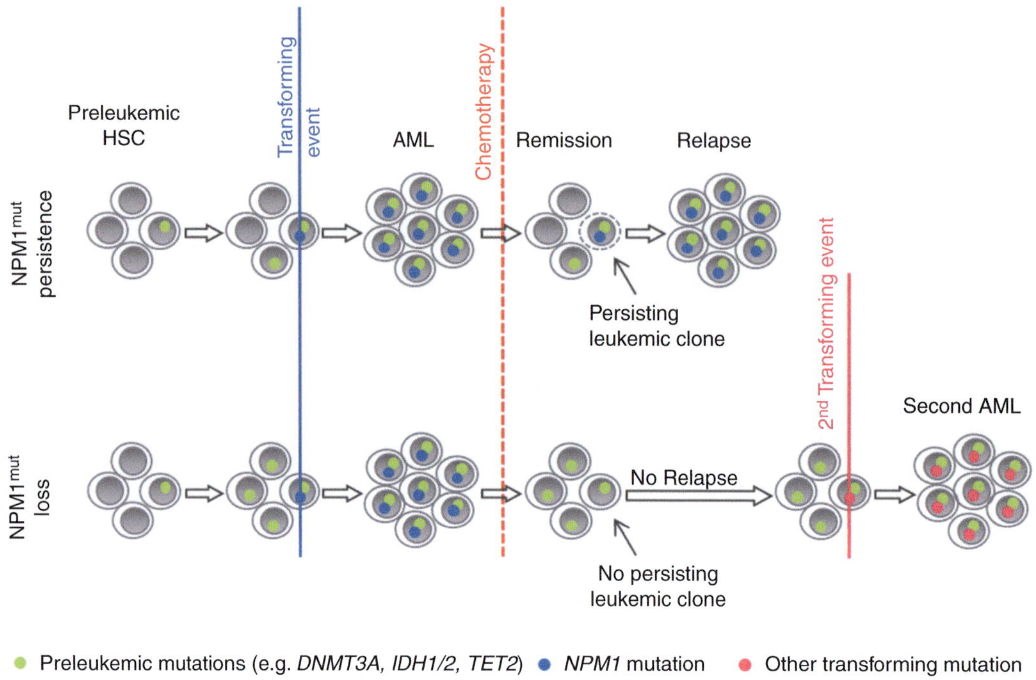


**Fig. 5.3** Mutational landscape in acute myeloid leukemia (AML): illustration of eight functional categories of genes commonly mutated in AML. (Adapted from Reference (Cocciardi et al. 2019)). Possible mechanisms of relapse in *NPM1*$^{mut}$ AML. Based on our mutation data, we postulate different mechanisms of relapse for *NPM1*$^{mut}$ loss and *NPM1*$^{mut}$ persistent pts

hematologic malignancy (Jaiswal et al. 2014; Genovese et al. 2014; Steensma et al. 2015; Xie et al. 2014). CHIP is associated with an increased risk of hematologic cancers, cardiovascular disease, and death from coronary heart disease collectively leading to an increased overall mortality (Jaiswal et al. 2017). CHIP most likely derives from mutated Lin$^{-}$CD34$^{+}$CD38$^{-}$ hematopoietic stem cells (HSCs) and may precede many hematologic disorders with a significantly increased risk for hematologic malignancies (hazard ratio 12.9) (Shlush et al. 2014; Arends et al. 2018; Yoshizato et al. 2015; Damm et al. 2014b; Woll et al. 2014; Schmidt et al. 2014; Quivoron et al. 2011). The estimated transformation rate of CHIP into myeloid and lymphoid cancers with 0.5–1% per year, may be similar to the rate of progression of other premalignant states, such as monoclonal gammopathy of undetermined significance (MGUS) to multiple myeloma or to other plasma or lymphoid malignancies (Kyle et al. 2018). Recent studies have also demonstrated an increased risk for therapy-related myeloid neoplasms in individuals that had CHIP at the diagnosis of their primary cancer (Takahashi et al. 2017; Gillis et al. 2017). However, in the vast majority of healthy individuals, mutated HSCs have been shown to be stable over many years without causing disease signs or symptoms making individual predictions of the malignant transformation potential highly challenging (Young et al. 2016).

The risk factors for progression of CHIP into overt hematologic neoplasms remain largely obscure. Nagase and colleagues recently described a mouse model, in which they conditionally introduced a common "dominant-negative" mutation of the *ASXL1* gene, resulting in a mutant protein that also inhibits the wildtype protein (Nagase et al. 2018). These mice showed myeloid skewing, anemia, and thrombocytosis, features that are also seen in patients with CHIP, but mutated *ASXL1* alone did not result in the development of leukemia in an 18-month timeframe. However, *ASXL1*-mutated mice had an altered epigenome with increased susceptibility to leukemic transformation as demonstrated by viral insertional mutagenesis or overexpression of *RUNX1*. Future studies are warranted to explore the impact of stochastic, environmental (e.g., chronic inflammation, drugs, and toxicity exposures), or hereditary effects on a genomic and epigenomic level that may lead to the development and progression of CHIP before implementation as a biomarker in clinical practice. Likewise, the role of persisting CHIP following leukemia treatment will have to be better understood by monitoring of measurable residual disease (MRD) for both pre-leukemic and leukemic markers, as well as the role of donor CHIP in the setting of allogeneic hematopoietic stem cell transplantation (HSCT) (Frick et al. 2019).

## 5.6 Molecular Genetic Testing and Measurable Residual Disease (MRD)

Depending on a variety of clinical and disease-related factors, about half of AML patients in morphologic remission (as defined by <5% bone marrow blasts) will eventually relapse. This has led scientist to develop ways to trace the presence of leukemic cells down to levels of $1{:}10^4$ to $1{:}10^6$ white blood cells. These low quantities of persisting leukemic cells have been termed minimal, or recently, more appropriately, measurable residual disease (MRD). MRD detection methods are already indispensable tools in AML for risk-stratification and monitoring disease in conjunction with other diagnostic tools such as clinical, cytogenetic, and molecular data. Different techniques can be used for the assessment of MRD in AML such as multiparameter flow cytometry (MFC) or real-time quantitative polymerase chain reaction (qPCR). A number of studies has been investigating the prognostic value of MRD assessed by MFC in AML, and showed that MRD negativity is highly prognostic for outcome (Schuurhuis et al. 2018).

Today, conventional cytogenetic analysis remains mandatory for the initial AML workup, although molecular testing by reverse transcriptase–polymerase chain reaction (RT-PCR) for recurring rearrangements and fluorescent in situ hybridization (FISH) can be useful if cytogenetic analysis fails. In the future, whole genome sequencing approaches might fill in. The current ELN guidelines recommend molecular genetic testing for aberrations that mainly guide treatment decisions and have prognostic impact; some of them may also be used for molecular disease monitoring (Dohner et al. 2017). This includes screening for *NPM1*, *CEBPA*, and *RUNX1*, mutations in *FLT3* (both for internal tandem duplications [ITDs] together with mutant-to-wildtype allelic ratio and *FLT3*$^{D835/I836}$), as well as mutations in *TP53* and *ASXL1* as they confer poor prognosis. While it is time consuming and cost ineffective to capture these aberrations by conventional sequencing strategies, the list of molecular markers informing clinical practice is growing and testing will have to be replaced by gene panel diagnostics. Currently, a number of commercial and custom-designed gene panels is available (Kuo and Dong 2015), but it will be crucial to invest in flexible platforms and to develop diagnostic tools that can simultaneously test for both gene mutations and gene rearrangements (He et al. 2016; McKerrell et al. 2016).

The assessment of molecular MRD in AML is well established for qPCR-based quantification of *NPM1*, that has proved as a powerful independent prognosticator in the trials of the British National Cancer Research Institute and the German and Austrian AML study group (Ivey et al. 2016; Kronke et al. 2011), and for the fusion genes *RUNX1-RUNXT1*, *CBFB-MYH11*, and *PML-RARA*, as their presence following therapy is a strong predictor for relapse, as recently again nicely demonstrated for *RUNX1-RUNXT1* (Rucker et al. 2019). As we face rapid NGS and other technical advances, such as digital PCR, these techniques might allow for more accurate MRD assessment in the future and even offer the possibility to capture leukemia heterogeneity at the single-cell level (Zhang et al. 2016; Wang and Navin 2015). For now, these approaches are reserved for research questions. As mentioned earlier, NGS allows detection of at least one driver mutation in >95% of de novo AML (Papaemmanuil et al. 2016a), and thus can, theoretically, be applied for MRD assessment following treatment. However, a constantly growing list of disease-relevant genes in AML, the lack of knowledge about the role of MRD negativity for each individual or a set of genes, and a lack of international quality and quantity standards are currently limiting the use of molecular MRD in clinical practice. A recent study by Jongen-Lavrience et al. showed that in patients with previously untreated AML who received intensive induction therapy and were in complete morphological remission, the presence of MRD as assessed by targeted sequencing was detectable in 51% of 430 patients (Jongen-Lavrencic et al. 2018). Importantly, in patients with mutations in genes associated with CHIP (and likewise believed to represent disease-initiating events in AML, e.g., *DNMT3A*, *TET2*, and *ASXL1*), the detection of these mutations during morphological remission did not have value for predicting relapse and lacked prognostic significance. In contrast, the detection of MRD for mutations other than *DNMT3A*, *TET2*, and *ASXL1* had indeed a negative prognostic value. Two other groups independently confirmed the value of persisting MRD in complete remission (CR) as an important marker for risk-adapted treatment approaches at relapse (Morita et al. 2018; Rothenberg-Thurley et al. 2018). The MRD working party of the European LeukemiaNet developed a consensus paper for the current and future use of MRD in clinical practice (Schuurhuis et al. 2018). The authors suggest that the combination of several markers for MRD assessment might overcome limitations due to subclonal heterogeneity of AML and to CHIP. For instance, if a patient with mutations in *TP53*, *ASXL1*, and *PTPN11* will stay *ASXL1* positive at a high VAF during remission, further *ASXL1* assessment may not be helpful. However, if the *PTPN11* clone is eradicated and there is persistent MRD for *TP53* at the same time, *TP53* may represent the MRD clone. Thus, the analysis of several molecular MRD markers might prove more useful and may increase the likelihood for prediction of relapse (Thol et al. 2018). However, the clinically most useful MRD test and targets are yet to be determined.

## 5.7 Prognostic Impact of Genetic Characteristics/Genomics Informed Patient Care

With novel insights into the genomic landscape of AML and the increasing knowledge about leukemia-initiating events and driver mutations, it is important to acknowledge that there is a distinction of classifying AML patients for diagnostic or prognostic purposes. A diagnostic classification should be stable and durable, emphasizing differences in the underlying biology of the disease. Prognostic systems should be flexible and adjustable, especially to changing outcomes in the advent of targeted therapies in AML (Dohner et al. 2017). For instance, an effective treatment with FLT3 and RAS-pathway kinase inhibitors will lead to changes in outcome predictions but will not alter their assignment to class-defining genetic lesions (Papaemmanuil et al. 2016b). In addition, characterization of epigenetic, proteomic, or miRNA profiles have begun to play an important role in how the disease can be approached and might alter the prognosis of distinct AML subgroups in the future. Table 5.1 gives an overview about the three prognostic risk groups defined by the ELN 2017. However, one has to keep in mind that the prognostic impact of a single genetic lesion will largely depend on the genomic context in which they occur. For instance, the effect of $FLT3^{ITD}$ in the context of concomitant *NPM1* and *DNMT3A* mutations confers a significantly worse prognosis than the additive prognostic effects conferred by these genes. On the other hand, the effect of $FLT3^{ITD}$ on survival is considerably less pronounced in *NPM1* or $DNMT3A^{wt}$ patients (Papaemmanuil et al. 2016a). In addition, for patients in the *NPM1* cohort, with *NPM1* being one of the most favorable prognostic markers in AML (Cancer Genome Atlas Research Network 2013; Papaemmanuil et al. 2016b; Thiede et al. 2006), clinical outcomes for patients are largely predicted by other co-occurring mutations (i.e., *NRAS*, *IDH*, *PTPN11*, *FLT3*, and chromatin–spliceosome mutations).

Recent advances proved also that novel genetic information can be successfully applied to inform clinical practice. For example, a large knowledge bank of matched genomic–clinical AML data could be devised to accurately predict likelihoods of remission, relapse, and mortality with findings being validated on independent TCGA data (Gerstung et al. 2017). Future models based on increased patient numbers will allow to further reduce the error rate of such personalized treatment predictions, and European initiatives like HARMONY—Healthcare Alliance for Resourceful Medicines Offensive against Neoplasms in HematologY—are currently capturing, integrating, and harmonizing patient data from large AML cohorts to gain valuable novel insights (Bullinger et al. 2020). Similarly, as mentioned earlier, genomic knowledge can facilitate follow-up monitoring of MRD. The NGS-based identification of molecular markers in almost 100% of diagnostic AML cases provides a prerequisite for comprehensive and individualized MRD assessment to identify patients at high relapse risk at early time points. With further understanding of AML genetics and on the verge of targeted therapies in AML, we are given the opportunity to refine post-remission strategies depending on molecular information, the individual patient's characteristics, and the therapy administered. In addition, future developments will ultimately allow genome-wide unbiased tests at high quality, based on which individualized treatment approaches can be further advanced. These platforms need careful validation and standards have to be set qualitatively as well as quantitatively prior to implementation in daily clinical routine.

Future molecular targeted treatment designs will have to take clonal relationships into account, and treatment strategies should be adjusted based on longitudinal clonal monitoring and might even selectively or longitudinally target multiple clones.

## References


Arber DA et al (2016) The 2016 revision to the World Health Organization classification of myeloid neoplasms and acute leukemia. Blood 127(20):2391–2405

Arends CM et al (2018) Hematopoietic lineage distribution and evolutionary dynamics of clonal hematopoiesis. Leukemia

Baccin C et al (2020) Combined single-cell and spatial transcriptomics reveal the molecular, cellular and spatial bone marrow niche organization. Nat Cell Biol 22(1):38–48

Bennett JM et al (1976) Proposals for the classification of the acute leukaemias. French-American-British (FAB) Co-operative Group. Br J Haematol 33(4):451–458

Bennett JM et al (1985a) Proposed revised criteria for the classification of acute myeloid leukemia. A report of the French-American-British Cooperative Group. Ann Intern Med 103(4):620–625

Bennett JM et al (1985b) Criteria for the diagnosis of acute leukemia of megakaryocyte lineage (M7). A report of the French-American-British Cooperative Group. Ann Intern Med 103(3):460–462

Bonnet D, Dick JE (1997) Human acute myeloid leukemia is organized as a hierarchy that originates from a primitive hematopoietic cell. Nat Med 3(7): 730–737

Bullinger L, Dohner K, Dohner H (2017) Genomics of acute myeloid leukemia diagnosis and pathways. J Clin Oncol 35(9):934–946

Bullinger L, et al (2020) Novel insights into genomic classification and prognosis in acute myeloid leukemia based on a Pan-European public-private partnership, the harmony alliance. EHA Library (294950), p S130

Cancer Genome Atlas Research Network et al (2013) Genomic and epigenomic landscapes of adult de novo acute myeloid leukemia. N Engl J Med 368(22):2059–2074

Cocciardi S et al (2019) Clonal evolution patterns in acute myeloid leukemia with NPM1 mutation. Nat Commun 10(1):2031

Cortes JE et al (2019) Randomized comparison of low dose cytarabine with or without glasdegib in patients with newly diagnosed acute myeloid leukemia or high-risk myelodysplastic syndrome. Leukemia 33(2).379–389

Damm F et al (2013) BCOR and BCORL1 mutations in myelodysplastic syndromes and related disorders. Blood 122(18):3169–3177

Damm F et al (2014a) TET2 mutations in cytogenetically normal acute myeloid leukemia: clinical implications and evolutionary patterns. Genes Chromosomes Cancer 53(10):824–832

Damm F et al (2014b) Acquired initiating mutations in early hematopoietic cells of CLL patients. Cancer Discov 4(9):1088–1101

Delhommeau F et al (2009) Mutation in TET2 in myeloid cancers. N Engl J Med 360(22):2289–2301

DiNardo CD et al (2018) Durable remissions with Ivosidenib in IDH1-mutated relapsed or refractory AML. N Engl J Med 378(25):2386–2398

Ding L et al (2012) Clonal evolution in relapsed acute myeloid leukaemia revealed by whole-genome sequencing. Nature 481(7382):506–510

Dohner H, Weisdorf DJ, Bloomfield CD (2015) Acute myeloid leukemia. N Engl J Med 373(12):1136–1152

Dohner H et al (2017) Diagnosis and management of AML in adults: 2017 ELN recommendations from an international expert panel. Blood 129(4):424–447

Dufour A et al (2010) Acute myeloid leukemia with biallelic CEBPA gene mutations and normal karyotype represents a distinct genetic entity associated with a favorable clinical outcome. J Clin Oncol 28(4):570–577

Falini B et al (2005) Cytoplasmic nucleophosmin in acute myelogenous leukemia with a normal karyotype. N Engl J Med 352(3):254–266

Falini B et al (2007) Aberrant cytoplasmic expression of C-terminal-truncated NPM leukaemic mutant is dictated by tryptophans loss and a new NES motif. Leukemia 21(9):2052–2054; author reply 2054; discussion 2055-6

Federici L, Falini B (2013) Nucleophosmin mutations in acute myeloid leukemia: a tale of protein unfolding and mislocalization. Protein Sci 22(5):545–556

Frick M et al (2019) Role of donor clonal hematopoiesis in allogeneic hematopoietic stem-cell transplantation. J Clin Oncol 37(5):375–385

Gaidzik VI et al (2018) DNMT3A mutant transcript levels persist in remission and do not predict outcome in patients with acute myeloid leukemia. Leukemia 32(1):30–37

Genovese G et al (2014) Clonal hematopoiesis and blood-cancer risk inferred from blood DNA sequence. N Engl J Med 371(26):2477–2487

Gerstung M et al (2017) Precision oncology for acute myeloid leukemia using a knowledge bank approach. Nat Genet 49(3):332–340

Gillis NK et al (2017) Clonal haemopoiesis and therapy-related myeloid malignancies in elderly patients: a proof-of-concept, case-control study. Lancet Oncol 18(1):112–121

Golub TR et al (1999) Molecular classification of cancer: class discovery and class prediction by gene expression monitoring. Science 286(5439):531–537

Greaves M, Maley CC (2012) Clonal evolution in cancer. Nature 481(7381):306–313

Green CL et al (2010) Prognostic significance of CEBPA mutations in a large cohort of younger adult patients with acute myeloid leukemia: impact of double CEBPA mutations and the interaction with FLT3 and NPM1 mutations. J Clin Oncol 28(16):2739–2747

Green CL et al (2011) The prognostic significance of IDH2 mutations in AML depends on the location of the mutation. Blood 118(2):409–412

Grimwade D et al (1998) The importance of diagnostic cytogenetics on outcome in AML: analysis of 1,612 patients entered into the MRC AML 10 trial. The Medical Research Council Adult and Children's Leukaemia Working Parties. Blood 92(7):2322–2333

Grimwade D et al (2001) The predictive value of hierarchical cytogenetic classification in older adults with acute myeloid leukemia (AML): analysis of 1065 patients entered into the United Kingdom Medical Research Council AML11 trial. Blood 98(5):1312–1320

Haferlach T et al (2016) The new provisional WHO entity 'RUNX1 mutated AML' shows specific genetics but no prognostic influence of dysplasia. Leukemia 30(10):2109–2112

Hanahan D, Weinberg RA (2000) The hallmarks of cancer. Cell 100(1):57–70

Hanahan D, Weinberg RA (2011) Hallmarks of cancer: the next generation. Cell 144(5):646–674

He J et al (2016) Integrated genomic DNA/RNA profiling of hematologic malignancies in the clinical setting. Blood 127(24):3004–3014

Hughes AE et al (2014) Clonal architecture of secondary acute myeloid leukemia defined by single-cell sequencing. PLoS Genet 10(7):e1004462

Ivey A et al (2016) Assessment of minimal residual disease in standard-risk AML. N Engl J Med 374(5):422–433

Jaiswal S et al (2014) Age-related clonal hematopoiesis associated with adverse outcomes. N Engl J Med 371(26):2488–2498

Jaiswal S et al (2017) Clonal hematopoiesis and risk of atherosclerotic cardiovascular disease. N Engl J Med 377(2):111–121

Jan M et al (2012) Clonal evolution of preleukemic hematopoietic stem cells precedes human acute myeloid leukemia. Sci Transl Med 4(149):149ra118

Jongen-Lavrencic M et al (2018) Molecular minimal residual disease in acute myeloid leukemia. N Engl J Med 378(13):1189–1199

Kronke J et al (2011) Monitoring of minimal residual disease in NPM1-mutated acute myeloid leukemia: a study from the German-Austrian Acute Myeloid Leukemia Study Group. J Clin Oncol 29(19):2709–2716

Kronke J et al (2013) Clonal evolution in relapsed NPM1-mutated acute myeloid leukemia. Blood 122(1):100–108

Kuo FC, Dong F (2015) Next-generation sequencing-based panel testing for myeloid neoplasms. Curr Hematol Malig Rep 10(2):104–111

Kyle RA et al (2018) Long-term follow-up of monoclonal gammopathy of undetermined significance. N Engl J Med 378(3):241–249

Ley TJ et al (2008) DNA sequencing of a cytogenetically normal acute myeloid leukaemia genome. Nature 456(7218):66–72

Ley TJ et al (2010) DNMT3A mutations in acute myeloid leukemia. N Engl J Med 363(25):2424–2433

Lindstrom MS (2011) NPM1/B23: a multifunctional chaperone in ribosome biogenesis and chromatin remodeling. Biochem Res Int 2011:195209

Mardis ER et al (2009) Recurring mutations found by sequencing an acute myeloid leukemia genome. N Engl J Med 361(11):1058–1066

McKerrell T et al (2016) Development and validation of a comprehensive genomic diagnostic tool for myeloid malignancies. Blood 128(1):e1–e9

Mead AJ et al (2007) FLT3 tyrosine kinase domain mutations are biologically distinct from and have a significantly more favorable prognosis than FLT3 internal tandem duplications in patients with acute myeloid leukemia. Blood 110(4):1262–1270

Metzeler KH et al (2016) Spectrum and prognostic relevance of driver gene mutations in acute myeloid leukemia. Blood 128(5):686–698

Miller CA, Wilson RK, Ley TJ (2013) Genomic landscapes and clonality of de novo AML. N Engl J Med 369(15):1473
Morita K et al (2018) Clearance of somatic mutations at remission and the risk of relapse in acute myeloid leukemia. J Clin Oncol 36(18):1788–1797
Mrozek K, Heerema NA, Bloomfield CD (2004) Cytogenetics in acute leukemia. Blood Rev 18(2):115–136
Nagase R et al (2018) Expression of mutant Asxl1 perturbs hematopoiesis and promotes susceptibility to leukemic transformation. J Exp Med 215(6):1729–1747
Papaemmanuil E, Dohner H, Campbell PJ (2016a) Genomic classification in acute myeloid leukemia. N Engl J Med 375(9):900–901
Papaemmanuil E et al (2016b) Genomic classification and prognosis in acute myeloid leukemia. N Engl J Med 374(23):2209–2221
Paschka P et al (2010) IDH1 and IDH2 mutations are frequent genetic alterations in acute myeloid leukemia and confer adverse prognosis in cytogenetically normal acute myeloid leukemia with NPM1 mutation without FLT3 internal tandem duplication. J Clin Oncol 28(22):3636–3643
Patel JP et al (2012) Prognostic relevance of integrated genetic profiling in acute myeloid leukemia. N Engl J Med 366(12):1079–1089
Pellegrino M et al (2018) High-throughput single-cell DNA sequencing of acute myeloid leukemia tumors with droplet microfluidics. Genome Res 28(9):1345–1352
Ploen GG et al (2014) Persistence of DNMT3A mutations at long-term remission in adult patients with AML. Br J Haematol 167(4):478–486
Quek L et al (2018) Clonal heterogeneity of acute myeloid leukemia treated with the IDH2 inhibitor enasidenib. Nat Med 24(8):1167–1177
Quivoron C et al (2011) TET2 inactivation results in pleiotropic hematopoietic abnormalities in mouse and is a recurrent event during human lymphomagenesis. Cancer Cell 20(1):25–38
Richard-Carpentier G, DiNardo CD (2019) Single-agent and combination biologics in acute myeloid leukemia. Hematology Am Soc Hematol Educ Program 2019(1):548–556
Rothenberg-Thurley M et al (2018) Persistence of pre-leukemic clones during first remission and risk of relapse in acute myeloid leukemia. Leukemia 32(7):1598–1608
Rowley JD (1973) Identificaton of a translocation with quinacrine fluorescence in a patient with acute leukemia. Ann Genet 16(2):109–112
Rucker FG et al (2019) Measurable residual disease monitoring in acute myeloid leukemia with t(8;21)(q22;q22.1): results from the AML Study Group. Blood 134(19):1608–1618
Schmidt M et al (2014) Molecular-defined clonal evolution in patients with chronic myeloid leukemia independent of the BCR-ABL status. Leukemia 28(12):2292–2299
Schuurhuis GJ et al (2018) Minimal/measurable residual disease in AML: a consensus document from the European LeukemiaNet MRD Working Party. Blood 131(12):1275–1291
Shlush LI, Hershkovitz D (2015) Clonal evolution models of tumor heterogeneity. Am Soc Clin Oncol Educ Book, e662–e665
Shlush LI et al (2014) Identification of pre-leukaemic haematopoietic stem cells in acute leukaemia. Nature 506(7488):328–333
Steensma DP et al (2015) Clonal hematopoiesis of indeterminate potential and its distinction from myelodysplastic syndromes. Blood 126(1):9–16
Stirewalt DL, Radich JP (2003) The role of FLT3 in haematopoietic malignancies. Nat Rev Cancer 3(9):650–665
Stone RM et al (2017) Midostaurin plus chemotherapy for acute myeloid leukemia with a FLT3 mutation. N Engl J Med 377(5):454–464
Suela J, Alvarez S, Cigudosa JC (2007) DNA profiling by arrayCGH in acute myeloid leukemia and myelodysplastic syndromes. Cytogenet Genome Res 118(2–4):304–309
Takahashi K et al (2017) Preleukaemic clonal haemopoiesis and risk of therapy-related myeloid neoplasms: a case-control study. Lancet Oncol 18(1):100–111
Tarlock K, Meshinchi S (2015) Pediatric acute myeloid leukemia: biology and therapeutic implications of genomic variants. Pediatr Clin North Am 62(1):75–93
Taskesen E et al (2011) Prognostic impact, concurrent genetic mutations, and gene expression features of AML with CEBPA mutations in a cohort of 1182 cytogenetically normal AML patients: further evidence for CEBPA double mutant AML as a distinctive disease entity. Blood 117(8):2469–2475
Thiede C et al (2006) Prevalence and prognostic impact of NPM1 mutations in 1485 adult patients with acute myeloid leukemia (AML). Blood 107(10):4011–4020
Thol F et al (2011) Incidence and prognostic influence of DNMT3A mutations in acute myeloid leukemia. J Clin Oncol 29(21):2889–2896
Thol F et al (2018) Measurable residual disease monitoring by NGS before allogeneic hematopoietic cell transplantation in AML. Blood 132(16):1703–1713
Vardiman JW, Harris NL, Brunning RD (2002) The World Health Organization (WHO) classification of the myeloid neoplasms. Blood 100(7):2292–2302
Vardiman JW et al (2009) The 2008 revision of the World Health Organization (WHO) classification of myeloid neoplasms and acute leukemia: rationale and important changes. Blood 114(5):937–951
Walter MJ et al (2011) Recurrent DNMT3A mutations in patients with myelodysplastic syndromes. Leukemia 25(7):1153–1158
Walter MJ et al (2012) Clonal architecture of secondary acute myeloid leukemia. N Engl J Med 366(12):1090–1098
Wang ZY, Chen Z (2008) Acute promyelocytic leukemia: from highly fatal to highly curable. Blood 111(5):2505–2515

Wang Y, Navin NE (2015) Advances and applications of single-cell sequencing technologies. Mol Cell 58(4):598–609
Wang K et al (2017) Patient-derived xenotransplants can recapitulate the genetic driver landscape of acute leukemias. Leukemia 31(1):151–158
Ward PS et al (2013) The potential for isocitrate dehydrogenase mutations to produce 2-hydroxyglutarate depends on allele specificity and subcellular compartmentalization. J Biol Chem 288(6):3804–3815
Welch JS et al (2012) The origin and evolution of mutations in acute myeloid leukemia. Cell 150(2):264–278
Woll PS et al (2014) Myelodysplastic syndromes are propagated by rare and distinct human cancer stem cells in vivo. Cancer Cell 25(6):794–808
Wong TN et al (2015) Role of TP53 mutations in the origin and evolution of therapy-related acute myeloid leukaemia. Nature 518(7540):552–555
Wouters BJ et al (2009) Double CEBPA mutations, but not single CEBPA mutations, define a subgroup of acute myeloid leukemia with a distinctive gene expression profile that is uniquely associated with a favorable outcome. Blood 113(13):3088–3091
Xie M et al (2014) Age-related mutations associated with clonal hematopoietic expansion and malignancies. Nat Med 20(12):1472–1478
Yoshizato T et al (2015) Somatic mutations and clonal hematopoiesis in aplastic Anemia. N Engl J Med 373(1):35–47
Young AL et al (2016) Clonal haematopoiesis harbouring AML-associated mutations is ubiquitous in healthy adults. Nat Commun 7:12484
Zhang X et al (2016) Single-cell sequencing for precise cancer research: progress and prospects. Cancer Res 76(6):1305–1312

# 6 Clinical Manifestation and Diagnostic Workup

Agnieszka Wierzbowska
and Magdalena Czemerska

## 6.1 Clinical Manifestation of AML

Patients with acute myeloid leukemia (AML) usually present with signs and symptoms resulting from bone marrow (BM) failure, circulation of blasts in peripheral blood, and organ infiltration with leukemic cells. The time course of leukemia symptoms is variable. In some patients, particularly younger ones, clinical symptoms develop rapidly, over a few days to 1–2 weeks. Others have a longer course, with fatigue or other symptoms preceding the proper diagnosis by 1 or 2 months. A longer course is more frequently observed in elderly patients and may suggest an antecedent hematologic disorder, such as myelodysplastic syndrome (MDS). The initial signs and symptoms of AML are usually nonspecific and may mimic those of the common chronic diseases or of casual infections like cold or flu. Patients may present with lethargy and fatigue, loss of appetite and weight, fever, or night sweats (Metzeler 2016).

### 6.1.1 Symptoms Related to Bone Marrow Failure

The clonal proliferation of leukemic blasts ultimately leads to the failure of normal hematopoiesis. The symptoms of bone marrow failure are related to anemia, neutropenia, and thrombocytopenia, and may vary based on the type of blood cell affected (Metzeler 2016).

The most common symptom of anemia is fatigue. Patients usually complain of a decreased energy level and deterioration of exercise tolerance over previous weeks. Underproduction of red blood cells may lead to weakness, headache, or dizziness. Anemia also causes shortness of breath, dyspnea, heart palpitation, or chest pain. Severe cardiac complications may be observed as the first symptoms of AML, especially in patients with a history of cardiovascular disease or in elderly patients.

AML patients frequently demonstrate decreased neutrophil level, regardless of white blood cell (WBC) count. The level of neutropenia correlates with the risk of infections. Patients often present with fever, which may occur with or without specific documentation of an infection. Medical history usually reveals the occurrence of frequent infections of varied clinical localization and presentation that have not improved despite treatment with oral antibiotics.

Patients with thrombocytopenia often complain of easily bruised skin, ecchymoses, and

A. Wierzbowska (✉) · M. Czemerska
Department of Hematology, Medical University of Lodz, Copernicus Memorial Hospital, Lodz, Poland



C. Röllig, G. J. Ossenkoppele (eds.), *Acute Myeloid Leukemia*, Hematologic Malignancies,
https://doi.org/10.1007/978-3-030-72676-8_6

unusual bleeding, such as frequent nosebleeds and bleeding from the gums. In women, menorrhagia is commonly observed. In some cases, especially those with co-existing coagulopathy due to disseminated intravascular coagulation (DIC), life-threatening hemorrhagic complications such as gastrointestinal, respiratory, intracranial, or subdural bleeding may occur. DIC is most commonly observed in acute promyelocytic leukemia (APL).

### 6.1.2 Symptoms Related to Circulation of Blasts in Peripheral Blood

Leukemic blasts may be present in the peripheral blood, resulting in an increased WBC count. About 10% of AML patients demonstrate hyperleukocytosis, defined as WBC >100 × $10^9$/L. Such patients, with markedly elevated WBC counts, can present with symptoms of leukostasis such as dizziness, blurred vision, headache, confusion, somnolence, and dyspnea, resulting in both respiratory and neurological distress. Leukostasis is a medical emergency that requires an urgent intervention (Metzeler 2016).

Patients with high leukemic cell burden often complain of bone pain related to increased pressure in the bone marrow.

### 6.1.3 Symptoms Related to Organ Infiltration with Leukemic Cells

Extramedullary infiltration is usually diagnosed simultaneously with overt AML. In rare cases, it precedes the bone marrow involvement (myeloid sarcoma). It may occur at any site and varied clinical presentation is possible. Extramedullary disease is most frequently observed in AML of monocytic origin. The most common sites of infiltration include the spleen, liver, gums, and skin. Cutaneous manifestations of AML are usually described as multiple papules. Gingival infiltration results in hypertrophy and swollen gums. In the case of spleen or liver involvement, patients may report abdominal discomfort or feelings of fullness and early satiety. In rare cases, AML can spread to the lymph nodes, leading to their enlargement (Metzeler 2016).

Central nervous system (CNS) involvement at presentation is rare in adult AML patients. The typical symptoms of overt CNS infiltration consist of headache, cranial nerve palsies, visual changes, and balance problems.

### 6.1.4 Physical Examination

Patients usually present with pallor of the skin, conjunctiva, and oral mucosa. Examination of the mouth and pharynx may reveal mucositis, neutropenic ulcers, gum hypertrophy, gingivitis, or bleeding gums. Petechiae, a small, punctate hemorrhagic rash that is not palpable, can be detected, especially on the lower limbs. Moreover, bruises or hematoma can be seen on the skin, particularly in patients with concomitant coagulopathy. The symptoms of infection can be detected by respiratory tract auscultation, and cardiac flow murmur, heart rhythm disorder, or extrasystole may be revealed by heart examination. Moreover, in cases with extramedullary involvement, lymphadenopathy, splenomegaly, hepatomegaly or substantial reddish or purple red, firm papules, plaques, or nodules in the skin may be observed (Metzeler 2016).

## 6.2 Diagnostic Workup of Patients with Suspected AML

The diagnostic evaluation of patients with suspected acute leukemia has two objectives: firstly, to confirm a diagnosis, and secondly, to characterize disease-specific and patient-specific factors to provide important information for risk stratification and treatment decisions. The schema of initial diagnostic workup of acute leukemia is shown in Fig. 6.1.

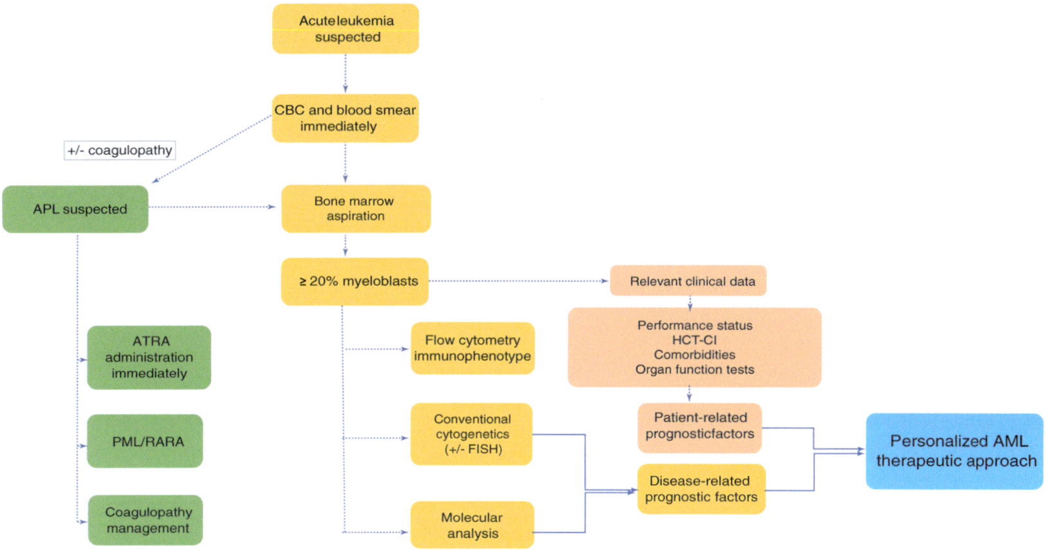


**Fig. 6.1** The initial diagnostic workup of acute leukemia. *APL* acute promyelocytic leukemia, *AML* acute myeloid leukemia, *ATRA* all-trans retinoid acid, *CBC* complete blood count, *FISH* fluorenscence in situ hybridization, *HCT-CI* hematopoietic cell transplantation-comorbidity index

The diagnosis of AML requires a comprehensive medical history and physical examination as well as detailed morphologic, cytochemical, immunophenotypic, cytogenetic, and molecular evaluation of bone marrow samples; this demands close collaboration between the treating physician and the pathologist (Döhner et al. 2017).

A comprehensive clinical assessment should include the age, sex, and ethnicity of the patient; history of any hematologic disorder; any prior malignancy; smoking status; exposure to cytotoxic therapy, immunotherapy, radiotherapy or other possibly toxic substances, such as benzene or pesticides. Any past medical history regarding known predisposing conditions or syndromes should be carefully reviewed to avoid overlooking any myeloid neoplasms with germline predisposition (Döhner et al. 2017).

Clinical symptoms related to anemia, thrombocytopenia, and neutropenia, as well as the presence of tumor masses; other tissue lesions; the presence of organomegaly and findings from neurologic examination should be elaborately collected. Immediate evaluation of symptoms related to potentially life-threatening leukostasis, coagulopathy, and tumor lysis syndrome is of particular importance.

## 6.3 Blood and Bone Marrow Morphology

### 6.3.1 Complete Blood Count

A complete blood count (CBC) with differential demonstrates anemia, neutropenia, and thrombocytopenia of varying degrees. Anemia is usually normocytic but macrocytosis is also a common finding in AML with myelodysplasia related changes (AML-MRC). Patients with AML often display high, normal, or low WBC counts. A review of a peripheral blood smear can confirm the any findings from a CBC count and usually also the presence of circulating blasts. According to European LeukemiaNet (ELN) recommendations, at least 200 leukocytes on blood smears should be counted (Döhner et al. 2010, 2017). Dysplastic changes can be found in granulocytes and erythrocytes. Schistocytes are occasionally seen in patients with DIC.

### 6.3.2 Bone Marrow Morphology

Bone marrow aspiration is obligatory to establish AML diagnosis. According to WHO 2016 classification, AML is defined based on the presence of a myeloid blast count of ≥20% out of 500 nucleated cells on spiculated marrow smears following morphological BM evaluation (Vardiman et al. 2009). Counting fewer BM cells may be sufficient in patients with a high blast count (Abdulrahman et al. 2018). Myeloblasts, monoblasts, and megakaryoblasts are included in the blast count. In AML with monocytic or myelomonocytic differentiation, promonocytes are also considered as blast equivalents (Arber et al. 2016; Döhner et al. 2017). Sometimes, linear groupings of primary granules (Auer rods) may be observed in myeloblasts. Bone marrow evaluation should always include the level of dysplasia (≥ 50% or <50% of cells) in erythroid, granulocytic, and megakaryocytic line, which is required for diagnosis of AML-MRC.

The bone marrow biopsy is always mandatory in patients with a dry tap, but it can be also used to provide correct blast enumeration and to avoid "undercounts" in the aspirate due to spotty cellularity, fatty marrows, or fibrosis (Döhner et al. 2017). Bone marrow biopsy yields useful information for differential diagnosis of AML associated with marrow fibrosis (e.g., acute megakaryoblastic leukemia and acute panmyelosis with myelofibrosis) or in several other diagnostic settings.

## 6.4 Cytochemistry and Immunophenotyping

Although multiparameter flow cytometry (MFC) is the recommended method for determining the lineage involvement in patients with suspected AML, cytochemical staining with myeloperoxidase (MPO), Sudan Black B (SBB), or nonspecific esterase (NSE) may also be useful in the early period of diagnosis, when the MFC results are not available or when bone marrow aspirate or peripheral blood material is not available for flow cytometry study. Immunophenotyping by MFC of bone marrow or peripheral blood samples can be used to distinguish AML from acute lymphoblastic leukemia (ALL); it can also be used to further classify the subtype of AML, and also to evaluate a panel of leukemia-associated immunophenotypes (LAIP) as a background for further monitoring of measurable residual disease (MRD). At least 3-colour MFC is recommended by ELN (Béné et al. 2011; Döhner et al. 2017) for routine diagnostic workup in AML; however, a minimum of six colors is required for the diagnosis of specific diagnostic entities, such as mixed phenotype acute leukemia (MPAL), AML not otherwise specified with minimal differentiation, acute megakaryoblastic leukemia, or blastic plasmacytoid dendritic cell neoplasm (BPDCN) (Johansson et al. 2014; van Dongen et al. 2012). A minimal panel of antigens recommended for AML diagnosis is presented in Table 6.1. Because MRD is an important post-diagnosis prognostic factor in AML, included as a new response criterion (i.e., complete response (CR) with/without MRD), MRD monitoring should be considered as a part of the standard of care of AML patients (Döhner et al. 2017; Schuurhuis et al. 2018). ELN experts recommend MFC with at least eight colors to be used at diagnosis and further MRD monitoring in AML patients (Schuurhuis et al. 2018).

## 6.5 Genetic Analysis

### 6.5.1 Cytogenetic and FISH

Cytogenetic testing is a mandatory part of any diagnostic workup of patients with AML that provides important information for prognosis and is needed for the WHO classification of "AML with recurrent genetic abnormalities" as well as "AML with myelodysplasia-related changes." In the presence of t(15;17), t(8;21) and inv(16) or t(16;16), a diagnosis of AML can be made even with less than 20% of blasts in BM (Arber et al. 2016). Cytogenetic abnormalities can also guide further treatment in selected cases (i.e., t(15;17); t(9;22); MDS-like cytogenetic abnormalities). In conventional cytogenetic analysis using karyotyping of G-banded metaphase chromosomes, at least 20 metaphases should be evaluated (Döhner et al. 2017). An abnormal clone can be reported if at least two of 20 cells carry the same karyotypic

**Table 6.1** Procedures recommended for AML diagnosis and classification according to WHO 2016 classification, ELN 2017 recommendations and ELN-MRD 2019 recommendations

| Diagnostic workup | Recommended |
|---|---|
| Cytological assessment | Peripheral blood smear (at least 200 leukocytes to be assessed)<br>Bone marrow aspiration (at least 500 nucleated cells + dysplastic changes to be assessed)<br>Bone marrow biopsy (if dry tap in bone marrow aspiration) |
| Flow cytometry (FC) immunophenotype | At least 3-colour FC, optimal at least 8-colour FC<br>*Markers recommended for diagnosis of AML*<br>– Precursors markers: CD34, CD117, CD33, CD13, HLA-DR<br>– Granulocytic markers: CD65, cytoplasmic MPO<br>– Monocytic markers: CD14, CD36, CD64<br>– Megakaryocytic markers: CD41 (glycoprotein IIb/IIIa), CD61 (glycoprotein IIIa)<br>– Erythroid markers: CD235a (glycophorin A), CD36<br>Assessment of LAIPs for further MRD evaluation<br>LSC assessment |
| | *Markers recommended for diagnosis of MPAL*<br>– Myeloid lineage: MPO or at least 2 monocytic markers (NE, CD11c, CD14, CD64, lysozyme)<br>– T-lineage: strong cytoplasmatic or surface CD3<br>B-lineage: strong CD19 + at least 1 of: cytoplasmatic CD79a, CD22, CD10 or weak CD19 and at least 2 of: CD79a, CD22, CD10 |
| Cytogenetics | Conventional cytogenetics with GTG banding technique (at least 20 metaphases to be assessed)<br>FISH (if conventional cytogenetics fails) – to detect: *RUNX1-RUNX1T1*, *CBFB-MYH11*, *KMT2A* (*MLL*), *MECOM* (*EVI1*), loss of chromosome 5q, 7q or 17p |
| Molecular genetic | *Gene mutations:*<br>*NPM1*, *FLT3-ITD* with allelic ratio data, *FLT3-TKD* (mutations at codons D835 and I836), *CEBPA*, *TP53*, *ASXL1*, *IDH1*, *IDH2*, *RUNX1*, *cKIT* in CBF-AML<br>*Gene rearrangements:*<br>*PML-RARA*, *RUNX1-RUNX1T1*, *CBFB-MYH11*, *BCR/ABL1* |

*MPAL* mixed phenotype acute leukemia, *LSC* leukemic stem cells, *LAIPs* leukemia associated immunophenotypes, *FISH* fluorescence in situ hybridization

abnormality. Fluorescence in situ hybridization (FISH) assays are helpful to define chromosomal aberrations in patients with complex karyotype, or partner fusion chromosomes in 11q23 translocations. FISH is always mandatory when conventional cytogenetic fails. An example of initial workup in patient with AML is presented in Fig. 6.2.

### 6.5.2 Molecular Genetic Testing (PCR, NGS)

The field of genomics in AML and related implications are evolving rapidly (Lindsley et al. 2015; Papaemmanuil et al. 2016). In AML, a variety of gene mutations (*NPM1*, biallelic *CEBPA*, *FLT3-ITD*, *RUNX1*, *TP53*, and *ALXL1*) are associated with specific prognoses and may guide the intensity of post-remission treatment (see Chap. 9) (Döhner et al. 2017). Molecular genetic testing for *NPM1*, biallelic *CEBPA* and *RUNX1* mutations is also required for WHO classification of "AML with recurrent genetic abnormalities." Other mutations, such as *FLT3-ITD*, *FLT3-TKD*, *IDH1/2* may have therapeutic implications. The panel of molecular genetic tests recommended in the diagnostic workup of newly-diagnosed AML patients is presented in Table 6.1. Screening for single

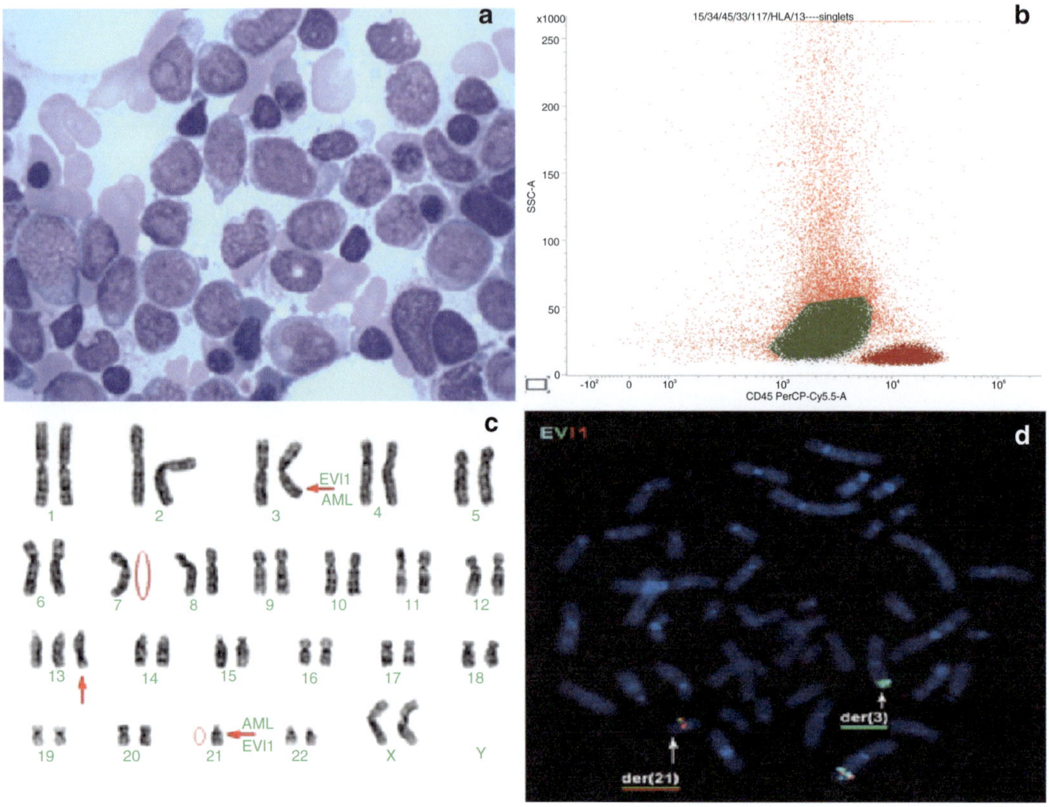


**Fig. 6.2** The initial acute leukemia workup which contains cytological assessment of AML blasts (**a**), flow cytometry immunophenotyping (**b**), conventional cytogenetics that revealed complex katyotype (**c**) with MECOM (EVI1) abnormality confirmed by FISH (**d**). (Courtesy of Ewa Wawrzyniak and Agata Majchrzak)

genes may be replaced by multiplex gene panels and next-generation sequencing (NGS) analysis for a comprehensive prognostic assessment. Molecular testing by reverse transcriptase–polymerase chain reaction (RT-PCR) for recurring rearrangements can also be helpful if rapid information is needed for recommendation of suitable therapy (i.e., *PML-RARA*) or if chromosome morphology is of poor quality (Döhner et al. 2017). As midostaurin, the FLT3 inhibitor, is currently approved in AML treatment, molecular results confirming the presence of *FLT3* gene mutations should be available rapidly (optimally within 72 h from the diagnosis) in order to allow timely initiation of midostaurin treatment by day 8 (Stone et al. 2017). Procedures recommended for diagnosis and classification of AML are presented in Table 6.1.

## 6.6 Additional Procedures Recommended at Diagnosis of AML

As coagulopathy is common at presentation of AML, an evaluation of prothrombin time, activated partial thromboplastin time and fibrinogen activity is a part of the routine initial evaluation and is advisable before performing any invasive procedures.

Other laboratory tests frequently performed during the diagnostic workup in AML include a comprehensive metabolic panel, serum uric acid and lactate dehydrogenase, liver function tests, tumor lysis syndrome (TLS) panel, uric acid measurement, urine analysis and viral screening (i.e., evaluation of HBV, HCV, HIV, and CMV antibodies). In women of childbearing potential, a pregnancy test should be performed.

For patients with neurologic signs or symptoms at diagnosis, cranial magnetic resonance imaging (MRI) or computed tomography (CT) should be performed to detect meningeal disease or CNS hemorrhage. Lumbar puncture (LP) should be performed if no mass lesion is detected on the imaging study and a coagulopathy is excluded (Tallman et al. 2019). In APL with suspected CNS involvement, due to high hemorrhagic risk, LP should be postponed to the end of induction (Sanz et al. 2019).

If extramedullary disease is suspected, positron emission tomography (PET/CT) or CT of the relevant organ should be performed with a biopsy in rare cases of myeloid sarcoma without bone marrow involvement. Imaging technics (CT, X-ray) are also useful to diagnose and monitor concomitant pulmonary infections.

An ECG, echocardiogram or MUGA (multigated acquisition) scan evaluation is of particular importance in AML patients with a history or symptoms of cardiac disease or prior/planned exposure to cardiotoxic drugs or radiation to the thorax (Tallman et al. 2019). In case of pulmonary comorbidity, the function tests of respiratory track should be performed.

Human leukocyte antigen (HLA) typing and an early search for family or an alternative donor is recommended in all patients with newly-diagnosed AML for whom an allogenic hematopoietic cell transplantation (alloHCT) is being considered.

Sperm cryopreservation before starting chemotherapy (ChT), should be proposed to younger patients, particularly if they are planned for alloHCT. Cryopreservation of ovarian tissue is rarely feasible at diagnosis because of the urgent need for ChT and the possibility that ovarian fragments may be contaminated with leukemic cells (Shapira et al. 2014).

Because of the relationship between level of fitness and the treatment outcomes, an evaluation should be performed of the patient's performance status according to ECOG/WHO score as well as a careful assessment of their pre-existing comorbidities (i.e., based on hematopoietic cell transplantation-comorbidity index [HCT-CI] score) (Sorror et al. 2005; Sorror et al. 2017). In elderly patients (>65 years), a comprehensive geriatric assessment may provide additional information to determine eligibility to conventional chemotherapy (Klepin et al. 2020; Pettit and Odenike 2015).

## 6.7 Differential Diagnosis

It is crucial to quickly and accurately distinguish AML from less urgent hematological or other diseases, the most common being the following: infectious causes, such as mononucleosis, Plaut-Vincent angina, and severe infections such as sepsis or tuberculosis; other hematological disorders such as acute lymphoblastic leukemia, aplastic anemia, paroxysmal nocturnal hemoglobinuria, and MDS; other miscellaneous causes such as solid tumors metastases and bone marrow failure due to drug toxicity.

## References

Abdulrahman AA, Patel KH, Yang T et al (2018) Is a 500-cell count necessary for bone marrow differentials?: a proposed analytical method for validating a lower cutoff. Am J Clin Pathol 150(1):84–91

Arber DA, Orazi A, Hasserjian R et al (2016) The 2016 revision to the World Health Organization classification of myeloid neoplasms and acute leukemia. Blood 127(20):2391–2405

Béné MC, Nebe T, Bettelheim P et al (2011) Immunophenotyping of acute leukemia and lymphoproliferative disorders: a consensus proposal of the European LeukemiaNet work package 10. Leukemia 25(4):567–574

Döhner H, Estey EH, Amadori S et al (2010) Diagnosis and management of acute myeloid leukemia in adults: recommendations from an international expert panel, on behalf of the European LeukemiaNet. Blood 115(3):453–474

Döhner H, Estey E, Grimwade D et al (2017) Diagnosis and management of AML in adults: 2017 ELN recommendations from an international expert panel. Blood 129(4):424–447

Johansson U, Bloxham D, Couzens S et al (2014) Guidelines on the use of multicolour flow cytometry in the diagnosis of haematological neoplasms. British Committee for Standards in Haematology. Br J Haematol 165(4):455–488

Klepin HD, Ritchie E, Major-Elechi B et al (2020) Geriatric assessment among older adults receiving intensive therapy for acute myeloid leukemia:

report of CALGB 361006 (Alliance). J Geriatr Oncol 11(1):107–113
Lindsley RC, Mar BG, Mazzola E et al (2015) Acute myeloid leukemia ontogeny is defined by distinct somatic mutations. Blood 125(9):1367–1376
Metzeler K (2016) Clinical manifestations and diagnosis. In: Hiddemann W (ed) Handbook of acute leukemia. Springer International Publishing, Switzerland, pp 15–23
Papaemmanuil E, Gerstung M, Bullinger L et al (2016) Genomic classification and prognosis in acute myeloid leukemia. N Engl J Med 374(23):2209–2221
Pettit K, Odenike O (2015) Defining and treating older adults with acute myeloid leukemia who are ineligible for intensive therapies. Front Oncol 5:280
Sanz MA, Fenaux P, Tallman MS et al (2019) Management of acute promyelocytic leukemia: updated recommendations from an expert panel of the European LeukemiaNet. Blood 133(15):1630–1643
Schuurhuis GJ, Heuser M, Freeman S et al (2018) Minimal/measurable residual disease in AML: a consensus document from the European LeukemiaNet MRD working party. Blood 131(12):1275–1291
Shapira M, Raanani H, Cohen Y, Meirow D (2014) Fertility preservation in young females with hematological malignancies. Acta Haematol 132(3–4):400–413
Sorror ML, Maris MB, Storb R et al (2005) Hematopoietic cell transplantation (HCT)-specific comorbidity index: a new tool for risk assessment before allogeneic HCT. Blood 106(8):2912–2919
Sorror ML, Storer BE, Fathi AT et al (2017) Development and validation of a novel acute myeloid leukemia-composite model to estimate risks of mortality. JAMA Oncol 3(12):1675–1682
Stone RM, Mandrekar SJ, Sanford BL et al (2017) Midostaurin plus chemotherapy for acute myeloid leukemia with a FLT3 mutation. N Engl J Med 377(5):454–464
Tallman MS, Wang ES, Altman JK et al (2019) Acute myeloid leukemia, version 3.2019, NCCN clinical practice guidelines in oncology. J Natl Compr Cancer Netw 17(6):721–749
van Dongen JJ, Lhermitte L, Bottcher S et al (2012) EuroFlow antibody panels for standardized n-dimensional flow cytometric immunophenotyping of normal, reactive and malignant leukocytes. Leukemia 26(9):1908–1975
Vardiman JW, Thiele J, Arber DA et al (2009) The 2008 revision of the World Health Organization (WHO) classification of myeloid neoplasms and acute leukemia: rationale and important changes. Blood 114(5):937–951

# Prognostic Factors in AML

# 7

Raphael Itzykson, Marco Cerrano, and Jordi Esteve

## 7.1 Introduction

Prognostication in acute myeloid leukemia (AML) is the result of a multilayer, comprehensive assessment, comprising a wide diversity of variables, including patient-related features, disease manifestations at the time of presentation, and intrinsic disease-related genetic features, such as cytogenetic abnormalities and driver mutations (Table 7.1). Moreover, prognostic allocation of AML patients will depend not only on baseline variables, identifiable at diagnosis, but also on evolutive markers, such as measurable residual disease at different critical time points during treatment.

Disease outcome is a multistage function, including early death rate, treatment refractoriness, disease recurrence, outcome after salvage therapy, and mortality due to treatment-related complications. The impact of prognostic variables varies during disease and treatment phase. Thus, disease features at presentation and patient-related factors have a strong impact on the risk of early death, usually quantified as mortality rate at 30 days after diagnosis. On the other hand, AML genetic background is highly predictive of response to chemotherapy as well as relapse risk. Patient-related variables such as comorbidity or Eastern Cooperative Oncology Group (ECOG) have a high impact on treatment-related death, especially in the setting of hematopoietic cell transplantation (HCT). Outcome measures reported in AML studies can broadly be divided into short-term versus long-term and disease-specific versus global assessments. These metrics are now standardized for clinical trials (Table 7.2).

Importantly, the relative contribution of each prognostic factor is influenced by treatment, and many inconsistencies in the literature have been attributed to differences in treatment intensity or modalities, notably regarding post-remission therapy (e.g., autologous versus allogeneic transplant). Though intensive chemotherapy remains the mainstay of AML therapy, the addition of novel agents, or the development of novel therapy backbones in unfit patients, may impact the prognostic value of different patient- or disease-related factors. Accurate

R. Itzykson (✉)
Service Hématologie Adultes, Hôpital Saint-Louis, Assistance Publique-Hôpitaux de Paris, Paris, France

Université de Paris, Génomes, Biologie Cellulaire et Thérapeutique U944, INSERM, CNRS, Paris, France
e-mail: raphael.itzykson@aphp.fr

M. Cerrano
Service Hématologie Adultes, Hôpital Saint-Louis, Assistance Publique-Hôpitaux de Paris, Paris, France

Division of Hematology, Department of Molecular Biotechnology and Health Sciences, University of Turin, Turin, Italy

J. Esteve
Hematology Department, IDIBAPS, Hospital Clínic of Barcelona, Barcelona, Spain

University of Barcelona, Barcelona, Spain



C. Röllig, G. J. Ossenkoppele (eds.), *Acute Myeloid Leukemia*, Hematologic Malignancies,
https://doi.org/10.1007/978-3-030-72676-8_7

**Table 7.1** Prognostic factors in AML

| Prognostic factors | Evaluation measures & scales | References |
|---|---|---|
| ***Patient-related*** | | |
| Age | >75 years, or <75 years with significant comorbidity is a usual definition to define patients not candidate for intensive chemotherapy | Juliusson et al. (2009), Pulte et al. (2016), Bower et al. (2016), Appelbaum et al. (2006a) |
| Performance status | ECOG | Appelbaum et al. (2006a) |
| Comorbidity index | Hematopoietic cell transplantation-comorbidity index (HCT-CI score) | Sorror et al. (2007a, b, 2014) |
| Individual organ severe dysfunction (e.g., renal, cardiac, hepatic, pulmonary) | Renal insufficiency<br>LVEF<45% | Hupfer et al. (2018), Bhatt (2019), Klepin et al. (2013), Hshieh et al. (2018) |
| Geriatric assessment | Cumulative illness rating scale geriatrics (CIRS-G) | Kirkhus et al. (2016) |
| | Geriatric assessment for Hematology (GAH) | Bonanad et al. (2015) |
| ***Disease presentation*** | | |
| Severe infection | | Cannas et al. (2012) |
| AML-related coagulopathy | | Slichter (2004), Lad et al. (2017), De Stefano et al. (2005) |
| Leukostasis | | Giammarco et al. (2017) |
| Tumor lysis syndrome | | Cairo and Bishop (2004) |
| Hyperleukocytosis | | Canaani et al. (2017), Tien et al. (2018a) |
| Extramedullary disease | | Chang et al. (2004), Tallman et al. (2004), Tallman et al. (1993), Byrd et al. (1997), Kobayashi et al. (2007), Tsimberidou et al. (2008), Ganzel et al. (2016), Cheng et al. (2015), Del Principe et al. (2018), Rozovski et al. (2015) |
| ***Disease biology*** | | |
| AML ontogeny | De novo/primary vs Secondary AML arising from antecedent hematological disorders (MDS, MPN, MDS/MPN, BMF)<br>Therapy-related AML | Hulegårdh et al. (2015), Granfeldt Østgård et al. (2015), Lindsley et al. (2015), Kayser et al. (2011), Schmaelter et al. (2020) |
| Dysplastic features | | Devillier et al. (2015b), Armand et al. (2007), Ossenkoppele and Montesinos (2019) |
| Immunophenotypic markers | Leukemia-stem cell phenotype | Nakase et al. (1997), Fujiwara et al. (2017), Kauer et al. (2019), Märklin et al. (2020), Chisini et al. (2017), Costa et al. (2017), Repp et al. (2003), Mason et al. (2006), Minetto et al. (2018), van Solinge et al. (2018) |
| Cytogenetics (see Table 7.2) | | |
| Recurrent genetic mutations (see Table 7.3) | Individual gene mutation | Grimwade and Mrózek (2011), Döhner et al. (2017), Arber et al. (2016) |
| | Gene-gene interactions (e.g., *NPM1-FLT3-DNMT3A*) | Papaemmanuil et al. (2016), Loghavi et al. (2014), Wang et al. (2016), Bezerra et al. (2020) |
| | European LeukemiaNet classification | (Döhner et al. 2017) |

**Table 7.1** (continued)

| Prognostic factors | Evaluation measures & scales | References |
|---|---|---|
| Gene-expression profile | Leukemia stem-cell-like signature | Gentles et al. (2010), Jung et al. (2015), Levine et al. (2015), Metzeler et al. (2008), Eppert et al. (2011), Marcucci et al. (2014), Bullinger et al. (2004), Li et al. (2013), Ng et al. (2016), Duployez et al. (2019), Bill et al. (2020) |
| Non-coding RNA expression pattern & signature | | Schwind et al. (2010b), Marcucci et al. (2013), Díaz-Beyá et al. (2014), Beck et al. (2018) |
| DNA methylation status | | Bullinger et al. (2010), Figueroa et al. (2010), Deneberg et al. (2010), Li et al. (2016), Lin et al. (2011), Yang et al. (2019), Deneberg et al. (2011), Jost et al. (2014), Kroeze et al. (2014), Luskin et al. (2016), DiNardo et al. (2017) |
| ***Treatment administered*** | | See Chaps. 8–10 |
| Treatment intensity | Intensive chemotherapy vs. low intensity | |
| Post-remission therapy | AlloHCT (CR1) | |
| | Maintenance therapy | |
| ***Response to therapy*** | | See Chap. 18 |
| No. of cycles to achieve complete remission | >1 course | |
| Measurable residual disease | Early evaluation (after induction/two courses) | |
| | Pre-allogeneic stem cell transplantation | |
| | Follow-up measurement | |
| ***Appropriate management and access to health resources*** | | See Chaps. 8–10 |
| Adequate supportive treatment | Transfusional support | |
| | Prophylactic & treatment of infections | |
| Access to allogeneic HCT | | |
| ***Integrative multilayer scores*** | | |
| Risk classification integrations clinical, genetic and treatment data | https://cancer.sanger.ac.uk/aml-multistage | Gerstung et al. (2017), Huet et al. (2018), Fenwarth et al. (2019) |

prognostic evaluation plays a key role in treatment choice. Specifically, the benefit of allogeneic hematopoietic cell transplantation (HCT) is mostly restricted to patients predicted to have the highest risk of relapse without HCT. However, it must be emphasized that prognostic assessment in a given therapeutic context is methodologically distinct from the study of interactions between a "theranostic" factor and different treatment options. The present chapter thus focuses on prognosis, and how prognostic factors influence treatment choice in newly diagnosed AML is presented in Chaps. 8–10.

Biology-driven prognostication of AML has long relied on cytogenetics. A limited number of gene mutations were then included, initially to refine the prognosis of patients with normal karyotype. They are now used in all patients regardless of cytogenetics. The broader panel of recurrent gene mutations uncovered in the genomics era occurring, along with cytogenetic alterations, in a myriad of combinations, challenges conventional risk stratification approaches. Baseline gene expression data have also been proposed to refine prognosis in

**Table 7.2** Outcome metrics

| Outcome | Definition | Comments |
|---|---|---|
| **Response to treatment** | | |
| Complete remission (CR) | BM blasts <5%; absence of circulating blasts and blasts with Auer rods; absence of extramedullary disease; ANC ≥1.0*10^9/L; PLT ≥1.0*10^9/L | According to NCCN, patients should be independent of transfusions |
| CR with incomplete hematologic recovery (CRi) | All CR criteria except for residual neutropenia (ANC < 1.0*10^9/L) or thrombocytopenia (PLT <1.0*10^9/L) | According to NCCN, patients should be independent of transfusions |
| Morphologic leukemia-freestate (MLFS) | BM blasts <5%; absence of blasts with Auer rods;absence of extramedullary disease; no hematologic recovery required | BM not merely “aplastic”; at least 200 cells should be enumerated or cellularity should be at least 10% |
| Partial remission (PR) | All hematologic criteria of CR; decrease of BM blast percentage to 5–25% and decrease of pretreatment BM blast percentage by at least 50% | Especially important in the context of phase 1–2 clinical trials |
| Primary refractory disease | No CR or CRi after 2 courses of intensive induction treatment; excluding patients with death in aplasia or death due to indeterminate cause | 1. primary refractory disease is also called primary induction failure<br>2. death in aplasia is used for deaths occurring >7 days following completion of initial treatment while cytopenic without evidence of persistent leukemia; death due to indeterminate cause refers to cases occurring before 7 days after the end of treatment or in cases without BM examination |
| CR without minimal residualdisease (CRmrd-) | If studied pretreatment, CR with negativity for a genetic marker by RT-qPCR, or CR with negativity by MFC | 1. test used and sensitivity of the assay should be reported; analyses should be done in experienced laboratories<br>2. according to NCCN, cytogenetic CR can also be defined (in patients with a previous abnormality) and molecular CR is firmly established for clinical use only in for APL and Ph positive leukemias |
| Hematologic relapse | BM blasts ≥5%; or reappearance of blasts in the blood; or development of extramedullary disease | After CRmrd-, CR, CRi |
| Molecular relapse | Reoccurrence of MRD as assessed by RT-qPCR or by MFC | After CRmrd-; test applied, sensitivity of the assay, and cutoff values used must be reported; analyses should be done in experienced laboratories |
| **Survival measures** | | |
| Overall survival (OS) | Measured from the date of entry into a clinical trial or from the date of diagnosis to the date of death from any cause | Defined for all patients of a trial; patients not known to have died at last follow-up are censored on the date they were last known to be alive |
| Event-free survival (EFS) | Measured from the date of entry into a clinical trial or from the date of diagnosis to the date of primary refractory disease, or relapse from CR (or CRi), or death from any cause | Defined for all patients of a trial; patients not known to have died at last follow-up are censored on the date they were last known to be alive |

**Table 7.2** (continued)

| Outcome | Definition | Comments |
|---|---|---|
| Relapse-free survival (RFS) | Measured from the date of achievement of a remission until the date of relapse or death from any cause | Defined only for patients achieving CR, or CRi; patients not known to have relapsed or died at last follow-up are censored on the date they were last examined; clinical trials in which the response criterion CRmrd-, should include molecular relapse as a criterion for relapse |
| Cumulative incidence of relapse (CIR) | Measured from the date of achievement of a remission until the date of relapse; patients who died without relapse are counted as a competing cause of failure | Defined for all patients achieving CR, CRi; patients not known to have relapsed are censored on the date they were last examined; clinical trials in which the response criterion CRmrd-, should include molecular relapse as a criterion for relapse; it is important to provide estimates of cumulative incidence o f death as well |
| Time to neutrophil recovery | No. of days from day 1 of commencing induction therapy to first day ANC 0.5 ≥ 1.0*10^9/L | And to first day ANC ≥1.0*10^9/L |
| Time to platelet recovery | No. of days from day 1 of commencing inductiontherapy to first day PLTS ≥50*10^9/L | And to first day PLTS ≥100*10^9/L |

*APL* acute promyelocytic leukemia, *ANC* absolute neutrophil count, *BM* Bone marrow, *MFC* multiparameter flow cytometry, *NCCN* national comprehensive cancer network, *PLTS* platelets, *PH* Philadelphia, *RT-qPCR* real-time polymerase chain reaction

Adapted from Dohner, Blood 2017 and NCCN V3 2020, AML

AML. Initially focused on a limited set of genes, they are now expanding to gene expression signatures, leading to further issues related to standardization. Unbiased, systematic integration of these different prognostic factors into personalized predictions is only beginning. Finally, the relative contribution of baseline prognostic factors, compared to dynamic assessment of Measurable Residual Disease (Chap. 18), is another area of future investigation in AML. Here we review the prognostic contribution of recurrent molecular lesions. For further insight into the pathophysiologic role of these lesions or to their diagnostic tools, we refer the reader to Chaps. 2 and 5, respectively.

## 7.2 Host-Related Factors

### 7.2.1 Age

Age is a major determinant of patient outcome in AML, for different reasons. First, the distribution of AML genetic characteristics differs markedly with age, with an increasing incidence of high-risk cytogenetics subtypes and genetic features in older patients accounting for treatment resistance. Specifically, the incidence of MDS-related cytogenetics such as chromosomal aneuploidies with loss of 5q, 7q, and 17p regions surpasses 30 (×100.000 inhabitants/years), an almost ten-fold increase compared to individuals younger than 60 years of age (Lazarevic et al. 2014). Moreover, incidence of many high-risk mutations such as those in *RUNX1*, *ASXL1*, *TP53*, or spliceosome genes (e.g., *SRSF2*, *U2AF1*) is markedly age-dependent (The Cancer Genome Atlas Research Network 2013). Overall, virtually half of elderly patients are diagnosed with an unfavorable subtype of AML according to European LeukemiaNet (ELN) classification (Nagel et al. 2017). Second, older age is associated with poorer performance status (PS), and higher incidence of frailty and comorbidity. Thus, the proportion of PS ≥ 2 according to the ECOG scale is ≥50% over 70 years (Juliusson et al. 2009). The prognostic relevance of age is reflected on the modest improvement on patient outcome observed in elderly patients in recent years, compared to a higher improvement in younger individuals.

Thus, median survival and 5-year survival remain inferior to 1 year and 20% in individuals over 70, with limited improvement in recent years (Pulte et al. 2016; Bower et al. 2016).

### 7.2.2 Performance Status, Comorbidity, and Frailty

Performance status (PS), as an instantaneous picture of general condition, and comorbidity are two important prognostic factors, with a clear impact on early death rate, chance to achieve complete response, and long-term outcome (Appelbaum et al. 2006a). Although PS is clearly related to age and coexistent chronic diseases, PS might be largely determined by disease presentation, and improve with disease treatment. Comorbidity assessment is evaluated using different scales aimed to identify relevant acute and chronic illnesses that impact patient outcome. The Hematopoietic Cell Transplantation-Comorbidity Index (HCT-CI score), initially designed for predicting risk of non-relapse mortality in patients undergoing allogeneic HCT, evaluates 17 different items, including pre-existing renal, liver, pulmonary, cardiac, endocrine, and digestive diseases (Sorror et al. 2005). This score has also demonstrated predictive value among patients receiving intensive induction chemotherapy (Sorror et al. 2007a, b, 2014). Individual organ dysfunction might constitute a limitation for specific antileukemic agents, such as use of anthracyclines in patients with depressed cardiac contractility or standard chemotherapy in patients with impaired renal function.

The choice of an adequate therapy in elderly patients is a difficult exercise, which may require the use of integrative geriatric scales, aimed to assess frailty and autonomy of these patients (Hupfer et al. 2018; Bhatt 2019). These scales analyze different functional spheres, including comorbidity, cognitive function, mobility capability, autonomy, emotional status, nutritional status, or concomitant medication, which can interact with antileukemic agents (Klepin et al. 2013; Hshieh et al. 2018). Some of the most used geriatric scales are CIRS-G (Cumulative Illness Rating Scale Geriatrics) and GAH Geriatric Assessment for Hematology (GAH) (Bonanad et al. 2015; Kirkhus et al. 2016).

### 7.2.3 Disease Presentation

Hyperleukocytosis, defined by a WBC count >50–100 * $10^9$/L in different studies, is present in 5–13% of AML. Risk factors for hyperleukocytosis include younger age, myelomonocytic/monoblastic morphology, microgranular APL variant, 11q23 rearrangements, inv(16), and *FLT3*-ITD mutations (Ganzel et al. 2012).

Hyperleukocytosis is associated with a high risk of early mortality due to associated complications (see *infra*). However, higher WBC remains associated with higher risk of relapse and inferior overall survival beyond remission, even when adjusting for confounding oncogenetic factors, such as *FLT3*-ITD mutations (Canaani et al. 2017; Tien et al. 2018a).

Extramedullary disease (EMD) is present at diagnosis in 2–30% of AML patients, notably those with high WBC count. This wide distribution is explained by the lack of standardized evaluation, for example, with $^{18}$Fluorodesoxy-glucose positron emission tomography/computed tomography ($^{18}$FDG-PET/CT) imaging, which reveals EMD in ~20% of unselected AML patients (Stölzel et al. 2014). EMD frequently involves the gingiva, liver, spleen, skin, and lymph nodes but can affect any organ, manifesting as a mass ("chloroma," or myeloid sarcoma) or diffuse organ infiltration. EMD is more frequent in AML with t(8;21) and in patients with high WBC count. The prognostic value of EMD is debated (Chang et al. 2004; Tallman et al. 2004; Tallman et al. 1993; Byrd et al. 1997; Kobayashi et al. 2007; Tsimberidou et al. 2008), but in the largest study published so far, lacked independent prognostic value when accounting for the poor prognostic value of higher WBC count (Ganzel et al. 2016).

Central nervous system (CNS) involvement as a specific form of EMD is reported in 5–30% of AML patients, based on the presence of blasts in the Cerebrospinal fluid (CSF) detected by cytomorphology and/or multiparameter flow cytometry, the presence of neurological symptoms, or both. Some studies indicate an adverse prognostic value of CNS involvement, mostly in pediatric cohorts where diagnostic lumbar puncture remains standard of care (Chang et al. 2004; Kobayashi et al. 2007; Cheng et al. 2015; Del Principe et al. 2018; Rozovski et al. 2015). Lack of systematic CSF evaluation in adults with AML in the era of high-dose cytarabine makes it difficult to ascertain this prognostic value independent of other clinical and oncogenetic features.

### 7.2.4 Initial Complications

Determined complications at presentation constitute a real threat for a fatal outcome. Among these, severe infection, coagulation disorders including disseminated intravascular coagulation (DIC), leukostasis, or tumor lysis syndrome (TLS) should be evaluated and rapidly reverted.

First, due to the hematopoietic impairment caused by AML, patients can present with a concomitant severe infection that needs to be properly and quickly assessed. However, infectious complications normally appear during the treatment course due to the usage of cytotoxic agents. Cannas et al. analyzed the frequency of infectious complications in AML patients included in the multicenter Acute Leukemia French Association (ALFA)-9802 trial and found that 18% of patients presented with fever of unknown origin and 16% with a documented infection at the time of diagnosis, most often involving the ear-nose-throat area (Cannas et al. 2012).

Second, coagulation disorders at presentation are common in AML, clinically evident in 40–70% of patients at diagnosis. Underlying mechanisms can be multiple, highlighting platelet abnormalities and coagulopathic situations (DIC, excessive fibrinolysis, liver dysfunction). Thrombocytopenia at presentation is common, although it is unlikely to present spontaneous bleeding with a platelet count >20 * $10^9$/L. (Slichter 2004) DIC is biologically present in all APL patients, being the most common cause of death of these patients due to intracranial hemorrhage. In non-APL AML, DIC can be also present (10–50%), depending upon the subtype of leukemia (Lad et al. 2017). Thrombotic events, most often deep vein thrombosis, can also be present at the time of presentation (3.9%) (De Stefano et al. 2005).

Hyperleukocytosis is the most important risk factor for leukostasis, which is the mechanical obstruction of the microcirculation due to blast accumulation, affecting pronominally brain, lungs, and kidney vessels (Giammarco et al. 2017). Finally, TLS occurs at disease presentation or in the early therapeutic phase, caused by the massive death of malignant cells. Currently, the Cairo–Bishop definition and grading criteria are widely used for TLS diagnosis, taking into account analytic and clinical variables (Cairo and Bishop 2004). In a study conducted by Montesinos et al., the incidence of TLS and clinical TLS in AML patients was 17% and 5%, respectively (Montesinos et al. 2008). In a single-center study, patients having required intense care during the induction phase had comparable disease-free survival (Schellongowski et al. 2011). Further studies are required to determine the long-term impact of such early complications on relapse incidence.

## 7.3 AML Ontogeny

Secondary AML (sAML), as opposed to de novo or primary AML presentation, is a well-recognized unfavorable prognostic factor in multiple studies. The concept of secondary AML is often vague and has received multiple definitions, referring to patients with an antecedent hematological disorder (AHD) on complete blood counts available before AML diagnosis, patients with a bona fide antecedent myeloid neoplasm before transformation such as MDS, MPN, or MDS/MPN (including CMML), patients with an antecedent congenital bone marrow failure syndrome, and therapy-related AML (tAML), that is, AML arising in a patient with a previous exposure to genotoxic agents (mainly chemo-radiotherapy for lymphoma and solid tumors) or immunosuppressants. Regardless of the precise definition, the inferior outcome of sAML has been confirmed in population-based studies, with a lower response rate after intensive treatment and inferior overall survival compare to de novo AML, especially among younger patients (Hulegårdh et al. 2015; Granfeldt Østgård et al. 2015). The proportion of AHD-AML and tAML in both studies was similar, comprising approximately 20% and 7%, respectively, of all AML registered cases. Since patients with AHD-AML are older and harbor a higher proportion of adverse cytogenetics and worse mutational profile, the independent value of AML ontogeny per se has been debated. Patients with sAML more often present with complex karyotype, mutations of genes involved in RNA splicing (e.g., *SF3B1*, *SRSF2*, *U2AF1*, and *ZRSR2*), epigenetic regulation, chromatin modification (e.g., *ASXL1*, *EZH2*, *BCOR*), RAS signaling, myeloid transcription, and cohesion complex such as *STAG2*, typically found in MDS, and often lack oncogenetic events characteristic of de novo AML such as *NPM1*, *KMT2A*, or core-binding factor rearrangements (Lindsley et al. 2015). Moreover, patients with tAML, who have received chemotherapy or radiation therapy for a preceding cancer, can present with a poorer PS and higher comorbidity and eventual immune impairment as a consequence of cumulated toxicity derived from treatment received. Consequently, higher non-relapse mortality has been reported in tAML patients treated intensively, especially among those undergoing allogeneic HCT (Kayser et al. 2011). Indeed, sAML remains an adverse prognostic factor beyond CR in patients receiving an allogeneic transplant, independent of cytogenetic risk (Schmaelter et al. 2020). Novel therapeutic options in these patients, including the liposomal chemotherapeutic formulation CPX-351 in fit patients, or the combination of azacitidine and venetoclax in unfit patients, may challenge the prognostic value of AML ontogeny in these populations (Lancet et al. 2016; DiNardo et al. 2019).

## 7.4 Cytogenetic Abnormalities

Cytogenetic abnormalities are present in 55–60% of AML patients and are essential elements both for the classification and the prognostic stratification of AML (Grimwade and Mrózek 2011; Döhner et al. 2017; Arber et al. 2016). Indeed, recurrent cytogenetic abnormalities have been the cornerstone of biology-driven prognostic classifications in AML (Byrd et al. 2002; Grimwade et al. 1998; Slovak et al. 2000; Grimwade et al. 2001) and their prognostic stratification has now been consolidated by European (ELN 2017) (Döhner et al. 2017) and US (NCCN 2020) (Tallman et al. 2019) guidelines thanks to large-scale cohorts. Cytogenetic alterations contribute both to the risk of induction failure and to post-remission outcome (Slovak et al. 2000). The recurrence of cytogenetic alterations is crucial to robustly capture their prognostic role, explaining the "intermediate" risk value attributed to most rare lesions. Below we summarize the prognostic role of the most frequent translocations and copy number of alterations. For their role in the pathophysiology of AML, we refer the reader to Chap. 5. The interactions between specific factors and treatment modalities, hence their contribution to the choice of upfront (e.g., intensive chemotherapy versus non-intensive approaches) or post-remission therapy, are discussed in Chaps. 11–13.

### 7.4.1 Favorable-Risk Translocations

The best example of cytogenetic-defined AML entity is represented by acute promyelocytic leukemia (APL), which is almost exclusively characterized by the t(15;17)(q22;q21) leading to the *PML-RARA* fusion gene and which can be cured in the vast majority of the cases with specific arsenic trioxide-ATRA-based treatment protocols (Sanz et al. 2019). Given its unique nature, APL is now considered as a separate entity and is discussed elsewhere (Chap. 8).

Approximately 10–15% of AMLs belong to the group of core-binding factor (CBF) leukemias, which include AML with t(8;21)(q22;q22), and inv(16)(p13.1q22), or t(16;16)(p13.1;q22), leading to the *RUNX1-RUNX1T1* and *CBFB-MYH11* fusion genes, respectively (Grimwade and Mrózek 2011; Kuykendall et al. 2018). Those entities, which are more common in children and younger adults (Creutzig et al. 2016), respond well to intensive chemotherapy, with complete remission (CR) rate usually above 85–90%, and are associated with generally favorable long-term overall survival (OS), exceeding 60% in recent reports (Jourdan et al. 2013; Schlenk et al. 2004; Marcucci et al. 2005a; Burnett et al. 2013; Boddu et al. 2018). Even though often grouped together, these two entities are biologically distinct (Faber et al. 2016). Some reports have shown superior results for *CBFB-MYH11* compared to *RUNX1-RUNX1T1* leukemias (Schlenk et al. 2004; Papaemmanuil et al. 2016; Mosna et al. 2015; Appelbaum et al. 2006b; Vasu et al. 2018; Fröhling et al. 2006; Herold et al. 2020). Other studies did not find differences in outcomes between these two entities (Jourdan et al. 2013; Boddu et al. 2018; Ishikawa et al. 2020; Opatz et al. 2020; Cher et al. 2016). Additional chromosomal abnormalities are frequently seen in CBF leukemias (Faber et al. 2016; Duployez et al. 2018), but their prognostic impact, with the possible exception of trisomy 22 in *CBFB-MYH11* patients as a favorable prognostic factor, has been inconsistent among different reports (Byrd et al. 2002; Schlenk et al. 2004; Marcucci et al. 2005a; Papaemmanuil et al. 2016; Appelbaum et al. 2006b; Ishikawa et al. 2020; Opatz et al. 2020; Duployez et al. 2018; Paschka et al. 2013; Shin et al. 2019; Zhou et al. 2020; Grimwade et al. 2010; Krauth et al. 2014; Christen et al. 2019). Thus, the impact of these aberrations is not taken into account by current guidelines (Döhner et al. 2017; Tallman et al. 2019). Elderly (i.e., >60 years old) patients with CBF leukemias can achieve CR in the vast majority of cases as well, but their long-term outcomes have been historically poorer, at least in part because intensive consolidation could be administered to only a fraction of the cases (Appelbaum et al. 2006b; Fröhling et al. 2006; Prébet et al. 2009; Farag et al. 2006).

### 7.4.2 Intermediate and Adverse-Risk Translocations

Balanced translocations involving the *KMT2A* gene (formerly *MLL*) at 11q23 are found in up to 5% of AML cases (Grimwade et al. 2010, 2016). *KMT2A* gene fusions involve multiple partners (Meyer et al. 2018), are frequently found in therapy-related AML (Bloomfield et al. 2002), most commonly after topoisomerase II inhibitors exposure, and are generally associated with unfavorable outcomes (Papaemmanuil et al. 2016; Schoch et al. 2003). Some subgroups, however, seem to achieve slightly better outcomes. Patients with t(9;11)(p22;q23), the most frequent translocation which leads to the *KMT2A-MLLT3* fusion gene, show relatively acceptable results with intensive chemotherapy (Grimwade et al. 2010; Mrózek et al. 1997; Stölzel et al. 2016; Chen et al. 2013; Pigneux et al. 2015), placing them in the intermediate risk group according to ELN 2017 classification (Döhner et al. 2017), while patients with t(11;19)(q23;p13) were considered at intermediate risk by some (Grimwade et al. 2010; Pigneux et al. 2015), but not all (Döhner et al. 2017; Chen et al. 2013; Bhatnagar et al. 2016), studies. Of note, associated (cyto)genetic lesions should not be accounted for in the context of *KMT2A* gene fusions. For instance, t(9;11)(p22;q23) can be found along with additional cytogenetic alterations in a "complex" karyotype, but should still be considered of intermediate prognostic value in this case (Grimwade et al. 2010).

Among recurrent translocations associated with unfavorable outcomes, t(6;9)(p23;q34.1) leading to the *DEK-NUP214* fusion gene occurs roughly in 1% of AML patients. This entity has been associated with relatively younger age, bone marrow dysplasia, high incidence of *FLT3*-ITD, and high relapse risk (Papaemmanuil et al. 2016; Grimwade et al. 2010; Slovak et al. 2006). It is thus regarded as an adverse risk entity (Döhner et al. 2017). Additional cytogenetic aberrations occur in 10–20% of the cases, without a clear prognostic impact.

Inv(3;3)(q21.3q26.2) or t(3;3)(q21.3;q26.2) is a rare entity representing 1–2% of AMLs, driven by the repositioning of the *GATA2* enhancer (located at 3q21), which leads to the overexpression of *MECOM* (*EVI1*) (located at 3q26) and to the haploinsufficiency of *GATA2*. Consequently,

*EVI1* overexpression can be found in virtually all these patients, but also in the majority of cases with other 3q abnormalities and in up to 10% cases without any 3q aberrations, with significant prognostic implications (see *below*) (Hinai and Valk 2016).

Inv(3;3)/t(3;3) AML has been uniformly associated with very low CR rate after intensive chemotherapy (usually <30–40%) and dismal prognosis (Papaemmanuil et al. 2016; Grimwade et al. 2010; Lugthart et al. 2010; Sitges et al. 2020). Conversely, although often associated with poor outcomes, the impact of other 3q aberrations has been less firmly established, possibly due to their heterogeneity (Lugthart et al. 2010). Thus, 3q aberrations other than inv(3;3)/t(3;3) are not incorporated in the ELN 2017 classification (Döhner et al. 2017), but are considered high-risk alterations according to the Medical Research Council (MRC) classification (Table 7.3) (Grimwade et al. 2010). Recently, atypical 3q26 rearrangements have been shown to be biologically very similar to inv(3)/t(3;3) AML, suggesting that these cases could be incorporated with inv(3;3)/t(3;3) AML in the broader 3q26-rearranged AML group, and treated consequently (Ottema et al. 2020). The most frequent additional chromosomal aberration in inv(3;3)/t(3;3) patients is monosomy 7, which does not seem to independently worsen prognosis (Grimwade et al. 2010), unless in the context of a monosomal karyotype (Lugthart et al. 2010; Sitges et al. 2020).

*BCR-ABL1*-positive AML was recently introduced as a provisional entity in the 2016 WHO classification (Arber et al. 2016), distinguishing it from myeloid blast crisis of chronic myeloid leukemia (Neuendorff et al. 2016). Although ELN guidelines place this entity in the adverse risk category (Döhner et al. 2017), it has been suggested that its prognosis largely depends on co-occurring genetic abnormalities. Besides, the incorporation of TKIs in the treatment strategy is likely to change its natural history and alloHCT was associated with favorable long-term survival in some reports (Lazarevic et al. 2018; Neuendorff et al. 2018). Further effort is required to define more accurately this entity.

### 7.4.3 Adverse-Risk Aneuploidies

Among patients with an abnormal karyotype lacking recurrent translocations, the adverse prognostic role of deletion 5q/−5, deletion 7q/−7, and deletion 17p/−17 is well established (Byrd et al. 2002; Slovak et al. 2000; Seifert et al. 2009; Nahi et al. 2008). Of note, despite being grouped together in some reports (Slovak et al. 2000; Grimwade et al. 2010), the majority of studies have shown that patients harboring monosomy 7 have a worse outcome compared to those with del(7q) (Byrd et al. 2002; Grimwade et al. 1998, 2010), which is consistent with data in MDS (Greenberg et al. 2012; Schanz et al. 2012). These results were also confirmed for patients undergoing alloHCT (Poiré et al. 2020; Canaani et al. 2019). Thus, only monosomy 7 is regarded as an adverse risk abnormality according to ELN 2017 classification (Döhner et al. 2017) (Table 7.3).

The role of other aneuploidies or rare translocations has been more controversial. The MRC group performed a detailed analysis including 5876 intensively treated younger AML patients, in order to clarify their impact. The authors derived a revised cytogenetic classification (Grimwade et al. 2010) that has largely, but not entirely, been incorporated into the current ELN risk stratification (Döhner et al. 2017). As a matter of fact, del(7q) and the abnormalities of 3(q) are defined as high risk by the MRC classification only, which conversely excludes from this category patients with t(11;19) and those with three unrelated abnormalities (see *below* and Table 7.3).

The presence of a complex karyotype (CK), currently defined by the 2017 ELN guidelines as the presence of at least 3 unrelated chromosome abnormalities—whether or not in the same clone—in the absence of one of the WHO-designated recurrent translocations or inversions (Döhner et al. 2017; Byrd et al. 2002; Slovak et al. 2000; Schoch et al. 2001), occurs in 10–15% of AML patients. Its incidence increases with age. CK has invariably been associated with unfavorable outcomes in AML (Byrd et al. 2002; Grimwade et al. 2001; Creutzig et al. 2016;

**Table 7.3** Current prognostic classifications

| Risk category | Genetic abnormality | Comments |
|---|---|---|
| **Favorable** | t(8;21)(q22;q22.1); *RUNX1-RUNX1T1* | According to NCCN only, alloHCT should be considered for t(8;21) in case of *KIT* mutations. Favorable risk irrespective of additional cytogenetic abnormalities |
| | Inv(16)(p13.1q22) or t(16;16)(p13.1;q22); *CBFB-MYH11* | Favorable risk irrespective of additional cytogenetic abnormalities |
| | Mutated *NPM1* without *FLT3*-ITD or with *FLT3*-ITDlow* | If allelic ratio is not available, *FLT3*-ITD pos patients are high risk, or intermediate if also *NPM1* positive (NCCN)<br>ELN states that *NPM1* positive cases (without *FLT3*-ITD or with *FLT3*-ITDlow) are considered favorable risk regardless of cytogenetics. However, a recent large multinational report suggests this might not be true if an adverse risk cytogenetic aberration is present.§ |
| | Biallelic mutated *CEBPA* | ELN states that biallelic mutated *CEBPA* positive cases are considered favorable risk regardless of cytogenetics |
| **Intermediate** | Mutated *NPM1* and *FLT3*-ITDhigh* | |
| | Wild-type *NPM1* without *FLT3*-ITD or with *FLT3*-ITDlow* | In the absence of adverse-risk genetic lesions |
| | t(9;11)(p21.3;q23.3); *MLLT3-KMT2A* | The presence of t(9;11)) takes precedence over rare, concurrent adverse-risk gene mutations. According to the MRC cytogenetic classification, t(11;19)(q23;p13) is also an intermediate risk abnormality |
| | Cytogenetic abnormalities not favorable or adverse | Very large consortium data may be necessary to assign prognostic value to rare entities |
| **Adverse** | t(6;9)(p23;q34.1); *DEK-NUP214* | |
| | t(v;11q23.3); *KMT2A*-rearranged | According to the MRC cytogenetic classification, t(11;19)(q23;p13) is an intermediate risk abnormality |
| | t(9;22)(q34.1;q11.2); *BCR-ABL1* | |
| | Inv(3)(q21.3q26.2) or t(3;3)(q21.3;q26.2); *GATA2,MECOM(EVI1)* | According to the MRC cytogenetic classification, all abn(3q), excluding t(3;5)(q21 25,q31 35), are adverse risk |
| | Monosomy 5 or del(5q) | |
| | Monosmy 7 | According to the MRC cytogenetic classification, del(7p) is also a high risk abnormality |
| | Monosmy 17/abn(17p) | |
| | Complex karyotype | Three or more unrelated chromosome abnormalities in the absence of 1 of the WHO-designated recurring translocations or inversions. According to the MRC cytogenetic classification, at least 4 abnormalities are required |
| | Monosomal karyotype | One single monosomy (excluding loss of X or Y) with at least 1 additional monosomy or structural chromosome abnormality |
| | Wild-type *NPM1* and *FLT3*-ITDhigh* | |
| | Mutated *RUNX1* | Not an adverse prognostic marker if co-occurring with favorable-risk AML subtypes |
| | Mutated *ASXL1* | Not an adverse prognostic marker if co-occurring with favorable-risk AML subtypes |
| | Mutated *TP53* | |

* Low (<0.5) or high (≥0.5) allelic ratio is derived by semi-quantitative assessment using DNA fragment analysis and is determined as ratio of the area under the curve "*FLT3*-ITD" divided by area under the curve "FLT3-wild type".
§ Angenendt et al. (2019).
Adapted from Dohner, Blood 2017, NCCN V3 2020 AML and Grimwade Blood 2010 NCCN national comprehensive cancer network; MRC Medical Research Council

Stölzel et al. 2016). It is important to stress that CK should not be considered as an unfavorable feature in patients with favorable or intermediate risk translocations, including t(8;21), inv(16), or t(9;11) (Grimwade et al. 2010). This suggests that, in the absence of these recurrent founder lesions, CK is only an indirect surrogate of an unfavorable disease subtype. Several attempts have thus been made to define more accurately this subgroup.

Authors initially stressed the importance of the number of cytogenetic alterations. According to the MRC classification, 4 abnormalities (Grimwade et al. 2010) (or, formerly, 5) (Grimwade et al. 2001) were necessary to define CK. Stölzel and colleagues analyzed the outcome of 3526 AML patients included in three prospective trials of the Study Alliance Leukemia. They found that patients with ≥4 abnormalities have an adverse risk per se, while patients with 3 abnormalities have a borderline intermediate-adverse outcome, in the absence of individual abnormalities of strong influence (Stölzel et al. 2016). However, irrespectively of the cutoff chosen, each additional aberration worsens prognosis (Papaemmanuil et al. 2016; Grimwade et al. 2010).

Others studied the respective contribution of complexity and aneuploidy, given the strong correlation between CK and chromosome 5, 7, and 17 complete or partial monosomy. Indeed, patients with monosomies had unfavorable outcomes, with long-term survival not exceeding 15% (Breems et al. 2008). Among those cases, Breems and colleagues identified a group with extremely poor outcomes, with 4-year OS of less than 5%, characterized by a monosomal karyotype (MK). They defined MK as the presence of two or more distinct autosomal chromosome monosomies or one single autosomal monosomy in the presence of at least one structural abnormality. Thus defined, MK showed a greater prognostic impact than CK, as patients with CK but lacking MK had relatively better outcomes. The negative prognostic value of MK was confirmed in the following reports analyzing independent patient cohorts (Grimwade et al. 2010; Kayser et al. 2012; Medeiros et al. 2010; Weinberg et al. 2014; Wierzbowska et al. 2017). Further studies indicated that CK defined by exactly 3 alterations, in the absence of MK, was associated with a better outcome than MK and/or CK with 4 or more abnormalities (Haferlach et al. 2012). Consistently (Slovak et al. 2000; Breems et al. 2008; Chilton et al. 2014), Mrózek and colleagues recently reported that atypical CK, that is, lacking 5q, 7q, and/or 17p loss, represents a biologically distinct entity and it is associated with a relatively superior prognosis compared to typical CK (Mrózek et al. 2019).

Hyperdiploidy (i.e., ≥49 chromosomes) is infrequent in AML (less than 2% of AML). Its prognosis appears heterogeneous, with a poor prognosis restricted in most (Chilton et al. 2014; Lazarevic et al. 2015; Abaza et al. 2018), but not all (Stölzel et al. 2016), reports to patients also harboring adverse risk abnormalities (i.e., chromosome 5, 7, or 17 abnormalities), while those with pure hyperdiploid karyotype showed an intermediate risk.

In an attempt to define the biological process underlying the poor prognosis of MK and CK, authors have turned to indirect markers of chromothripsis, a term coined to describe a phenomenon of multiple chromosome fragmentation in a single catastrophic event, and initially identified in cancers through whole genome sequencing rather than karyotyping (Stephens et al. 2011). These authors could show that presence of marker chromosomes, which reflects gross structural chromosomal damage and is sometimes seen in patients with CK, was associated with chromothripsis, defined by array of comparative genomic hybridization, and with poor outcomes independently of adverse-risk karyotype according to MRC or ELN. A strong association of chromothripsis with *TP53* mutations was found, but whether both exert an independent prognostic impact remains to be established (Bochtler et al. 2017; Fontana et al. 2018).

## 7.5 Gene Mutations

Knowledge on the biological implications, prognostic relevance, and clinical impact of recurrent gene mutations has greatly expanded in recent years. Extensive molecular characterization at diagnosis has become standard practice in AML (The Cancer Genome Atlas Research Network 2013; Papaemmanuil et al. 2016; Grimwade et al. 2016; Metzeler et al. 2016; Bullinger et al. 2017; Patel et al. 2012). Below we describe the prognostic relevance of the most frequent gene mutations (Table 7.4). Importantly, only a few (*NPM1*, *CEBPA*) can be considered as "founder," class-defining lesions in AML on the basis of their near complete exclusivity one from another and from the recurrent translocations listed above (Papaemmanuil et al. 2016).

### 7.5.1 FLT3

*FLT3* is the most commonly mutated gene in younger AML patients (Papaemmanuil et al. 2016; Nakao et al. 1996). It is associated with cytogenetically normal AML (CN-AML), APL, and t(6;9)(p23;q34.1) (Thiede et al. 2002), and the prognostic relevance of its aberrations has been extensively explored. Point mutations in the Tyrosine Kinases Domain (TKD), more frequently in the D835 residue, occur in 7–10% of the patients and do not exert a significant independent prognostic role (Döhner et al. 2017; Tallman et al. 2019; Grimwade et al. 2016), with some conflicting results (Bacher et al. 2008; Mead et al. 2007; Fröhling et al. 2002). *FLT3-TKD* mutations could exert distinct prognostic impact depending on the context (i.e., CBF, *NPM1* vs. *KMT2A*-PTD-positive AML, see also *below*) (Papaemmanuil et al. 2016; Eisfeld et al. 2018; Boddu et al. 2017; Perry et al. 2018). Conversely, Internal Tandem Duplications (ITDs), which occur in the juxtamembrane (JM) domain and/or first tyrosine kinase domain (TKD1) of the FLT3 receptor, have been consistently associated with unfavorable outcomes (Kiyoi et al. 1999; Kottaridis et al. 2001; Port et al. 2014; Whitman et al. 2010). *FLT3*-ITD can be categorized based on allelic ratio, size of the insertion, and location of the insertion. In several reports, the adverse prognostic value of *FLT3*-ITD seemed mostly restricted to patients with high ITD/wild-type allelic ratios (Thiede et al. 2002; Blau et al. 2013; Gale et al. 2008; Chen et al. 2019; Schnittger et al. 2011a; Schlenk et al. 2014; Whitman et al. 2001). *FLT3*-ITD allelic ratio is defined as the ratio of the area under the curve of the *FLT3*-ITD signal divided by the area under the curve of the wild-type signal in conventional DNA fragment analysis. Thus defined, allelic ratio differs from Variant Allele Frequencies (VAF) for other genetic lesions, which report the relative abundance of the mutated allele over the total (mutant + wild type) allele burden. Among the different cutoffs reported in the literature (Thiede et al. 2002; Cornelissen and Blaise 2016; Ho et al. 2016; de Jonge et al. 2011), the current version of the ELN guidelines adopted the value of 0.5 to define low (<0.5) and high (≥0.5) *FLT3*-ITD allelic ratios (Döhner et al. 2017). Of note, in some patients, multiple ITDs may coexist, presumably in independent clones. In those cases, the sum of allelic ratios should be compared to the 0.5 threshold. An important effort has yet to be done to guarantee the inter-laboratory reproducibility of such allelic ratio results, which currently rely on partly standardized PCR assays (Daver et al. 2019). Finally, though the length and site of the insertion may also play a prognostic role, with longer ITDs being associated with the insertion in the TKD1 domain, and potentially with a more unfavorable outcome in several reports (Chen et al. 2019; Schlenk et al. 2014; Kayser et al. 2009; Stirewalt et al. 2006; Kim et al. 2015; Arreba-Tutusaus et al. 2016; Liu et al. 2019; Fischer et al. 2017), these parameters are currently not used to stratify patients according to current guidelines (Döhner et al. 2017; Tallman et al. 2019), because of conflicting results (Blau et al. 2013; Gale et al. 2008; Ponziani et al. 2006; Kusec et al. 2006), and of ongoing efforts to standardize the detailed molecular assessment of *FLT3*-ITDs (Schwartz et al. 2019).

### 7.5.2 NPM1

*NPM1* mutations are also common in AML, with an overall incidence around 30%. They are mostly detected in patients with normal karyotype. *NPM1* mutations have overall been associated with favorable outcomes and good response to intensive chemotherapy in most, but

**Table 7.4** Prognostic role of recurrent gene mutations

| Gene | Mutation | Prognostic significance | Subset and interactions | References |
|---|---|---|---|---|
| ***FLT3*** | **ITD** | Unfavorable | Independently worse OS | Kiyoi et al. (1999) |
| | | | Independently worse EFS, RFS, OS | Kottaridis et al. (2001) |
| | | | Independently worse RFS and OS only if high mutant level | Thiede et al. (2002) |
| | | | Independently worsen OS | Fröhling et al. (2002) |
| | | | Independently worse RFS and OS, worsening with increasing mutant level | Gale et al. (2008) |
| | | | Independently worse RFS and OS in AML > 60 years | Whitman et al. (2010) |
| | | | Only high AR adverse prognostic impact in *NPM1*-mutated AML | Schnittger et al. (2011a, b) |
| | | | *FLT3*-ITD worsen prognosis in *NPM1* mutated AML, especially if high AR | Schneider et al. (2012) |
| | | | Independently worsen OS | How et al. (2012) |
| | | | *FLT3*-ITD worsen OS, EFS, RFS but only if high AR in *NPM1*-mutated AML | Pratcorona et al. (2013) |
| | | | Independently worsen RFS | Metzeler et al. (2016) |
| | | | Independently worsen OS | Papaemmanuil et al. (2016) |
| | **TKD** | Controversial | Improved EFS in AML with *NPM1*- or *CEBPA* mutations | Bacher et al. (2008) |
| | | | Improved OS (only if mutant level >25%) | Mead et al. (2007) |
| | | | Improved RFS and a trend for OS in *NPM1*-mutated AML | Boddu (2017) |
| | | | Independently improved CR rate, no impact on OS and RFS | Metzeler et al. (2016) |
| | | | Impact strongly dependent on the presence of *KMT2A*-PTD | Papaemmanuil et al. (2016) |
| | | | Improved OS in *NPM1*-mutated AML > 60 years | Eisfeld et al. (2018) |
| | | | Improved OS in *NPM1*-mutated AML | Perry et al. (2018) |
| ***NPM1*** | | Favorable | Improve CR rate | Falini et al. (2005) |
| | | | No impact on CR and OS in IR-AML | Boissel et al. (2005) |
| | | | Improved CR rate and RFS | Suzuki et al. (2005) |
| | | | Improved CR rate, OS, RFS in absence *FLT3*-ITD | Thiede et al. (2006) |
| | | | Improved CR rate and OS in absence *FLT3*-ITD | Döhner et al. (2005) |
| | | | Improved CR rate, EFS, OS in the absence of *FLT3*-ITD | Schnittger et al. (2005) |
| | | | Improved EFS, OS, RFS in the absence of *FLT3*-ITD | Verhaak et al. (2005) |
| | | | Improved OS and RFS | Gale et al. (2008) |

**Table 7.4** (continued)

| Gene | Mutation | Prognostic significance | Subset and interactions | References |
|---|---|---|---|---|
| | | | Improved CR rate, OS, RFS in absence *FLT3*-ITD | Schlenk et al. (2008) |
| | | | Improved CR rate, OS, RFS in absence *FLT3*-ITD | Büchner et al. (2009) |
| | | | Improved CR rate, OS, RFS in>60 years CN AML | Becker et al. (2010) |
| | | | Favorable OS in absence FLT3 ITD | How et al. (2012) |
| | | | Favorable OS and EFS in absence FLT3 ITD | Grossmann et al. (2012) |
| | | | Favorable OS and EFS in absence FLT3 ITD, intermediate if FLT3 low AR | Schneider et al. (2012) |
| | | | Favorable OS and EFS in absence FLT3 ITD or if *FLT3*-ITD with low AR | Pratcorona et al. (2013) |
| | | | Improved CR rate and, in de absence of *FLT3*-ITD, improved OS | Kihara et al. (2014) |
| | | | Improved OS for in absence of *FLT3*-ITD only 55-65y, not >65 years | Ostronoff et al. (2015) |
| | | | Improved CR rate and favorable OS (in the absence of *FLT3*-ITD) | Metzeler et al. (2016) |
| | | | Favorable impact on OS | Papaemmanuil et al. (2016) |
| ***DNMT3A*** | **Globally** | Controversial, mostly unfavorable | Independently reduce OS, irrespectively of age an type of mutations | Ley et al. (2010) |
| | | | Independently reduce OS but not CR or RFS globally, lower OS and CR in CN-AML | Thol et al. (2011) |
| | | | Independently reduced OS and RFS | Hou et al. (2012) |
| | | | Independently reduced OS and EFS in CN AML | Shen et al. (2011) |
| | | | Independently reduced OS and RFS < 60 years | Ribeiro et al. (2012) |
| | | | Independently reduced for EFS and OS in CN AML <60 years | Renneville et al. (2012) |
| | | | Independently worse RFS and, only in AML <60 years, OS and CR rate | Metzeler et al. (2016) |
| | | | No clear independent prognostic value (only with some co-mutational patterns) | Papaemmanuil et al. (2016) |
| | | | Worse OS in each ELN2017 defined subgroup | Herold et al. (2020) |
| | **R882** | | Shorted DFS, not independently worse OS. Different impact R882 vs others according to age | Marcucci et al. (2012) |
| | | | No effect on OS and EFS globally; negative only in unfavorable ELN risk and for R882 mutation | Gaidzik et al. (2013) |
| | | | R822 mutations worsen OS, DFS and increase CIR; particularly bad with *FLT3*-ITD and *NPM1* | Bezerra et al. (2020) |
| | | | Non-R882 mutations worsen CIR and RFS in *NPM1*-mutated AML | Peterlin et al. (2015) |
| ***CEBPA*** | **Globally** | Favorable (restricted to bi-allelic) | First study reporting the favorable clinical impact of *CEBPA* mutations on OS | Preudhomme et al. (2002) |

(continued)

**Table 7.4** (continued)

| Gene | Mutation | Prognostic significance | Subset and interactions | References |
|---|---|---|---|---|
| | | | *CEBPA* independently improve OS | Schlenk et al. (2008) |
| | **Biallelic** | | Only bi*CEBPA* independent favorable effect on OS and EFS | Wouters et al. (2009) |
| | | | Only bi*CEBPA* independent favorable effect on OS and EFS | Shen et al. (2011) |
| | | | Only bi*CEBPA* independent favorable effect on OS and EFS | Rockova et al. (2011) |
| | | | Only bi*CEBPA* independent favorable effect on OS and RFS | Pabst et al. (2009) |
| | | | Only bi*CEBPA* independent favorable effect on OS; *FLT3*-ITD abolish this favorable effect | Green et al. (2010) |
| | | | Only bi*CEBPA* independent favorable effect on OS and EFS | Dufour et al. (2010) |
| | | | Only bi*CEBPA* independent favorable effect on OS and EFS | Taskesen et al. (2011) |
| | | | bi*CEBPA* favorable impact on OS | Grossmann et al. (2012) |
| | | | Only bi*CEBPA* independent favorable effect on OS, *TET2* worsen outcomes while *GATA2* has positive effect | Fasan et al. (2014) |
| | | | bi*CEBPA* better OS compared to monoallelic mutation only at univariate analysis | Marceau-Renaut et al. (2015) |
| | | | bi*CEBPA* favorable long-term OS compared to monoallelic mutation | Pastore et al. (2014a, b) |
| | | | bi*CEBPA* favorable long-term OS | Papaemmanuil et al. (2016) |
| | | | bi*CEBPA* favorable long-term OS (borderline significance) | Metzeler et al. (2016) |
| | | | bi*CEBPA* increased CR, OS, RFS; concomitant *WT1* mutations worsen OS and RSF | Tien et al. (2018a, b) |
| ***KMT2A*** | **PTD** | Controversial, mostly unfavorable | OS and RFS significantly worse in CN-AML | Schnittger et al. (2000) |
| | | | Independently worsen RFS | Döhner et al. (2002) |
| | | | Worsen OS | Shiah et al. (2002) |
| | | | Independently worse RFS | Schlenk et al. (2008) |
| | | | Only worsen RFS in <60 years, not OS | Steudel et al. (2003) |
| | | | Independently worse EFS | Grossmann et al. (2012) |
| | | | Independently worsen OS | Kihara et al. (2014) |
| | | | Worsen EFS and OS only at univariate analysis | Fasan et al. (2014) |
| | | | No clear impact on any survival outcomes | Metzeler et al. (2016) |

**Table 7.4** (continued)

| Gene | Mutation | Prognostic significance | Subset and interactions | References |
|---|---|---|---|---|
| | | | Impact on OS mainly if *FLT3*-TKD co-occurs | Papaemmanuil et al. (2016) |
| | | | No impact on OS and EFS. Unfavorable outcome restricted to *DNMT3A* and *NRAS* comutated | Hinai et al. (2019) |
| ***RUNX1*** | | Unfavorable (mostly) | Independently worsen OS | Tang et al. (2009) |
| | | | Independently worsen EFS | Gaidzik et al. (2011) |
| | | | Independently worsen OS | Schnittger et al. (2011a, b) |
| | | | Independently worsen OS in CN-AML | Greif et al. (2012) |
| | | | Independently worsen CR rate, EFS, OS RFS | Mendler et al. (2012) |
| | | | Independently worsen OS | Kihara et al. (2014) |
| | | | Worsen EFS and OS only at univariate analysis | Fasan et al. (2014) |
| | | | Independently worsen EFS | Gaidzik et al. (2016) |
| | | | No independent prognostic impact in AML-NOS | Weinberg et al. (2017) |
| | | | Independently worse RFS and, only in AML <60 years, OS and CR rate | Metzeler et al. (2016) |
| | | | No independent prognostic value | Papaemmanuil et al. (2016) |
| | | | Worse prognosis of multiple versus single *RUNX1* mutation (loss of wt allele) | Stengel et al. (2018) |
| | | | No independent prognostic impact in de novo AML | Quesada et al. (2020) |
| | | | Impact on OS more pronounced in AML with MDS-related changes | Nguyen et al. (2020) |
| ***ASXL1*** | | Unfavorable (mostly) | Detrimental effect on OS lost at multivariate analysis | Chou et al. (2010) |
| | | | Independent effect on OS in CN-AML only | Patel et al. (2012) |
| | | | Worse CR rate, RFS, OS and EFS among ELN2010 favorable patients | Metzeler et al. (2011a, b) |
| | | | Independently worse OS | Grossmann et al. (2012) |
| | | | Independently worse OS | Pratcorona et al. (2012) |
| | | | Independently worse OS in intermediate-risk AML | Schnittger et al. (2013) |
| | | | Worsen EFS and OS only at univariate analysis | Fasan et al. (2014) |
| | | | Independently worsen OS only when co-occur with *RUNX1* | Paschka et al. (2015) |
| | | | Independently worsen OS in AML-MRC | Devillier et al. (2015) |
| | | | No independent prognostic value | Metzeler et al. (2016) |

(continued)

**Table 7.4** (continued)

| Gene | Mutation | Prognostic significance | Subset and interactions | References |
|---|---|---|---|---|
| | | | Independently worse OS | Papaemmanuil et al. (2016) |
| ***TET2*** | | Controversial | No prognostic impact | Nibourel et al. (2010) |
| | | | Impact on OS lost at multivariable analysis | Chou et al. (2011a, b) |
| | | | Shorter EFS, lower CR rate, and shorter RFS only among favorable-risk CN-AML | Metzeler et al. (2011a, b) |
| | | | Shorter EFS in favorable-risk de novo CN-AML | Weissmann et al. (2012) |
| | | | Impact on OS lost at multivariable analysis | Gaidzik et al. (2012) |
| | | | Worse OS in CN-AML | Patel et al. (2012) |
| | | | No significant prognostic impact | Metzeler et al. (2016) |
| ***IDH*** | **Grouped *IDH1/2*** | Controversial | Impact on OS lost at multivariable analysis | Gaidzik et al. (2012) |
| | | | Worse OS and RFS only in *NPM1*-mutated *FLT3*-ITD negative AML | Paschka et al. (2010) |
| | ***IDH1*** | | Favorable OS in *NPM1*-mutated AML | Patel et al. (2012) |
| | | | No prognostic impact | Metzeler et al. (2016) |
| | | | Inferior CR rate and OS in intensively treated AML over 75 years | Prassek et al. (2018) |
| | | | Worse OS and RFS only in *NPM1*-mutated *FLT3*-ITD negative AML | Marcucci et al. (2010) |
| | | | Worse OS and RFS only in *NPM1*-mutated *FLT3*-ITD negative AML | Boissel et al. (2010) |
| | | | No prognostic impact in CN AML | Wagner et al. (2010) |
| | | | Worse OS and EFS only in NPM1wt FLT3wt AML | Abbas et al. (2010) |
| | | | Independently worse EFS | Schnittger et al. (2010) |
| | | | No prognostic impact | Green et al. (2011) |
| | | | No prognostic impact | Shenet et al. (2011) |
| | | | Worse RFS and higher CIR in *NPM1*-mutated AML | Peterlin et al. (2015) |
| | ***IDH2* (all)** | | No prognostic impact | Metzeler et al. (2016) |
| | | | No prognostic impact | Thol et al. (2010) |
| | | | No prognostic impact | Shen et al. (2011) |
| | | | No prognostic impact | Abbas et al. (2010) |
| | **R140** | | Favorable OS, especially in *NPM1*-mutated CN AML | Patel et al. (2012) |
| | | | No independent impact, strongly dependent on co-mutations | Papaemmanuil et al. (2016) |
| | | | Worse OS and RFS only in *NPM1*-mutated *FLT3*-ITD negative AML | Marcucci et al. (2010) |

**Table 7.4** (continued)

| Gene | Mutation | Prognostic significance | Subset and interactions | References |
|---|---|---|---|---|
| | | | Favorable OS and reduced CIR | Green et al. (2011) |
| | | | Favorable OS | Chou et al. (2011a, b) |
| | | | No prognostic impact | Boissel et al. (2011) |
| | **R172** | | Trend for better outcomes | Papaemmanuil et al. (2016) |
| | | | Lower CR rate and trend for lower OS in older AML | Marcucci et al. (2010) |
| | | | Worse OS and higher CIR | Green et al. (2011) |
| | | | Independently worse OS and RFS | Boissel et al. (2010) |
| | | | Favorable OS | Chou et al. (2011a, b) |
| ***WT1*** | | Controversial | Independently worse CR rate, CIR, RFS and OS | Virappane et al. (2008) |
| | | | Independently worse OS and RFS | Paschka et al. (2008) |
| | | | No independent prognostic impact in CN-AML | Gaidzik et al. (2009) |
| | | | Independently worse RFS in CN-AML | Renneville et al. (2009a, b) |
| | | | Independently worse OS in CN-AML | Patel et al. (2012) |
| | | | No significant prognostic impact.. | Metzeler et al. (2016) |
| ***TP53*** | | Unfavorable | Independently worse OS in AML > 55 years | Stirewalt et al. (2001) |
| | | | Independently worse OS and EFS | Grossmann et al. (2012) |
| | | | Independently worse OS, RFS and CR rate AML with adverse risk cytogenetics | Bowen et al. (2009) |
| | | | Independently worse EFS, RFS, OS in AML with CK | Rücker et al. (2012) |
| | | | Independently worse OS | Kihara et al. (2014) |
| | | | Independently worse OS in therapy-related AML | Ok et al. (2015) |
| | | | Worse OS irrespective of age and treatment intensity (only univariate data) | Kadia et al. (2016) |
| | | | Independently worse OS and RFS | Metzeler et al. (2016) |
| | | | Independently worse OS | Papaemmanuil et al. (2016) |
| | | | Independently worse OS in AML > 60 years | Yanada et al. (2016) |
| | | | Independently worse OS | Stengel et al. (2017) |
| | | | Significantly shorter RSF in AML > 75 treated intensively | Prassek et al. (2018) |

(continued)

**Table 7.4** (continued)

| Gene | Mutation | Prognostic significance | Subset and interactions | References |
|---|---|---|---|---|
| ***KIT*** | | Controversial, mostly unfavorable in t(8;21) | Exon 8 mutations increased CIR in inv(16) | Care et al. (2003) |
| | | | Shorter EFS and RFS in t(8;21) but not inv(16) | Boissel et al. (2006) |
| | | | Worse OS and higher CIR in inv(16); Higher CIR similar OS in t(8;21) | Paschka et al. (2006) |
| | | | Worse OS and higher CIR in t(8;21); no impact in inv(16) | Cairoli et al. (2006) |
| | | | Lower OS and EFS in patients with t(8;21) (D816 Mut at exon 17) | Schnittger et al. (2006) |
| | | | Worse OS and EFS in adult t(8;21) for exon 17 Mut; no impact in inv(16) and pediatric | Park et al. (2011) |
| | | | Worse OS and EFS t(8;21) for mutations D816 at exon 17 | Kim et al. (2013) |
| | | | Worse RFS in inv(16), mainly if exon 8 mutations | Paschka et al. (2013) |
| | | | No significant prognostic impact | Riera et al. (2013) |
| | | | Higher CIR (if mutant level > 25%) in t(8;21) | Allen et al. (2013) |
| | | | Higher CIR, worse DFS and OS in adult t(8;21) AML; no impact inv(16) and pediatric AML | Qin et al. (2014) |
| | | | D816 mutations negatively impacted on OS in t(8;21) | Krauth et al. (2014) |
| | | | No impact in pediatric t(8;21) | Klein et al. (2015) |
| | | | Exon 17 mutations worsen RFS and OS | Cher et al. (2016) |
| | | | Exon 17 mutations worsen OS and EFS | Faber et al. (2016) |
| | | | Higher CIR (if mutant level > 35%) in t(8;21) | Duployez et al. (2016) |
| | | | No independent prognostic impact in any subgroup | Itzykson et al. (2018a, b) |
| | | | Lower CR,EFS,OS, RFS in t(8;21), but outperformed by MRD | Rücker et al. (2019) |
| | | | Inferior RFS and OS (if mutant level > 25%) in t(8;21) | Christen et al. (2019) |
| | | | D816 mutation negatively impacted on RFS in t(8;21) | Opatz et al. (2020) |
| | | | Exon 17 mutations worsen RFS in t(8;21) but not inv(16) | Ishikawa et al. (2020) |

not all, studies (Falini et al. 2005; Boissel et al. 2005; Suzuki et al. 2005). These discrepancies were soon found to reflect the strong interaction between *NPM1* and *FLT3*-ITD statuses to determine outcome. *NPM1* mutations and *FLT3*-ITD co-occur in 40–45% of the cases. The favorable outcome of *NPM1*-mutated patients is mostly restricted to those not harboring *FLT3*-ITD (Thiede et al. 2006; Döhner et al. 2005; Schlenk et al. 2008; Schnittger et al. 2005; Verhaak et al. 2005), as initially outlined by the ELN 2010 classification (Döhner et al. 2010; Mrózek et al. 2012; Röllig et al. 2011), or to those with low allelic ratios *FLT3*-ITDs as defined above (Döhner et al. 2017), while *NPM1*-mutated patients with *FLT3*-ITD with high allelic ratio (*FLT3*-ITD$^{high}$) have an outcome comparable to *NPM1*wt patients with intermediate risk disease

(Table 7.2) (Schnittger et al. 2011a; Schneider et al. 2012; Pratcorona et al. 2013).

The role of *FLT3*-ITD allelic ratio and its interaction with *NPM1* status remain an area of controversy (Daver et al. 2019; Pratz and Levis 2017; Straube et al. 2018; Boddu et al. 2019; Versluis and Hout 2017; Harada et al. 2018; How et al. 2012). The MRC group reported that *NPM1*-mutated patients with *FLT3*-ITD have an increased relapse risk and decreased survival, irrespective of the allelic ratio (Linch et al. 2014), and a recent Japanese study showed that patients with *NPM1*-mutated AML with *FLT3*-ITD$^{low}$ experienced unfavorable long-term outcomes when alloHCT was not performed in CR1 (Sakaguchi et al. 2018). Conversely, a recent analysis on the RATIFY trial, which demonstrated the beneficial effect of midostaurin added to chemotherapy for *FLT3*-mutated patients, confirmed the ELN 2017 approach on *FLT3*-ITD allelic ratio and its interaction with *NPM1* mutations. As a matter of fact, patients belonging to the three prognostic subgroups showed markedly different OS, EFS, and CIR, both in the midostaurin and in the placebo arm (Döhner et al. 2020).

Another controversial topic is the prognostic relevance of cytogenetic lesions in *NPM1*-mutated patients. These cytogenetic lesions can be found in 15–20% of patients and are typically nonrecurrent, except for trisomy 8 (Thiede et al. 2006; Verhaak et al. 2005; Haferlach et al. 2009). Most (Thiede et al. 2006; Haferlach et al. 2009) but not all (Harada et al. 2018; Micol et al. 2009; Balsat et al. 2017) studies initially suggested that these infrequent cases with abnormal karyotype behaved similarly to *NPM1*-mutated CN-AML. This led to discard normal cytogenetics as a prerequisite to class *NPM1*-mutated patients in the 2017 ELN classification (Döhner et al. 2017). However, a recent meta-analysis of 2426 *NPM1*-mutated *FLT3*-ITD$^{neg/low}$ patients showed that those with adverse-risk chromosomal abnormalities (3.4%) had significantly worse CR rate, OS, and increased relapse incidence, independently of other risk factors, thus challenging this modification (Angenendt et al. 2019).

Finally, additional co-mutation such as *IDH1/2* and *DNMT3A* plays a major role, which has yet to be fully explored (Papaemmanuil et al. 2016; Eisfeld et al. 2018) (*see below*).

### 7.5.3 CEBPA

CCAAT/enhancer binding protein α (*CEBPA*) gene mutations occur in around 10% AML of patients and have been initially associated with a favorable prognostic value (Schlenk et al. 2008; Fröhling et al. 2004; Pabst et al. 2001; Preudhomme et al. 2002; Renneville et al. 2009a). However, several reports have subsequently clarified that only patients harboring biallelic *CEBPA* (bi*CEBPA*) mutations, generally involving an N-terminal frameshift on one allele and an in-frame C-terminal mutation in the C-terminal bZIP domains, showed favorable outcomes (i.e., classical bi*CEBPA*), with 5-year OS often reaching 60–70% after intensive treatments. Conversely, single allele mutations had no prognostic impact (Metzeler et al. 2016; Wouters et al. 2009; Green et al. 2010; Fasan et al. 2014; Pastore et al. 2014a; Marceau-Renaut et al. 2015; Pabst et al. 2009; Tien et al. 2018b; Li et al. 2015; Rockova et al. 2011). Besides, single *CEBPA* mutations frequently co-occur in other well-defined AML entities, while biallelic ones define a specific AML genetic subgroup (Papaemmanuil et al. 2016; Fasan et al. 2014; Dufour et al. 2010; Konstandin et al. 2018; Taskesen et al. 2011; Grossmann et al. 2012). It should be considered that patients with atypical bi*CEBPA* mutations might not achieve results as favorable as classical cases (El-Sharkawi et al. 2018), although further validation of these findings is required. So far, no significant impact of karyotype abnormalities has emerged in this context (Fasan et al. 2014; Schlenk et al. 2013).

### 7.5.4 TP53

*TP53* mutations occur in 10–15% of AML patients. Their incidence increases with age and they are strongly associated with previous chemo-radiotherapy exposure, CK/MK, poor response to intensive chemotherapy, and dismal prognosis (Papaemmanuil et al. 2016; Herold et al. 2020; Metzeler et al. 2016; Grossmann et al. 2012; Prassek et al. 2018; Rücker et al. 2012; Bowen et al. 2009; Haferlach et al. 2008; Kadia et al. 2016; Christiansen et al. 2016; Kihara et al. 2014; Yanada et al. 2016; Stengel et al. 2017; Ok et al. 2015; Stirewalt et al. 2001). Among patients with CK, *TP53* aberrations occur in up to 70% of the cases and worsen survival, even outweighing the role of MK (Rücker et al. 2012). This observation was recently confirmed in a large cohort of patients with myelodysplastic syndromes, including a few low blast count AMLs (International Working Group for MDS Molecular Prognostic Committee et al. 2019). As previously discussed, del(17p), leading to *TP53* inactivation, is associated with poor outcomes in AML and often co-occurs with a *TP53* mutations (Seifert et al. 2009; Rücker et al. 2012). Several studies are focusing on the impact of mono vs. biallelic *TP53* alterations, but, unlike in MDS, data available so far do not clearly demonstrate a worse outcome of patients with *TP53* biallelic involvement (Rücker et al. 2012; Stengel et al. 2017), possibly due to epigenetic mechanisms for bi-allelic TP53 silencing in patients with mono-allelic genetic inactivation (Moison et al. 2019).

Survival of *TP53*-mutated AML remains poor after alloHCT, not exceeding 10–20% at 3–5 years (Qin et al. 2017; Middeke et al. 2016; Della Porta et al. 2016). Interestingly, a recent Japanese study on a vast cohort of MDS and secondary AML patients who underwent alloHCT suggested that patients with *TP53* mutations without CK can experience fairly good long-term outcomes, while those with both aberrations have dismal results (Yoshizato et al. 2017), as already seen in the general intensively treated AML population (Papaemmanuil et al. 2016). Additional observations suggest that highly select subgroups of patients (i.e., very fit and in CR before alloHCT) can achieve long-term survival (Ciurea et al. 2018). It should be noted, however, that the majority of data come from patients with MDS and secondary AML, and it remains to be fully proven that these observations hold true in de novo AML.

### 7.5.5 *RUNX1* and *ASXL1*

*RUNX1* mutations are found in roughly 10% of AML patients—more frequently in the elderly—and have been associated with male gender, secondary AML, and intermediate-risk cytogenetics. Several studies have assessed their prognostic implications, consistently showing reduced CR rate, EFS, and OS (Kihara et al. 2014; Mendler et al. 2012; Tang et al. 2009; Gaidzik et al. 2011, 2016; Schnittger et al. 2011b; Greif et al. 2012). However, recent data suggest that the negative impact of *RUNX1* mutations might be more pronounced in secondary AML and AML with myelodysplasia-related changes, while truly de novo cases could achieve better results despite harboring this abnormality (Quesada et al. 2020; Nguyen et al. 2020; Weinberg et al. 2017). Interestingly, in the two largest studies which explored the impact of an extensive panel of somatic mutations in AML, Papaemmanuil et al. did not find an independent detrimental effect of *RUNX1* mutations on OS (Papaemmanuil et al. 2016), which conversely was significant—but only in patients <60 years—in the report by Metzeler et al. (2016) Of note, a recent study showed that multiple *RUNX1* mutations and loss of wild-type *RUNX1* are associated with a worse prognosis compared to a single mutation (Stengel et al. 2018).

*ASXL1* mutations are also more common in older age, male sex, and secondary AML and have been associated with the presence of trisomy 8. Several studies have linked this aberration with poor otcomes (Papaemmanuil et al. 2016; Grossmann et al. 2012; Devillier et al. 2015a; Pratcorona et al. 2012; Schnittger et al. 2013), although in some cases its impact was not confirmed in multivariate analyses (Metzeler et al. 2016; Fasan et al. 2014; Chou et al. 2010) or was limited to selected subgroups (Patel et al. 2012; Metzeler et al. 2011a).

Given the vast majority of studies showed an independent unfavorable prognostic impact of *RUNX1* and *ASXL1* mutations, particularly when they co-occur (Papaemmanuil et al. 2016; Stengel et al. 2018; Paschka et al. 2015), they were both incorporated in the 2017 ELN classification as adverse risk mutations, except in cases with favorable risk abnormalities (Table 7.2) (Döhner et al. 2017).

### 7.5.6 Other Genes

A partial tandem duplication (PTD) in *KMT2A* is detected in roughly 5% of AML patients. *KMT2A*-PTDs are associated with older age and several reports have shown that this lesion is associated with unfavorable outcome (Schlenk et al. 2008; Kihara et al. 2014; Vetro et al. 2020; Schnittger et al. 2000; Döhner et al. 2002; Shiah et al. 2002; Dicker et al. 2010). However, it has not been uniformly accepted as an independent prognostic marker (Döhner et al. 2017; Grimwade et al. 2016; Bullinger et al. 2017), possibly because of the discordant result of some studies (Metzeler et al. 2016; Fasan et al. 2014; Steudel et al. 2003; Hinai et al. 2019) and the importance of the co-mutation patterns (Papaemmanuil et al. 2016; Hinai et al. 2019).

*DNMT3A* mutations, which are strongly associated with age and clonal hematopoiesis, were shown to be independently associated with unfavorable outcomes (Herold et al. 2020; Grimwade et al. 2016; Ley et al. 2010; Hou et al. 2012; Renneville et al. 2012; Thol et al. 2011; Shen et al. 2011; Ribeiro et al. 2012), but their role was not consistent among all studies as their prognostic role could be influenced by age, co-occurring molecular alterations, and possibly the type of mutations (i.e., R882 versus others) (Papaemmanuil et al. 2016; Metzeler et al. 2016; Bullinger et al. 2017; Gaidzik et al. 2013; Ahn et al. 2016; Marcucci et al. 2012). Likewise, the prognostic role of *TET2 (*Metzeler et al. 2016*;* Patel et al. 2012*;* Chou et al. 2011a*;* Gaidzik et al. 2012*;* Metzeler et al. 2011b*;* Weissmann et al. 2012*;* Nibourel et al. 2010*)* or *WT1 (*Metzeler et al. 2016*;* Patel et al. 2012*;* Virappane et al. 2008*;* Paschka et al. 2008*;* Gaidzik et al. 2009*;* Renneville et al. 2009b*)* mutations has been controversial (Döhner et al. 2017).

The clinical implications of *IDH1* and *IDH2* mutations have been debated as well (Papaemmanuil et al. 2016; Metzeler et al. 2016; Patel et al. 2012; Prassek et al. 2018; Paschka et al. 2010; Marcucci et al. 2010; Peterlin et al. 2015; Boissel et al. 2010, 2011; Chou et al. 2011b; Thol et al. 2010; Abbas et al. 2010), with a recent meta-analysis suggesting a detrimental effect of *IDH1* R132 mutations and a positive impact of *IDH2* aberrations (Xu et al. 2017). However, *IDH2* R140 and R172 mutations should not be grouped together, because they are associated with different co-mutations and clinical outcomes (Papaemmanuil et al. 2016; Boissel et al. 2011; Green et al. 2011). Of note, the role of *IDH1* single nucleotide polymorphism rs11554137 has not been consistent among different reports (Wagner et al. 2010; Ho et al. 2011). The impact of many more recurrently mutated genes in AML has been explored, but results among studies have been globally inconsistent and they do not presently have a recognized prognostic relevance (Bullinger et al. 2017). However, it should be noted that patients belonging to the genetic chromatin-spliceosome group, that is, harboring at least one mutations in splicing (*SRSF2, SF3B1,U2AF1*, and *ZRSR2*), chromatin (*STAG2, BCOR, EZH2*, *PHF6* in addition to *ASXL1*, and *KMT2A-PTD*), or in *RUNX1* in the absence of other class defining lesions, showed very unfavorable outcomes in large patient cohorts (Papaemmanuil et al. 2016; Ahn et al. 2018). Besides, several of these mutations (namely, *SRSF2, SF3B1, U2AF1, ZRSR2, ASXL1, EZH2, BCOR,* and *STAG2*) were shown to be highly specific for secondary AML and define an entity with poor clinical results (Lindsley et al. 2015; Gardin et al. 2020). Nonetheless, more data are required before firm recommendations can be made for these patients.

## 7.6 Integration of Prognostic Factors

Historically, the integration of the prognostic value of cytogenetic and genetic lesions in AML has been done in a hierarchical manner. For instance, gene mutations were initially considered only in patients with normal cytogenetics. Currently, used prognostic classifications rely on a limited number of well-identified, empirically determined pairwise interactions between (cyto) genetic lesions, as exemplified by *NPM1* and *FLT3*-ITD. The identification of mutually exclusive, class-defining "founder" cytogenetic, or molecular lesions, such as CBF translocations, or *NPM1* mutations, has set the ground for the proposal of many class-specific prognostic systems. Indeed, the pattern of co-mutations in AML is particularly complex to decipher and the prognostic impact of different genetic driver combinations is only partially known so far. Thus, with the exception of the NCCN (but not ELN) proposal to account for *KIT* status in CBF leukemias (Döhner et al. 2017; Tallman et al. 2019), none has been sufficiently validated to be implemented in routine practice (Table 7.2).

### 7.6.1 In Specific Molecular Groups

#### 7.6.1.1 CBF-AML

In the cytogenetic subgroup of CBF leukemias, the role of signaling genes has been explored in several studies, most of which have focused on the prognostic influence of *KIT* aberrations, which occur in up to 20–35% of the cases (Faber et al. 2016; Ishikawa et al. 2020; Opatz et al. 2020; Duployez et al. 2016; Itzykson et al. 2018a; Eisfeld et al. 2017). The impact of *KIT* mutations has been globally inconsistent in *CBFB-MYH11* AML (Paschka et al. 2013; Care et al. 2003; Boissel et al. 2006; Riera et al. 2013; Qin et al. 2014; Paschka et al. 2006; Park et al. 2011), while they have been associated with increased relapse risk and worse OS in *RUNX1-RUNX1T1* patients in several (Boissel et al. 2006; Paschka et al. 2006; Park et al. 2011; Cairoli et al. 2006; Schnittger et al. 2006; Rücker et al. 2019; Chen et al. 2016; Kim et al. 2013), but not all (Itzykson et al. 2018a; Klein et al. 2015), reports, including some in which their impact was restricted to a subgroup of *KIT* mutations (e.g., above a certain VAF cutoff or only when present in a specific exon of the gene (Faber et al. 2016; Ishikawa et al. 2020; Opatz et al. 2020; Krauth et al. 2014; Christen et al. 2019; Duployez et al. 2016; Kim et al. 2013; Allen et al. 2013)). While NCCN recommendations take *KIT* mutations into account for *RUNX1-RUNX1T1* patients, suggesting that those cases should be entered in clinical trials and considered for alloHCT in CR1 (Tallman et al. 2019), ELN 2017 guidelines do not account for *KIT* mutations in CBF patients, since their impact is outperformed by measurable residual disease (MRD) (Döhner et al. 2017), as detailed in Chap. 18. *FLT3* aberrations are present in 10–20% of CBF leukemias (Paschka et al. 2013; Christen et al. 2019; Duployez et al. 2016) and there is some evidence (Paschka et al. 2013; Boissel et al. 2006), possibly restricted to *FLT3*-ITD$^{high}$ (Christen et al. 2019), of a negative prognostic role of these alterations. Indeed, a recent international survey on 65 AML patients with CBF-AML and *FLT3*-ITD showed inferior results compared to the general CBF population, with 4-year OS around 50% (Kayser et al. 2019). Nonetheless, this has not been consistently seen (Itzykson et al. 2018a; Santos et al. 2011). Further studies are needed to better understand the impact of *FLT3* aberrations in CBF leukemias, which could be influenced by treatments such as FLT3 inhibitors or gemtuzumab ozogamicin (Cerrano and Itzykson 2019). A few reports also suggested that *JAK2* V617F mutations might be detrimental (Christen et al. 2019; Illmer et al. 2007).

Recently, researchers have focused on the impact of additional genetic lesions belonging to chromatin modifiers/cohesin pathway, which are more prevalent in *RUNX1-RUNX1T1* compared to *CBFB-MYH11* patients (Faber et al. 2016; Duployez et al. 2016) Although these aberrations did not show an independent prognostic impact per se, (Faber et al. 2016; Duployez et al. 2016) they were associated with a poor prognosis in patients with concurrent signaling mutations, hinting at synergic cooperation between these events (Duployez et al. 2016).

#### 7.6.1.2 *NPM1*-Mutated AML

The impact of the co-mutation pattern in the large group of *NPM1*-mutated AML has been extensively studied, and is emerging as one of the most important factors to define the outcome of these patients. As already discussed (see *above*), *FLT3*-ITD plays a major role, while the role of *FLT3*-TKD is debated.

The implications of the presence of *DNMT3A* mutations have been thoroughly studied by Papaemmanuil and colleagues, who found that the adverse prognostic impact of *FLT3*-ITD in *NPM1*-mutated patients was restricted to those with concurrent *DNMT3A* mutations (Papaemmanuil et al. 2016), as suggested in other reports (Patel et al. 2018; Loghavi et al. 2014; Wang et al. 2016; Bezerra et al. 2020). *DNMT3A* was able to influence the prognostic impact of other genetic profiles as well, including *NPM1:NRAS*$^{G12/13}$. Besides, Dunlap and colleagues showed that a reduced OS was associated with the combination *NPM1:DNMT3A:IDH1–2* (Dunlap et al. 2019) and Papaemmanuil et al. found that *NPM1:IDH2* patients had reduced CR and increased relapse rates (Papaemmanuil et al. 2016), consistent with some (Paschka et al. 2010), but not all (Patel et al. 2012), previous observations.

#### 7.6.1.3 bi*CEBPA* AML

Frequent co-mutations in bi*CEBPA*-mutated patients affect the *GATA2* (Greif et al. 2012) and *CSF3R* (Lavallée et al. 2016) genes, while mutations in chromatin, cohesin, and splicing genes are less frequent (Wilhelmson and Porse 2020). Mutations of the latter groups, in particular of *WT1* (Tien et al. 2018b) or *TET2* (Fasan et al. 2014; Grossmann et al. 2013a), have been associated with lower response and survival rates (Konstandin et al. 2018). Besides, some evidence suggests that the presence of *FLT3*-ITD, which is rarely found in bi*CEBPA* AML, could impact on the favorable outcomes of this entity (Green et al. 2010; Zhang et al. 2019), but this finding was not consistent in all reports (Tien et al. 2018b; Grossmann et al. 2013a). The unfavorable impact of other signaling mutations, including *CSF3R*, is even more controversial (Konstandin et al. 2018; Zhang et al. 2019; Su et al. 2018, 2019). Conversely, *GATA2* mutations were shown to exert a favorable impact in earlier reports (Grossmann et al. 2013a; Fasan et al. 2013, 2014), but this finding was not confirmed in recent studies (Su et al. 2018; Theis et al. 2016).

#### 7.6.1.4 *KMT2A*-Rearranged AML

The signaling/RAS pathway is the most frequently mutated in *KMT2A*-rearranged AML and its alterations have been shown to be associated with chemotherapy residence in experimental models (Esposito 2019). However, unlike in *KMT2A*-rearranged infant ALL (Driessen et al. 2013), no clear prognostic impact has been observed in AML (Vetro et al. 2020; Grossmann et al. 2013b). Conversely, concurrent *TP53* mutations might be associated with reduced OS (Grossmann et al. 2013b).

#### 7.6.1.5 *DEK-NUP214* AML

*FLT3*-ITD is present in roughly 70% of patients harboring *DEK-NUP214*, but its prognostic impact has been controversial in this context. While earlier data suggested a detrimental effect (Thiede et al. 2007), additional studies could not confirm this finding (Díaz-Beyá et al. 2020; Sandahl et al. 2014; Tarlock et al. 2014).

### 7.6.2 In Specific Clinical Groups

Most of our knowledge on the prognostic impact of genetic aberrations come from cohorts of younger AML patients enrolled in clinical trials. However, things might be different in biologically distinct subgroups, which are underrepresented in most studies.

#### 7.6.2.1 Older Patients

Median age of AML diagnosis isabove 65 years, but data on the prognostic impact of genetic aberrations are less abundant in older patients.The favorable prognostic role of *NPM1* mutations has been challenged in this context (Straube et al. 2018; Prassek et al. 2018; Becker et al. 2010; Lazenby et al. 2014; Juliusson et al. 2020). Some reports confirmed the relatively favorable outcome of these patients, although they rarely reached a long-term survival plateau indicative of cure (Hefazi et al. 2015; Daver et al. 2013; Büchner et al. 2009; Scholl et al. 2008). Data from the Southwest Oncology Group (SWOG) showed that isolated *NPM1*-mutated patients >65 years had unfavorable results even early after diagnosis (2 year-OS around 30%) (Ostronoff et al. 2015).The relatively favorable outcome of *NPM1*-mutated AML thus results fromtheir chemosensitivity, andis thus dependent on treatment intensity. This illustrates the need to interpret prognosis in a given therapeutic context. This becomes challenging in a dynamic therapeutic landscape (see Chap 12).

In addition, the impact of other mutations has been controversial, including *FLT3-ITD* (Straube et al. 2018; Prassek et al. 2018; Juliusson et al. 2020; Heiblig et al. 2019). Differences in the patterns of co-mutations between older and younger patients could contribute to these differences (Prassek et al. 2018; Silva et al. 2017).

Globally, the applicability of current prognostic stratifications has been weaker in patients above 60 years (Mrózek et al. 2012; Röllig et al. 2011). Thus, specific prognostic classification systems have been developed in this population (Eisfeld et al. 2018; Itzykson et al. 2018b; Tsai et al. 2016). Recently, in a large cohort of intensively treated patients above 60 years, the ALFA group showed that the presence of secondary AML-type mutations (as defined by Lindsley et al. (2015), excluding *ASXL1*) could refine the 2017 ELN classification, identifying among intermediate-risk patients those with worse outcome whocould possibly benefit from alloHCT (Gardin et al. 2020). These new classification systems have yet to be validated in independent cohorts.

#### 7.6.2.2 Childhood AML

AML is a rare disease in children, with significant biological and clinical differences compared to adult disease. The molecular landscape of pediatric AML is different, lacking almost entirely certain aberrations relevant for adults (e.g., *DNMT3A* mutations (Bolouri et al. 2018)), but being enriched for other entities virtually absent in adults.

Acute megakaryoblast leukemia (AMKL) is not uncommon in infants and young children. While in patients with Down Syndrome (DS)—generally experiencing positive results—this entity has been associated with *GATA1* mutations and excellent long-term OS (around 90%) in recent studies (Taub et al. 2017), clinical results in non-DS patients is more heterogeneous. AMKL patients with t(1;22)(p13;q13) leading to the *RBM15-MKL1* translocation (Ma et al. 2001) generally show intermediate-to-favorable outcomes. Those harboring the *CBFA2T3-GLIS2* fusion gene, which characterizes an extremely aggressive subtype—frequent in non-DS AMKL leukemia but not limited to this entity—experience dismal outcomes (de Rooij et al. 2017; Masetti et al. 2019; Inaba et al. 2015).

CBF leukemias, which are more common among older children and adolescents, are associated with favorable prognosis, like in the adult population (Harrison et al. 2010; von Neuhoff et al. 2010). Recently, a rare entity characterized by the t(16;21)(q24;q22), resulting in the *RUNX1-CBFA2T3* fusion and whose gene expression profile resembles that of *RUNX1-RUNX1T1* AML, was shown to be associated with favorable outcomes. Conversely, a completely different entity characterized by the t(16;21)(p11;q22) translocation resulting in the fusion *FUS-ERG* has been associated with very poor survival (Noort et al. 2018).

*KMT2A* rearrangements are significantly more common in children than adults, being observed in roughly 20% of AML cases, especially in infants and young children. Globally, the outcome of *KMT2A*-rearranged AML is considered similar to that of patients not harboring this abnormality, thus intermediate (Harrison et al. 2010; von Neuhoff et al. 2010; Marceau-Renaut et al. 2018). However, this subgroup is quite heterogeneous, with some entities such as t(10;11)(p12;q23) and t(6;11) (q27;q23) being associated with poor prognosis, while others, such as t(1;11)(q21;q23), showing favorable outcomes. Of note, the positive results reported in some studies for t(9;11)(p22;q23), the most common *KMT2A* translocation, were not confirmed in a large retrospective international report (Balgobind et al. 2009, 2011).

*NPM1* mutations, which are less frequent in children compared to adults, are also relatively favorable in this context (Bolouri et al. 2018; Hollink et al. 2009). Conversely, the prognostic role of *FLT3*-ITD has been more controversial, although a detrimental effect was demonstrated in the majority of reports, especially in cases with *FLT3*-ITD$^{high}$ (Marceau-Renaut et al. 2018; Meshinchi et al. 2006; Manara et al. 2017; Shimada et al. 2018; Wu et al. 2016). The *NUP98-*

*NSD1* fusion gene, which is cryptic at conventional karyotype analysis and more frequent in children and young adults (Hollink et al. 2011; Thol et al. 2013), exerts a negative prognostic role which is significantly increased by the presence of *FLT3*-ITD, leading to CR rates below 30% and dismal long-term OS (Ostronoff et al. 2014). Indeed, this was recently confirmed by Bolouri and colleagues, who demonstrated that *FLT3*-ITD positive patients' prognosis could be stratified according to co-occurring aberrations: while those with concomitant *NPM1* mutations were confirmed to experience rather favorable outcomes, *FLT3*-ITD in association with *NUP98-NSD1* (or *WT1* mutations) was associated with reduced CR rate and dismal EFS (Bolouri et al. 2018). The role of another *NUP98* rearrangement, *NUP98-KDM5A*, which demonstrated a trend toward poor outcomes in non-DS AMKL (de Rooij et al. 2017), was explored in a recent large multinational pediatric study outside AMKL. *NUP98-KDM5A* was associated with different clinical features compared to *NUP98-NSD1,* but retained an adverse prognosis (Noort et al. 2021).

Although the impact of several—but not all—adult AML prognostic factors was often confirmed in children, including recent data on *RUNX1* mutations (Yamato et al. 2018), the performance of stratification systems developed in the adult population is less robust in pediatric patients. Recently, the French group showed that ELN 2017 classification was able to identify good risk patients but failed to separate intermediate from adverse risk ones. Conversely, the presence of *NUP98* fusions, *WT1*, *RUNX1*, and *PHF6* mutations were able to identify a poor molecular subgroup with 3-year OS below 50%, underling the need of larger studies to better clarify the impact of gene mutations in pediatric AML and to improve patients' stratification (Marceau-Renaut et al. 2018).

#### 7.6.2.3 Secondary AML

Secondary AML (sAML) occurring after an antecedent MDS (or more rarely MPN or MDS/MPN) is an entity distinct from WHO-defined therapy-related myeloid neoplasms (t-MN, when blasts are $\geq$20%). The WHO classification proposed to group sAML along with de novo AML presenting with myelodysplasia-related cytogenetic or morphologic changes (Arber et al. 2016), while others have attempted to identify a molecular portrait of sAML (notably mutations in *SRSF2, SF3B1, U2AF1, ZRSR2, ASXL1, EZH2, BCOR,* and *STAG2*) that could then be applied to de novo AML to define "secondary-type" AML (Lindsley et al. 2015).

Secondary AML has historically been associated with unfavorable outcome (Arber et al. 2016; Kuykendall et al. 2018), but this category is heterogeneous. Response to treatment and prognosis can vary considerably among patients. Along with clinical differences (e.g., s-AML arising from myeloproliferative neoplasms is associated with worse outcome compared to AML secondary to MDS (Granfeldt Østgård et al. 2015)), the genetic profile plays a major role. Cytogenetic risk stratification remains a major determinant of outcome in sAML, although unfavorable subtypes are overrepresented compared to de novo cases. Most, but not all (Schoch et al. 2004), studies suggested that the clinical prognostic factors of AML with myelodysplasia-related changes or t-MN could lose their significance when cytogenetic risk is taken into account, outlining the importance of this parameter in this context (Devillier et al. 2015b; Armand et al. 2007; Ossenkoppele and Montesinos 2019). Specifically, favorable translocations such as t(15;17) or CBF translocations induced by anthracyclines/epipodophyllotoxins exposures retain their favorable prognosis in t-MNs (Braun et al. 2015; Heuser 2016). Other therapy-related AML, notably those induced by alkylating agents, are characterized by a high frequency of *TP53* mutations (Ok et al. 2015; Christiansen et al. 2001). Globally, adverse risk mutations have been shown to maintain their adverse impact in sAML and t-AML (Rücker et al. 2012; Devillier et al. 2015a).

#### 7.6.2.4 Relapsed AML

Even though the impact of genetic aberrations at AML relapse has not been completely explored so far, it is emerging as one of the most important predictors of response to treatment and patients' long-term outcomes (Montesinos et al. 2019). In intensively treated patients, the role of cytogenetics has been confirmed, with patients with CBF leukemias, especially those with *CBFB-MYH11,* showing relatively high salvage rates, adverse cytogenetic abnormalities being associated with poor prognosis (Breems et al. 2005; Chevallier et al. 2011). Among gene mutations, bi*CEBPA* have been associated with relatively good salvage rates while *NPM1* mutations do not seem to exert a positive impact in this context (Schlenk et al. 2017; Bergua et al. 2016). Relapsed patients with *FLT3*-ITD have been consistently shown to obtain dismal results with conventional treatments and *IDH1* mutations have emerged as a negative prognostic factor in a recent report as well (Wattad et al. 2017). This picture will probably change with the advent of novel targeted therapies (Cerrano and Itzykson 2019). Indeed, considering the frequent changes in the molecular landscape compared to diagnosis (Greif et al. 2018), obtaining a detailed genetic reassessment at relapse before choosing the therapeutic approach is now mandatory (detailed in Chaps. 11–12).

## 7.7 Clonal Architecture

Despite significant progresses, the extensive cytogenetic and mutational characterization routinely obtained at AML diagnosis cannot comprehensively depict its biological basis, and it is not always able to accurately estimate disease behavior and response to treatments in individual patients. Thus, other aspects of AML are being explored to improve patients' stratification.

As discussed *supra, FLT3*-ITD impact strongly depends on its mutated/wild-type ratio, prompting its integration in current guidelines (Döhner et al. 2017). Besides, the clinical implications of mutational burden are emerging for several candidate genes in specific contexts. Several studies found that *KIT* and *FLT3*-ITD prognostic impact in CBF leukemias was restricted to those above a certain burden threshold (Christen et al. 2019; Duployez et al. 2016; Allen et al. 2013), likewise *FLT3*-TKD or *NRAS/KRAS* mutations in other reports (Mead et al. 2007; Duployez et al. 2016). A recent study by Patel and colleagues suggested that *NPM1* mutational burden could also be important. The authors showed that patients with *NPM1* mutations having a variant allele frequency (VAF) above the upper quartile had a significantly reduced OS, independently of other baseline known prognostic variables (Patel et al. 2018). However, this finding has been mitigated (Linch et al. 2020), or infirmed (Abbas et al. 2019), in the following reports, suggesting that *NPM1* VAF impact might be mostly due to co-mutations and/or a reflection of higher leukemia burden. Several reports explored the impact of the allele burden of other mutations, including *DNMT3A* (Yuan et al. 2019), *TP53* (Prochazka et al. 2019), and *ASXL1* (Sasaki et al. 2020), without being validated so far. With the possible exception of *FLT3*-ITD, further validation and better standardization methods (Touw and Sanders 2020) are thus necessary to account for mutational burden for daily prognostic purposes.

Mounting evidence suggests that a better understanding of clonal architecture may refine risk stratification. Intra-tumor heterogeneity is associated with unfavorable outcomes in many cancers (Andor et al. 2016), but its precise role remains to be defined in AML. Indeed, a higher number of driver lesions has been proven to be a marker of poor prognosis (Papaemmanuil et al. 2016; Wakita et al. 2016). However, whether this unfavorable outcome has to be attributed to the additive fitness of driver lesions accumulated in a single clone or to the presence of clonal heterogeneity is not clear. In CBF leukemias, the presence of clonal interference, that is, the co-existence of clones sharing a common ancestor and harboring independent lesions targeting the same pathway—signaling in this case—was associated with reduced event-free survival, independent of other baseline clinical variables and MRD (Itzykson et al. 2018a). Besides, a higher number of clones, as assessed by conventional cytogenetic, was shown to worsen prognosis in AML, but mainly in the context of complex karyotype (Bochtler et al. 2013; Medeiros et al. 2015), while clonal dominance, as assessed by the Shannon diversity Index (Maley et al. 2017), may worsen prognosis (Cerrano et al. 2021). Further efforts are needed to fully understand the impact of clonal architecture and dynamics on AML behavior.

## 7.8 Other Biological Risk Factors

Additional biological factors have been explored in AML, with a vast number of studies outlying their prognostic implications. Although the majority of the data we present below do not affect the clinical management of AML patients in current practice, with the implementation of more comprehensive diagnostic platforms some of the risk factors described below might soon be integrated in prognostic stratification algorithms.

### 7.8.1 Gene Expression

Several studies have focused on the impact of the over-expression of certain genes. One of the most extensively studied is *MECOM* (or *EVI1*), the hallmark of inv(3)/t(3;3), which is overexpressed also in up to 10% of AML cases that do not carry any 3q aberrations, most commonly in those harboring monosomy 7 and 11q23 abnormalitis (Hinai and Valk 2016). High *MECOM* expression was associated with unfavorable outcomes in several studies, especially in CN (Barjesteh van Waalwijk van Doorn-Khosrovani et al. 2003; Gröschel et al. 2010; Lugthart et al. 2008; Valk et al. 2004) and *KMT2A*-rearranged AML (Gröschel et al. 2013), thus assigning patients to the adverse risk group according to some authors (Cornelissen and Blaise 2016). The overexpression of other genes (Damm et al. 2011), including *BAALC* (Weber et al. 2014; Torrebadell et al. 2018; Schwind et al. 2010a; Baldus et al. 2006; Langer et al. 2008), *ERG* (Schwind et al. 2010a; Metzeler et al. 2009; Marcucci et al. 2005b, 2007), and *MN1* (Langer et al. 2009), has been linked to adverse outcome as well, but their independent prognostic value has been questioned due to the correlations with relevant genetic alterations (Weber et al. 2016). They are not employed to stratify patients' risk by current guidelines (Döhner et al. 2017; Tallman et al. 2019).

Additional efforts have been made to derive gene expression profiles (GEP) to stratify AML patients. Among many signatures and scores proposed (Gentles et al. 2010; Jung et al. 2015; Levine et al. 2015; Metzeler et al. 2008; Eppert et al. 2011; Marcucci et al. 2014; Bullinger et al. 2004; Li et al. 2013), Ng and colleagues established a panel of 17 genes defining a "stemness" signature called LSC17 (i.e., indicating overrepresented gene sets with stem cell-like properties), the expression of which was highly indicative of poor clinical outcomes in multiple AML cohorts (Ng et al. 2016; Duployez et al. 2019), even in the context of ELN 2017 classification (Bill et al. 2020). In this regard, it has been suggested the applicability and performance of genetic signatures might be improved if restricted to defined patient subgroups (Wiggers et al. 2019). Interestingly, Herold and colleagues recently validated a score integrating 29 gene expression markers and the MRC cytogenetic risk groups. This score which was able to accurately predict resistance to induction chemotherapy, outperforming currently available models (Herold et al. 2018).

In addition, also microRNA expression might play a role in CN-AML stratification (Marcucci et al. 2008). The up-regulation of miR-181a was shown to be associated with favorable prognosis, whereas higher expression of miR-155, miR-196b, and miR-644 was independently associated with shorter overall survival (Schwind et al. 2010b; Marcucci et al. 2013; Díaz-Beyá et al. 2014). Expression signatures of large non-coding RNAs, such as long intergenic non-coding RNAs (lincRNA) involved in gene expression regulation and cell lineage and differentiation, have demonstrated added prognostic value to standard cytogenetic and genetic molecular stratification (Beck et al. 2018).

### 7.8.2 Flow Cytometry

Flow cytometry has entered routine clinical practice in AML diagnosis, almost completely replacing cytochemical stains. Besides, the prognostic implications of the immunophenotypic characterization of AML blasts have been extensively explored.

For instance, the expression of CD25 (IL-2 receptor alpha) has been associated with reduced response to chemotherapy and inferior survival (Nakase et al. 1997; Fujiwara et al. 2017) and CD105 was shown to be associated with unfavorable outcomes in AML (Kauer et al. 2019), including in the HCT setting (Märklin et al. 2020). Many additional immunophenotypic markers have been shown to exert a meaningful prognostic impact, including but not limited to CD7, CD56, CD82, CD93, CXCR4, CD262, CD120a, hMICL, CD96,CD11b, CD117, CD34, CD13, CD14, CD15 (Chisini et al. 2017), some of these recently reviewed by Costa et al. (2017), but these and the aforementioned findings have neither been consistent nor been robustly validated in adequately sized independent cohorts.

The combination of multiple immunophenotypic markers could also be prognostically informative. Initial studies suggested that patterns of myeloid lineage differentiation could impact on outcomes (Repp et al. 2003); however, results have been inconsistent (Mason et al. 2006). Recently, the co-expression of CD56, CD123, CD4 was shown to identify a subgroup of *NPM1*-mutated patients with blastic plasmacytoid dendritic cell neoplasm (BPDCN)-like AML with poor prognosis, an intriguing finding which needs to be validated (Minetto et al. 2018).

Globally, the prognostic value of immunophenotype has been difficult to reproduce, probably because of the size and heterogeneity of patient cohorts, and difficulties to standardize MFC in a multicentric way. Besides, the association of immunophenotypic markers with relevant genetic alterations interferes with their prognostic impact (van Solinge et al. 2018), which has not been firmly proven to add independent information so far.

### 7.8.3 Proteomic

The impact of protein expression in AML has been studied for more the 20 years, with earlier reports focusing mostly on the impact of proteins involved in chemotherapy resistance, such as P-glycoprotein (the *MDR1* gene product), MRP1 (multidrug resistance-associated protein 1), and LRP (lung resistance protein). The majority of these reports associated the hyperexpression of these proteins with worse prognosis, especially for P-glycoprotein, albeit with some inconsistencies (Pirker et al. 1991; Leith et al. 1997, 1999; Tsuji et al. 2000; Legrand et al. 1998; Laupeze et al. 2002).

In addition, several studies assessed the impact of the hyperexpression of anti-apoptotic proteins (e.g., BCL-2 and survivin) or pro-apoptotic ones (e.g., measuring BAX levels or BAX/BCL2 ratio) suggesting they can affect outcomes in opposite ways, although with some contrasting results (Ong et al. 2000; Lauria et al. 1997; Del Poeta et al. 2003; Karakas et al. 2002; Carter et al. 2012; Venditti et al. 2004; Zhou et al. 2019a).

Subsequent functional protein studies showed that signal transduction pathways activation had an adverse effect on prognosis (Kornblau et al. 2006), and that specific functional proteomic profiles correlated with known morphologic features, cytogenetics, and outcome (Kornblau et al. 2009, 2010a, 2011).

Investigators also explored the role of circulating cytokines and chemokines, which were shown to be differently expressed in AML compared to healthy controls and whose patterns of expression might have prognostic relevance (Kornblau et al. 2010b). Many of these studies were performed before the genomics era. Thus, the independence prognostic value of protein expression in AML remains to be determined.

### 7.8.4 DNA Methylation

Deregulation of DNA methylation plays a key role in AML pathogenesis, and genes involved in its regulations (i.e., *DNMT3A, TET2, IDH1/2*) are among the most frequently mutated in AML. Along with these gene mutations (discussed *supra*), several studies have explored the clinical and prognostic implications of DNA methylation patterns. Unsupervised clustering analysis demonstrated that some cytogenetic subgroups (e.g., CBF leukemias) are associated with distinct epigenetic modifications. Besides, DNA methylation signatures could also sub-stratify large genetic groups, such as *NPM1*-mutated AML, possibly identifying new clinically relevant disease entities (The Cancer Genome Atlas Research Network 2013; Bullinger et al. 2010; Figueroa et al. 2010).

Aberrant DNA methylation was shown to be independently associated with outcomes (Deneberg et al. 2010; Li et al. 2016), and specific quantitative methylation patterns could give significant prognostic information. Further studies suggested that aberrant methylation of individual (Deneberg et al. 2010; Lin et al. 2011; Yang et al. 2019) or multiple genes (Marcucci et al. 2014; Figueroa et al. 2010; Deneberg et al. 2011; Jost et al. 2014) was associated with clinical outcomes.

In addition, the level of hydroxy-methylation, measured by 5-hydroxymethylcytosine levels, was shown to offer meaningful prognostic information (Kroeze et al. 2014), although these findings need validation.

Beyond clinical validation, simple and reliable methylation assays are warranted before these potential biomarkers enter yet clinical practice. Recently, Luskin and colleagues developed a microsphere-based assay for simultaneous assessment of DNA methylation status at multiple loci and generated, in relatively large AML cohort, a methylation-based risk score (M-score), which was independently associated with CR and OS probability, and validated in independent cohorts (Luskin et al. 2016; DiNardo et al. 2017). This approach, if confirmed robust in additional studies, might be implemented in routine AML diagnostic panels.

## 7.9 Global Risk Assessment Strategies

Currently available (cyto)genetic prognostic stratification models are simple and provide reliable prognostic stratification (Table 7.2). Their performance has improved over time. Indeed, ELN 2017 classification has been validated, and was shown to be globally superior to previous stratification models (Döhner et al. 2017; Boddu et al. 2019; Harada et al. 2018). Further improvements to ELN 2017 could be brought by the inclusion of additional genes on its backbone (Herold et al. 2020; Gardin et al. 2020).

However, clinical parameters, such as age, WBC count, performance status, or previous hematologic malignancies, exert a meaningful prognostic impact and interact with genetic parameters to influence patients' outcome (Papaemmanuil et al. 2016). Recommendations for alloHCT in CR1 are starting to incorporate most of these factors and weighting them against the risk of non-relapse mortality in an integrated system aiming to develop a tailored approach to the individual patient (Cornelissen and Blaise 2016; Cornelissen et al. 2012).

To integrate cytogenetic, molecular, and clinical factors in a more objective way, different scoring systems have been proposed (Pastore et al. 2014b; Stölzel et al. 2011; Zhou et al. 2019b; Malagola et al. 2011), but they are not able to keep up with complex and frequently changing molecular data and their use is not widespread. Indeed, the comparison of various risk stratification tools based on genetics and/or gene expression profiling revealed that several of them can add significantly to the current prognostic models (Wang et al. 2017), but it has been difficult to incorporate them in clinical practice.

It is now clear that approaches based on a hierarchical, step-by-step integration of (cyto)genetic lesions are currently reaching their limit. First, not all gene lesions may have the same impact. This is well known for *FLT3* (ITD vs TKD) or *KMT2A* (fusions vs PTD, fusion depending on partner). Other examples may include *DNMT3A* (R882 vs others) (Peterlin et al. 2015) or *KIT* (exon 8 vs 17) (Paschka et al. 2013). Second, three-gene interactions have recently been reported to be of major importance in patients stratification (Papaemmanuil et al. 2016; Bezerra et al. 2020).

To overcome these limitations, two approaches have been undertaken, the first relying on the integration of (cyto)genetic lesions into a global "clonal architecture" of each AML to derive prognosis (see *supra*). The second relies on machine learning approaches to integrate all available prognostic information layers, agnostic to biological studies on specific genetic interactions. Gerstung and colleagues recently reported on a "knowledge bank approach" (Gerstung et al. 2017) able to improve OS prediction compared to current risk classifications, thanks to the use of matched genomic–clinical data derived from over 1500 AML patients (Papaemmanuil et al. 2016). Importantly, this multistage model was able to predict the probability of different causes of mortality in each patient (i.e., death without remission, death after relapse, death without relapse), and to weight the impact of alloHCT on these probabilities. The use of this system might significantly impact on patients' care, and the authors estimated that this tailored approach could reduce the number of alloHCT by 20–25%, while maintaining OS rates. An online tool, which allows an accurate prediction even if some of the data originally used for the development of the model are missing, was also developed (https://cancer.sanger.ac.uk/aml-multistage). The performance of this "knowledge bank" approach was recently validated in the real life setting (Huet et al. 2018) and could possibly be combined with ELN2017 risk stratification to optimize indications of alloHCT in CR1 (Fenwarth et al. 2019). Knowledge banks could optimize personally tailored therapeutic decisions; however, they require frequent updating. As new effective drugs are becoming available (Cerrano and Itzykson 2019), the survival estimation of a given patient might become inaccurate if the knowledge bank relies only on data of patients treated with "3 + 7" like traditional chemotherapy program. Besides, inclusive cohorts are necessary, not to underrepresent certain subgroups (e.g., elderly patients less often enrolled in clinical trials) and all the important prognostic factors identified should ideally be considered, including recently discovered ones (Walker et al. 2019; Nibourel et al. 2017), stressing the need for constant update. Finally, such global risk assessment strategies will increasingly rely on MRD (see Chap. 18), which have yet to be implemented in these models (Schuurhuis et al. 2018; Estey and Gale 2017; Patkar et al. 2019). Large cohorts are required to accurately estimate the impact of rare co-mutational patterns, as discussed *supra*. International consortia, such as the European Union funded HARMONY project, will likely be instrumental to that prospect (Bullinger et al. 2019). Such "big data" analyses including many layers of information are hoped to be a turning point on the road toward precision medicine in AML.

## References

Abaza Y, Cortes J, Ravandi F et al (2018) Prognostic significance of hyperdiploidy in adult acute myeloid leukemia. Am J Hematol 93(11):E357–E360

Abbas S, Lugthart S, Kavelaars FG et al (2010) Acquired mutations in the genes encoding IDH1 and IDH2 both are recurrent aberrations in acute myeloid leukemia: prevalence and prognostic value. Blood 116(12):2122–2126

Abbas HA, Ravandi F, Loghavi S et al (2019) NPM1 mutant variant allele frequency correlates with leukemia burden but does not provide prognostic information in NPM1-mutated acute myeloid leukemia. Am J Hematol 94(6):E158–E160

Ahn J-S, Kim H-J, Kim Y-K et al (2016) DNMT3A R882 mutation with FLT3-ITD positivity is an extremely poor prognostic factor in patients with normal-karyotype acute myeloid leukemia after allogeneic hematopoietic cell transplantation. Biol Blood Marrow Transplant 22(1):61–70

Ahn J-S, Kim H-J, Kim Y-K et al (2018) Assessment of a new genomic classification system in acute myeloid leukemia with a normal karyotype. Oncotarget 9(4):4961–4968

Allen C, Hills RK, Lamb K et al (2013) The importance of relative mutant level for evaluating impact on outcome of KIT, FLT3 and CBL mutations in core-binding factor acute myeloid leukemia. Leukemia 27(9):1891–1901

Andor N, Graham TA, Jansen M et al (2016) Pan-cancer analysis of the extent and consequences of intratumor heterogeneity. Nat Med 22(1):105–113

Angenendt L, Röllig C, Montesinos P et al (2019) Chromosomal abnormalities and prognosis in NPM1-mutated acute myeloid Leukemia: a pooled analysis of individual patient data from nine international cohorts. JCO. 37(29):2632–2642

Appelbaum FR, Gundacker H, Head DR et al (2006a) Age and acute myeloid leukemia. Blood 107(9):3481–3485

Appelbaum FR, Kopecky KJ, Tallman MS et al (2006b) The clinical spectrum of adult acute myeloid leukaemia associated with core binding factor translocations. Br J Haematol 135(2):165–173

Arber DA, Orazi A, Hasserjian R et al (2016) The 2016 revision to the World Health Organization classification of myeloid neoplasms and acute leukemia. Blood 127(20):2391–2405

Armand P, Kim HT, DeAngelo DJ et al (2007) Impact of cytogenetics on outcome of de novo and therapy-related AML and MDS after allogeneic transplantation. Biol Blood Marrow Transplant 13(6):655–664

Arreba-Tutusaus P, Mack T, Bullinger L et al (2016) Impact of FLT3-ITD location on sensitivity to TKI-therapy in vitro and in vivo. Leukemia 30(5):1220–1225

Bacher U, Haferlach C, Kern W, Haferlach T, Schnittger S (2008) Prognostic relevance of FLT3-TKD mutations in AML: the combination matters—an analysis of 3082 patients. Blood 111(5):2527–2537

Baldus CD, Thiede C, Soucek S et al (2006) BAALC expression and FLT3 internal tandem duplication mutations in acute myeloid leukemia patients with normal cytogenetics: prognostic implications. J Clin Oncol 24(5):790–797

Balgobind BV, Raimondi SC, Harbott J et al (2009) Novel prognostic subgroups in childhood 11q23/MLL-rearranged acute myeloid leukemia: results of an international retrospective study. Blood 114(12):2489–2496

Balgobind BV, Zwaan CM, Pieters R, Van den Heuvel-Eibrink MM (2011) The heterogeneity of pediatric MLL-rearranged acute myeloid leukemia. Leukemia 25(8):1239–1248

Balsat M, Renneville A, Thomas X et al (2017) Postinduction minimal residual disease predicts outcome and benefit from allogeneic stem cell transplantation in acute myeloid leukemia with *NPM1* mutation: a study by the Acute Leukemia French Association Group. J Clin Oncol 35(2):185–193

Barjesteh van Waalwijk van Doorn-Khosrovani S, Erpelinck C, van Putten WLJ et al (2003) High EVI1 expression predicts poor survival in acute myeloid leukemia: a study of 319 de novo AML patients. Blood 101(3):837–845

Beck D, Thoms JAI, Palu C et al (2018) A four-gene LincRNA expression signature predicts risk in multiple cohorts of acute myeloid leukemia patients. Leukemia 32(2):263–272

Becker H, Marcucci G, Maharry K et al (2010) Favorable prognostic impact of NPM1 mutations in older patients with cytogenetically normal de novo acute myeloid leukemia and associated gene- and microRNA-expression signatures: a Cancer and Leukemia Group B study. J Clin Oncol 28(4):596–604

Bergua JM, Montesinos P, Martinez-Cuadrón D et al (2016) A prognostic model for survival after salvage treatment with FLAG-Ida +/− gemtuzumab-ozogamicine in adult patients with refractory/relapsed acute myeloid leukaemia. Br J Haematol 174(5):700–710

Bezerra MF, Lima AS, Piqué-Borràs M-R et al (2020) Co-occurrence of DNMT3A, NPM1, FLT3 mutations identifies a subset of acute myeloid leukemia with adverse prognosis. Blood 135(11):870–875

Bhatnagar B, Blachly JS, Kohlschmidt J et al (2016) Clinical features and gene- and microRNA-expression patterns in adult acute leukemia patients with t(11;19)(q23;p13.1) and t(11;19)(q23;p13.3). Leukemia 30(7):1586–1589

Bhatt VR (2019) Personalizing therapy for older adults with acute myeloid leukemia: role of geriatric assessment and genetic profiling. Cancer Treat Rev 75:52–61

Bill M, Nicolet D, Kohlschmidt J et al (2020) Mutations associated with a 17-gene leukemia stem cell score and the score's prognostic relevance in the context of the European LeukemiaNet classification of acute myeloid leukemia. Haematologica 105(3):721–729

Blau O, Berenstein R, Sindram A, Blau IW (2013) Molecular analysis of different FLT3-ITD mutations in acute myeloid leukemia. Leuk Lymphoma 54(1):145–152

Bloomfield CD, Archer KJ, Mrózek K et al (2002) 11q23 balanced chromosome aberrations in treatment-related myelodysplastic syndromes and acute leukemia: report from an international workshop. Genes Chromosomes Cancer 33(4):362–378

Bochtler T, Stölzel F, Heilig CE et al (2013) Clonal heterogeneity as detected by metaphase karyotyping is an indicator of poor prognosis in acute myeloid leukemia. J Clin Oncol 31(31):3898–3905

Bochtler T, Granzow M, Stölzel F et al (2017) Marker chromosomes can arise from chromothripsis and predict adverse prognosis in acute myeloid leukemia. Blood 129(10):1333–1342

Boddu P, Kantarjian H, Borthakur G et al (2017) Co-occurrence of FLT3-TKD and NPM1 mutations defines a highly favorable prognostic AML group. Blood Adv 1(19):1546–1550

Boddu P, Gurguis C, Sanford D et al (2018) Response kinetics and factors predicting survival in core-binding factor leukemia. Leukemia 32(12):2698–2701

Boddu PC, Kadia TM, Garcia-Manero G et al (2019) Validation of the 2017 European LeukemiaNet classification for acute myeloid leukemia with NPM1 and FLT3-internal tandem duplication genotypes. Cancer 125(7):1091–1100

Boissel N, Renneville A, Biggio V et al (2005) Prevalence, clinical profile, and prognosis of NPM mutations in AML with normal karyotype. Blood 106(10):3618–3620

Boissel N, Leroy H, Brethon B et al (2006) Incidence and prognostic impact of c-kit, FLT3, and Ras gene mutations in core binding factor acute myeloid leukemia (CBF-AML). Leukemia 20(6):965–970

Boissel N, Nibourel O, Renneville A et al (2010) Prognostic impact of isocitrate dehydrogenase enzyme isoforms 1 and 2 mutations in acute myeloid leukemia: a study by the Acute Leukemia French Association Group. J Clin Oncol 28(23):3717–3723

Boissel N, Nibourel O, Renneville A et al (2011) Differential prognosis impact of IDH2 mutations in cytogenetically normal acute myeloid leukemia. Blood 117(13):3696–3697

Bolouri H, Farrar JE, Triche T et al (2018) The molecular landscape of pediatric acute myeloid leukemia reveals

recurrent structural alterations and age-specific mutational interactions. Nat Med 24(1):103–112
Bonanad S, De la Rubia J, Gironella M et al (2015) Development and psychometric validation of a brief comprehensive health status assessment scale in older patients with hematological malignancies: the GAH scale. J Geriatr Oncol 6(5):353–361
Bowen D, Groves MJ, Burnett AK et al (2009) TP53 gene mutation is frequent in patients with acute myeloid leukemia and complex karyotype, and is associated with very poor prognosis. Leukemia 23(1):203–206
Bower H, Andersson TM-L, Björkholm M et al (2016) Continued improvement in survival of acute myeloid leukemia patients: an application of the loss in expectation of life. Blood Cancer J 6(2):e390
Braun T, Cereja S, Chevret S et al (2015) Evolving characteristics and outcome of secondary acute promyelocytic leukemia (APL): a prospective analysis by the French-Belgian-Swiss APL Group. Cancer 121(14):2393–2399
Breems DA, Van Putten WLJ, Huijgens PC et al (2005) Prognostic index for adult patients with acute myeloid leukemia in first relapse. J Clin Oncol 23(9):1969–1978
Breems DA, Van Putten WLJ, De Greef GE et al (2008) Monosomal karyotype in acute myeloid leukemia: a better indicator of poor prognosis than a complex karyotype. J Clin Oncol 26(29):4791–4797
Büchner T, Berdel WE, Haferlach C et al (2009) Age-related risk profile and chemotherapy dose response in acute myeloid leukemia: a study by the German Acute Myeloid Leukemia Cooperative Group. J Clin Oncol 27(1):61–69
Bullinger L, Döhner K, Bair E et al (2004) Use of gene-expression profiling to identify prognostic subclasses in adult acute myeloid leukemia. N Engl J Med 350(16):1605–1616
Bullinger L, Ehrich M, Döhner K et al (2010) Quantitative DNA methylation predicts survival in adult acute myeloid leukemia. Blood 115(3):636–642
Bullinger L, Döhner K, Döhner H (2017) Genomics of acute myeloid leukemia diagnosis and pathways. J Clin Oncol 35(9):934–946
Bullinger L, Valk P, Versluis J et al (2019) Harmony alliance: European public-private data collection leads the way—first results of the "proof-of-principle" study in acute myeloid leukemia: PS1003. HemaSphere 3:451
Burnett AK, Russell NH, Hills RK et al (2013) Optimization of chemotherapy for younger patients with acute myeloid leukemia: results of the Medical Research Council AML15 trial. J Clin Oncol 31(27):3360–3368
Byrd JC, Weiss RB, Arthur DC et al (1997) Extramedullary leukemia adversely affects hematologic complete remission rate and overall survival in patients with t(8;21)(q22;q22): results from Cancer and Leukemia Group B 8461. J Clin Oncol 15(2):466–475
Byrd JC, Mrózek K, Dodge RK et al (2002) Pretreatment cytogenetic abnormalities are predictive of induction success, cumulative incidence of relapse, and overall survival in adult patients with de novo acute myeloid leukemia: results from Cancer and Leukemia Group B (CALGB 8461) presented in part at the 43rd annual meeting of the American Society of Hematology, Orlando, FL, December 10, 2001, and published in abstract form.59. Blood 100(13):4325–4336
Cairo MS, Bishop M (2004) Tumour lysis syndrome: new therapeutic strategies and classification. Br J Haematol 127(1):3–11
Cairoli R, Beghini A, Grillo G et al (2006) Prognostic impact of c-KIT mutations in core binding factor leukemias: an Italian retrospective study. Blood 107(9):3463–3468
Canaani J, Labopin M, Socié G et al (2017) Long term impact of hyperleukocytosis in newly diagnosed acute myeloid leukemia patients undergoing allogeneic stem cell transplantation: an analysis from the acute leukemia working party of the EBMT: Canaani et al. Am J Hematol 92(7):653–659
Canaani J, Labopin M, Itälä-Remes M et al (2019) Prognostic significance of recurring chromosomal abnormalities in transplanted patients with acute myeloid leukemia. Leukemia 33(8):1944–1952
Cannas G, Pautas C, Raffoux E et al (2012) Infectious complications in adult acute myeloid leukemia: analysis of the Acute Leukemia French Association-9802 prospective multicenter clinical trial. Leuk Lymphoma 53(6):1068–1076
Care RS, Valk PJM, Goodeve AC et al (2003) Incidence and prognosis of c-KIT and FLT3 mutations in core binding factor (CBF) acute myeloid leukaemias. Br J Haematol 121(5):775–777
Carter BZ, Qiu Y, Huang X et al (2012) Survivin is highly expressed in CD34+38− leukemic stem/progenitor cells and predicts poor clinical outcomes in AML. Blood 120(1):173–180
Cerrano M, Itzykson R (2019) New treatment options for acute myeloid leukemia in 2019. Curr Oncol Rep 21(2):16
Cerrano M, Duchmann M, Kim R et al (2021) Clonal dominance is an adverse prognostic factor in acute myeloid leukemia treated with intensive chemotherapy. Leukemia 35(3):712–723
Chang H, Brandwein J, Yi Q-L et al (2004) Extramedullary infiltrates of AML are associated with CD56 expression, 11q23 abnormalities and inferior clinical outcome. Leuk Res 28(10):1007–1011
Chen Y, Kantarjian H, Pierce S et al (2013) Prognostic significance of 11q23 aberrations in adult acute myeloid leukemia and the role of allogeneic stem cell transplantation. Leukemia 27(4):836–842
Chen W, Xie H, Wang H et al (2016) Prognostic significance of KIT mutations in core-binding factor acute myeloid leukemia: a systematic review and meta-analysis. PLoS One 11(1):e0146614
Chen F, Sun J, Yin C et al (2019) Impact of FLT3-ITD allele ratio and ITD length on therapeutic outcome in cytogenetically normal AML patients without NPM1 mutation. Bone Marrow Transplant 55(4):740–748
Cheng C-L, Li C-C, Hou H-A et al (2015) Risk factors and clinical outcomes of acute myeloid leukaemia

with central nervous system involvement in adults. BMC Cancer 15(1):344
Cher CY, Leung GMK, Au CH et al (2016) Next-generation sequencing with a myeloid gene panel in core-binding factor AML showed KIT activation loop and TET2 mutations predictive of outcome. Blood Cancer J 6(7):e442
Chevallier P, Labopin M, Turlure P et al (2011) A new leukemia prognostic scoring system for refractory/relapsed adult acute myelogeneous leukaemia patients: a GOELAMS study. Leukemia 25(6):939–944
Chilton L, Hills RK, Harrison CJ et al (2014) Hyperdiploidy with 49-65 chromosomes represents a heterogeneous cytogenetic subgroup of acute myeloid leukemia with differential outcome. Leukemia 28(2):321–328
Chisini M, Stefanizzi C, Ceglie T et al (2017) Independent prognostic impact of CD15 on complete remission achievement in patients with acute myeloid leukemia. Hematol Oncol 35(4):804–809
Chou W-C, Huang H-H, Hou H-A et al (2010) Distinct clinical and biological features of de novo acute myeloid leukemia with additional sex comb-like 1 (ASXL1) mutations. Blood 116(20):4086–4094
Chou W-C, Chou S-C, Liu C-Y et al (2011a) TET2 mutation is an unfavorable prognostic factor in acute myeloid leukemia patients with intermediate-risk cytogenetics. Blood 118(14):3803–3810
Chou W-C, Lei W-C, Ko B-S et al (2011b) The prognostic impact and stability of isocitrate dehydrogenase 2 mutation in adult patients with acute myeloid leukemia. Leukemia 25(2):246–253
Christen F, Hoyer K, Yoshida K et al (2019) Genomic landscape and clonal evolution of acute myeloid leukemia with t(8;21): an international study on 331 patients. Blood 133(10):1140–1151
Christiansen DH, Andersen MK, Pedersen-Bjergaard J (2001) Mutations with loss of heterozygosity of p53 are common in therapy-related myelodysplasia and acute myeloid leukemia after exposure to alkylating agents and significantly associated with deletion or loss of 5q, a complex karyotype, and a poor prognosis. J Clin Oncol 19(5):1405–1413
Christiansen DH, Andersen MK, Pedersen-Bjergaard J (2016) Mutations with loss of heterozygosity of p53 are common in therapy-related myelodysplasia and acute myeloid leukemia after exposure to alkylating agents and significantly associated with deletion or loss of 5q, a complex karyotype, and a poor prognosis. J Clin Oncol 19(5):1405–1413
Ciurea SO, Chilkulwar A, Saliba RM et al (2018) Prognostic factors influencing survival after allogeneic transplantation for AML/MDS patients with TP53 mutations. Blood 131(26):2989–2992
Cornelissen JJ, Blaise D (2016) Hematopoietic stem cell transplantation for patients with AML in first complete remission. Blood 127(1):62–70
Cornelissen JJ, Gratwohl A, Schlenk RF et al (2012) The European LeukemiaNet AML working party consensus statement on allogeneic HCT for patients with AML in remission: an integrated-risk adapted approach. Nat Rev Clin Oncol 9(10):579–590
Costa AFO, Menezes DL, Pinheiro LHS et al (2017) Role of new Immunophenotypic markers on prognostic and overall survival of acute myeloid leukemia: a systematic review and meta-analysis. Sci Rep 7(1):4138
Creutzig U, Zimmermann M, Reinhardt D et al (2016) Changes in cytogenetics and molecular genetics in acute myeloid leukemia from childhood to adult age groups. Cancer 122(24):3821–3830
Damm F, Heuser M, Morgan M et al (2011) Integrative prognostic risk score in acute myeloid leukemia with normal karyotype. Blood 117(17):4561–4568
Daver N, Liu Dumlao T, Ravandi F et al (2013) Effect of NPM1 and FLT3 mutations on the outcomes of elderly patients with acute myeloid leukemia receiving standard chemotherapy. Clin Lymphoma Myeloma Leuk 13(4):435–440
Daver N, Schlenk RF, Russell NH, Levis MJ (2019) Targeting FLT3 mutations in AML: review of current knowledge and evidence. Leukemia 33(2):299–312
de Jonge HJM, Valk PJM, de Bont ESJM et al (2011) Prognostic impact of white blood cell count in intermediate risk acute myeloid leukemia: relevance of mutated NPM1 and FLT3-ITD. Haematologica 96(9):1310–1317
de Rooij JDE, Branstetter C, Ma J et al (2017) Pediatric non–Down syndrome acute megakaryoblastic leukemia is characterized by distinct genomic subsets with varying outcomes. Nat Genet 49(3):451–456
De Stefano V, Sorà F, Rossi E et al (2005) The risk of thrombosis in patients with acute leukemia: occurrence of thrombosis at diagnosis and during treatment. J Thromb Haemost 3(9):1985–1992
Del Poeta G, Venditti A, Del Principe MI et al (2003) Amount of spontaneous apoptosis detected by Bax/Bcl-2 ratio predicts outcome in acute myeloid leukemia (AML). Blood 101(6):2125–2131
Del Principe MI, Buccisano F, Soddu S et al (2018) Involvement of central nervous system in adult patients with acute myeloid leukemia: incidence and impact on outcome. Semin Hematol 55(4):209–214
Della Porta MG, Gallì A, Bacigalupo A et al (2016) Clinical effects of driver somatic mutations on the outcomes of patients with myelodysplastic syndromes treated with allogeneic hematopoietic stem-cell transplantation. J Clin Oncol 34(30):3627–3637
Deneberg S, Grövdal M, Karimi M et al (2010) Gene-specific and global methylation patterns predict outcome in patients with acute myeloid leukemia. Leukemia 24(5):932–941
Deneberg S, Guardiola P, Lennartsson A et al (2011) Prognostic DNA methylation patterns in cytogenetically normal acute myeloid leukemia are predefined by stem cell chromatin marks. Blood 118(20):5573–5582
Devillier R, Mansat-De Mas V, Gelsi-Boyer V et al (2015a) Role of ASXL1 and TP53 mutations in the molecular classification and prognosis of acute myeloid leuke-

mias with myelodysplasia-related changes. Oncotarget 6(10):8388–8396
Devillier R, Gelsi-Boyer V, Murati A et al (2015b) Prognostic significance of myelodysplasia-related changes according to the WHO classification among ELN-intermediate-risk AML patients. Am J Hematol 90(1):E22–E24
Díaz-Beyá M, Brunet S, Nomdedéu J et al (2014) MicroRNA expression at diagnosis adds relevant prognostic information to molecular categorization in patients with intermediate-risk cytogenetic acute myeloid leukemia. Leukemia 28(4):804–812
Díaz-Beyá M, Labopin M, Maertens J et al (2020) Allogeneic stem cell transplantation in AML with t(6;9)(p23;q34);DEK-NUP214 shows a favourable outcome when performed in first complete remission. Br J Haematol 189(5):920–925
Dicker F, Haferlach C, Sundermann J et al (2010) Mutation analysis for RUNX1, MLL-PTD, FLT3-ITD, NPM1 and NRAS in 269 patients with MDS or secondary AML. Leukemia 24(8):1528–1532
DiNardo CD, Luskin MR, Carroll M et al (2017) Validation of a clinical assay of multi-locus DNA methylation for prognosis of newly diagnosed AML. Am J Hematol 92(2):E14–E15
DiNardo CD, Pratz K, Pullarkat V et al (2019) Venetoclax combined with decitabine or azacitidine in treatment-naive, elderly patients with acute myeloid leukemia. Blood 133(1):7–17
Döhner K, Tobis K, Ulrich R et al (2002) Prognostic significance of partial tandem duplications of the MLL gene in adult patients 16 to 60 years old with acute myeloid leukemia and normal cytogenetics: a study of the Acute Myeloid Leukemia Study Group Ulm. J Clin Oncol 20(15):3254–3261
Döhner K, Schlenk RF, Habdank M et al (2005) Mutant nucleophosmin (NPM1) predicts favorable prognosis in younger adults with acute myeloid leukemia and normal cytogenetics: interaction with other gene mutations. Blood 106(12):3740–3746
Döhner H, Estey EH, Amadori S et al (2010) Diagnosis and management of acute myeloid leukemia in adults: recommendations from an international expert panel, on behalf of the European LeukemiaNet. Blood 115(3):453–474
Döhner H, Estey E, Grimwade D et al (2017) Diagnosis and management of AML in adults: 2017 ELN recommendations from an international expert panel. Blood 129(4):424–447
Döhner K, Thiede C, Jahn N et al (2020) Impact of NPM1/FLT3-ITD genotypes defined by the 2017 European LeukemiaNet in patients with acute myeloid leukemia. Blood 135(5):371–380
Driessen EMC, van Roon EHJ, Spijkers-Hagelstein JAP et al (2013) Frequencies and prognostic impact of RAS mutations in MLL-rearranged acute lymphoblastic leukemia in infants. Haematologica 98(6):937–944
Dufour A, Schneider F, Metzeler KH et al (2010) Acute myeloid leukemia with biallelic CEBPA gene mutations and normal karyotype represents a distinct genetic entity associated with a favorable clinical outcome. J Clin Oncol 28(4):570–577
Dunlap JB, Leonard J, Rosenberg M et al (2019) The combination of NPM1, DNMT3A, and IDH1/2 mutations leads to inferior overall survival in AML. Am J Hematol 94(8):913–920
Duployez N, Marceau-Renaut A, Boissel N et al (2016) Comprehensive mutational profiling of core binding factor acute myeloid leukemia. Blood 127(20):2451–2459
Duployez N, Boudry-Labis E, Roumier C et al (2018) SNP-array lesions in core binding factor acute myeloid leukemia. Oncotarget 9(5):6478–6489
Duployez N, Marceau-Renaut A, Villenet C et al (2019) The stem cell-associated gene expression signature allows risk stratification in pediatric acute myeloid leukemia. Leukemia 33(2):348–357
Eisfeld A-K, Mrózek K, Kohlschmidt J et al (2017) The mutational oncoprint of recurrent cytogenetic abnormalities in adult patients with de novo acute myeloid leukemia. Leukemia 31(10):2211–2218
Eisfeld A-K, Kohlschmidt J, Mrózek K et al (2018) Mutation patterns identify adult patients with de novo acute myeloid leukemia aged 60 years or older who respond favorably to standard chemotherapy: an analysis of alliance studies. Leukemia 32(6):1338–1348
El-Sharkawi D, Sproul D, Allen CG et al (2018) Variable outcome and methylation status according to CEBPA mutant type in double-mutated acute myeloid leukemia patients and the possible implications for treatment. Haematologica 103(1):91–100
Eppert K, Takenaka K, Lechman ER et al (2011) Stem cell gene expression programs influence clinical outcome in human leukemia. Nat Med 17(9):1086–1093
Esposito MT (2019) The impact of PI3-kinase/RAS pathway cooperating mutations in the evolution of KMT2A-rearranged leukemia. Hemasphere 3(3):e195
Estey E, Gale RP (2017) How good are we at predicting the fate of someone with acute myeloid leukaemia? Leukemia 31(6):1255–1258
Faber ZJ, Chen X, Gedman AL et al (2016) The genomic landscape of core-binding factor acute myeloid leukemias. Nat Genet 48(12):1551–1556
Falini B, Mecucci C, Tiacci E et al (2005) Cytoplasmic nucleophosmin in acute myelogenous leukemia with a normal karyotype. N Engl J Med 352(3):254–266
Farag SS, Archer KJ, Mrózek K et al (2006) Pretreatment cytogenetics add to other prognostic factors predicting complete remission and long-term outcome in patients 60 years of age or older with acute myeloid leukemia: results from Cancer and Leukemia Group B 8461. Blood 108(1):63–73
Fasan A, Eder C, Haferlach C et al (2013) GATA2 mutations are frequent in intermediate-risk karyotype AML with biallelic CEBPA mutations and are associated with favorable prognosis. Leukemia 27(2):482–485
Fasan A, Haferlach C, Alpermann T et al (2014) The role of different genetic subtypes of CEBPA mutated AML. Leukemia 28(4):794–803

Fenwarth L, Itzykson R, De Botton S et al (2019) Integrating ELN criteria and a "knowledge bank" approach to guide allogeneic stem cell transplantation (SCT) indication in younger adults with acute myeloid leukemia (AML): an Acute Leukemia French Association Study. Blood 134(Suppl_1):1423
Figueroa ME, Lugthart S, Li Y et al (2010) DNA methylation signatures identify biologically distinct subtypes in acute myeloid leukemia. Cancer Cell 17(1):13–27
Fischer M, Schnetzke U, Spies-Weisshart B et al (2017) Impact of FLT3-ITD diversity on response to induction chemotherapy in patients with acute myeloid leukemia. Haematologica 102(4):e129–e131
Fontana MC, Marconi G, Feenstra JDM et al (2018) Chromothripsis in acute myeloid leukemia: biological features and impact on survival. Leukemia 32(7):1609–1620
Fröhling S, Schlenk RF, Breitruck J et al (2002) Prognostic significance of activating FLT3 mutations in younger adults (16 to 60 years) with acute myeloid leukemia and normal cytogenetics: a study of the AML Study Group Ulm. Blood 100(13):4372–4380
Fröhling S, Schlenk RF, Stolze I et al (2004) CEBPA mutations in younger adults with acute myeloid leukemia and normal cytogenetics: prognostic relevance and analysis of cooperating mutations. J Clin Oncol 22(4):624–633
Fröhling S, Schlenk RF, Kayser S et al (2006) Cytogenetics and age are major determinants of outcome in intensively treated acute myeloid leukemia patients older than 60 years: results from AMLSG trial AML HD98-B. Blood 108(10):3280–3288
Fujiwara S, Muroi K, Yamamoto C et al (2017) CD25 as an adverse prognostic factor in elderly patients with acute myeloid leukemia. Hematology 22(6):347–353
Gaidzik VI, Schlenk RF, Moschny S et al (2009) Prognostic impact of WT1 mutations in cytogenetically normal acute myeloid leukemia: a study of the German-Austrian AML Study Group. Blood 113(19):4505–4511
Gaidzik VI, Bullinger L, Schlenk RF et al (2011) RUNX1 mutations in acute myeloid leukemia: results from a comprehensive genetic and clinical analysis from the AML Study Group. J Clin Oncol 29(10):1364–1372
Gaidzik VI, Paschka P, Späth D et al (2012) TET2 mutations in acute myeloid leukemia (AML): results from a comprehensive genetic and clinical analysis of the AML Study Group. J Clin Oncol 30(12):1350–1357
Gaidzik VI, Schlenk RF, Paschka P et al (2013) Clinical impact of DNMT3A mutations in younger adult patients with acute myeloid leukemia: results of the AML Study Group (AMLSG). Blood 121(23):4769–4777
Gaidzik VI, Teleanu V, Papaemmanuil E et al (2016) RUNX1 mutations in acute myeloid leukemia are associated with distinct clinico-pathologic and genetic features. Leukemia 30(11):2160–2168
Gale RE, Green C, Allen C et al (2008) The impact of FLT3 internal tandem duplication mutant level, number, size, and interaction with NPM1 mutations in a large cohort of young adult patients with acute myeloid leukemia. Blood 111(5):2776–2784
Ganzel C, Becker J, Mintz PD, Lazarus HM, Rowe JM (2012) Hyperleukocytosis, leukostasis and leukapheresis: practice management. Blood Rev 26(3):117–122
Ganzel C, Manola J, Douer D et al (2016) Extramedullary disease in adult acute myeloid leukemia is common but lacks independent significance: analysis of patients in ECOG-ACRIN Cancer research group trials, 1980-2008. J Clin Oncol 34(29):3544–3553
Gardin C, Pautas C, Fournier E et al (2020) Added prognostic value of secondary AML-like gene mutations in ELN intermediate-risk older AML: ALFA-1200 study results. Blood Adv 4(9):1942–1949
Gentles AJ, Plevritis SK, Majeti R, Alizadeh AA (2010) Association of a leukemic stem cell gene expression signature with clinical outcomes in acute myeloid leukemia. JAMA 304(24):2706–2715
Gerstung M, Papaemmanuil E, Martincorena I et al (2017) Precision oncology for acute myeloid leukemia using a knowledge bank approach. Nat Genet 49(3):332–340
Giammarco S, Chiusolo P, Piccirillo N et al (2017) Hyperleukocytosis and leukostasis: management of a medical emergency. Expert Rev Hematol 10(2):147–154
Granfeldt Østgård LS, Medeiros BC, Sengeløv H et al (2015) Epidemiology and clinical significance of secondary and therapy-related acute myeloid Leukemia: a National Population-Based Cohort Study. JCO 33(31):3641–3649
Green CL, Koo KK, Hills RK et al (2010) Prognostic significance of CEBPA mutations in a large cohort of younger adult patients with acute myeloid leukemia: impact of double CEBPA mutations and the interaction with FLT3 and NPM1 mutations. J Clin Oncol 28(16):2739–2747
Green CL, Evans CM, Zhao L et al (2011) The prognostic significance of IDH2 mutations in AML depends on the location of the mutation. Blood 118(2):409–412
Greenberg PL, Tuechler H, Schanz J et al (2012) Revised international prognostic scoring system for myelodysplastic syndromes. Blood 120(12):2454–2465
Greif PA, Konstandin NP, Metzeler KH et al (2012) RUNX1 mutations in cytogenetically normal acute myeloid leukemia are associated with a poor prognosis and up-regulation of lymphoid genes. Haematologica 97(12):1909–1915
Greif PA, Hartmann L, Vosberg S et al (2018) Evolution of cytogenetically normal acute myeloid Leukemia during therapy and relapse: an exome sequencing study of 50 patients. Clin Cancer Res 24(7):1716–1726
Grimwade D, Mrózek K (2011) Diagnostic and prognostic value of cytogenetics in acute myeloid Leukemia. Hematol Oncol Clin North Am 25(6):1135–1161
Grimwade D, Walker H, Oliver F et al (1998) The importance of diagnostic cytogenetics on outcome in AML: analysis of 1,612 patients entered into the MRC AML 10 trial. The Medical Research Council Adult and Children's Leukaemia Working Parties. Blood 92(7):2322–2333

Grimwade D, Walker H, Harrison G et al (2001) The predictive value of hierarchical cytogenetic classification in older adults with acute myeloid leukemia (AML): analysis of 1065 patients entered into the United Kingdom Medical Research Council AML11 trial. Blood 98(5):1312–1320

Grimwade D, Hills RK, Moorman AV et al (2010) Refinement of cytogenetic classification in acute myeloid leukemia: determination of prognostic significance of rare recurring chromosomal abnormalities among 5876 younger adult patients treated in the United Kingdom Medical Research Council trials. Blood 116(3):354–365

Grimwade D, Ivey A, Huntly BJP (2016) Molecular landscape of acute myeloid leukemia in younger adults and its clinical relevance. Blood 127(1):29–41

Gröschel S, Lugthart S, Schlenk RF et al (2010) High EVI1 expression predicts outcome in younger adult patients with acute myeloid leukemia and is associated with distinct cytogenetic abnormalities. J Clin Oncol 28(12):2101–2107

Gröschel S, Schlenk RF, Engelmann J et al (2013) Deregulated expression of EVI1 defines a poor prognostic subset of MLL-rearranged acute myeloid leukemias: a study of the German-Austrian Acute Myeloid Leukemia Study Group and the Dutch-Belgian-Swiss HOVON/SAKK Cooperative Group. J Clin Oncol 31(1):95–103

Grossmann V, Schnittger S, Kohlmann A et al (2012) A novel hierarchical prognostic model of AML solely based on molecular mutations. Blood 120(15):2963–2972

Grossmann V, Haferlach C, Nadarajah N et al (2013a) CEBPA double-mutated acute myeloid leukaemia harbours concomitant molecular mutations in 76·8% of cases with TET2 and GATA2 alterations impacting prognosis. Br J Haematol 161(5):649–658

Grossmann V, Schnittger S, Poetzinger F et al (2013b) High incidence of RAS signalling pathway mutations in MLL-rearranged acute myeloid leukemia. Leukemia 27(9):1933–1936

Haferlach C, Dicker F, Herholz H et al (2008) Mutations of the TP53 gene in acute myeloid leukemia are strongly associated with a complex aberrant karyotype. Leukemia 22(8):1539–1541

Haferlach C, Mecucci C, Schnittger S et al (2009) AML with mutated NPM1 carrying a normal or aberrant karyotype show overlapping biologic, pathologic, immunophenotypic, and prognostic features. Blood 114(14):3024–3032

Haferlach C, Alpermann T, Schnittger S et al (2012) Prognostic value of monosomal karyotype in comparison to complex aberrant karyotype in acute myeloid leukemia: a study on 824 cases with aberrant karyotype. Blood 119(9):2122–2125

Harada Y, Nagata Y, Kihara R et al (2018) Prognostic analysis according to the 2017 ELN risk stratification by genetics in adult acute myeloid leukemia patients treated in the Japan Adult Leukemia Study Group (JALSG) AML201 study. Leuk Res 66:20–27

Harrison CJ, Hills RK, Moorman AV et al (2010) Cytogenetics of childhood acute myeloid leukemia: United Kingdom Medical Research Council treatment trials AML 10 and 12. J Clin Oncol 28(16):2674–2681

Hefazi M, Siddiqui M, Patnaik M et al (2015) Prognostic impact of combined NPM1+/FLT3− genotype in patients with acute myeloid leukemia with intermediate risk cytogenetics stratified by age and treatment modalities. Leuk Res 39(11):1207–1213

Heiblig M, Labussière-Wallet H, Nicolini FE et al (2019) Prognostic value of genetic alterations in elderly patients with acute myeloid leukemia: a single institution experience. Cancers (Basel) 11(4):570

Herold T, Jurinovic V, Batcha AMN et al (2018) A 29-gene and cytogenetic score for the prediction of resistance to induction treatment in acute myeloid leukemia. Haematologica 103(3):456–465

Herold T, Rothenberg-Thurley M, Grunwald VV et al (2020) Validation and refinement of the revised 2017 European LeukemiaNet genetic risk stratification of acute myeloid leukemia. Leukemia 34:3161–3172

Heuser M (2016) Therapy-related myeloid neoplasms: does knowing the origin help to guide treatment? Hematology Am Soc Hematol Educ Program 2016(1):24–32

Hinai AA, Valk PJM (2016) Review: aberrant EVI1 expression in acute myeloid leukaemia. Br J Haematol 172(6):870–878

Hinai ASAA, Pratcorona M, Grob T et al (2019) The landscape of KMT2A-PTD AML: concurrent mutations, gene expression signatures, and clinical outcome. Hemasphere 3(2):e181

Ho PA, Kopecky KJ, Alonzo TA et al (2011) Prognostic implications of the IDH1 synonymous SNP rs11554137 in pediatric and adult AML: a report from the Children's Oncology Group and SWOG. Blood 118(17):4561–4566

Ho AD, Schetelig J, Bochtler T et al (2016) Allogeneic stem cell transplantation improves survival in patients with acute myeloid Leukemia characterized by a high allelic ratio of mutant FLT3-ITD. Biol Blood Marrow Transplant 22(3):462–469

Hollink IHIM, Zwaan CM, Zimmermann M et al (2009) Favorable prognostic impact of NPM1 gene mutations in childhood acute myeloid leukemia, with emphasis on cytogenetically normal AML. Leukemia 23(2):262–270

Hollink IHIM, van den Heuvel-Eibrink MM, Arentsen-Peters STCJM et al (2011) NUP98/NSD1 characterizes a novel poor prognostic group in acute myeloid leukemia with a distinct HOX gene expression pattern. Blood 118(13):3645–3656

Hou H-A, Kuo Y-Y, Liu C-Y et al (2012) DNMT3A mutations in acute myeloid leukemia: stability during disease evolution and clinical implications. Blood 119(2):559–568

How J, Sykes J, Gupta V et al (2012) Influence of FLT3-internal tandem duplication allele burden and white blood cell count on the outcome in patients with intermediate-risk karyotype acute myeloid leukemia. Cancer 118(24):6110–6117

Hshieh TT, Jung WF, Grande LJ et al (2018) Prevalence of cognitive impairment and association with survival among older patients with hematologic cancers. JAMA Oncol 4(5):686–693

Huet S, Paubelle E, Lours C et al (2018) Validation of the prognostic value of the knowledge bank approach to determine AML prognosis in real life. Blood 132(8):865–867

Hulegårdh E, Nilsson C, Lazarevic V et al (2015) Characterization and prognostic features of secondary acute myeloid leukemia in a population-based setting: a report from the Swedish acute Leukemia registry. Am J Hematol 90(3):208–214

Hupfer V, Grishina O, Schmoor C et al (2018) Validation of a frailty score predicting survival of elderly, non-fit aml patients receiving hypomethylating therapy: results of the decider trial. Blood 132(Suppl 1):720

Illmer T, Schaich M, Ehninger G, Thiede C (2007) Tyrosine kinase mutations of JAK2 are rare events in AML but influence prognosis of patients with CBF-leukemias. Haematologica 92(1):137–138

Inaba H, Zhou Y, Abla O et al (2015) Heterogeneous cytogenetic subgroups and outcomes in childhood acute megakaryoblastic leukemia: a retrospective international study. Blood 126(13):1575–1584

International Working Group for MDS Molecular Prognostic Committee, Haase D, Stevenson KE et al (2019) TP53 mutation status divides myelodysplastic syndromes with complex karyotypes into distinct prognostic subgroups. Leukemia 33(7):1747–1758

Ishikawa Y, Kawashima N, Atsuta Y et al (2020) Prospective evaluation of prognostic impact of KIT mutations on acute myeloid leukemia with RUNX1-RUNX1T1 and CBFB-MYH11. Blood Adv 4(1):66–75

Itzykson R, Duployez N, Fasan A et al (2018a) Clonal interference of signaling mutations worsens prognosis in core-binding factor acute myeloid leukemia. Blood 132(2):187–196

Itzykson R, Fournier E, Braun T et al (2018b) Oncogenic predictors of outcome in older AML patients treated intensively. Analysis of the ALFA-1200 trial. Blood 132(Suppl 1):993

Jost E, Lin Q, Weidner CI et al (2014) Epimutations mimic genomic mutations of DNMT3A in acute myeloid leukemia. Leukemia 28(6):1227–1234

Jourdan E, Boissel N, Chevret S et al (2013) Prospective evaluation of gene mutations and minimal residual disease in patients with core binding factor acute myeloid leukemia. Blood 121(12):2213–2223

Juliusson G, Antunovic P, Derolf Å et al (2009) Age and acute myeloid leukemia: real world data on decision to treat and outcomes from the Swedish Acute Leukemia Registry. Blood 113(18):4179–4187

Juliusson G, Jädersten M, Deneberg S et al (2020) The prognostic impact of FLT3-ITD and NPM1 mutation in adult AML is age-dependent in the population-based setting. Blood Adv 4(6):1094–1101

Jung N, Dai B, Gentles AJ, Majeti R, Feinberg AP (2015) An LSC epigenetic signature is largely mutation independent and implicates the HOXA cluster in AML pathogenesis. Nat Commun 6(1):1–12

Kadia TM, Jain P, Ravandi F et al (2016) TP53 mutations in newly diagnosed acute myeloid leukemia: clinicomolecular characteristics, response to therapy, and outcomes. Cancer 122(22):3484–3491

Karakas T, Miething CC, Maurer U et al (2002) The coexpression of the apoptosis-related genes bcl-2 and wt1 in predicting survival in adult acute myeloid leukemia. Leukemia 16(5):846–854

Kauer J, Schwartz K, Tandler C et al (2019) CD105 (Endoglin) as negative prognostic factor in AML. Sci Rep 9(1):1–11

Kayser S, Schlenk RF, Londono MC et al (2009) Insertion of FLT3 internal tandem duplication in the tyrosine kinase domain-1 is associated with resistance to chemotherapy and inferior outcome. Blood 114(12):2386–2392

Kayser S, Döhner K, Krauter J et al (2011) The impact of therapy-related acute myeloid leukemia (AML) on outcome in 2853 adult patients with newly diagnosed AML. Blood 117(7):2137–2145

Kayser S, Zucknick M, Döhner K et al (2012) Monosomal karyotype in adult acute myeloid leukemia: prognostic impact and outcome after different treatment strategies. Blood 119(2):551–558

Kayser S, Elliott MA, Luskin M et al (2019) Characteristics and outcome of patients with core binding factor acute myeloid leukemia and FLT3-ITD: results from an international collaboration. Blood 134(Suppl_1):2693

Kihara R, Nagata Y, Kiyoi H et al (2014) Comprehensive analysis of genetic alterations and their prognostic impacts in adult acute myeloid leukemia patients. Leukemia 28(8):1586–1595

Kim H-J, Ahn HK, Jung CW et al (2013) KIT D816 mutation associates with adverse outcomes in core binding factor acute myeloid leukemia, especially in the subgroup with RUNX1/RUNX1T1 rearrangement. Ann Hematol 92(2):163–171

Kim Y, Lee GD, Park J et al (2015) Quantitative fragment analysis of FLT3-ITD efficiently identifying poor prognostic group with high mutant allele burden or long ITD length. Blood Cancer J 5(8):e336

Kirkhus L, Jordhøy M, Šaltytė Benth J et al (2016) Comparing comorbidity scales: attending physician score versus the cumulative illness rating scale for geriatrics. J Geriatr Oncol 7(2):90–98

Kiyoi H, Naoe T, Nakano Y et al (1999) Prognostic implication of FLT3 and N-RAS gene mutations in acute myeloid leukemia. Blood 93(9):3074–3080

Klein K, Kaspers G, Harrison CJ et al (2015) Clinical impact of additional cytogenetic aberrations, cKIT and RAS mutations, and treatment elements in Pediatric t(8;21)-AML: results from an international retrospective study by the International Berlin-Frankfurt-Münster Study group. J Clin Oncol 33(36):4247–4258

Klepin HD, Geiger AM, Tooze JA et al (2013) Geriatric assessment predicts survival for older adults receiving induction chemotherapy for acute myelogenous leukemia. Blood 121(21):4287–4294

Kobayashi R, Tawa A, Hanada R et al (2007) Extramedullary infiltration at diagnosis and prognosis in children with acute myelogenous leukemia. Pediatr Blood Cancer 48(4):393–398

Konstandin NP, Pastore F, Herold T et al (2018) Genetic heterogeneity of cytogenetically normal AML with mutations of CEBPA. Blood Adv 2(20):2724–2731

Kornblau SM, Womble M, Qiu YH et al (2006) Simultaneous activation of multiple signal transduction pathways confers poor prognosis in acute myelogenous leukemia. Blood 108(7):2358–2365

Kornblau SM, Tibes R, Qiu YH et al (2009) Functional proteomic profiling of AML predicts response and survival. Blood 113(1):154–164

Kornblau SM, Singh N, Qiu Y et al (2010a) Highly phosphorylated FOXO3A is an adverse prognostic factor in acute myeloid leukemia. Clin Cancer Res 16(6):1865–1874

Kornblau SM, McCue D, Singh N et al (2010b) Recurrent expression signatures of cytokines and chemokines are present and are independently prognostic in acute myelogenous leukemia and myelodysplasia. Blood 116(20):4251–4261

Kornblau SM, Qiu YH, Zhang N et al (2011) Abnormal expression of FLI1 protein is an adverse prognostic factor in acute myeloid leukemia. Blood 118(20):5604–5612

Kottaridis PD, Gale RE, Frew ME et al (2001) The presence of a FLT3 internal tandem duplication in patients with acute myeloid leukemia (AML) adds important prognostic information to cytogenetic risk group and response to the first cycle of chemotherapy: analysis of 854 patients from the United Kingdom Medical Research Council AML 10 and 12 trials. Blood 98(6):1752–1759

Krauth M-T, Eder C, Alpermann T et al (2014) High number of additional genetic lesions in acute myeloid leukemia with t(8;21)/RUNX1-RUNX1T1: frequency and impact on clinical outcome. Leukemia 28(7):1449–1458

Kroeze LI, Aslanyan MG, van Rooij A et al (2014) Characterization of acute myeloid leukemia based on levels of global hydroxymethylation. Blood 124(7):1110–1118

Kusec R, Jaksic O, Ostojic S et al (2006) More on prognostic significance of FLT3/ITD size in acute myeloid leukemia (AML). Blood 108(1):405–406

Kuykendall A, Duployez N, Boissel N, Lancet JE, Welch JS (2018) Acute myeloid Leukemia: the good, the bad, and the ugly. Am Soc Clin Oncol Educ Book 38:555–573

Lad D, Jain A, Varma S (2017) Complications and management of coagulation disorders in leukemia patients. Blood Lymphat Cancer 7:61–72

Lancet JE, Uy GL, Cortes JE et al (2016) Final results of a phase III randomized trial of CPX-351 versus 7+3 in older patients with newly diagnosed high risk (secondary) AML. JCO 34(15_suppl):7000

Langer C, Radmacher MD, Ruppert AS et al (2008) High BAALC expression associates with other molecular prognostic markers, poor outcome, and a distinct gene-expression signature in cytogenetically normal patients younger than 60 years with acute myeloid leukemia: a Cancer and Leukemia Group B (CALGB) study. Blood 111(11):5371–5379

Langer C, Marcucci G, Holland KB et al (2009) Prognostic importance of MN1 transcript levels, and biologic insights from MN1-associated gene and microRNA expression signatures in cytogenetically normal acute myeloid leukemia: a Cancer and Leukemia Group B study. J Clin Oncol 27(19):3198–3204

Laupeze B, Amiot L, Drenou B et al (2002) High multidrug resistance protein activity in acute myeloid leukaemias is associated with poor response to chemotherapy and reduced patient survival. Br J Haematol 116(4):834–838

Lauria F, Raspadori D, Rondelli D et al (1997) High bcl-2 expression in acute myeloid leukemia cells correlates with CD34 positivity and complete remission rate. Leukemia 11(12):2075–2078

Lavallée V-P, Krosl J, Lemieux S et al (2016) Chemo-genomic interrogation of CEBPA mutated AML reveals recurrent CSF3R mutations and subgroup sensitivity to JAK inhibitors. Blood 127(24):3054–3061

Lazarevic V, Hörstedt A-S, Johansson B et al (2014) Incidence and prognostic significance of karyotypic subgroups in older patients with acute myeloid leukemia: the Swedish population-based experience. Blood Cancer J 4(2):e188–e188

Lazarevic V, Rosso A, Juliusson G et al (2015) Prognostic significance of high hyperdiploid and triploid/tetraploid adult acute myeloid leukemia. Am J Hematol 90(9):800–805

Lazarevic VL, Labopin M, Depei W et al (2018) Relatively favorable outcome after allogeneic stem cell transplantation for BCR-ABL1-positive AML: a survey from the acute leukemia working party of the European Society for Blood and Marrow Transplantation (EBMT). Am J Hematol 93(1):31–39

Lazenby M, Gilkes AF, Marrin C et al (2014) The prognostic relevance of flt3 and npm1 mutations on older patients treated intensively or non-intensively: a study of 1312 patients in the UK NCRI AML16 trial. Leukemia 28(10):1953–1959

Legrand O, Simonin G, Perrot JY, Zittoun R, Marie JP (1998) Pgp and MRP activities using calcein-AM are prognostic factors in adult acute myeloid leukemia patients. Blood 91(12):4480–4488

Leith CP, Kopecky KJ, Godwin J et al (1997) Acute myeloid leukemia in the elderly: assessment of multidrug resistance (MDR1) and cytogenetics distinguishes biologic subgroups with remarkably distinct responses to standard chemotherapy. A Southwest Oncology Group study. Blood 89(9):3323–3329

Leith CP, Kopecky KJ, Chen IM et al (1999) Frequency and clinical significance of the expression of the multidrug resistance proteins MDR1/P-glycoprotein, MRP1, and LRP in acute myeloid leukemia: a Southwest Oncology Group study. Blood 94(3):1086–1099

Levine JH, Simonds EF, Bendall SC et al (2015) Data-driven phenotypic dissection of AML reveals progenitor-like cells that correlate with prognosis. Cell 162(1):184–197

Ley TJ, Ding L, Walter MJ et al (2010) DNMT3A mutations in acute myeloid leukemia. N Engl J Med 363(25):2424–2433

Li Z, Herold T, He C et al (2013) Identification of a 24-gene prognostic signature that improves the European LeukemiaNet risk classification of acute myeloid leukemia: an international collaborative study. J Clin Oncol 31(9):1172–1181

Li H-Y, Deng D-H, Huang Y et al (2015) Favorable prognosis of biallelic CEBPA gene mutations in acute myeloid leukemia patients: a meta-analysis. Eur J Haematol 94(5):439–448

Li S, Garrett-Bakelman FE, Chung SS et al (2016) Distinct evolution and dynamics of epigenetic and genetic heterogeneity in acute myeloid leukemia. Nat Med 22(7):792–799

Lin T-C, Hou H-A, Chou W-C et al (2011) CEBPA methylation as a prognostic biomarker in patients with de novo acute myeloid leukemia. Leukemia 25(1):32–40

Linch DC, Hills RK, Burnett AK, Khwaja A, Gale RE (2014) Impact of FLT3(ITD) mutant allele level on relapse risk in intermediate-risk acute myeloid leukemia. Blood 124(2):273–276

Linch DC, Hills RK, Burnett AK, Russell N, Gale RE (2020) Analysis of the clinical impact of NPM1 mutant allele burden in a large cohort of younger adult patients with acute myeloid leukaemia. Br J Haematol 188(6):852–859

Lindsley RC, Mar BG, Mazzola E et al (2015) Acute myeloid leukemia ontogeny is defined by distinct somatic mutations. Blood 125(9):1367–1376

Liu S-B, Dong H-J, Bao X-B et al (2019) Impact of FLT3-ITD length on prognosis of acute myeloid leukemia. Haematologica 104(1):e9–e12

Loghavi S, Zuo Z, Ravandi F et al (2014) Clinical features of de novo acute myeloid leukemia with concurrent DNMT3A, FLT3 and NPM1 mutations. J Hematol Oncol 7(1):74

Lugthart S, van Drunen E, van Norden Y et al (2008) High EVI1 levels predict adverse outcome in acute myeloid leukemia: prevalence of EVI1 overexpression and chromosome 3q26 abnormalities underestimated. Blood 111(8):4329–4337

Lugthart S, Gröschel S, Beverloo HB et al (2010) Clinical, molecular, and prognostic significance of WHO type inv(3)(q21q26.2)/t(3;3)(q21;q26.2) and various other 3q abnormalities in acute myeloid leukemia. J Clin Oncol 28(24):3890–3898

Luskin MR, Gimotty PA, Smith C et al (2016) A clinical measure of DNA methylation predicts outcome in de novo acute myeloid leukemia. JCI Insight 1(9):e87323

Ma Z, Morris SW, Valentine V et al (2001) Fusion of two novel genes, RBM15 and MKL1, in the t(1;22)(p13;q13) of acute megakaryoblastic leukemia. Nat Genet 28(3):220–221

Malagola M, Skert C, Vignetti M et al (2011) A simple prognostic scoring system for newly diagnosed cytogenetically normal acute myeloid leukemia: retrospective analysis of 530 patients. Leuk Lymphoma 52(12):2329–2335

Maley CC, Aktipis A, Graham TA et al (2017) Classifying the evolutionary and ecological features of neoplasms. Nat Rev Cancer 17(10):605–619

Manara E, Basso G, Zampini M et al (2017) Characterization of children with FLT3-ITD acute myeloid leukemia: a report from the AIEOP AML-2002 Study Group. Leukemia 31(1):18–25

Marceau-Renaut A, Guihard S, Castaigne S et al (2015) Classification of CEBPA mutated acute myeloid leukemia by GATA2 mutations. Am J Hematol 90(5):E93–E94

Marceau-Renaut A, Duployez N, Ducourneau B et al (2018) Molecular profiling defines distinct prognostic subgroups in childhood AML: a report from the French ELAM02 study group. HemaSphere 2(1):e31

Marcucci G, Mrózek K, Ruppert AS et al (2005a) Prognostic factors and outcome of core binding factor acute myeloid leukemia patients with t(8;21) differ from those of patients with inv(16): a Cancer and Leukemia Group B study. J Clin Oncol 23(24):5705–5717

Marcucci G, Baldus CD, Ruppert AS et al (2005b) Overexpression of the ETS-related gene, ERG, predicts a worse outcome in acute myeloid leukemia with normal karyotype: a Cancer and Leukemia Group B study. J Clin Oncol 23(36):9234–9242

Marcucci G, Maharry K, Whitman SP et al (2007) High expression levels of the ETS-related gene, ERG, predict adverse outcome and improve molecular risk-based classification of cytogenetically normal acute myeloid leukemia: a Cancer and Leukemia Group B study. J Clin Oncol 25(22):3337–3343

Marcucci G, Radmacher MD, Maharry K et al (2008) MicroRNA expression in cytogenetically normal acute myeloid leukemia. N Engl J Med 358(18):1919–1928

Marcucci G, Maharry K, Wu Y-Z et al (2010) IDH1 and IDH2 gene mutations identify novel molecular subsets within de novo cytogenetically normal acute myeloid leukemia: a Cancer and Leukemia Group B study. J Clin Oncol 28(14):2348–2355

Marcucci G, Metzeler KH, Schwind S et al (2012) Age-related prognostic impact of different types of DNMT3A mutations in adults with primary cytogenetically normal acute myeloid leukemia. J Clin Oncol 30(7):742–750

Marcucci G, Maharry KS, Metzeler KH et al (2013) Clinical role of microRNAs in cytogenetically normal acute myeloid leukemia: miR-155 upregulation independently identifies high-risk patients. J Clin Oncol 31(17):2086–2093

Marcucci G, Yan P, Maharry K et al (2014) Epigenetics meets genetics in acute myeloid leukemia: clinical impact of a novel seven-gene score. J Clin Oncol 32(6):548–556

Märklin M, Hagelstein I, Hinterleitner C et al (2020) CD105 (Endoglin) as risk marker in AML patients undergoing stem cell transplantation. Int J Hematol 112(1):57–64

Masetti R, Bertuccio SN, Pession A, Locatelli F (2019) CBFA2T3-GLIS2-positive acute myeloid leukaemia. A peculiar paediatric entity. Br J Haematol 184(3):337–347

Mason KD, Juneja SK, Szer J (2006) The immunophenotype of acute myeloid leukemia: is there a relationship with prognosis? Blood Rev 20(2):71–82

Mead AJ, Linch DC, Hills RK et al (2007) FLT3 tyrosine kinase domain mutations are biologically distinct from and have a significantly more favorable prognosis than FLT3 internal tandem duplications in patients with acute myeloid leukemia. Blood 110(4):1262–1270

Medeiros BC, Othus M, Fang M, Roulston D, Appelbaum FR (2010) Prognostic impact of monosomal karyotype in young adult and elderly acute myeloid leukemia: the southwest oncology group (SWOG) experience. Blood 116(13):2224–2228

Medeiros BC, Othus M, Fang M, Appelbaum FR, Erba HP (2015) Cytogenetic heterogeneity negatively impacts outcomes in patients with acute myeloid leukemia. Haematologica 100(3):331–335

Mendler JH, Maharry K, Radmacher MD et al (2012) RUNX1 mutations are associated with poor outcome in younger and older patients with cytogenetically normal acute myeloid leukemia and with distinct gene and MicroRNA expression signatures. J Clin Oncol 30(25):3109–3118

Meshinchi S, Alonzo TA, Stirewalt DL et al (2006) Clinical implications of FLT3 mutations in pediatric AML. Blood 108(12):3654–3661

Metzeler KH, Hummel M, Bloomfield CD et al (2008) An 86-probe-set gene-expression signature predicts survival in cytogenetically normal acute myeloid leukemia. Blood 112(10):4193–4201

Metzeler KH, Dufour A, Benthaus T et al (2009) ERG expression is an independent prognostic factor and allows refined risk stratification in cytogenetically normal acute myeloid leukemia: a comprehensive analysis of ERG, MN1, and BAALC transcript levels using oligonucleotide microarrays. J Clin Oncol 27(30):5031–5038

Metzeler KH, Becker H, Maharry K et al (2011a) ASXL1 mutations identify a high-risk subgroup of older patients with primary cytogenetically normal AML within the ELN favorable genetic category. Blood 118(26):6920–6929

Metzeler KH, Maharry K, Radmacher MD et al (2011b) TET2 mutations improve the new European LeukemiaNet risk classification of acute myeloid leukemia: a Cancer and Leukemia Group B study. J Clin Oncol 29(10):1373–1381

Metzeler KH, Herold T, Rothenberg-Thurley M et al (2016) Spectrum and prognostic relevance of driver gene mutations in acute myeloid leukemia. Blood 128(5):686–698

Meyer C, Burmeister T, Gröger D et al (2018) The MLL recombinome of acute leukemias in 2017. Leukemia 32(2):273–284

Micol JB, Boissel N, Renneville A et al (2009) The role of cytogenetic abnormalities in acute myeloid leukemia with NPM1 mutations and no FLT3 internal tandem duplication. Blood 114(20):4601–4602

Middeke JM, Herold S, Rücker-Braun E et al (2016) TP53 mutation in patients with high-risk acute myeloid leukaemia treated with allogeneic haematopoietic stem cell transplantation. Br J Haematol 172(6):914–922

Minetto P, Guolo F, Clavio M et al (2018) A blastic plasmacytoid dendritic cell neoplasm-like phenotype identifies a subgroup of npm1-mutated acute myeloid leukemia patients with worse prognosis. Am J Hematol 93(2):E33–E35

Moison C, Lavallée V-P, Thiollier C et al (2019) Complex karyotype AML displays G2/M signature and hypersensitivity to PLK1 inhibition. Blood Adv 3(4):552–563

Montesinos P, Lorenzo I, Martín G et al (2008) Tumor lysis syndrome in patients with acute myeloid leukemia: identification of risk factors and development of a predictive model. Haematologica 93(1):67 LP–74 LP

Montesinos P, Bergua J, Infante J et al (2019) Update on management and progress of novel therapeutics for R/R AML: an Iberian expert panel consensus. Ann Hematol 98(11):2467–2483

Mosna F, Papayannidis C, Martinelli G et al (2015) Complex karyotype, older age, and reduced first-line dose intensity determine poor survival in core binding factor acute myeloid leukemia patients with long-term follow-up. Am J Hematol 90(6):515–523

Mrózek K, Heinonen K, Lawrence D et al (1997) Adult patients with de novo acute myeloid leukemia and t(9; 11)(p22; q23) have a superior outcome to patients with other translocations involving band 11q23: a Cancer and Leukemia Group B study. Blood 90(11):4532–4538

Mrózek K, Marcucci G, Nicolet D et al (2012) Prognostic significance of the European LeukemiaNet standardized system for reporting cytogenetic and molecular alterations in adults with acute myeloid leukemia. J Clin Oncol 30(36):4515–4523

Mrózek K, Eisfeld A-K, Kohlschmidt J et al (2019) Complex karyotype in de novo acute myeloid leukemia: typical and atypical subtypes differ molecularly and clinically. Leukemia 33(7):1620–1634

Nagel G, Weber D, Fromm E et al (2017) Epidemiological, genetic, and clinical characterization by age of newly diagnosed acute myeloid leukemia based on an academic population-based registry study (AMLSG BiO). Ann Hematol 96(12):1993–2003

Nahi H, Lehmann S, Bengtzen S et al (2008) Chromosomal aberrations in 17p predict in vitro drug resistance and short overall survival in acute myeloid leukemia. Leuk Lymphoma 49(3):508–516
Nakao M, Yokota S, Iwai T et al (1996) Internal tandem duplication of the flt3 gene found in acute myeloid leukemia. Leukemia 10(12):1911–1918
Nakase K, Kita K, Kageyama S et al (1997) Clinical importance of interleukin-2 receptor alpha-chain expression in acute leukemia. The Japan Cooperative Group of Leukemia/Lymphoma. Cancer Detect Prev 21(3):273–279
Neuendorff NR, Burmeister T, Dörken B, Westermann J (2016) BCR-ABL-positive acute myeloid leukemia: a new entity? Analysis of clinical and molecular features. Ann Hematol 95(8):1211–1221
Neuendorff NR, Hemmati P, Arnold R et al (2018) BCR-ABL+ acute myeloid leukemia: are we always dealing with a high-risk disease? Blood Adv 2(12):1409–1411
Ng SWK, Mitchell A, Kennedy JA et al (2016) A 17-gene stemness score for rapid determination of risk in acute leukaemia. Nature 540(7633):433–437
Nguyen L, Zhang X, Roberts E et al (2020) Comparison of mutational profiles and clinical outcomes in patients with acute myeloid leukemia with mutated RUNX1 versus acute myeloid leukemia with myelodysplasia-related changes with mutated RUNX1. Leuk Lymphoma 61(6):1395–1405
Nibourel O, Kosmider O, Cheok M et al (2010) Incidence and prognostic value of TET2 alterations in de novo acute myeloid leukemia achieving complete remission. Blood 116(7):1132–1135
Nibourel O, Guihard S, Roumier C et al (2017) Copy-number analysis identified new prognostic marker in acute myeloid leukemia. Leukemia 31(3):555–564
Noort S, Zimmermann M, Reinhardt D et al (2018) Prognostic impact of t(16;21)(p11;q22) and t(16;21)(q24;q22) in pediatric AML: a retrospective study by the I-BFM study group. Blood 132(15):1584–1592
Noort S, Wander P, Alonzo TA et al (2021) The clinical and biological characteristics of NUP98-KDM5A in pediatric acute myeloid leukemia. Haematologica 106(2):630–634
Ok CY, Patel KP, Garcia-Manero G et al (2015) TP53 mutation characteristics in therapy-related myelodysplastic syndromes and acute myeloid leukemia is similar to de novo diseases. J Hematol Oncol 8:45
Ong YL, McMullin MF, Bailie KE et al (2000) High bax expression is a good prognostic indicator in acute myeloid leukaemia. Br J Haematol 111(1):182–189
Opatz S, Bamopoulos SA, Metzeler KH et al (2020) The clinical mutatome of core binding factor leukemia. Leukemia:1–10
Ossenkoppele G, Montesinos P (2019) Challenges in the diagnosis and treatment of secondary acute myeloid leukemia. Crit Rev Oncol Hematol 138:6–13
Ostronoff F, Othus M, Gerbing RB et al (2014) NUP98/NSD1 and FLT3/ITD coexpression is more prevalent in younger AML patients and leads to induction failure: a COG and SWOG report. Blood 124(15):2400–2407
Ostronoff F, Othus M, Lazenby M et al (2015) Prognostic significance of NPM1 mutations in the absence of FLT3-internal tandem duplication in older patients with acute myeloid leukemia: a SWOG and UK National Cancer Research Institute/Medical Research Council report. J Clin Oncol 33(10):1157–1164
Ottema S, Mulet-Lazaro R, Beverloo HB et al (2020) Atypical 3q26/MECOM rearrangements genocopy inv(3)/t(3;3) in acute myeloid leukemia. Blood 136(2):224–234
Pabst T, Mueller BU, Zhang P et al (2001) Dominant-negative mutations of CEBPA, encoding CCAAT/enhancer binding protein-alpha (C/EBPalpha), in acute myeloid leukemia. Nat Genet 27(3):263–270
Pabst T, Eyholzer M, Fos J, Mueller BU (2009) Heterogeneity within AML with CEBPA mutations; only CEBPA double mutations, but not single CEBPA mutations are associated with favourable prognosis. Br J Cancer 100(8):1343–1346
Papaemmanuil E, Gerstung M, Bullinger L et al (2016) Genomic classification and prognosis in acute myeloid leukemia. N Engl J Med 374(23):2209–2221
Park SH, Chi H-S, Min S-K et al (2011) Prognostic impact of c-KIT mutations in core binding factor acute myeloid leukemia. Leuk Res 35(10):1376–1383
Paschka P, Marcucci G, Ruppert AS et al (2006) Adverse prognostic significance of KIT mutations in adult acute myeloid leukemia with inv(16) and t(8;21): a Cancer and Leukemia Group B study. J Clin Oncol 24(24):3904–3911
Paschka P, Marcucci G, Ruppert AS et al (2008) Wilms' tumor 1 gene mutations independently predict poor outcome in adults with cytogenetically normal acute myeloid leukemia: a Cancer and Leukemia Group B study. J Clin Oncol 26(28):4595–4602
Paschka P, Schlenk RF, Gaidzik VI et al (2010) IDH1 and IDH2 mutations are frequent genetic alterations in acute myeloid leukemia and confer adverse prognosis in cytogenetically normal acute myeloid leukemia with NPM1 mutation without FLT3 internal tandem duplication. J Clin Oncol 28(22):3636–3643
Paschka P, Du J, Schlenk RF et al (2013) Secondary genetic lesions in acute myeloid leukemia with inv(16) or t(16;16): a study of the German-Austrian AML study group (AMLSG). Blood 121(1):170–177
Paschka P, Schlenk RF, Gaidzik VI et al (2015) ASXL1 mutations in younger adult patients with acute myeloid leukemia: a study by the German-Austrian Acute Myeloid Leukemia Study Group. Haematologica 100(3):324–330
Pastore F, Kling D, Hoster E et al (2014a) Long-term follow-up of cytogenetically normal CEBPA-mutated AML. J Hematol Oncol 7(1):55
Pastore F, Dufour A, Benthaus T et al (2014b) Combined molecular and clinical prognostic index for relapse and survival in cytogenetically normal acute myeloid leukemia. J Clin Oncol 32(15):1586–1594

Patel JP, Gönen M, Figueroa ME et al (2012) Prognostic relevance of integrated genetic profiling in acute myeloid leukemia. N Engl J Med 366(12):1079–1089
Patel SS, Kuo FC, Gibson CJ et al (2018) High NPM1-mutant allele burden at diagnosis predicts unfavorable outcomes in de novo AML. Blood 131(25):2816–2825
Patkar N, Shaikh AF, Kakirde C et al (2019) A novel machine-learning-derived genetic score correlates with measurable residual disease and is highly predictive of outcome in acute myeloid leukemia with mutated NPM1. Blood Cancer J 9(10):1–4
Perry M, Bertoli S, Rocher C et al (2018) FLT3-TKD mutations associated with NPM1 mutations define a favorable-risk group in patients with acute myeloid Leukemia. Clin Lymph Myeloma Leukemia 18(12):e545–e550
Peterlin P, Renneville A, Abdelali RB et al (2015) Impact of additional genetic alterations on the outcome of patients with NPM1-mutated cytogenetically normal acute myeloid leukemia. Haematologica 100(5):e196–e199
Pigneux A, Labopin M, Maertens J et al (2015) Outcome of allogeneic hematopoietic stem-cell transplantation for adult patients with AML and 11q23/MLL rearrangement (MLL-r AML). Leukemia 29(12):2375–2381
Pirker R, Wallner J, Geissler K et al (1991) MDR1 gene expression and treatment outcome in acute myeloid leukemia. J Natl Cancer Inst 83(10):708–712
Poiré X, Labopin M, Polge E et al (2020) The impact of concomitant cytogenetic abnormalities on acute myeloid leukemia with monosomy 7 or deletion 7q after HLA-matched allogeneic stem cell transplantation. Am J Hematol 95(3):282–294
Ponziani V, Gianfaldoni G, Mannelli F et al (2006) The size of duplication does not add to the prognostic significance of FLT3 internal tandem duplication in acute myeloid leukemia patients. Leukemia 20(11):2074–2076
Port M, Böttcher M, Thol F et al (2014) Prognostic significance of FLT3 internal tandem duplication, nucleophosmin 1, and CEBPA gene mutations for acute myeloid leukemia patients with normal karyotype and younger than 60 years: a systematic review and meta-analysis. Ann Hematol 93(8):1279–1286
Prassek VV, Rothenberg-Thurley M, Sauerland MC et al (2018) Genetics of acute myeloid leukemia in the elderly: mutation spectrum and clinical impact in intensively treated patients aged 75 years or older. Haematologica 103(11):1853–1861
Pratcorona M, Abbas S, Sanders MA et al (2012) Acquired mutations in ASXL1 in acute myeloid leukemia: prevalence and prognostic value. Haematologica 97(3):388–392
Pratcorona M, Brunet S, Nomdedéu J et al (2013) Favorable outcome of patients with acute myeloid leukemia harboring a low-allelic burden FLT3-ITD mutation and concomitant NPM1 mutation: relevance to post-remission therapy. Blood 121(14):2734–2738
Pratz KW, Levis M (2017) How I treat FLT3-mutated AML. Blood 129(5):565–571
Prébet T, Boissel N, Reutenauer S et al (2009) Acute myeloid leukemia with translocation (8;21) or inversion (16) in elderly patients treated with conventional chemotherapy: a collaborative study of the French CBF-AML Intergroup. J Clin Oncol 27(28):4747–4753
Preudhomme C, Sagot C, Boissel N et al (2002) Favorable prognostic significance of CEBPA mutations in patients with de novo acute myeloid leukemia: a study from the Acute Leukemia French Association (ALFA). Blood 100(8):2717–2723
Prochazka KT, Pregartner G, Rücker FG et al (2019) Clinical implications of subclonal TP53 mutations in acute myeloid leukemia. Haematologica 104(3):516–523
Pulte D, Jansen L, Castro FA et al (2016) Survival in patients with acute myeloblastic leukemia in Germany and the United States: major differences in survival in young adults. Int J Cancer 139(6):1289–1296
Qin Y-Z, Zhu H-H, Jiang Q et al (2014) Prevalence and prognostic significance of c-KIT mutations in core binding factor acute myeloid leukemia: a comprehensive large-scale study from a single Chinese center. Leuk Res 38(12):1435–1440
Qin T, Wu S, Zhao H et al (2017) Molecular predictors of post-transplant survival in acute myeloid leukemia. Blood Cancer J 7(12):1–5
Quesada AE, Montalban-Bravo G, Luthra R et al (2020) Clinico-pathologic characteristics and outcomes of the World Health Organization (WHO) provisional entity de novo acute myeloid leukemia with mutated RUNX1. Mod Pathol 33(9):1678–1689
Renneville A, Boissel N, Gachard N et al (2009a) The favorable impact of CEBPA mutations in patients with acute myeloid leukemia is only observed in the absence of associated cytogenetic abnormalities and FLT3 internal duplication. Blood 113(21):5090–5093
Renneville A, Boissel N, Zurawski V et al (2009b) Wilms tumor 1 gene mutations are associated with a higher risk of recurrence in young adults with acute myeloid leukemia: a study from the Acute Leukemia French Association. Cancer 115(16):3719–3727
Renneville A, Boissel N, Nibourel O et al (2012) Prognostic significance of DNA methyltransferase 3A mutations in cytogenetically normal acute myeloid leukemia: a study by the Acute Leukemia French Association. Leukemia 26(6):1247–1254
Repp R, Schaekel U, Helm G et al (2003) Immunophenotyping is an independent factor for risk stratification in AML. Cytometry B Clin Cytom 53(1):11–19
Ribeiro AFT, Pratcorona M, Erpelinck-Verschueren C et al (2012) Mutant DNMT3A: a marker of poor prognosis in acute myeloid leukemia. Blood 119(24):5824–5831
Riera L, Marmont F, Toppino D et al (2013) Core binding factor acute myeloid leukaemia and c-KIT mutations. Oncol Rep 29(5):1867–1872
Rockova V, Abbas S, Wouters BJ et al (2011) Risk stratification of intermediate-risk acute myeloid leukemia: integrative analysis of a multitude of gene mutation

and gene expression markers. Blood 118(4):1069–1076
Röllig C, Bornhäuser M, Thiede C et al (2011) Long-term prognosis of acute myeloid Leukemia according to the new genetic risk classification of the European LeukemiaNet recommendations: evaluation of the proposed reporting system. JCO 29(20):2758–2765
Rozovski U, Ohanian M, Ravandi F et al (2015) Incidence of and risk factors for involvement of the central nervous system in acute myeloid leukemia. Leuk Lymphoma 56(5):1392–1397
Rücker FG, Schlenk RF, Bullinger L et al (2012) TP53 alterations in acute myeloid leukemia with complex karyotype correlate with specific copy number alterations, monosomal karyotype, and dismal outcome. Blood 119(9):2114–2121
Rücker FG, Agrawal M, Corbacioglu A et al (2019) Measurable residual disease monitoring in acute myeloid leukemia with t(8;21)(q22;q22.1): results from the AML Study Group. Blood 134(19):1608–1618
Sakaguchi M, Yamaguchi H, Najima Y et al (2018) Prognostic impact of low allelic ratio FLT3-ITD and NPM1 mutation in acute myeloid leukemia. Blood Adv 2(20):2744–2754
Sandahl JD, Coenen EA, Forestier E et al (2014) t(6;9)(p22;q34)/DEK-NUP214-rearranged pediatric myeloid leukemia: an international study of 62 patients. Haematologica 99(5):865–872
Santos FPS, Jones D, Qiao W et al (2011) Prognostic value of FLT3 mutations among different cytogenetic subgroups in acute myeloid leukemia. Cancer 117(10):2145–2155
Sanz MA, Fenaux P, Tallman MS et al (2019) Management of acute promyelocytic leukemia: updated recommendations from an expert panel of the European LeukemiaNet. Blood 133(15):1630–1643
Sasaki K, Kanagal-Shamanna R, Montalban-Bravo G et al (2020) Impact of the variant allele frequency of ASXL1, DNMT3A, JAK2, TET2, TP53, and NPM1 on the outcomes of patients with newly diagnosed acute myeloid leukemia. Cancer 126(4):765–774
Schanz J, Tüchler H, Solé F et al (2012) New comprehensive cytogenetic scoring system for primary myelodysplastic syndromes (MDS) and oligoblastic acute myeloid leukemia after MDS derived from an international database merge. J Clin Oncol 30(8):820–829
Schellongowski P, Staudinger T, Kundi M et al (2011) Prognostic factors for intensive care unit admission, intensive care outcome, and post-intensive care survival in patients with de novo acute myeloid leukemia: a single center experience. Haematologica 96(2):231–237
Schlenk RF, Benner A, Krauter J et al (2004) Individual patient data-based meta-analysis of patients aged 16 to 60 years with core binding factor acute myeloid leukemia: a survey of the German Acute Myeloid Leukemia Intergroup. J Clin Oncol 22(18):3741–3750
Schlenk RF, Döhner K, Krauter J et al (2008) Mutations and treatment outcome in cytogenetically normal acute myeloid leukemia. N Engl J Med 358(18):1909–1918
Schlenk RF, Taskesen E, van Norden Y et al (2013) The value of allogeneic and autologous hematopoietic stem cell transplantation in prognostically favorable acute myeloid leukemia with double mutant CEBPA. Blood 122(9):1576–1582
Schlenk RF, Kayser S, Bullinger L et al (2014) Differential impact of allelic ratio and insertion site in FLT3-ITD-positive AML with respect to allogeneic transplantation. Blood 124(23):3441–3449
Schlenk RF, Frech P, Weber D et al (2017) Impact of pretreatment characteristics and salvage strategy on outcome in patients with relapsed acute myeloid leukemia. Leukemia 31(5):1217–1220
Schmaelter A-K, Labopin M, Socié G et al (2020) Inferior outcome of allogeneic stem cell transplantation for secondary acute myeloid leukemia in first complete remission as compared to de novo acute myeloid leukemia. Blood Cancer J 10(3):26–26
Schneider F, Hoster E, Unterhalt M et al (2012) The FLT3ITD mRNA level has a high prognostic impact in NPM1 mutated, but not in NPM1 unmutated, AML with a normal karyotype. Blood 119(19):4383–4386
Schnittger S, Kinkelin U, Schoch C et al (2000) Screening for MLL tandem duplication in 387 unselected patients with AML identify a prognostically unfavorable subset of AML. Leukemia 14(5):796–804
Schnittger S, Schoch C, Kern W et al (2005) Nucleophosmin gene mutations are predictors of favorable prognosis in acute myelogenous leukemia with a normal karyotype. Blood 106(12):3733–3739
Schnittger S, Kohl TM, Haferlach T et al (2006) KIT-D816 mutations in AML1-ETO-positive AML are associated with impaired event-free and overall survival. Blood 107(5):1791–1799
Schnittger S, Haferlach C, Ulke M, Alpermann T, Kern W, Haferlach T. IDH1 mutations are detected in 6.6% of 1414 AML patients and are associated with intermediate risk karyotype and unfavorable prognosis in adults younger than 60 years and unmutated NPM1 status. Blood. 2010;116(25):5486–96.
Schnittger S, Bacher U, Kern W et al (2011a) Prognostic impact of FLT3-ITD load in NPM1 mutated acute myeloid leukemia. Leukemia 25(8):1297–1304
Schnittger S, Dicker F, Kern W et al (2011b) RUNX1 mutations are frequent in de novo AML with noncomplex karyotype and confer an unfavorable prognosis. Blood 117(8):2348–2357
Schnittger S, Eder C, Jeromin S et al (2013) ASXL1 exon 12 mutations are frequent in AML with intermediate risk karyotype and are independently associated with an adverse outcome. Leukemia 27(1):82–91
Schoch C, Haferlach T, Haase D et al (2001) Patients with de novo acute myeloid leukaemia and complex karyotype aberrations show a poor prognosis despite intensive treatment: a study of 90 patients. Br J Haematol 112(1):118–126
Schoch C, Schnittger S, Klaus M et al (2003) AML with 11q23/MLL abnormalities as defined by the WHO classification: incidence, partner chromosomes, FAB

subtype, age distribution, and prognostic impact in an unselected series of 1897 cytogenetically analyzed AML cases. Blood 102(7):2395–2402
Schoch C, Kern W, Schnittger S, Hiddemann W, Haferlach T (2004) Karyotype is an independent prognostic parameter in therapy-related acute myeloid leukemia (t-AML): an analysis of 93 patients with t-AML in comparison to 1091 patients with de novo AML. Leukemia 18(1):120–125
Scholl S, Theuer C, Scheble V et al (2008) Clinical impact of nucleophosmin mutations and Flt3 internal tandem duplications in patients older than 60 yr with acute myeloid leukaemia. Eur J Haematol 80(3):208–215
Schuurhuis GJ, Heuser M, Freeman S et al (2018) Minimal/measurable residual disease in AML: a consensus document from the European LeukemiaNet MRD working party. Blood 131(12):1275–1291
Schwartz GW, Manning B, Zhou Y et al (2019) Classes of ITD predict outcomes in AML patients treated with FLT3 inhibitors. Clin Cancer Res 25(2):573–583
Schwind S, Marcucci G, Maharry K et al (2010a) BAALC and ERG expression levels are associated with outcome and distinct gene and microRNA expression profiles in older patients with de novo cytogenetically normal acute myeloid leukemia: a Cancer and Leukemia Group B study. Blood 116(25):5660–5669
Schwind S, Maharry K, Radmacher MD et al (2010b) Prognostic significance of expression of a single microRNA, miR-181a, in cytogenetically normal acute myeloid leukemia: a Cancer and Leukemia Group B study. J Clin Oncol 28(36):5257–5264
Seifert H, Mohr B, Thiede C et al (2009) The prognostic impact of 17p (p53) deletion in 2272 adults with acute myeloid leukemia. Leukemia 23(4):656–663
Shen Y, Zhu Y-M, Fan X et al (2011) Gene mutation patterns and their prognostic impact in a cohort of 1185 patients with acute myeloid leukemia. Blood 118(20):5593–5603
Shiah H-S, Kuo Y-Y, Tang J-L et al (2002) Clinical and biological implications of partial tandem duplication of the MLL gene in acute myeloid leukemia without chromosomal abnormalities at 11q23. Leukemia 16(2):196–202
Shimada A, Iijima-Yamashita Y, Tawa A et al (2018) Risk-stratified therapy for children with FLT3-ITD-positive acute myeloid leukemia: results from the JPLSG AML-05 study. Int J Hematol 107(5):586–595
Shin H-J, Min W-S, Min YH et al (2019) Different prognostic effects of core-binding factor positive AML with Korean AML registry data. Ann Hematol 98(5):1135–1147
Silva P, Neumann M, Schroeder MP et al (2017) Acute myeloid leukemia in the elderly is characterized by a distinct genetic and epigenetic landscape. Leukemia 31(7):1640–1644
Sitges M, Boluda B, Garrido A et al (2020) Scute myeloid leukemia with inv(3)(q21q26.2)/t(3;3)(q21;q26.2): study of 61 patients treated with intensive protocols. Eur J Haematol 105(2):138–147
Slichter SJ (2004) Relationship between platelet count and bleeding risk in thrombocytopenic patients. Transfus Med Rev 18(3):153–167
Slovak ML, Kopecky KJ, Cassileth PA et al (2000) Karyotypic analysis predicts outcome of preremission and postremission therapy in adult acute myeloid leukemia: a Southwest Oncology Group/Eastern Cooperative Oncology Group Study. Blood 96(13):4075–4083
Slovak ML, Gundacker H, Bloomfield CD et al (2006) A retrospective study of 69 patients with t(6;9)(p23;q34) AML emphasizes the need for a prospective, multicenter initiative for rare 'poor prognosis' myeloid malignancies. Leukemia 20(7):1295–1297
Sorror ML, Maris MB, Storb R et al (2005) Hematopoietic cell transplantation (HCT)-specific comorbidity index: a new tool for risk assessment before allogeneic HCT. Blood 106(8):2912–2919
Sorror ML, Giralt S, Sandmaier BM et al (2007a) Hematopoietic cell transplantation–specific comorbidity index as an outcome predictor for patients with acute myeloid leukemia in first remission: combined FHCRC and MDACC experiences. Blood 110(13):4606–4613
Sorror ML, Sandmaier BM, Storer BE et al (2007b) Comorbidity and disease status–based risk stratification of outcomes among patients with acute myeloid leukemia or myelodysplasia receiving allogeneic hematopoietic cell transplantation. J Clin Oncol 25(27):4246–4254
Sorror ML, Storb RF, Sandmaier BM et al (2014) Comorbidity-age index: a clinical measure of biologic age before allogeneic hematopoietic cell transplantation. J Clin Oncol 32(29):3249–3256
Stengel A, Kern W, Haferlach T et al (2017) The impact of TP53 mutations and TP53 deletions on survival varies between AML, ALL, MDS and CLL: an analysis of 3307 cases. Leukemia 31(3):705–711
Stengel A, Kern W, Meggendorfer M et al (2018) Number of RUNX1 mutations, wild-type allele loss and additional mutations impact on prognosis in adult RUNX1-mutated AML. Leukemia 32(2):295–302
Stephens PJ, Greenman CD, Fu B et al (2011) Massive genomic rearrangement acquired in a single catastrophic event during cancer development. Cell 144(1):27–40
Steudel C, Wermke M, Schaich M et al (2003) Comparative analysis of MLL partial tandem duplication and FLT3 internal tandem duplication mutations in 956 adult patients with acute myeloid leukemia. Genes Chromosomes Cancer 37(3):237–251
Stirewalt DL, Kopecky KJ, Meshinchi S et al (2001) FLT3, RAS, and TP53 mutations in elderly patients with acute myeloid leukemia. Blood 97(11):3589–3595
Stirewalt DL, Kopecky KJ, Meshinchi S et al (2006) Size of FLT3 internal tandem duplication has prognostic significance in patients with acute myeloid leukemia. Blood 107(9):3724–3726
Stölzel F, Pfirrmann M, Aulitzky WE et al (2011) Risk stratification using a new prognostic score for patients

with secondary acute myeloid leukemia: results of the prospective AML96 trial. Leukemia 25(3):420–428
Stölzel F, Lüer T, Parmentier SB et al (2014) The prevalence of extramedullary AML detected by 18-FDG/PET-CT: results from the prospective PET-AML trial. Blood 124(21):2270–2270
Stölzel F, Mohr B, Kramer M et al (2016) Karyotype complexity and prognosis in acute myeloid leukemia. Blood Cancer J 6(1):e386
Straube J, Ling VY, Hill GR, Lane SW (2018) The impact of age, NPM1mut, and FLT3ITD allelic ratio in patients with acute myeloid leukemia. Blood 131(10):1148–1153
Su L, Tan Y, Lin H et al (2018) Mutational spectrum of acute myeloid leukemia patients with double CEBPA mutations based on next-generation sequencing and its prognostic significance. Oncotarget 9(38):24970–24979
Su L, Gao S, Tan Y et al (2019) CSF3R mutations were associated with an unfavorable prognosis in patients with acute myeloid leukemia with CEBPA double mutations. Ann Hematol 98(7):1641–1646
Suzuki T, Kiyoi H, Ozeki K et al (2005) Clinical characteristics and prognostic implications of NPM1 mutations in acute myeloid leukemia. Blood 106(8):2854–2861
Tallman MS, Hakimian D, Shaw JM et al (1993) Granulocytic sarcoma is associated with the 8;21 translocation in acute myeloid leukemia. J Clin Oncol 11(4):690–697
Tallman MS, Kim HT, Paietta E et al (2004) Acute monocytic leukemia (French-American-British classification M5) does not have a worse prognosis than other subtypes of acute myeloid leukemia: a report from the Eastern Cooperative Oncology Group. J Clin Oncol 22(7):1276–1286
Tallman MS, Wang ES, Altman JK et al (2019) Acute myeloid Leukemia, version 3.2019, NCCN clinical practice guidelines in oncology. J Natl Compr Cancer Netw 17(6):721–749
Tang J-L, Hou H-A, Chen C-Y et al (2009) AML1/RUNX1 mutations in 470 adult patients with de novo acute myeloid leukemia: prognostic implication and interaction with other gene alterations. Blood 114(26):5352–5361
Tarlock K, Alonzo TA, Moraleda PP et al (2014) Acute myeloid leukaemia (AML) with t(6;9)(p23;q34) is associated with poor outcome in childhood AML regardless of FLT3-ITD status: a report from the Children's Oncology Group. Br J Haematol 166(2):254–259
Taskesen E, Bullinger L, Corbacioglu A et al (2011) Prognostic impact, concurrent genetic mutations, and gene expression features of AML with CEBPA mutations in a cohort of 1182 cytogenetically normal AML patients: further evidence for CEBPA double mutant AML as a distinctive disease entity. Blood 117(8):2469–2475
Taub JW, Berman JN, Hitzler JK et al (2017) Improved outcomes for myeloid leukemia of Down syndrome: a report from the Children's Oncology Group AAML0431 trial. Blood 129(25):3304–3313
The Cancer Genome Atlas Research Network (2013) Genomic and epigenomic landscapes of adult de novo acute myeloid leukemia. N Engl J Med 368(22):2059–2074
Theis F, Corbacioglu A, Gaidzik VI et al (2016) Clinical impact of GATA2 mutations in acute myeloid leukemia patients harboring CEBPA mutations: a study of the AML study group. Leukemia 30(11):2248–2250
Thiede C, Steudel C, Mohr B et al (2002) Analysis of FLT3-activating mutations in 979 patients with acute myelogenous leukemia: association with FAB subtypes and identification of subgroups with poor prognosis. Blood 99(12):4326–4335
Thiede C, Koch S, Creutzig E et al (2006) Prevalence and prognostic impact of NPM1 mutations in 1485 adult patients with acute myeloid leukemia (AML). Blood 107(10):4011–4020
Thiede C, Bloomfield CD, Coco FL et al (2007) The high prevalence of FLT3-ITD mutations is associated with the poor outcome in adult patients with t(6;9)(p23;q34) positive AML—results of an international metaanalysis. Blood 110(11):761–761
Thol F, Damm F, Wagner K et al (2010) Prognostic impact of IDH2 mutations in cytogenetically normal acute myeloid leukemia. Blood 116(4):614–616
Thol F, Damm F, Lüdeking A et al (2011) Incidence and prognostic influence of DNMT3A mutations in acute myeloid leukemia. J Clin Oncol 29(21):2889–2896
Thol F, Kölking B, Hollink IHI et al (2013) Analysis of NUP98/NSD1 translocations in adult AML and MDS patients. Leukemia 27(3):750–754
Tien F-M, Hou H-A, Tsai C-H et al (2018a) Hyperleukocytosis is associated with distinct genetic alterations and is an independent poor-risk factor in de novo acute myeloid leukemia patients. Eur J Haematol 101(1):86–94
Tien F-M, Hou H-A, Tang J-L et al (2018b) Concomitant WT1 mutations predict poor prognosis in acute myeloid leukemia patients with double mutant CEBPA. Haematologica 103(11):e510–e513
Torrebadell M, Díaz-Beyá M, Kalko SG et al (2018) A 4-gene expression prognostic signature might guide post-remission therapy in patients with intermediate-risk cytogenetic acute myeloid leukemia. Leuk Lymphoma 59(10):2394–2404
Touw IP, Sanders MA (2020) Mutant allelic burden in acute myeloid leukaemia: why bother? Br J Haematol 188(6):817–818
Tsai C-H, Hou H-A, Tang J-L et al (2016) Genetic alterations and their clinical implications in older patients with acute myeloid leukemia. Leukemia 30(7):1485–1492
Tsimberidou A-M, Kantarjian HM, Wen S et al (2008) Myeloid sarcoma is associated with superior event-free survival and overall survival compared with acute myeloid leukemia. Cancer 113(6):1370–1378
Tsuji K, Motoji T, Sugawara I et al (2000) Significance of lung resistance-related protein in the clinical outcome of acute leukaemic patients with reference to P-glycoprotein. Br J Haematol 110(2):370–378

Valk PJM, Verhaak RGW, Beijen MA et al (2004) Prognostically useful gene-expression profiles in acute myeloid leukemia. N Engl J Med 350:1617–1628. https://doi.org/10.1056/NEJMoa040465
van Solinge TS, Zeijlemaker W, Ossenkoppele GJ, Cloos J, Schuurhuis GJ (2018) The interference of genetic associations in establishing the prognostic value of the immunophenotype in acute myeloid leukemia. Cytometry B Clin Cytom 94(1):151–158
Vasu S, Kohlschmidt J, Mrózek K et al (2018) Ten-year outcome of patients with acute myeloid leukemia not treated with allogeneic transplantation in first complete remission. Blood Adv 2(13):1645–1650
Venditti A, Poeta GD, Maurillo L et al (2004) Combined analysis of bcl-2 and MDR1 proteins in 256 cases of acute myeloid leukemia. Haematologica 89(8):934–939
Verhaak RGW, Goudswaard CS, van Putten W et al (2005) Mutations in nucleophosmin (NPM1) in acute myeloid leukemia (AML): association with other gene abnormalities and previously established gene expression signatures and their favorable prognostic significance. Blood 106(12):3747–3754
Versluis J, Hout FEM (2017) In ‘t, Devillier R, et al. Comparative value of post-remission treatment in cytogenetically normal AML subclassified by NPM1 and FLT3 -ITD allelic ratio. Leukemia 31(1):26–33
Vetro C, Haferlach T, Meggendorfer M et al (2020) Cytogenetic and molecular genetic characterization of KMT2A-PTD positive acute myeloid leukemia in comparison to KMT2A-rearranged acute myeloid leukemia. Cancer Genet 240:15–22
Virappane P, Gale R, Hills R et al (2008) Mutation of the Wilms’ tumor 1 gene is a poor prognostic factor associated with chemotherapy resistance in normal karyotype acute myeloid leukemia: the United Kingdom Medical Research Council Adult Leukaemia Working Party. J Clin Oncol 26(33):5429–5435
von Neuhoff C, Reinhardt D, Sander A et al (2010) Prognostic impact of specific chromosomal aberrations in a large group of pediatric patients with acute myeloid leukemia treated uniformly according to trial AML-BFM 98. J Clin Oncol 28(16):2682–2689
Wagner K, Damm F, Göhring G et al (2010) Impact of IDH1 R132 mutations and an IDH1 single nucleotide polymorphism in cytogenetically normal acute myeloid leukemia: SNP rs11554137 is an adverse prognostic factor. J Clin Oncol 28(14):2356–2364
Wakita S, Yamaguchi H, Ueki T et al (2016) Complex molecular genetic abnormalities involving three or more genetic mutations are important prognostic factors for acute myeloid leukemia. Leukemia 30(3):545–554
Walker CJ, Kohlschmidt J, Eisfeld A-K et al (2019) Genetic characterization and prognostic relevance of acquired uniparental disomies in cytogenetically normal acute myeloid leukemia. Clin Cancer Res 25(21):6524–6531
Wang B, Liu Y, Hou G et al (2016) Mutational spectrum and risk stratification of intermediate-risk acute myeloid leukemia patients based on next-generation sequencing. Oncotarget 7(22):32065–32078
Wang M, Lindberg J, Klevebring D et al (2017) Validation of risk stratification models in acute myeloid leukemia using sequencing-based molecular profiling. Leukemia 31(10):2029–2036
Wattad M, Weber D, Döhner K et al (2017) Impact of salvage regimens on response and overall survival in acute myeloid leukemia with induction failure. Leukemia 31(6):1306–1313
Weber S, Alpermann T, Dicker F et al (2014) BAALC expression: a suitable marker for prognostic risk stratification and detection of residual disease in cytogenetically normal acute myeloid leukemia. Blood Cancer J 4(1):e173
Weber S, Haferlach T, Haferlach C, Kern W (2016) Comprehensive study on ERG gene expression in normal karyotype acute myeloid leukemia: ERG expression is of limited prognostic value, whereas the accumulation of adverse prognostic markers stepwise worsens the prognosis. Blood Cancer J 6(12):e507
Weinberg OK, Ohgami RS, Ma L et al (2014) Acute myeloid leukemia with monosomal karyotype: morphologic, immunophenotypic, and molecular findings. Am J Clin Pathol 142(2):190–195
Weinberg OK, Gibson CJ, Blonquist TM et al (2017) NPM1 mutation but not RUNX1 mutation or multilineage dysplasia defines a prognostic subgroup within de novo acute myeloid leukemia lacking recurrent cytogenetic abnormalities in the revised 2016 WHO classification. Am J Hematol 92(7):E123–E124
Weissmann S, Alpermann T, Grossmann V et al (2012) Landscape of TET2 mutations in acute myeloid leukemia. Leukemia 26(5):934–942
Whitman SP, Archer KJ, Feng L et al (2001) Absence of the wild-type allele predicts poor prognosis in adult de novo acute myeloid leukemia with normal cytogenetics and the internal tandem duplication of FLT3: a Cancer and Leukemia Group B study. Cancer Res 61(19):7233–7239
Whitman SP, Maharry K, Radmacher MD et al (2010) FLT3 internal tandem duplication associates with adverse outcome and gene- and microRNA-expression signatures in patients 60 years of age or older with primary cytogenetically normal acute myeloid leukemia: a Cancer and Leukemia Group B study. Blood 116(18):3622–3626
Wierzbowska A, Wawrzyniak E, Siemieniuk-Rys M et al (2017) Concomitance of monosomal karyotype with at least 5 chromosomal abnormalities is associated with dismal treatment outcome of AML patients with complex karyotype—retrospective analysis of Polish Adult Leukemia Group (PALG). Leuk Lymphoma 58(4):889–897
Wiggers CRM, Baak ML, Sonneveld E et al (2019) AML subtype is a major determinant of the association between prognostic gene expression signatures and

their clinical significance. Cell Rep 28(11):2866–2877.e5
Wilhelmson AS, Porse BT (2020) CCAAT enhancer binding protein alpha (CEBPA) biallelic acute myeloid leukaemia: cooperating lesions, molecular mechanisms and clinical relevance. Br J Haematol 190(4):495–507
Wouters BJ, Löwenberg B, Erpelinck-Verschueren CAJ et al (2009) Double CEBPA mutations, but not single CEBPA mutations, define a subgroup of acute myeloid leukemia with a distinctive gene expression profile that is uniquely associated with a favorable outcome. Blood 113(13):3088–3091
Wu X, Feng X, Zhao X et al (2016) Prognostic significance of FLT3-ITD in pediatric acute myeloid leukemia: a meta-analysis of cohort studies. Mol Cell Biochem 420(1–2):121–128
Xu Q, Li Y, Lv N et al (2017) Correlation between isocitrate dehydrogenase gene aberrations and prognosis of patients with acute myeloid leukemia: a systematic review and meta-analysis. Clin Cancer Res 23(15):4511–4522
Yamato G, Shiba N, Yoshida K et al (2018) RUNX1 mutations in pediatric acute myeloid leukemia are associated with distinct genetic features and an inferior prognosis. Blood 131(20):2266–2270
Yanada M, Yamamoto Y, Iba S et al (2016) TP53 mutations in older adults with acute myeloid leukemia. Int J Hematol 103(4):429–435
Yang X, Wong MPM, Ng RK (2019) Aberrant DNA methylation in acute myeloid leukemia and its clinical implications. Int J Mol Sci 20(18):4576
Yoshizato T, Nannya Y, Atsuta Y et al (2017) Genetic abnormalities in myelodysplasia and secondary acute myeloid leukemia: impact on outcome of stem cell transplantation. Blood 129(17):2347–2358
Yuan X-Q, Chen P, Du Y-X et al (2019) Influence of DNMT3A R882 mutations on AML prognosis determined by the allele ratio in Chinese patients. J Transl Med 17(1):220
Zhang Y, Wang F, Chen X et al (2019) Companion gene mutations and their clinical significance in AML with double mutant CEBPA. Cancer Gene Ther 27(7-8):599–606
Zhou J, Zhang T, Xu Z et al (2019a) BCL2 overexpression: clinical implication and biological insights in acute myeloid leukemia. Diagn Pathol 14:68
Zhou F, Zhou F, Du M et al (2019b) Comprehensive prognostic scoring systems could improve the prognosis of adult acute myeloid leukemia patients. Int J Hematol 110(5):575–583
Zhou W, Chen G, Gong D et al (2020) Loss of the Y chromosome predicts a high relapse risk in younger adult male patients with t(8;21) acute myeloid leukemia on high-dose cytarabine consolidation therapy: a retrospective multicenter study. Leuk Lymphoma 61(4):820–830

# Management of Acute Promyelocytic Leukemia

**8**

Sabine Kayser and Uwe Platzbecker

## 8.1 Introduction

Acute promyelocytic leukemia (APL), characterized by the balanced translocation t(15;17)(q22;q12) resulting in the fusion transcript *PML-RARA,* is a rare entity of acute myeloid leukemia (AML), accounting for roughly 5–8% of AML patients (Swerdlow et al. 2017). According to the prior French-American-British (FAB) classification, APL was designated as "M3 leukemia"(Bennett et al. 1985) and is now assigned to the World Health Organization (WHO) defined type of AML with recurrent cytogenetic abnormalities, "acute promyelocytic leukemia with t(15;17)(q22;q12), (*PML-RARA*) and variants" (Swerdlow et al. 2017). According to the current WHO classification, patients with specific cytogenetic and molecular genetic abnormalities such as t(15;17)(q22;q12)/*PML-RARA* are classified as AML independently of the percentage of blast cells in the bone marrow and peripheral blood (Swerdlow et al. 2017).

Detection of the *PML-RARA* fusion is carried out by conventional cytogenetics including fluorescence in situ hybridization (FISH) and/or reverse transcriptase polymerase chain reaction (RT-PCR). Alternative fusion partners are the zinc finger gene (*PLZF*), the nucleophosmin gene (*NPM*), the nuclear mitotic apparatus (*NUMA*) or the *STAT5b* gene (Grimwade et al. 2000). These fusion partners are therapeutically relevant, since the alternative fusion partner involving the *PLZF* gene (t(11;17)(q23;q21)) is not sensitive to all-trans retinoic acid (ATRA) (Redner 2002).

## 8.2 Diagnostic Work-Up

The vast majority of APL patients mostly display a characteristic abnormal hypergranulation of blast cells and or promyelocytes (Fig. 8.1a) (Swerdlow et al. 2017). Thus, rapid morphological evaluation of peripheral blood as well as bone marrow is mandatory if an APL is suspected. The nuclei of the cells vary in shape and size, being often bilobulated and kidney-shaped (Fig. 8.1b). The cytoplasm of the cells is completely filled with dense and partially condensed granulation. In some cells the cytoplasm is filled with dust granulation. Cells with characteristic bundles of Auer rods are found in the bone marrow or in the peripheral blood, the so-called

S. Kayser (✉)
Medical Clinic and Policlinic I, Hematology and Cellular Therapy, University Hospital Leipzig, Leipzig, Germany

German Cancer Research Center (DKFZ), Heidelberg, Germany
e-mail: sabine.kayser@medizin.uni-leipzig.de

U. Platzbecker
Medical Clinic and Policlinic I, Hematology and Cellular Therapy, University Hospital Leipzig, Leipzig, Germany



C. Röllig, G. J. Ossenkoppele (eds.), *Acute Myeloid Leukemia*, Hematologic Malignancies,
https://doi.org/10.1007/978-3-030-72676-8_8

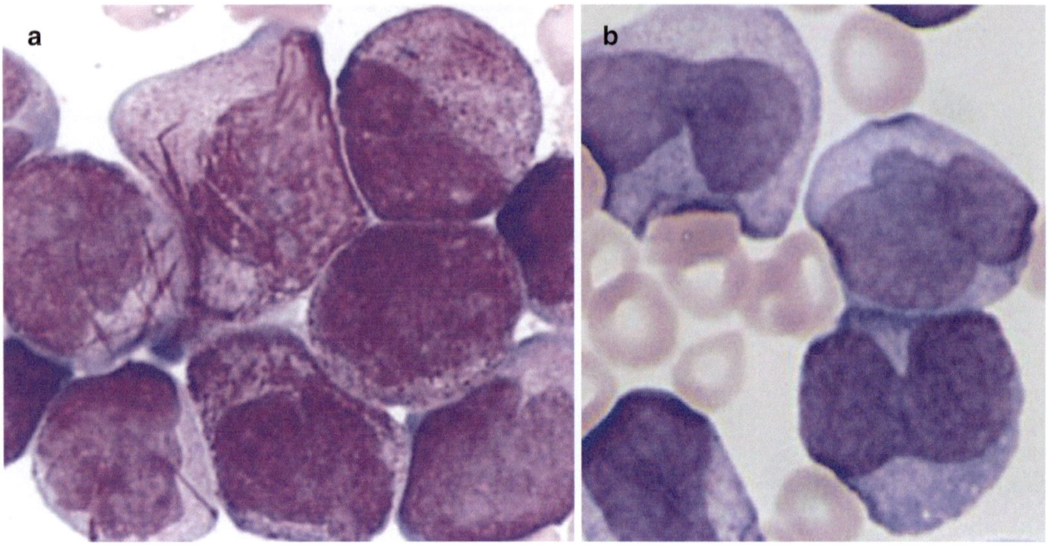


**Fig. 8.1** (**a**) Promyelocytes with characteristic Auer rods/Fagott cells in the cytoplasm. Faggot cells are cells normally found in the hypergranular form of APL (FAB-M3). The promyelocytes have numerous Auer rods in the cytoplasm which gives the appearance of a bundle of sticks. (**b**) Bilobulated and kidney-shaped blast cells which are characteristic for the microgranular variant (FAB M3v) of APL

**Table 8.1** Overview of the characteristics of the two APL variants

| Morphology | FAB M3 hypergranular | FAB M3v microgranular variant |
|---|---|---|
| Relative incidence (%) | 90–95 | 5–10 |
| Morphology | • Large blast cells<br>• Auer rods, often in bundles<br>• Faggot cells | • Micrograpular<br>• Bilobulated and kidney-shaped blast cells |
| Immunophenotype | CD2–,CD13+,CD33+,**CD34–**,CD117+,**HLA-DR–** | CD2+,CD13+,CD33+,**CD34–/+**,CD117+,**HLA-DR–** |

Faggot cells. The M3 variant (M3v), however, contains fewer cells with hypergranulations or bundles of Auer rods.

Hypergranulated promyelocytes strongly react with POX, SSB, and chloroacetate esterase. The expression of CD33, CD117, and absence of HLA-DR and CD34 on the surface of APL blasts is characteristic of the disease (Table 8.1). The t(15;17) translocation and the respective *PML-RARA* fusion transcript are diagnostically conclusive and represent definitive hallmarks of APL diagnosis (Swerdlow et al. 2017). The molecular analysis for the detection of *PML-RARA* is carried out by either RT-PCR or by FISH. Whereas both methods are used as a fast and highly sensitive verification of the initial diagnosis, only RT-qPCR is sensitive enough for the measurement of measurable residual disease (MRD) in the course of APL therapy. The results of several independent studies have shown that RT-qPCR positivity for *PML-RARA* transcripts during morphological remission within consolidation cycles is a predictive factor for an early hematological recurrence, whereas RT-qPCR negativity in the bone marrow is usually associated with long-term survival and cure after therapy (also in patients with relapse) (Burnett et al. 1999; Mandelli et al. 1997; Schnittger et al. 2003; Cicconi et al. 2018).

### 8.2.1 Diagnostic Examination Schedule

Morphological analyses of bone marrow and peripheral blood are recommended at the following time points:

- at initial diagnosis
- after induction
- prior to the second and following consolidation therapy
- after the last consolidation therapy
- quarterly during maintenance therapy in high-risk patients
- after therapy quarterly during a 3 years follow-up from start of therapy
- At suspected relapse

Cytogenetic and immunophenotypic analyses should be performed at diagnosis and in case of relapse.

Molecular analyses with RT-qPCR for evaluation of MRD are recommended according to the risk-status at diagnosis as indicated in Table 8.2.

## 8.3 Treatment

APL must be classified as an emergency with immediate initiation of treatment with all-rans retinoic acid (ATRA) 45 mg/m$^2$/day as well as supportive therapy. Even when APL is only suspected based on clinical and morphological findings, therapy must be started immediately before a genetic diagnosis is available due to the potential lethal complications and the potential for cure. Prior to therapy, bone marrow and blood diagnostics are essential. Treatment with ATRA has revolutionized~~improved~~ therapeutic success in APL, providing the prime example of molecularly targeted treatment (Huang et al. 1988; Tallman et al. 1997). ATRA causes differentiation of abnormal promyelocytes to mature neutrophils in vitro and in vivo. Complete remissions (CR) were achieved with single-agent ATRA in up to 80–90% of newly diagnosed and relapsed APL patients (Huang et al. 1988; Tallman et al. 1997; Ablain and de The 2011; Castaigne et al. 1990; Chen et al. 1991; Chomienne et al. 1990). Additionally, treatment with ATRA abrogates the disturbed coagulation cascade. However, the accelerated differentiation to mature neutrophils often induces a rapid WBC increase. In fact, in 15–20% of patients, the so-called "differentiation-syndrome" (DS) occurs, consisting of, for example, weight gain, respiratory distress, unexplained fever, interstitial pulmonary infiltrates, pleural or pericardial effusions with or without leukocytosis. This syndrome is associated with a high mortality rate (Fenaux et al. 1992; Frankel et al. 1992, 1994; Warrell et al. 1994); specific treatment to overcome DS is discussed in Chap. 4.

Unfortunately, remissions after single agent treatment with ATRA in most of the patients were not sustained (Huang et al. 1988; Tallman et al. 1997; Ablain and de The 2011; Castaigne et al. 1990; Chen et al. 1991; Chomienne et al. 1990). These findings led to the concurrent use of ATRA with chemotherapy (CTX; either an anthracycline plus cytarabine or an anthracycline alone) as the standard of care for induction in newly diagnosed APL (Coombs et al.

**Table 8.2** Molecular analyses with RT-qPCR for evaluation of measureable residual disease according to the risk-status at diagnosis

| Time point | Low-/intermediate-risk (WBC $\leq 10 \times 10^9$/L) | High-risk (WBC $> 10 \times 10^9$/L) |
|---|---|---|
| At initial diagnosis | ✓ | ✓ |
| After induction | – | ✓ |
| Prior to the second and following consolidation therapy | – | ✓ |
| After the last consolidation therapy | ✓ | ✓ |
| Quarterly during maintenance therapy[a] | – | ✓ |
| After therapy quarterly during a 3 year follow-up from start of therapy[a] | – | ✓ |
| At suspected relapse | ✓ | ✓ |

*Abbreviation: WBC*, white blood cell count

[a]Peripheral blood is sufficient for measureable residual disease analysis

2015). More recently, the combination of arsenic trioxide (ATO) with ATRA has been shown to be a very effective CTX-free treatment strategy in de novo, low-/intermediate-risk (low-/intermediate-risk: WBC ≤ 10.0 × 10⁹/l; high-risk: WBC > 10.0 × 10⁹/l) APL (Estey et al. 2006).

In addition, published data of a large multicenter phase 3 randomized trial on the direct comparison of ATO/ATRA vs ATRA in combination with idarubicin (AIDA) or mitoxantrone in adult patients with de novo, non-high-risk APL showed very promising results in favor of ATO/ATRA, with a 2-year event-free survival (EFS) rate of 97 vs 86% ($P = 0.02$) (Lo-Coco et al. 2013). Within this trial, early mortality as well as hematological toxicities were significantly lower in patients treated with ATO/ATRA as compared to AIDA. Particularly, the cumulative incidence of relapse (CIR) after 50 months was only 1.9% after ATO/ATRA as compared to 13.9% after CTX + ATRA (Platzbecker et al. 2016). Moreover, none of the patients treated with ATO/ATRA developed a therapy-related myeloid neoplasm as compared to two patients in the CTX/ATRA arm (Platzbecker et al. 2016). Another publication of the Medical Research Council supports these results, with a 4-year EFS rate of 91% after ATO/ATRA as compared to 70% after CTX/ATRA ($P = 0.002$) (Burnett et al. 2015). However, the regimen with ATO/ATRA was associated with a higher frequency of grade 3 or 4 hepatic toxicity as compared to CTX/ATRA (44% vs 3%; $P < 0.001$). In all cases, the toxic effects resolved with temporary discontinuation of ATO and/or ATRA (Platzbecker et al. 2016). Taken together, the CTX-free regimen with ATO/ATRA has become standard first-line therapy in non-high-risk de novo APL. Figure 8.2 and Table 8.3 give an overview of the treatment schedule and dosages. We recommend the following approach:

- prophylaxis of differentiation syndrome with prednisone 0.5 mg/kg/day p.o. from day 1 of ATO application to the end of induction therapy as well as hydroxyurea (see Chap. 4, Sect. 4.3) if WBC count raises up to >10 × 10⁹/L)
- bone marrow evaluation on day 28
- induction therapy should be terminated on the basis of morphological criteria (if CR or CRi is reached on day 28)
- in case CR or CRi is not achieved by day 28, ATO/ATRA therapy should be continued up to max. day 60 until terminal differentiation is reached; this should be accompanied by serial bone marrow assessments to definitively demonstrate CR

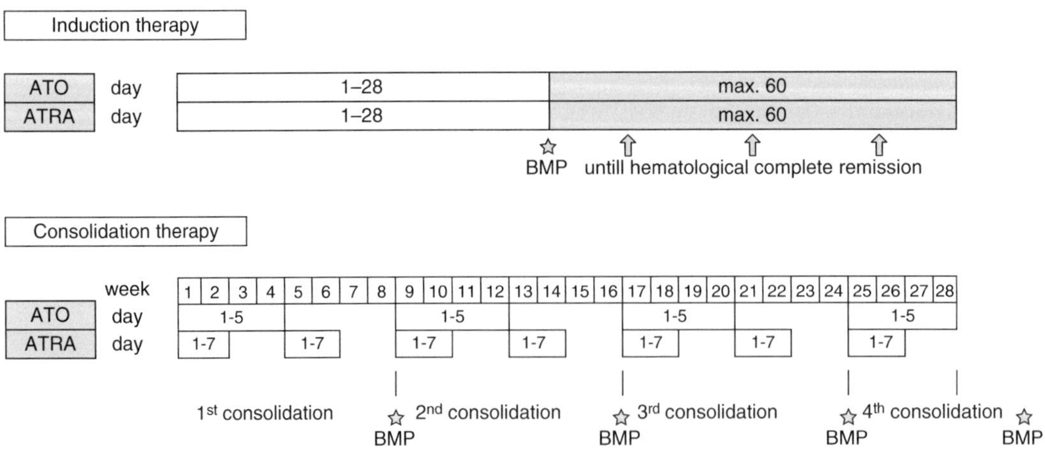


**Fig. 8.2** Treatment recommendation for non-high-risk APL (WBC ≤10 × 10⁹ at diagnosis) according to the APL0406 study

**Table 8.3** Treatment schedule and dosages of arsenic trioxide and all-trans retinoic acid as first-line therapy in non-high-risk acute promyelocytic leukemia

| Drug | Dose | Route | Administration |
|---|---|---|---|
| *Induction* | | | |
| ATO | 0.15 mg/kg | Intravenously | Over 2 h daily starting on day 1, until CR, maximally 60 days |
| ATRA | 45 mg/m$^2$ | Per os | In two single doses daily starting on day 1, until CR, maximally 60 days; doses will be rounded-up to next 10 mg increment |
| *Consolidation* | | | |
| ATO | 0.15 mg/kg | Intravenously | Over 2 h daily for 5 days a week; treatment break on day 6 and 7<br>4 weeks on 4 weeks off for a total of 4 courses;<br>last cycles will be administered on week 25–28 |
| ATRA | 45 mg/m$^2$ | Per os | In two single doses daily 14 days on, 14 days off for a total of 7 courses; doses will be rounded-up to next 10 mg increment |

*ATO* arsenic trioxide, *ATRA* all-trans retinoic acid

- cytogenetic and molecular assessment at the end of induction therapy has no value in case of CR. Molecular responses should be assessed after consolidation only

ATO/ATRA-based induction therapy is followed by 4 courses of ATO/ATRA-based consolidation. Start of consolidation cycles is considered after hematological recovery with neutrophils $\geq 1.0 \times 10^9$/L and platelets $\geq 100 \times 10^9$/L. In case of morphological CR and hematological recovery, consolidation therapy should be started within 4 weeks after documented CR. Each course of therapy should be initiated at hematological recovery from the previous course. The PCR status after the end of consolidation is an important stratification parameter for the subsequent therapy. However, it needs to be mentioned that the rate of molecular remission was 100% after ATO/ATRA in the pivotal study (Platzbecker et al. 2016).

During all consolidation cycles (Swerdlow et al. 2017; Bennett et al. 1985; Grimwade et al. 2000; Redner 2002) the following diagnostics are recommended:

- bone marrow samples should be collected after full hematological recovery prior to the start of the second, third, and fourth consolidation cycle as well as after the last consolidation cycle and should be tested for morphology and by RT-qPCR for assessment of molecular remission
- patients without molecular remission at the end of all consolidation cycles are very rare cases (<1%) and will be considered molecularly resistant and should be offered conventional chemotherapy (e.g., AIDA) followed by an autologous or allogeneic hematopoietic stem cell transplantation

In countries where ATO is not yet available AIDA-based CTX is still the standard.

### 8.3.1 Dose Modifications

In case of non-hematological toxicities (grade 3/4 toxicities according to CTCAE Version 4.03) of ATO and ATRA (e.g., QT prolongation, differentiation syndrome, hepatotoxicity, pseudotumor cerebri) dose modifications according to Table 8.4 are recommended. As soon as the symptoms and the patients' clinical conditions improve, treatment with ATRA and/or ATO should be resumed at 50% of the previous dose during the first 7 days after the disappearance of the symptoms. Thereafter, in the absence of

**Table 8.4** Dose modifications in case of non-hematological toxicities

| Dose level | 0 (Start level) | −1 | −2 | −3 |
|---|---|---|---|---|
| ATO (mg/kg) | **0.15** | **0.11** | **0.10** | **0.075** |
| ATRA (mg/m$^2$) | **45** | **37.5** | **25** | **20** |

*ATO* arsenic trioxide, *ATRA* all-trans retinoic acid

worsening of the previous toxicity, ATRA and/or ATO should be resumed at full dosage. In case of the reappearance of symptoms, ATRA and ATO should be reduced to the previous dosage.

## 8.4 Supportive Measures and Management of Complications

### 8.4.1 Treatment of Coagulopathy

APL is typically associated with frequently life-threatening hemorrhagic diathesis, which is attributed to a disseminated intravascular coagulation-like coagulopathy (Swerdlow et al. 2017; Tallman and Kwaan 1992; Sanz and Montesinos 2010). The pathogenesis of hemorrhagic complications in patients with APL is complex, often triggered by higher white blood cell (WBC) counts and includes factors of blood coagulation and fibrinolysis such as severe hypofibrinogenemia, increased levels of fibrin degradation products, or D-dimers combined with a prolonged prothrombin or activated partial thromboplastin time as well as thrombocytopenia (Mantha et al. 2016). The hemorrhagic diathesis is one of the main causes of early death (ED) in APL patients (Sanz and Montesinos 2010; Mantha et al. 2016). Release and exposure of tissue factor and annexin II by the leukemic blasts are triggering these processes. Thus, the absolute WBC count, reflecting the absolute leukemic mass, seems to correlate with the severity of bleeding complications (Mantha et al. 2016).

Before the ATRA era, the risk of early hemorrhagic death for newly diagnosed patients with APL was up to 20% and decreased to 5–10% after introduction of ATRA in 1988 (Rodeghiero et al. 1990). Therefore, current guidelines advise to start ATRA as soon as the diagnosis of APL is suspected to treat and prevent hemorrhagic complications (Sanz et al. 2009). However, it must be noted that the therapy with ATRA can result in a reversion of the clotting disorder into a thrombophilic constellation with thromboembolic events. The benefit of heparin, tranexamic acid, or other anticoagulant or anti-fibrinolytic therapy to attenuate the thrombohemorrhagic risk remains questionable. In a historical comparison of the LPA99 with the LPA96 trials, the use of tranexamic acid had no impact on decreasing the hemorrhagic mortality (Sanz and Montesinos 2010). Additionally, the role of factor VIIa or prothrombotic complex concentrates for treating life-threatening hemorrhages in APL remains uncertain. Although there are case reports in which the use of recombinant factor VIIa was effective for the treatment of life-threatening hemorrhage in patients with APL (Zver et al. 2004; Alimoghaddam et al. 2006), theoretically these agents may enhance the thrombotic risk (Mantha et al. 2016; Rodeghiero et al. 1990). Therefore, the prophylactic use of anticoagulant, antifibrinolytic, or procoagulant agents should be restricted to clinical trials. Finally, any invasive procedures, including the insertion of central intravenous catheters as well as other procedures (e.g., bronchoscopy or lumbar puncture), should be avoided until coagulopathy has resolved (Sanz et al. 2009). Supportive therapy to counteract the coagulopathy should be initiated in parallel to APL-specific treatment. This includes the application of fibrinogen as well as platelet transfusions to maintain fibrinogen concentration above 100 mg/dL and platelet count as high as possible (>50 × $10^9$/L) but at least above 30 × $10^9$/L, respectively (Sanz et al. 2009). In case of unavailability of pure fibrinogen preparation, a substitution with fresh frozen plasma is indicated.

Only limited data exist about the effect on hemorrhagic risk by the addition of ATO to induction therapy. There was no case of early hemorrhagic death in the ATO/ATRA-arm for patients with low-/intermediate-risk (pretreatment WBC ≤ 10 × $10^9$/L) disease within the APL0406 trial (Lo-Coco et al. 2013). Nevertheless, in high-risk patients, CTX (preferably idarubicin) in combination with ATRA should be initiated as early as possible to terminate the perilous bleeding cascade.

### 8.4.2 Therapy of Differentiation Syndrome

DS is a complication during induction caused by the differentiating effects of ATRA and/or ATO on leukemic blasts, which can be fatal if not treated (Sanz and Montesinos 2014). Symptoms may include unexplained fever, dyspnea, acute respiratory distress, interstitial pulmonary infiltrates, pleural or pericardial effusions, weight gain or peripheral edema, hypotension, and renal, hepatic, or multi-organ dysfunction. Leukocytosis frequently but not always accompanies DS and often precedes its clinical manifestations (Montesinos et al. 2009a).

If DS is suspected, 10 mg dexamethasone twice daily intravenously, concomitant diuretic therapy and hemodynamic monitoring should immediately be initiated until resolution of signs and symptoms. Temporary discontinuation of ATRA and/or ATO may be required in cases of severe DS (Sanz et al. 2009). Early transfer of patients to an intermediate care unit for improved monitoring of vital signs should be considered. As soon as the patients' clinical condition improves, the symptoms have disappeared and the WBC count is sustainably lowered to <10 × $10^9$/L, the APL treatment with ATRA and/or ATO can be resumed at 50% of the previous dose during the first 7 days. ATRA and/or ATO might be resumed at full dosage in the absence of worsening of the previous toxicity. In case of reappearance of the previous symptoms, ATRA and ATO should be reduced to the previous dosage. The evidence for the use of corticosteroids as a prophylactic approach to prevent DS, however, is limited. Within the APL2000 trial, the DS-related death rate decreased from 5.7 to 3.9% in high-risk patients after the prophylactic use of dexamethasone as compared to the earlier APL93 trial, in which prophylactic dexamethasone was not used (Sanz and Montesinos 2010; Kelaidi et al. 2009). Within the APL0406 trial, prednisone was given prophylactically at a dose of 0.5 mg/kg/day from day 1 until the end of induction therapy (Lo-Coco et al. 2013). DS developed in 19% in the ATO/ATRA group and in 16% in the CTX/ATRA group, but was fatal in only 2.5% assigned to CTX/ATRA (Lo-Coco et al. 2013). Based on these results, we recommend prednisone prophylaxis as done in the APL0406 trial.

### 8.4.3 Treatment of Leukocytosis During Induction

Leukocytosis commonly occurs, either at initial presentation or during therapy in patients treated with ATRA and/or ATO induction as a result of DS. Thus, in low-risk APL, hydroxyurea 500 mg once/daily for WBC between 10 and 20 × $10^9$/L, 500 mg twice/daily for WBC between 21 and 50 × $10^9$/L, and 1.000 mg twice daily above 50 × $10^9$/L should be used in case of leukocytosis and should be continued at a given dose to keep the WBC count <10 × $10^9$/L and subsequently tapered (Table 8.5) (Lo-Coco et al. 2013). Additionally, APL cells are sensitive to therapy with anthracyclines. Thus, treatment with anthracyclines such as idarubicin should be considered as early as possible during induction therapy of high-risk patients. ATO/ATRA in combination with idarubicin was used up-front within the phase 2 APML4 trial, in part to prevent hyperleukocytosis and DS (Iland et al. 2012). In this trial, no deaths from DS occurred. Furthermore, gemtuzumab ozogamicin (GO) was successfully used within the AML17 trial in high-risk patients to control leukocytosis (Burnett et al. 2015).

**Table 8.5** Treatment of leukocytosis in low-/intermediate-risk acute promyelocytic leukemia during induction therapy due to differentiation syndrome

| White blood cell count × $10^9$/L | Hydroxyurea |
|---|---|
| 10–20 | 500 mg/daily |
| 21–50 | 500 mg twice/daily |
| >50 | 1.000 mg twice/daily |

In contrast, leukapheresis has no role in upfront treatment, and may even be harmful in high-risk patients with leukocytosis, because this procedure may exacerbate the coagulopathy and was associated with a high risk of death (Vahdat et al. 1994).

### 8.4.4 QT Prolongation Associated with ATO

Treatment with ATO is associated with electrolyte abnormalities and prolongation of the QT interval corrected for the heart rate (QTc), which can lead to ventricular tachycardia with fatal outcome (Barbey et al. 2003; Unnikrishnan et al. 2004). Prolongation of the QTc interval occurred in 12 of 77 (16%) patients in the ATO/ATRA group within the APL0406 trial and was severe (QTc ≥ 501 ms) in one patient. Therefore, close monitoring of the electrocardiogram and electrolytes is necessary during treatment with ATO. Particularly, magnesium and potassium levels should always be kept within the upper-normal range. Concomitant therapy with drugs that are known to prolong the QTc interval should be discontinued. In patients with an absolute QTc interval > 500 ms, ATO should be discontinued, ideally together with any QTc prolonging medication, and electrolytes should be repleted. The time between discontinuing ATO and normalization of the QTc interval may take several days. Once QTc is normalized, ATO should be continued at 0.075 mg/kg (50%) for the first 7 days, and, if no further prolongation occurs, ATO should be escalated to 0.11 mg/kg for a second week. Thereafter, if no prolongation occurs, ATO could be continued at full dose (Lo-Coco et al. 2013).

### 8.4.5 Pseudotumor cerebri with ATRA Therapy

A "pseudotumor cerebri," manifesting with headaches, nausea, vomiting, and blurred vision, may occur during ATRA therapy, particularly in younger patients. It is recommended to discontinue ATRA treatment temporarily and to administer pain killers. As soon as the symptoms and the patients' clinical conditions improve, the treatment with ATRA should be resumed at 50% of the previous dose during the first 7 days. In the absence of worsening of the previous toxicity, ATRA should be resumed at full dosage thereafter.

### 8.4.6 Long-Term Toxicities with ATO/ATRA

The up-front use of ATO/ATRA is anticipated to reduce the long-term toxicities associated with anthracycline therapy. However, studies indicate that potential long-term complications exist. In one long-term follow-up study among 265 newly diagnosed APL patients treated with ATO/ATRA between 2001 and 2012, with a median follow-up of 83 months, higher rates of grade 1 liver dysfunction (15% vs 2%) and hepatic steatosis (43% vs 18%) were seen as compared to healthy controls (Zhu et al. 2016). Breast cancer developed in one patient 3 years after termination of ATO. Eight patients developed hyper-, or hypopigmentation, or hyperkeratosis/hyperplasia. All skin lesions occurred during maintenance therapy or within 6 months after treatment, and patients recovered within 2 to 18 months (Zhu et al. 2016). However, the common signs of chronic arseniasis, such as cardiovascular events, chronic renal insufficiency, diabetes, or neurological dysfunction, were not observed (Zhu et al. 2016). In some cases, peripheral neuropathy has been reported during and after treatment with ATO (Kühn et al. 2016; Shigeno et al. 2005). Symptoms are usually mild and reversible following discontinuation of treatment, but may be severe and irreversible in patients with coexistence of thiamine deficiency (Kühn et al. 2016).

Further evidence suggests a high frequency of varicella zoster virus (VZV) reactivation after ATO-based treatment. In a publication by Yamakura et al. VZV reactivation occurred in seven (46.7%) of 15 patients after ATO-based treatment as compared to none in ten patients treated with conventional CTX. All patients responded promptly to treatment with acyclovir or valacyclovir and did not develop postherpetic neuralgia. Thus, we recommend the prophylactic use of acyclovir or valacyclovir throughout ATO-based therapy (Yamakura et al. 2014).

Very recently, Norsworthy et al. reported data of 124 adult APL patients from the Surveillance, Epidemiology, and End Results (SEER) program of the National Cancer Institute who were diagnosed with APL between 2006 and 2015 (Norsworthy et al. 2019). The authors performed an exploratory population-based analysis of secondary malignancies in patients treated with or without ATO. This exploratory analysis revealed a higher incidence of second malignancies in APL patients treated with ATO, although the risk was not significantly increased compared to patients who received other APL therapies (9.9% vs 6.0% at 24 months, $P = 0.24$). Despite that, survival outcomes appeared better after ATO-based therapy (Norsworthy et al. 2019). However, the analyses were limited by a small sample size, short follow-up, potential selection and immortal time bias, and unaccounted for differences between comparator groups.

Based on this limited data, no firm conclusions can be drawn regarding the occurrence of comorbidities and organ toxicities. However, we suggest routine follow-up to monitor for and manage cardiovascular risk factors. Finally, age-appropriate cancer screening should be emphasized in all patients after completion of APL therapy.

## 8.5 Treatment of High-Risk APL

Patients with high-risk APL account for roughly 30% of patients. After induction treatment with AIDA, subsequent risk-guided consolidation cycles have shown to equalize the risk of relapse between both APL risk groups based on initial WBC counts (Sanz et al. 2000, 2004a). Due to its success in *de novo* non-high-risk APL (Lo-Coco et al. 2013), ATO/ATRA has also been explored as front-line use in high-risk APL. However, phase 2 studies have demonstrated lower CR rates with single agent ATO ± ATRA as compared to classical AIDA-based induction regimens in high-risk patients (Estey et al. 2006; Sanz et al. 2000, 2004a; Ghavamzadeh et al. 2011; Mathews et al. 2006; Ravandi et al. 2009).

Recently, Abaza et al. published outcome data on 187 APL patients, including 54 with high-risk APL (Abaza et al. 2017). In an attempt to improve outcomes in high-risk patients, they added GO ($n = 45$) or idarubicin ($n = 7$) to ATO/ATRA. Albeit results were drawn from a small cohort, 5-year overall survival (OS) were not significantly different between the two treatment arms (84% vs 100%; $P = 0.45$) and are in-line reported by others (Estey et al. 2006; Ravandi et al. 2009). Similar results were reported by Burnett et al. on the phase-3 AML17 trial comparing ATO/ATRA with CTX/ATRA in newly diagnosed patients with APL (Burnett et al. 2015). High-risk patients treated with ATO/ATRA received one initial dose of GO (6 mg/m$^2$). The 4-year EFS-rate was 91% after ATO/ATRA/GO as compared to 70% in the CTX/ATRA group. Furthermore, the cumulative incidence of morphological and molecular relapses were reduced from 18% and 27% in the CTX/ATRA group to 1% and 0% in the ATO/ATRA/GO group (Burnett et al. 2015). Currently, the European randomized intergroup study "APOLLO" investigates idarubicin 12 mg/m$^2$ on days 1 and 3 in addition to oral ATRA 45 mg/m$^2$ twice daily on days 1–28 and ATO 0.15 mg/kg/day intravenously on days 5–28 followed by four cycles of ATO/ATRA consolidation therapy as compared to the standard CTX/ATRA approach (ClinicalTrails.gov identifier: NCT02688140).

In patients with high-risk APL, treatment with idarubicin + ATRA should be started as soon as possible. After achieving a hematological CR, three consolidation cycles of ATRA plus either idarubicin/cytarabine (course 1 and 3) or plus mitoxantrone (course 2) are intended (Norsworthy et al. 2019). This approach is also supported by published data combining intensive CTX according to the 7 + 3 scheme and ATRA (Lengfelder et al. 2009). Moreover, a positive impact of adding ATO to consolidation regimens was reported for all risk groups of APL in the C9710 trial (Powell et al. 2010). The efficacy of

ATO as consolidation therapy was recently confirmed by Lou et al., who reported that treatment with ATO as post-remission therapy significantly improved long-term outcome as compared to standard CTX (Lou et al. 2014).

Thus, ATO as consolidation therapy in high-risk patients could be considered, although currently not authority approved.

## 8.6 Maintenance Therapy

### 8.6.1 Maintenance in Patients with High-Risk APL

The clinical benefit of maintenance therapy particularly in patients with negative MRD is still discussed controversial due to adverse side effects (AEs) including cytopenia and/or increase of the liver values. In the European APL-93 study, triple-agent maintenance therapy with ATRA, 6-mercaptopurine (6-MP) and methotrexate (MTX) resulted in a lower recurrence rate, particularly in patients with high-risk (Fenaux et al. 1999). However, this study did not differentiate between patients according to the MRD status after consolidation. Several other publications also demonstrated that an ATRA-based maintenance is needed after consolidation to ameliorate survival (Tallman et al. 1997, 2002; Kantarjian et al. 1987; Adès et al. 2010). In contrast, patients randomized to maintenance therapy with 6-MP and MTX in the LAP 0389 study did not have better outcomes than those randomized to observation, which is in line with recently published results (Avvisati et al. 2002, 2011; Asou et al. 2007). It is currently unclear, if maintenance therapy further enhances the risk for secondary malignancies, including therapy-related myeloid neoplasm. Within the recently published long-term follow-up data of the LPA96&99 as well as LPA2005 trials, 24 patients (11%) developed a secondary neoplasm in CR within a median time of 51 months (range, 6–112 months; 11 solid tumors and 7 therapy-related myeloid neoplasms within the LPA96&99 trials; 3 solid tumors and 3 therapy-related myeloid neoplasms within the LPA2005 trial, respectively) (Martínez-Cuadrón et al. 2018). Twenty-one patients died because of the secondary neoplasm. Cumulative incidence of secondary neoplasms at 5 and 10 years was 8% and 16%, respectively. However, the authors stated that no predictive factors for this event were found (Martínez-Cuadrón et al. 2018).

Taken together, maintenance therapy may still play a role in patients with high-risk receiving CTX/ATRA while its omission in the setting of ATRA and ATO is currently under investigation.

### 8.6.2 ATO as Maintenance Therapy

Treatment with oral ATO was shown to be well absorbed and to achieve a bioavailability of up to 95% of an equivalent dose of intravenous ATO (Kumana et al. 2002). Since slow oral absorption results in lower peak plasma arsenic levels compared with intravenous ATO, the oral formulation is associated with minimal prolongation of the QT interval (Siu et al. 2006; Kwong et al. 2001). Thus, a home-based treatment without the need of daily hospital visits and monitoring for QT prolongation or cardiac arrhythmias seems to be feasible.

Recently, Au et al. have published 10-year follow-up data on outcome after oral ATO-based maintenance therapy (Au et al. 2011). Seventy-six APL patients in first CR after induction and consolidation with daunorubicin/cytarabine received oral maintenance therapy with ATO ± ATRA or ATO/ATRA/ascorbic acid, given for 2 weeks every 2 months for 2 years. Prolonged oral ATO maintenance was feasible and safe and resulted in 3-year leukemia-free and OS of 87.7% and 90.6%, respectively (Au et al. 2011).

Taken together, maintenance treatment has been mainly used in CTX/ATRA regimen. Based on the results of the APL0406 trial, it seems that using the CTX-free regimen in low-risk APL, no maintenance was needed (Lo-Coco et al. 2013). In contrast, in high-risk APL treated with CTX/ATRA, maintenance might still play a role, particularly in MRD positive patients. Thus, maintenance therapy is included in the majority of protocols based on CTX/ATRA and, so far, still recommended for high-risk patients after an AIDA-based therapy in the absence of toxicities.

### 8.6.3 Treatment of Elderly Patients

Although it is generally noted that APL seems to be rather uncommon in elderly patients (Sanz et al. 2009), its true incidence in this age cohort is unclear, particularly in patients beyond the age of 70 years. According to a population-based report from the Swedish adult acute leukemia registry, the proportion of patients with APL decreased significantly with age from 17% in patients younger than 30 years to 0.9% in patients 80 years and older (Lehmann et al. 2011), In addition, since comorbidities are more common in elderly patients, these patients are less likely to be admitted to a hematological department. More importantly, ED rate after ATRA ± anthracycline-based induction therapy was 60% in patients above the age of 80 years as compared to 18.8% in patients aged 50–59 years. ED was associated with poor performance status, explaining the high rate in very elderly patients (Lehmann et al. 2011). A previous report on 104 elderly (median age, 68 years; range, 60–83 years) patients showed that older patients could be successfully treated using ATRA plus anthracycline for induction and consolidation (Sanz et al. 2004b). Patients who were MRD negative at the end of consolidation received oral 6-mercaptopurine (50 mg/m$^2$/day), intramuscular methotrexate (15 mg/m$^2$/week), and ATRA (45 mg/m$^2$/day for 15 days every 3 months) over 2 years as maintenance therapy. Overall, outcome was favorable with an ED-rate of 15%, CR-rate of 84%, a 6-year CIR of 8.5%, and disease-free survival (DFS) of 79%, respectively (Sanz et al. 2004b). However, the CR-rate was lower in patients older than 70 years as compared to patients aged 60–70 years (74% vs 89%) (Sanz et al. 2004b). These results had recently been confirmed by Martinez-Cuadrón et al. comparing the long-term outcome of older patients (median age, 67 years) with de novo APL treated within the LPA2005 vs LPA96&99 trials (Martínez-Cuadrón et al. 2018). The LPA2005 trial, which was based on an age- and risk-adapted therapy with reduced post-consolidation CTX, resulted in a higher 5-year DFS (87% vs 69%; $P = 0.04$) and 5-year OS (74% vs 60%; $P = 0.06$) as compared to the LPA96&99 trials (Martínez-Cuadrón et al. 2018).

However, contrary results were published recently by Lengfelder et al. who reported on 91 newly diagnosed APL patients (median age, 67 years) registered by the German AML Cooperative Group between 1994 and 2011 (Lengfelder et al. 2013). Overall, 75% of the patients were treated on clinical trials, but the 25% non-eligibility rate was remarkably high, attributable to multimorbidity and low performance status. Fifty-six patients received induction therapy with ATRA and 6-thioguanine, cytarabine, daunorubicin (TAD), and consolidation and maintenance therapy. Treatment intensification with a second induction cycle (high dose cytarabine and mitoxantrone, (HAM)) was optional ($n = 14$). The 7-year OS, EFS and relapse-free survival (RFS) were 45%, 40%, and 48%, respectively. In patients treated with TAD-HAM induction, 7-year RFS was superior (83%; $P = 0.006$) compared to TAD only, and no relapse was observed. Thus, intensified induction therapy seemed to be highly effective, but was restricted to a selection of those patients, who could be treated intensively, since elderly patients have a higher vulnerability to treatment toxicity (Lengfelder et al. 2013). Sanz et al. noted that 6 of 25 (24%) patients ≥70 years died in remission (Sanz et al. 2004b), while Ades et al. reported that 19% of patients ≥60 years died due to complications of myelosuppression during consolidation with daunorubicin/cytarabine (Ades et al. 2005). Therefore, a higher vulnerability to treatment toxicities in older patients may result in a higher treatment-related mortality.

Regarding the distribution of risk-category according to WBC count at diagnosis, published data are again contradictory (Sanz et al. 2004b; Lengfelder et al. 2013). Sanz et al. reported that older patients seem to be more likely to present with non-high-risk APL as compared to their younger counterparts (37% vs 18%), which in part may account for the low relapse rate observed in their publication (Sanz et al. 2004b). In contrast, Lengfelder et al. reported on 31% ($n$ = 28/91) of patients with high-risk APL (Lengfelder et al. 2013).

Regarding outcome after ATO/ATRA in elderly patients, data are scarce also since age limit in the pivotal APL0406 trial was 70 years and only a very low number of patients above 60 years were included (Lo-Coco et al. 2013). On the other side, there is no evidence to assume that the biology of non-high-risk APL in the elderly might be different as compared to younger APL patients. Zhang et al. reported on 33 *de novo* APL patients with a median age of 65 years (range, 60–79 years) treated with single-agent ATO for remission induction and consolidation therapy (Zhang et al. 2013). The CR-rate was 88% and the ED-rate 12%. The 10-year CIR-, OS-, and DFS-rates were 10.3%, 69.3%, and 64.8%, respectively. Overall, monotherapy with ATO was well tolerated with leukocytosis (64%) being the most common adverse event during induction, whereas non-hematological adverse events were all manageable and reversible. In addition, non-relapse mortality (NRM) was only 6.9% after monotherapy with ATO due to noninfectious diseases (Zhang et al. 2013) as compared to 10–18.6% despite reduced intensities of CTX in older patients, mainly due to infection (Ades et al. 2005; Mandelli et al. 2003; Disperati et al. 2007). None of the patients treated with ATO developed a secondary malignancy with the exception of one patient who had longstanding hepatitis B virus infection and hepatic cirrhosis, and died of liver cancer 117 months after achievement of CR (Zhang et al. 2013). Very recently, we have evaluated the outcome of 433 elderly patients (median age, 73.4 years) treated either with CTX/ATRA or ATO-based therapy (Kayser et al. 2020). CR was achieved in 92% after therapy with ATO/ATRA and in 82% after CTX/ATRA; induction death rates were 8% and 18%, respectively. CIR was significantly lower after ATO/ATRA ± CTX as compared to CTX/ATRA ($P < 0.001$) (Kayser et al. 2020). High ($>10 \times 10^9$/L) WBC counts at diagnosis were associated with higher CIR ($P < 0.001$) as compared to lower WBC in the CTX/ATRA group, but not in the ATO/ATRA ± CTX group ($P = 0.48$). Thus, it seems reasonable to offer ATO/ATRA ± CTX as first line treatment to older patients irrespective of the risk-group.

### 8.6.4 Treatment of APL During Pregnancy

The occurrence of APL during pregnancy seems to be rather rare with limited evidence-based information available limited to small retrospective series and case reports. Most reliable data are therefore only available of national and international cancer registry databases (Sanz et al. 2015). Miguel Sanz on behalf of the PETHEMA study group has reported so far on the largest cohort of 14 (0.8%) pregnant women of overall 1.744 APL patients, who had been registered in their database between 1996 and 2012 (Sanz et al. 2015). Besides supportive therapy, the initiation of effective APL treatment to stop coagulopathy is of utmost importance. Table 8.6 provides an overview of fetal and maternal outcome after treatment of pregnant APL patients.

#### 8.6.4.1 Treatment Options During the First Trimester

Overall, therapeutic options are extremely limited during the first or early second trimester in terms of successful outcome of the fetus. Isotretinoin (a compound comparable to ATRA) has been shown to be teratogenic, leading to a range of severe craniofacial, cardiac, and central nervous system abnormalities as well as increased rate of abortions (Lammer et al. 1985; Rosa 1983; Lynberg et al. 1990; Chalmers 1992). In a systematic review by Verma and colleagues of 71 APL patients diagnosed during pregnancy, 23% were diagnosed with APL in the first trimester and 69% of those were treated with ATRA (Verma et al. 2016). Abortion rate, either spontaneously or therapeutically induced, was very high (90%) during the first trimester. Moreover, women in the first trimester were more likely to experience obstetric and fetal

**Table 8.6** Fetal and maternal outcome of pregnant patients with acute promyelocytic patients

| No. of pregnant women | Treatment | Maternal outcome | Fetal outcome | Reference |
|---|---|---|---|---|
| 71 (systematic review)<br>First trim: 16<br>Second trim: 20<br>Third trim: 28<br>Unk: 7 | ATRA/anthracycline/AraC: $n = 9$<br>ATRA/anthracycline: $n = 30$ ATRA: $n = 16$<br>Anthracycline/AraC: $n = 10$<br>Others: $n = 6$ | CR: 93% (53/58)<br>Obstetric complications during first as compared to second/third trim: 86.7% vs 15.9%<br>Premature cesarean section or induction of labor: 41% (27/66)<br>Relapses: $n = 4$ after a median follow-up of 10.5 months; salvage with CTX ± ATRA, 2 deaths due to APL, 1 death due in second CR | Outcome reported of $n = 54$<br>Preterm: $n = 25$<br>Spontaneous or therapeutic abortion or intrauterine death: $n = 18$<br>Fetal complications during first as compared to second/third trim: 92.3% vs 37.5%<br>Complications included:<br>Respiratory distress syndrome: $n = 6$ oligohydramnios and intrauterine<br>growth retardation: $n = 4$<br>Arrhythmias or cardiac issues: $n = 3$<br>Mild intraventricular brain hemorrhage: $n = 1$ | Verma et al. *Leuk Lymphoma* 2016; 57: 616–622 |
| 14<br>First trim: 3<br>Second trim: 2<br>Third trim: 7<br>After delivery: 2 | AIDA: 12 | CR: 92% (11/12)<br>ED: 2 (due to hemorrhage) | First trim: 5 abortions<br>Second and third trim: Normal development in $n = 8$, 1 dead fetus (26th week of gestation) | Sanz et al. *Ann Hematol* 2015; 94: 1357–1361 |
| 1 (third trim) | ATRA mono | CR: 100% | Cesarean section after 30 weeks: $n = 1$ | Culligan et al. *Clinical Leukaemia* 2007; 1: 183–191 |
| 1 (second trim) | ATRA/CTX | CR: 100% | Normal, but premature (35th week of gestation) | Giagounidis et al. *Eur J Haematol* 2000; 64: 267–271 |
| 1 (second trim) | ATRA mono (30 days) | CR: 100% | Caesarean section (30 weeks of gestation)<br>Cardiac arrhythmia and sustained cardiac arrest | Harrison et al. *Br J Haematol* 1994; 86: 681–682 |
| 1 (third trim) | ATRA mono | CR: 100%<br>Massive bleeding during delivery (extensive vaginal and perineal rupture) | Normal development | Stentoft et al. *Leukemia* 1994; 8: 1585–1588 |
| 1 (third trim) | ATRA mono for 4 weeks until delivery<br>2 weeks postpartum: Consolidation cycles with daunorubicin/AraC | CR: 100% | Induced labor, vaginal delivery, normal development | Lipovsky et al. *Br J Haematol* 1996; 94: 699–701 |

(continued)

**Table 8.6** (continued)

| No. of pregnant women | Treatment | Maternal outcome | Fetal outcome | Reference |
|---|---|---|---|---|
| 1 (second trim) | 4 cycles AIDA | CR: 100% | Term delivery (36.7 weeks of gestation), transient mild respiratory distress during the peripartum period, moderate, non-persistent dilation of the right atrium and right ventricle with mildly depressed function, two small secundum atrial septal defects, and a small patent ductus arteriosus | Siu et al. *Int J Gynecol Cancer* 2002; 12: 399–402 |
| 1 (third trim) | ATRA mono until CR consolidation with daunorubicin/ AraC | CR: 100% | Elective cesarean section (33.6 weeks of gestation); retardation of growth and non-persistent blocked atrial premature contractions and arrhythmia, resolving at the next day | Terada et al. *Leukemia* 1997; 11: 454–455 |
| 3<br>First trim: 1<br>Third trim: 2 | First patient (first trim): AIDA after therapeutic abortion<br>Second patient (third trim): AIDA 1 week after cesarean section<br>Third patient (third trim): ATRA for 2 weeks before delivery | CR: 67%<br>ED: 33% due to ATRA syndrome 1 week after delivery | Normal development | Consoli et al. *Int J Hematol* 2004; 79: 31–36 |

*AIDA* all-trans retinoic acid and idarubicin, *AraC* cytarabine, *ATRA* all-trans retinoic acid, *CR* complete remission, *CTX* chemotherapy, *trim* trimester

complications as compared to the subsequent trimesters (Verma et al. 2016). Therefore, ATRA should not be offered to pregnant APL patients during the first trimester, particularly during organogenesis (~8–10 weeks following conception) given the teratogenic potential of ATRA (Lammer et al. 1985; Rosa 1983; Lynberg et al. 1990; Chalmers 1992). Cytarabine and/or anthracyclines are known to increase the risk of spontaneous abortions or cause major malformations by up to 20% (Lishner et al. 2016; Caligiuri 1992; Yang and Hladnik 2009; Williams and Schilsky 2000; Amant 2012).

Thus, the option of therapeutic abortion has to be discussed with the patient, in particular during the first trimester. In cases, in which an abortion is no option, treatment with an anthracycline should be given and combined with ATRA in early second trimester. Since idarubicin is more lipophilic and may therefore be associated with an increased placental transfer and possible fetotoxicity (Reynoso and Huerta 1994; Achtari and Hohlfeld 2000), daunorubicin 60 mg/m$^2$ should be used for a maximum of three consecutive days. The addition of cytarabine 100–200 mg/m$^2$ days 1–7 should be considered during induction and consolidation (Adès et al. 2006), particularly in patients with high-risk APL. CTX alone, however, increases the risk of hemorrhage due to the release of pro-coagulants and plasminogen activators from malignant cells (Sanz and Montesinos 2010).

Moreover, early labor or cesarean section has to be considered the best option as soon as the fetus can be delivered at a viable stage. In addition, CTX with an anthracycline in combination with ATRA or ATO/ATRA (non-high-risk APL) should be given as soon as possible after delivery.

#### 8.6.4.2 Treatment Options During the Second or Third Trimester

CTX/ATRA after the beginning of the second trimester results in a more successful outcome for the unborn as compared to therapy in the first trimester, since the risk of fetal malformations reduces with advanced stage of pregnancy (Sanz et al. 2015; Claahsen et al. 1998; Consoli et al. 2004; Giagounidis et al. 2000). A high CR-rate of 92% had been reported in 11 of 12 pregnant APL patients treated with AIDA-based induction therapy; one woman died 2 weeks after start of induction therapy due to a DS. All women proceeded to consolidation and maintenance therapy and were reported to be in an ongoing CR after a median follow-up time of 83 months (Verma et al. 2016). In addition, the rate of fetal complications was comparable between the ATRA as compared to the non-ATRA group. Similarly, receipt of consolidation therapy in the study population was not associated with obstetric or fetal complications (Verma et al. 2016). Moreover, CTX rather increases the risk of abortion, prematurity, low birth weight, neonatal neutropenia, and sepsis, than to cause congenital malformations (Culligan et al. 2007).

Potentially, ATRA could be given as single agent therapy with the addition of an anthracycline after delivery. In case presentations, equivalent remission rates of ATRA as compared to CTX/ATRA have been observed (Fadilah et al. 2001; Harrison et al. 1994; Stentoft et al. 1994; Lipovsky et al. 1996). However, in pregnancies with a gestation of at least 20 weeks, there is still a risk of major malformations with ATRA monotherapy (Lammer et al. 1985). Additionally, ATRA monotherapy increases the risk of DS and possible ATRA resistance (Fenaux et al. 1999). Thus, the *PML-RARA* transcript needs to be monitored carefully by quantitative reverse-transcriptase polymerase chain-reaction (RT-qPCR); rise of the *PML-RARA* transcript potentially indicates the need to introduce CTX (Culligan et al. 2007).

As a result, ATRA monotherapy seems to be a valid option during the second or third trimester and low/intermediate-risk APL. However, molecular remission should be monitored carefully by RT-qPCR. Alternatively, in spite of the limited clinical experience, ATRA in combination with an anthracycline, particularly daunorubicin, seem reasonably safe during the second or third trimester of pregnancy.

We recommend a combination of CTX/ATRA for high-risk patients, and where RT-qPCR monitoring for *PML-RARA* is not feasible. Figure 8.3 shows the suggested approach to APL during pregnancy.

In addition, stringent fetal monitoring, with particular emphasis on cardiac function, is recommended for patients receiving ATRA during pregnancy because some cases of reversible fetal arrhythmias have been reported (Culligan et al. 2007; Siu et al. 2002; Terada et al. 1997).

ATO has been shown to be embryotoxic and to induce teratogenicity in animal studies (Holson et al. 2000). Therefore, ATO cannot be recommended throughout pregnancy. Similarly, GO is not justifiable for use in pregnancy (Culligan et al. 2007).

Finally, men and women of childbearing potential should use effective contraception, and breastfeeding must be discontinued during CTX or treatment with ATO.

### 8.6.5 Treatment of Extramedullary Relapse

Relapse at extramedullary sites was reported to occur in 3–5% of patients after CTX/ATRA, particularly within the CNS (Tallman 2007). Predictive factors for an extramedullary relapse may include the development of an ATRA syndrome (Ko et al. 1999), the predominance of the *PML-RARA* breakpoint cluster region isoform 3 (de Botton et al. 2006) and high-risk APL (de Botton et al. 2006; Breccia et al. 2003; Montesinos et al. 2009b). Montesinos et al. have evaluated the incidence of CNS recurrence on a large group of 739 patients between 1996 and

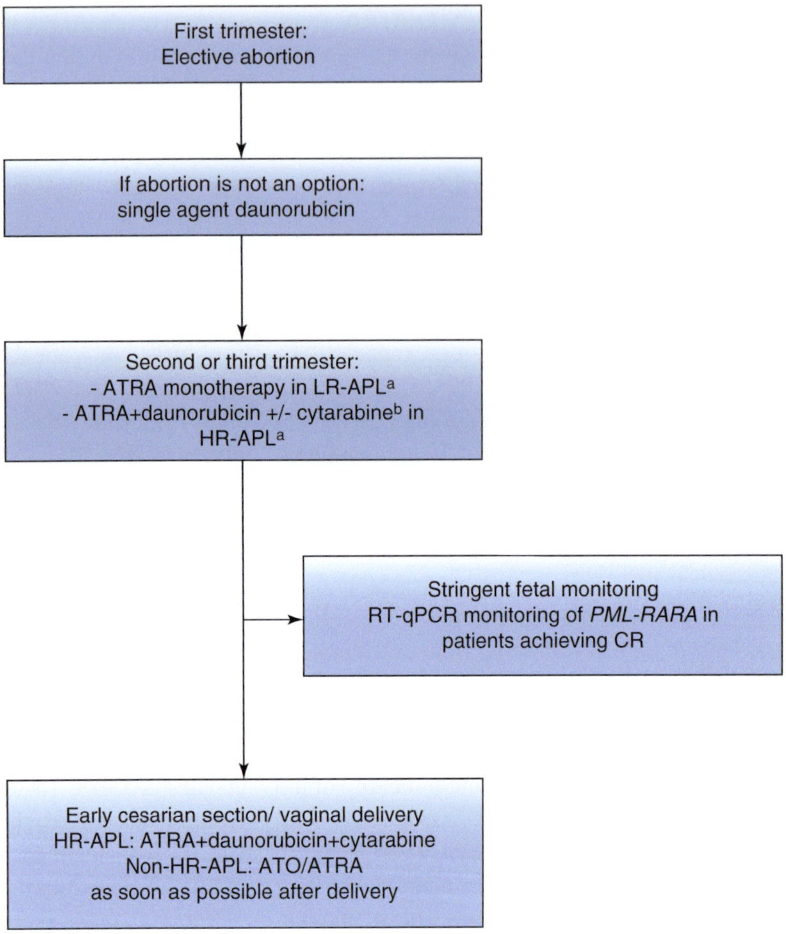


**Fig. 8.3** Suggested algorithm for management of pregnancy in acute promyelocytic leukemia. *APL* acute promyelocytic leukemia, *ATO* arsenic trioxide, *ATRA* all-trans retinoic acid, *HR* high-risk, *LR* low-risk, *PML* promyelocytic leukemia, *RARA* retinoic acid receptor alpha, *RT-qPCR* quantitative reverse-transcriptase polymerase chain-reaction, *WBC* white blood count. [a]Addition of cytarabine in high-risk APL; [b]Risk categorization based on WBC at diagnosis (low-/intermediate-risk: WBC $\leq 10.0 \times 10^9$/L; high-risk: WBC $>10.0 \times 10^9$/L)

2005 treated on the LPA96 and LPA99 PETHEMA trials (Montesinos et al. 2009b). No CNS prophylaxis was given in either protocol. Overall, CNS relapse was documented in 11 patients and the 5-year CIR within the CNS was 1.7% (Montesinos et al. 2009b). Of note, patients with high-risk had a CIR of 5.5% as compared to 0% and 0.8% in low- or intermediate-risk patients, respectively. Another independent risk factor was CNS hemorrhage during induction therapy (5-year CIR 18.7%, $P = 0.006$) (Montesinos et al. 2009b).

However, the strategy of an up-front CNS prophylaxis in high-risk patients is still a matter of debate. For low-risk patients, in whom the risk of CNS relapse is extremely low, there is a general consensus to avoid CNS prophylaxis (Sanz et al. 2019). Nevertheless, the possibility of CNS disease should be considered in any relapsed patient, particularly in those with neurological symptoms.

Data on the ability of ATO to cross the blood-brain barrier are derived from single case descriptions are fairly contradictory. Knipp et al. reported on a 42-year-old APL patient who developed a hematological relapse 1 year after AIDA-based therapy (Knipp et al. 2007). Since this patient had previously experienced an ATRA syndrome, he received ATO 10 mg daily for 30 days plus intrathecal therapy (40 mg cytarabine, 40 mg prednisone, and 15 mg MTX three times weekly for a total of nine treatments). In addition, his neuroaxis was irradiated with 30 Gy. Measurement of ATO in the cerebrospinal fluid (CSF) revealed a low CSF concentration of 0.11 μmol/L, representing only about 14% of blood levels. The authors concluded that ATO seems to cross the blood-CSF barrier when administered intravenously, but the concentration in CSF is probably not sufficient for treatment of meningeal leukemia (Knipp et al. 2007). Au et al. reported on a patient who relapsed 9 months after induction and consolidation therapy with ATRA, daunorubicin, and cytarabine (Au et al. 2000). Since reinduction with ATRA and cytarabine (four doses of 3 g/m$^2$) failed, he was treated with ATO at 10 mg/day. Eight months after achievement of a second CR, the patient experienced a second hematological relapse with involvement of the CNS. Despite urgent radiotherapy, the patient died of massive CNS bleeding 2 days later (Au et al. 2000). Hence, treatment with ATO seemed not sufficient to prevent CNS relapse. Contrary, Helwig et al. reported on a patient who was diagnosed with relapsed APL involving the CNS (Helwig et al. 2007). Treatment with ATO led to morphological changes in CNS cellularity consistent with the induction of a DS. Since ATO could be identified in the CNS, the authors concluded that the drug can cross the blood-brain barrier and could be used for treatment of extramedullary APL (Helwig et al. 2007).

Since the existing data are rather limited as well as contradictory, we recommend using triple intrathecal therapy with MTX, corticosteroids, and cytarabine until complete clearance of blasts in the CSF in case of a confirmed CNS relapse/involvement, followed by 6 to 10 more space out intrathecal therapies as consolidation therapy. Since a CNS relapse is almost invariably accompanied by a hematological or molecular relapse in the marrow, systemic therapy should also be given (Sanz et al. 2009).

## References


Abaza Y, Kantarjian HM, Garcia-Manero G, Estey E, Borthakur G, Jabbour E et al (2017) Long-term outcome of acute promyelocytic leukemia treated with all-transretinoic acid, arsenic trioxide, and gemtuzumab. Blood 129:1275–1283

Ablain J, de The H (2011) Revisiting the differentiation paradigm in acute promyelocytic leukemia. Blood 117:5795–5802

Achtari C, Hohlfeld P (2000) Cardiotoxic transplacental effect of idarubicin administered during the second trimester of pregnancy. Am J Obstet Gynecol 183:511–512

Ades L, Chevret S, De Botton S, Thomas X, Dombret H, Beve B et al (2005) Outcome of acute promyelocytic leukemia treated with all-trans retinoic acid and chemotherapy in elderly patients: the European group experience. Leukemia 19:230–233

Adès L, Chevret S, Raffoux E, de Botton S, Guerci A, Pigneux A et al (2006) Is cytarabine useful in the treatment of acute promyelocytic leukemia? Results of a randomized trial from the European Acute Promyelocytic Leukemia Group. J Clin Oncol 24:5703–5710

Adès L, Guerci A, Raffoux E, Sanz M, Chevallier P, Lapusan S et al (2010) Very long-term outcome of acute promyelocytic leukemia after treatment with all-trans retinoic acid and chemotherapy: the European APL Group experience. Blood 115:1690–1696

Alimoghaddam K, Ghavamzadeh A, Jahani M (2006) Use of NovoSevenR for arsenic trioxide-induced bleeding in PML. Am J Hematol 81:720

Amant F (2012) Safety of chemotherapy in pregnancy. Clin Adv Hematol Oncol 10:258–259

Asou N, Kishimoto Y, Kiyoi H, Okada M, Kawai Y, Tsuzuki M et al (2007) A randomized study with or without intensified maintenance chemotherapy in patients with acute promyelocytic leukemia who have become negative for PML-RARalpha transcript after consolidation therapy: the Japan Adult Leukemia Study Group (JALSG) APL97 study. Blood 110:59–66

Au WY, Ma SK, Ooi C, Liang R, Kwong YL (2000) Unusual manifestations of acute leukemia. J Clin Oncol 18:3435–3437

Au WY, Kumana CR, Lee HK, Lin SY, Liu H, Yeung DY et al (2011) Oral arsenic trioxide-based maintenance regimens for first complete remission of acute promyelocytic leukemia: a 10-year follow-up study. Blood 118:6535–6543

Avvisati G, Petti MC, Lo-Coco F, Vegna ML, Amadori S, Baccarani M et al (2002) Induction therapy with idarubicin alone significantly influences event-free survival duration in patients with newly diagnosed hypergranular acute promyelocytic leukemia: final results of the GIMEMA randomized study LAP 0389 with 7 years of minimal follow-up. Blood 100:3141–3146

Avvisati G, Lo-Coco F, Paoloni FP, Petti MC, Diverio D, Vignetti M et al (2011) AIDA 0493 protocol for newly diagnosed acute promyelocytic leukemia: very long-term results and role of maintenance. Blood 117:4716–4725

Barbey JT, Pezzullo JC, Soignet SL (2003) Effect of arsenic trioxide on QT interval in patients with advanced malignancies. J Clin Oncol 21:3609–3615

Bennett JM, Catovsky D, Daniel MT et al (1985) Proposed revised criteria for the classification of acute myeloid leukemia. A report of the French-American-British Cooperative Group. Ann Intern Med 103(4):620–625

Breccia M, Carmosino I, Diverio D, De Santis S, De Propris MS, Romano A et al (2003) Early detection of meningeal localization in acute promyelocytic leukaemia patients with high presenting leucocyte count. Br J Haematol 120:266–270

Burnett AK, Grimwade D, Solomon E, Wheatley K, Goldstone AH (1999) Presenting white blood cell count and kinetics of molecular remission predict prognosis in acute promyelocytic leukemia treated with all-trans retinoic acid: result of the randomized MRC trial. Blood 93:4131–4143

Burnett AK, Russell NH, Hills RK, Bowen D, Kell J, Knapper S et al (2015) Arsenic trioxide and all-trans retinoic acid treatment for acute promyelocytic leukaemia in all risk groups (AML17): results of a randomised, controlled, phase 3 trial. Lancet Oncol 16:1295–1305

Caligiuri MA (1992) Leukemia and pregnancy: treatment and outcome. Adv Oncol 8:10–17

Castaigne S, Chomienne C, Daniel MT, Ballerini P, Berger R, Fenaux P et al (1990) All-trans retinoic acid as a differentiation therapy for acute promyelocytic leukemia. I Clinical results. Blood 76:1704–1709

Chalmers RJ (1992) Retinoid therapy: a real hazard for the developing embryo. Br J Obstet Gynaecol 99:276–278

Chen ZX, Xue YQ, Zhang R, Tao RF, Xia XM, Li C et al (1991) A clinical and experimental study on all-trans retinoic acid-treated acute promyelocytic leukemia patients. Blood 78:1413–1419

Chomienne C, Ballerini P, Balitrand N, Daniel MT, Fenaux P, Castaigne S et al (1990) All-trans retinoic acid in acute promyelocytic leukemias. II. In vitro studies: structure-function relationship. Blood 76:1710–1717

Cicconi L, Fenaux P, Kantarjian H, Tallman M, Sanz MA, Lo-Coco F (2018) Molecular remission as a therapeutic objective in acute promyelocytic leukemia. Leukemia 32(8):1671–1678

Claahsen HL, Semmekrot BA, van Dongen PW, Mattijssen V (1998) Successful foetal outcome after exposure to idarubicin and cytosine-arabinoside during the second trimester of pregnancy-a case report. Am J Perinatol 15:295–297

Consoli U, Figuera A, Milone G, Meli CR, Guido G, Indelicato F et al (2004) Acute promyelocytic leukaemia during pregnancy: report of 3 cases. Int J Hematol 79:31–36

Coombs CC, Tavakkoli M, Tallman MS (2015) Acute promyelocytic leukemia: where did we start, where are we now, and the future. Blood Cancer J 5:e304

Culligan DJ, Merriman L, Kell J, Parker J, Jovanovic JV, Smith N et al (2007) The management of acute promyelocytic leukaemia presenting during pregnancy. Clin Leukaemia 1:183–191

de Botton S, Sanz MA, Chevret S, Dombret H, Martin G, Thomas X et al (2006) Extramedullary relapse in acute promyelocytic leukemia treated with all-trans retinoic acid and chemotherapy. Leukemia 20:35–41

Disperati P, Minden MD, Gupta V, Schimmer AD, Schuh AC, Yee KW et al (2007) Acute promyelocytic leukemia in patients aged 70 years and over—a single center experience of unselected patients. Leuk Lymphoma 48:1654–1658

Estey E, Garcia-Manero G, Ferrajoli A, Faderl S, Verstovsek S, Jones D et al (2006) Use of all-trans retinoic acid plus arsenic trioxide as an alternative to chemotherapy in untreated acute promyelocytic leukemia. Blood 107:3469–3473

Fadilah SA, Hatta AZ, Keng CS, Jamil MA, Singh S (2001) Successful treatment of acute promyelocytic leukemia in pregnancy with all-trans retinoic acid. Leukemia 15:1665–1666

Fenaux P, Castaigne S, Chomienne C, Dombret H, Degos L (1992) All trans-retinoic acid treatment for patients with acute promyelocytic leukemia. Leukemia 6:64–66

Fenaux P, Chastang C, Chevret S, Sanz M, Dombret H, Archimbaud E et al (1999) A randomized comparison of all transretinoic acid (ATRA) followed by chemotherapy and ATRA plus chemotherapy and the role of maintenance therapy in newly diagnosed acute promyelocytic leukemia. The European APL Group. Blood 94:1192–1200

Frankel SR, Eardley A, Lauwers G, Weiss M, Warrell RP (1992) The retinoic acid syndrome in acute promyelocytic leukemia. Ann Intern Med 117:292–296

Frankel SR, Eardley A, Heller G et al (1994) All-trans-retinoic acid for acute promyelocytic leukemia—results of the New-York study. Ann Intern Med 120:278–286

Ghavamzadeh A, Alimoghaddam K, Rostami S, Ghaffari SH, Jahani M, Iravani M et al (2011) Phase II study of single agent arsenic trioxide for the front-line therapy of acute promyelocytic leukemia. J Clin Oncol 29:2753–2757

Giagounidis AA, Beckmann MW, Giagounidis AS, Aivado M, Emde T, Germing U et al (2000) Acute promyelocytic leukemia and pregnancy. Eur J Haematol 64:267–271

Grimwade D, Biondi A, Mozziconacci MJ, Hagemeijer A, Berger R, Neat M et al (2000) Characterization of acute promyelocytic leukemia cases lacking the classic t(15;17): results of the European Working Party. Groupe Français de Cytogénétique Hématologique, Groupe de Français d'Hematologie Cellulaire, UK Cancer Cytogenetics Group and BIOMED 1 European Community-concerted action "molecular cytogenetic diagnosis in haematological malignancies". Blood 96(4):1297–1308

Harrison P, Chipping P, Fothergill GA (1994) Successful use of all-trans retinoic acid in acute promyelocytic leukaemia presenting during the second trimester of pregnancy. Br J Haematol 86:681–682

Helwig A, Klemm M, Schüttig R, Röllig C, Wassilew N, Ehninger G et al (2007) Arsenic-induced APL differentiation in cerebrospinal fluid. Leuk Res 31:703–705

Holson JF, Stump DG, Clevidence KJ, Knapp JF, Farr CH (2000) Evaluation of the prenatal developmental toxicity of orally administered arsenic trioxide in rats. Food Chem Toxicol 38:459–466

Huang ME, Ye YC, Chen SR, Chai JR, Lu JX, Zhoa L et al (1988) Use of all-trans retinoic acid in the treatment of acute promyelocytic leukemia. Blood 72:567–572

Iland HJ, Bradstock K, Supple SG, Catalano A, Collins M, Hertzberg M et al (2012) All-trans-retinoic acid, idarubicin, and IV arsenic trioxide as initial therapy in acute promyelocytic leukemia (APML4). Blood 120:1570–1580

Kantarjian HM, Keating MJ, Walters RS, Smith TL, McCredie KB, Freireich EJ (1987) Role of maintenance chemotherapy in acute promyelocytic leukemia. Cancer 59:1258–1263

Kayser S, Rahmé R, Martínez-Cuadrón D, Ghiaur G, Thomas X, Sobas M et al (2020) Outcome of older (≥70 years) APL patients frontline treated with or without arsenic trioxide-an International Collaborative Study. Leukemia 34(9):2333–2341. https://doi.org/10.1038/s41375-020-0758-4. [Epub ahead of print]

Kelaidi C, Chevret S, De Botton S, Raffoux E, Guerci A, Thomas X et al (2009) Improved outcome of acute promyelocytic leukemia with high WBC counts over the last 15 years: the European APL Group experience. J Clin Oncol 27:2668–2676

Knipp S, Gattermann N, Schapira M, Käferstein H, Germing U (2007) Arsenic in the cerebrospinal fluid of a patient receiving arsenic trioxide for relapsed acute promyelocytic leukemia with CNS involvement. Leuk Res 31:1585–1597

Ko BS, Tang JL, Chen YC, Yao M, Wang CH, Shen MC et al (1999) Extramedullary relapse after all-trans retinoic acid treatment in acute promyelocytic leukemia-the occurrence of retinoic acid syndrome is a risk factor. Leukemia 13:1406–1408

Kühn M, Sammartin K, Nabergoj M, Vianello F (2016) Severe acute axonal neuropathy following treatment with arsenic trioxide for acute promyelocytic leukemia: a case report. Mediterr J Hematol Infect Dis 8:e2016023

Kumana CR, Au WY, Lee NS, Kou M, Mak RW, Lam CW et al (2002) Systemic availability of arsenic from oral arsenic-trioxide used to treat patients with hematological malignancies. Eur J Clin Pharmacol 58:521–526

Kwong YL, Au WY, Chim CS, Pang A, Suen C, Liang R (2001) Arsenic trioxide- and idarubicin-induced remissions in relapsed acute promyelocytic leukaemia: clinicopathological and molecular features of a pilot study. Am J Hematol 66:274–279

Lammer EJ, Chen DT, Hoar RM, Agnish ND, Benke PJ, Braun JT et al (1985) Retinoic acid embryopathy. N Engl J Med 313:837–841

Lehmann S, Ravn A, Carlsson L, Antunovic P, Deneberg S, Möllgård L et al (2011) Continuing high early death rate in acute promyelocytic leukemia: a population-based report from the Swedish Adult Acute Leukemia Registry. Leukemia 25:1128–1134

Lengfelder E, Haferlach C, Saussele S, Haferlach T, Schultheis B, Schnittger S et al (2009) High dose ara-C in the treatment of newly diagnosed acute promyelocytic leukemia: long-term results of the German AMLCG. Leukemia 23:2248–2258

Lengfelder E, Hanfstein B, Haferlach C, Braess J, Krug U, Spiekermann K et al (2013) Outcome of elderly patients with acute promyelocytic leukemia: results of the German Acute Myeloid Leukemia Cooperative Group. Ann Hematol 92:41–52

Lipovsky MM, Biesma DH, Christiaens GC, Petersen EJ (1996) Successful treatment of acute promyelocytic leukaemia with all-trans-retinoic-acid during late pregnancy. Br J Haematol 94:699–701

Lishner M, Avivi I, Apperley JF, Dierickx D, Evens AM, Fumagalli M et al (2016) Hematologic malignancies in pregnancy: management guidelines from an international consensus meeting. J Clin Oncol 34:501–508

Lo-Coco F, Avvisati G, Vignetti M, Thiede C, Orlando SM, Iacobelli S et al (2013) Retinoic acid and arsenic trioxide for acute promyelocytic leukemia. N Engl J Med 369:111–121

Lou Y, Qian W, Meng H, Mai W, Tong H, Tong Y et al (2014) Long-term efficacy of low-dose all-trans retinoic acid plus minimal chemotherapy induction followed by the addition of intravenous arsenic trioxide post-remission therapy in newly diagnosed acute promyelocytic leukaemia. Hematol Oncol 32:40–46

Lynberg MC, Khoury MJ, Lammer EJ, Waller KO, Cordero JF, Erickson JD (1990) Sensitivity, specificity, and positive predictive value of multiple malformations in isotretinoin embryopathy surveillance. Teratology 42:513–519

Mandelli F, Diverio D, Avvisati G et al (1997) Molecular remission in PML/RAR alpha-positive acute promyelocytic leukemia by combined all-trans retinoic acid and Idarubicin (AIDA) therapy. Blood 90:1014–1021

Mandelli F, Latagliata R, Fazi P, Rodeghicro F, Leoni F et al (2003) Treatment of elderly patients (> or =60 years) with newly diagnosed acute promyelocytic leukemia. Results of the Italian multicenter group GIMEMA with ATRA and idarubicin (AIDA) protocols. Leukemia 17:1085–1090

Mantha S, Tallman MS, Soff GA (2016) What's new in the pathogenesis of the coagulopathy in acute promyelocytic leukemia? Curr Opin Hematol 23:121–126

Martínez-Cuadrón D, Montesinos P, Vellenga E, Bernal T, Salamero O, Holowiecka A et al (2018) Long-term outcome of older patients with newly diagnosed de novo acute promyelocytic leukemia treated with ATRA plus anthracycline-based therapy. Leukemia 32:21–29

Mathews V, George B, Lakshmi KM, Viswabandya A, Bajel A, Balasubramanian P et al (2006) Single-agent arsenic trioxide in the treatment of newly diagnosed acute promyelocytic leukemia: durable remissions with minimal toxicity. Blood 107:2627–3262

Montesinos P, Bergua JM, Vellenga E, Rayón C, Parody R, de la Serna J et al (2009a) Differentiation syndrome in patients with acute promyelocytic leukemia treated with all-trans retinoic acid and anthracycline chemotherapy: characteristics, outcome, and prognostic factors. Blood 113:775–783

Montesinos P, Díaz-Mediavilla J, Debén G, Prates V, Tormo M, Rubio V et al (2009b) Central nervous system involvement at first relapse in patients with acute promyelocytic leukemia treated with all-trans retinoic acid and anthracycline monochemotherapy without intrathecal prophylaxis. Haematologica 94:1242–1249

Norsworthy KJ, Bird T, Avagyan A, Li Y, Akhtar S, Liao J et al (2019) Second cancers in adults with acute promyelocytic leukemia (APL) treated with or without arsenic trioxide (ATO): a SEER-medicare analysis. Blood 134:3497. (abstract)

Platzbecker U, Avvisati G, Cicconi L, Thiede C, Paoloni F, Vignetti M et al (2016) Improved outcomes with retinoic acid and arsenic trioxide compared with retinoic acid and chemotherapy in non-high-risk acute promyelocytic leukemia: final results of the randomized Italian-German APL0406 trial. J Clin Oncol 35:605–612

Powell BL, Moser B, Stock W, Gallagher RE, Willman CL, Stone RM et al (2010) Arsenic trioxide improves event-free and overall survival for adults with acute promyelocytic leukemia: North American Leukemia Intergroup Study C9710. Blood 116:3751–3757

Ravandi F, Estey E, Jones D, Faderl S, O'Brien S, Fiorentino J et al (2009) Effective treatment of acute promyelocytic leukemia with all-trans-retinoic acid, arsenic trioxide, and gemtuzumab ozogamicin. J Clin Oncol 27:504–510

Redner RL (2002) Variations on a theme: the alternate translocations in APL. Leukemia 16(10):1927–1932

Reynoso EE, Huerta F (1994) Acute leukaemia and pregnancy-fatal foetal outcome after exposure to idarubicin during the second trimester. Acta Oncol 33:709–710

Rodeghiero F, Avvisati G, Castaman G, Barbui T, Mandelli F (1990) Early deaths and anti-hemorrhagic treatments in acute promyelocytic leukemia: a GIMEMA retrospective study in 268 consecutive patients. Blood 75:2112–2117

Rosa FW (1983) Teratogenicity of isotretinoin. Lancet 2:513

Sanz MA, Montesinos P (2010) Open issues on bleeding and thrombosis in acute promyelocytic leukemia. Thromb Res 125(Suppl 2):S51–S54

Sanz MA, Montesinos P (2014) How we prevent and treat differentiation syndrome in patients with acute promyelocytic leukemia. Blood 123:2777–2782

Sanz MA, Lo-Coco F, Martín G, Avvisati G, Rayón C, Barbui T et al (2000) Definition of relapse risk and role of nonanthracycline drugs for consolidation in patients with acute promyelocytic leukemia: a joint study of the PETHEMA and GIMEMA cooperative groups. Blood 96:1247–1253

Sanz MA, Martin G, Gonzalez M, Leon A, Rayon C, Rivas C et al (2004a) Risk-adapted treatment of acute promyelocytic leukemia with alltrans-retinoic acid and anthracycline monochemotherapy: a multicenter study by the PETHEMA group. Blood 103:1237–1243

Sanz MA, Vellenga E, Rayón C, Díaz-Mediavilla J, Rivas C, Amutio E et al (2004b) All-trans retinoic acid and anthracycline monochemotherapy for the treatment of elderly patients with acute promyelocytic leukemia. Blood 104:3490–3493

Sanz MA, Grimwade D, Tallman MS, Lowenberg B, Fenaux P, Estey EH et al (2009) Management of acute promyelocytic leukemia: recommendations from an expert panel on behalf of the European LeukemiaNet. Blood 113:1875–1891

Sanz MA, Montesinos P, Casale MF, Díaz-Mediavilla J, Jiménez S, Fernández I et al (2015) Maternal and fetal outcomes in pregnant women with acute promyelocytic leukemia. Ann Hematol 94:1357–1361

Sanz MA, Fenaux P, Tallman MS, Estey EH, Löwenberg B, Naoe T et al (2019) Management of acute promyelocytic leukemia: updated recommendations from an expert panel of the European LeukemiaNet. Blood 133(15):1630–1643

Schnittger S, Weisser M, Schoch C, Hiddemann W, Haferlach T, Kern W (2003) New score predicting for prognosis in PML-RARA+, AML1-ETO+, or CBFBMYH11+ acute myeloid leukemia based on quantification of fusion transcripts. Blood 102(8):2746–2755

Shigeno K, Naito K, Sahara N, Kobayashi M, Nakamura S, Fujisawa S et al (2005) Arsenic trioxide therapy in relapsed or refractory Japanese patients with acute promyelocytic leukemia: updated outcomes of the phase II study and postremission therapies. Int J Hematol 82:224–229

Siu BL, Alonzo MR, Vargo TA, Fenrich AL (2002) Transient dilated cardiomyopathy in a newborn exposed to idarubicin and all-trans-retinoic acid (ATRA) early in the second trimester of pregnancy. Int J Gynecol Cancer 12:399–402

Siu CW, Au WY, Yung C, Kumana CR, Lau CP, Kwong YL et al (2006) Effects of oral arsenic trioxide therapy on QT intervals in patients with acute promyelocytic leukemia: implications for long-term cardiac safety. Blood 108:103–106

Stentoft J, Nielsen JL, Hvidman LE (1994) All-trans retinoic acid in acute promyelocytic leukemia in late pregnancy. Leukemia 8:1585–1588

Swerdlow SH, Campo E, Harris NL, Jaffe ES, Pileri SA, Stein H, et al (2017) WHO classification of tumours of haematopoietic and lymphoid tissues, revised 4th edn. WHO Press, Geneva

Tallman MS (2007) Treatment of relapsed or refractory acute promyelocytic leukemia. Best Pract Res Clin Haematol 20:57–65

Tallman MS, Kwaan HC (1992) Reassessing the hemostatic disorder associated with acute promyelocytic leukemia. Blood 79:543–553

Tallman MS, Andersen JW, Schiffer CA, Appelbaum FR, Feusner JH, Ogden A et al (1997) All-trans-retinoic acid in acute promyelocytic leukemia. N Engl J Med 337:1021–1028

Tallman MS, Andersen JW, Schiffer CA, Appelbaum FR, Feusner JH, Woods WG et al (2002) All-trans retinoic acid in acute promyelocytic leukemia: long-term outcome and prognostic factor analysis from the North American Intergroup protocol. Blood 100:4298–4302

Terada Y, Shindo T, Endoh A, Watanabe M, Fukaya T, Yajima A (1997) Foetal arrhythmia during treatment of pregnancy-associated acute promyelocytic leukaemia with all-trans retinoic acid and favorable outcome. Leukemia 11:454–455

Unnikrishnan D, Dutcher JP, Garl S, Varshneya N, Lucariello R et al (2004) Cardiac monitoring of patients receiving arsenic trioxide therapy. Br J Haematol 124:610–617

Vahdat L, Maslak P, Miller WH Jr, Eardley A, Heller G, Scheinberg DA et al (1994) Early mortality and the retinoic acid syndrome in acute promyelocytic leukemia: impact of leukocytosis, low-dose chemotherapy, PMN/RAR-alpha isoform, and CD13 expression in patients treated with all-trans retinoic acid. Blood 84:3843–3849

Verma V, Giri S, Manandhar S, Pathak R, Bhatt VR (2016) Acute promyelocytic leukemia during pregnancy: a systematic analysis of outcome. Leuk Lymphoma 57:616–622

Warrell RP, Maslak P, Eardley A et al (1994) Treatment of acute promyelocytic leukemia with all-trans-retinoic acid—an update of the New-York experience. Leukemia 8:929–933

Williams SF, Schilsky RL (2000) Antineoplastic drugs administered during pregnancy. Semin Oncol 27:618–622

Yamakura M, Tsuda K, Ugai T, Sugihara H, Nisihida Y, Takeuchi M et al (2014) High frequency of varicella zoster virus reactivation associated with the use of arsenic trioxide in patients with acute promyelocytic leukemia. Acta Haematol 131(2):76–77

Yang D, Hladnik L (2009) Treatment of acute promyelocytic leukaemia during pregnancy. Pharmacotherapy 29(6):709–724

Zhang Y, Zhang Z, Li J, Li L, Han X, Han L et al (2013) Long-term efficacy and safety of arsenic trioxide for first-line treatment of elderly patients with newly diagnosed acute promyelocytic leukemia. Cancer 119:115–125

Zhu H, Hu J, Chen L, Zhou W, Li X, Wang L et al (2016) The 12-year follow-up of survival, chronic adverse effects, and retention of arsenic in patients with acute promyelocytic leukemia. Blood 128:1525–1528

Zver S, Andoljsek D, Cernelc P (2004) Effective treatment of life-threatening bleeding with recombinant activated factor VII in a patient with acute promyelocytic leukaemia. Eur J Haematol 72:455–456

# 9 Treatment of Newly Diagnosed AML in Fit Patients

Christoph Röllig and Gert J. Ossenkoppele

## 9.1 What Is Fit?

Untreated AML is a fatal disease. With the evolvement of treatment options beginning in the 1960s, it was demonstrated that a small proportion of patients can achieve long-term remissions, even beyond 5 years, indicating eradication of the disease and the potential of long-term cure. However, intensive cytoreductive treatment approaches had a rather high associated toxicity, in particular in old patients, leading to treatment-associated mortality during initial induction therapy around 20% (Atallah et al. 2007). In order to avoid that a potentially curative treatment results in a fatal outcome, researchers have continuously attempted to define and refine criteria and conditions associated with a high risk of life threatening complications such as severe infections and sepsis often resulting in multi-organ failure. Patients fulfilling these criteria would rather not benefit from intensive treatment and would be considered ineligible for intensive treatment, "unfit," or "frail." Best supportive care plus/minus low-intensity treatments are offered to these patients with the goal to reduce the leukemic burden and prolong life while maintaining a reasonable quality of life in an outpatient setting (see Chap. 10). Not in all instances, the decision is straightforward since treatment-related mortality rates have been going down during the last years and so far, and it is still a matter of debate which patients benefit from receiving low-intensive treatments rather than intensive chemotherapy (Michaelis 2018).

Over time, several retrospective analyses from clinical trials using intensive therapy have identified factors associated with the risk of early death. Additionally, the chances of achieving a CR and long-term remission can be estimated by scores in order to balance benefits and risks in a shared decision-making process (Appelbaum et al. 2006; Walter et al. 2011; Krug et al. 2010; Wheatley et al. 2009; Klepin et al. 2013; Ossenkoppele and Löwenberg 2015; Valcárcel et al. 2012). There is no prospective evaluation or intervention-based study to validate scores and determine their predictive potential. Instead, items of the scores have been used and variably combined in catalogs and lists to determine eligibility for intensive treatment in guidelines and position papers (Michaelis 2018; Ferrara et al. 2013). There is no internationally agreed general set of criteria defining frailness or ineligibility of intensive treatment. However, most sets of criteria include:

C. Röllig (✉)
Medizinische Klinik und Poliklinik I, Medizinische Fakultät Carl Gustav Carus, Universitätsklinikum Technische Universität Dresden, Dresden, Germany
e-mail: christoph.roellig@ukdd.de

G. J. Ossenkoppele
Amsterdam UMC Department of Haematology, VU University Medical Center,
Amsterdam, The Netherlands



C. Röllig, G. J. Ossenkoppele (eds.), *Acute Myeloid Leukemia*, Hematologic Malignancies,
https://doi.org/10.1007/978-3-030-72676-8_9

- age > 75–80 years,
- significant comorbidities such as severe cardiac insufficiency or pulmonary disease, late-stage diabetes mellitus with signs of end-organ damage or an HCT-CI score ≥3,
- geriatric assessment revealing high-risk features including poor cognitive function, and
- a general clinical performance not related to AML of WHO/ECOG >2.

## 9.2 Time from Diagnosis to Treatment

Untreated AML is in general associated with a very limited remaining life span of only a few weeks as known from historic data (Southam et al. 1951). As a result, it has been a long-standing treatment paradigm to consider AML a hematologic emergency and to start treatment immediately after the establishment of the diagnosis. This paradigm was reinforced by retrospective data from 2009 showing that in young patients up to the age of 60 years with a time interval from diagnosis to treatment (TDT) of ≥5 days, the overall survival was significantly worse than in patients with a TDT <5 days (Sekeres et al. 2009). However, in a different cohort of newly diagnosed AML patients receiving a more homogeneous induction treatment and including patients with hyperleukocytosis, no difference in the overall prognosis could be found by several statistical methods (Fig. 9.1; (Bertoli et al. 2013). This finding was confirmed in the most recent and largest analysis in more than 2200 uniformly treated AML patients, which again failed to show differences neither in remission rates, early death rates nor overall survival when analyzing TDT durations of 0–5, 6–10, 11–15, and >15 days (Röllig et al. 2019). Based on these findings, it seems reasonable to wait for the results of the diagnostic and genetic workup in a clinically stable patient as the prognosis and clinical course seem to be determined by other factors than TDT. Clearly, no evidence is necessary to recommend immediate treatment start in patients with AML-related complications such as leukostasis, neutropenic fever, or deranged coagulation. Close clinical observation and blood monitoring are necessary in patients with delayed treatment start in order to detect the onset of potential AML-related complications as early as possible.

## 9.3 Development of Current Standards

In 1971, James F. Holland, one of the pioneers of antineoplastic treatment in leukemias, stated three historic treatment phases of acute leukemia: (1) before 1947: the era of despair with no effective treatment; (2) from 1947 to 1963: the advent of chemotherapy, and with the failure to find a curative drug, the era of palliation; (3) since 1963, the appearance of new drugs, their use in

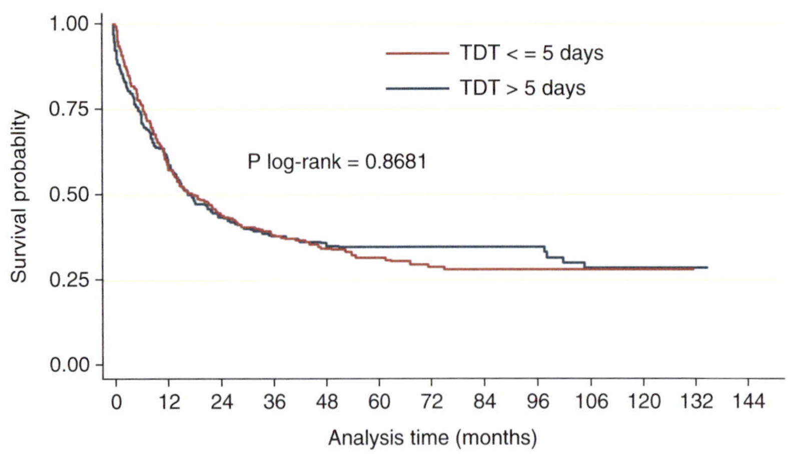


**Fig. 9.1** Association between overall survival (OS) and time from diagnosis to treatment (dichotomized at 5 days) (Bertoli et al. 2013)

intensive regimens and in combinations, which "have all made palliation too mean a goal" (Fairley 1971).

### 9.3.1 Induction

The first published attempts using cytarabine as a single agent in 1968 provided evidence of hematological remissions in 17–24% of patients (Ellison et al. 1968). Around the same time, daunorubicin was first used in pediatric and adult AML achieving hematologic remissions in 55% of patients (Boiron et al. 1969). Soon after, cytarabine and daunorubicin were combined in intermittent treatment intervals, followed by low-dose maintenance treatment with 6-MP and MTX or BCG. This first combination attempt was tested in 13 mostly younger patients aged 24–64 years and delivered a CR rate of 70% (Crowther et al. 1970). The combination of 7 days of cytarabine plus 3 days of daunorubicin was first published in 1973 (Yates et al. 1973). Later, four different variations of cytarabine (100 mg/m$^2$) plus daunorubicin (45 mg/m$^2$) combinations were prospectively evaluated in a randomized CALGB trial: 7 days of cytarabine continuous infusion plus 3 days of daunorubicin bolus versus delivered the highest CR rate (55%) and established the infusional 7 + 3 schema as a long-lasting treatment standard (Rai et al. 1981).

Continuous attempts were made to improve the efficacy of 7 + 3 by changing both the dose of its components, by substituting daunorubicin with other agents, by varying sequencing, and by the addition of other conventional cytoreductive agents.

The randomized comparison between 100 and 200 mg cytarabine provided no evidence of benefit in response or survival (Burnett et al. 2010a; Dillman et al. 1991). High doses of cytarabine (HDAC) delivered higher CR rates and prolonged RFS in randomized trials (Willemze et al. 2014; Burnett et al. 2013), whereas this could not be confirmed in other trials (Löwenberg et al. 2011; Röllig et al. 2018a; Niederwieser et al. 2016) or meta-analyses (Kern and Estey 2006). Subgroup analyses of one trial showed a survival benefit only in patients aged 15–45 years (Willemze et al. 2014). Apart from this, there is no significant evidence for an overall survival benefit associated with the use of HDAC in induction treatment in neither of these trials.

Doubling the traditional dose of daunorubicin to 90 mg/m$^2$ led to a significant increase both in remission rates and OS in three randomized trials in patients up to the age of 65 years, which led to a departure from using 45 mg/m$^2$. Two randomized comparisons of 60 mg versus 90 mg daunorubicin did not show significant differences in CR rates nor OS (Burnett et al. 2015; Röllig et al. 2018b). Subgroup analyses from one of these studies suggested a significant benefit of 90 mg daunorubicin in the subgroup of FLT3-ITD mutated patients (Burnett et al. 2016). Based on the mentioned results, most clinicians consider 60 mg daunorubicin as the standard dose. Furthermore, 7 + 3 containing 60 mg daunorubicin has been and is currently used as a backbone for the combination with novel agents (see Sect. 9.4).

The use of idarubicin as an alternative anthracycline instead of daunorubicin was associated with significantly higher remission rates, which did not translate into prolonged survival outcomes (Pautas et al. 2010). Other trials could not confirm a benefit in remission rates, and there is no evidence of a survival benefit by idarubicin (Lee et al. 2017; Gardin et al. 2013). In a meta-analysis, Teuffel et al. could show that the chances of remission are not different when the dose ratio of daunorubicin and idarubicin was ≥5 (Teuffel et al. 2013). Trials comparing the efficacy of mitoxantrone with daunorubicin showed no difference, neither in remission nor survival (Burnett et al. 2010a; Löwenberg et al. 1998; Mandelli et al. 2009).

A further 7 + 3 variation used a high-dose cytarabine–mitoxantrone combination and split it in two sequential halves (S-HAM) in order to increase efficacy and reduce toxicity. A comparison with two cycles of 7 + 3 showed a significantly reduced duration of leukopenia by S-HAM, but no difference in remission rates and no significant improvement in survival (Braess et al. 2018).

Various attempts have been made to improve the efficacy of 7 + 3 by the addition of other agents such as G-CSF or etoposide, but with no benefit (Krug et al. 2016; Burnett et al. 2010b; Estey et al. 1999). The addition of the purine analog cladribine to 7 + 3 in younger patients resulted in a significant OS benefit. It did not seem to benefit patients with poor-risk cytogenetics or age ≥50 years, and in general CR rates and OS in the control arm were relatively low (Holowiecki et al. 2012; Pluta et al. 2017).

### 9.3.2 Consolidation

After it had been shown that cytarabine and daunorubicin could induce complete hematologic remission as early as the late 1960s, it soon became clear that these remissions were not durable, even under low-dose cytarabine maintenance (Carey et al. 1975). Dose intensification of cytarabine to single doses of 3 g given repetitively over 5 days reduced the relapse rate significantly when compared with standard-dose cytarabine. However, this improvement was only seen in younger patients up to the age of 60 years (Mayer et al. 1994). Later it was shown that higher doses of cytarabine are able to significantly reduce the relapse rate also in patients older than 60 years (Röllig et al. 2018c). Attempts to improve the efficacy of consolidation treatment by adding other drugs were not superior to cytarabine alone, but associated with a higher risk of toxicity and no consistent survival benefit (Burnett et al. 2013; Schaich et al. 2013).

Whereas conventional consolidation treatment comprises 3–4 cycles of treatment, the administration of one cycle of myeloablative therapy followed by autologous stem cell rescue represents a more condensed and potentially equally effective treatment option. In comparative studies, autologous transplantation provided a benefit in RFS, mainly for favorable and intermediate risk patients. OS did not differ significantly between autologous transplantation and conventional high-dose cytarabine-based regimens (Vellenga et al. 2011; Pfirrmann et al. 2012; Cornelissen et al. 2015). The use of peripheral stem cells has reduced treatment-related mortality (TRM) enormously in comparison with bone marrow derived stem cells (SC), and hospital stay for one autologous transplantation is shorter than for 2–3 cycles of cytarabine.

There is evidence from several trials that a single dose of 1–1.5 g cytarabine may be equally effective as the original 3 g (Schaich et al. 2011). The only randomized comparison between 3 and 1.5 g shows a trend for better survival after 3 g in favorable and adverse and for 1.5 g in intermediate genetic risk (Burnett et al. 2013). Furthermore, data indicate that the third course of consolidation after double induction may not be necessary (Burnett et al. 2013; Löwenberg 2013).

### 9.3.3 Comparison of Standard Approaches for Induction and Consolidation

A large German intergroup study compared double induction chemotherapy using 7 + 3 (with 60 mg daunorubicin) followed by high-dose cytarabine consolidation with five different approaches for induction and consolidation including all variations of conventional induction and consolidation outlined above. The results of this 6-arm randomized trial assessing 3106 patients up to the age of 60 years showed significantly higher CR rates if patients with no response after one induction were treated with a combination of intermediate-dose cytarabine, idarubicin, and fludarabine (FLAG-Ida). However, as the main and sobering finding of the trial, no differences in relapse-free and overall survival were observed across all different induction-consolidation approaches (see Fig. 9.2) (Büchner et al. 2012).

The study gives a good overview of the results and the therapeutic potential of standard chemotherapy in a younger AML population with 70–82% CR/CRi rates, 5-year EFS of 27–39%, 5-year RFS of 35–47%, and a 5-year OS of 41–48%.

In elderly patients with intensive conventional treatment, trials produce 39–54% CR/CRi rates, a 5-year EFS of 10%, 5-year RFS of 10–25%,

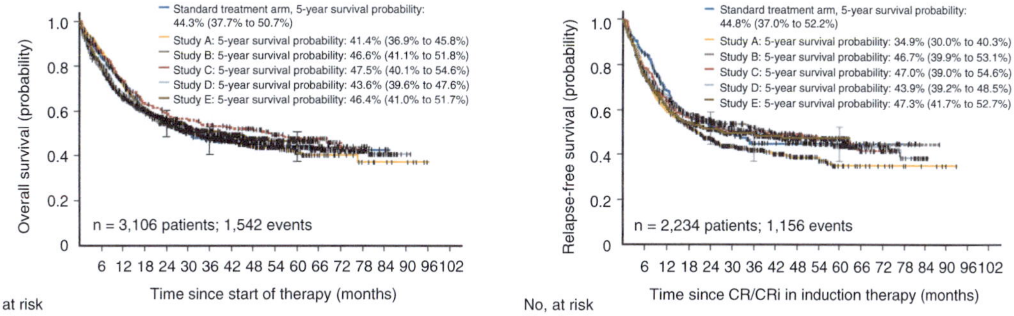


| No, at risk | | | | | | | |
|---|---|---|---|---|---|---|---|
| Standard treatment arm | 302 | 200 | 127 | 80 | 56 | 32 | 12 |
| Study A | 828 | 576 | 386 | 227 | 115 | 44 | 15 |
| Study B | 373 | 239 | 186 | 126 | 88 | 55 | 23 |
| Study C | 211 | 148 | 111 | 96 | 79 | 47 | 15 |
| Study D | 771 | 486 | 352 | 255 | 176 | 119 | 59 |
| Study E | 621 | 378 | 246 | 134 | 63 | 14 | 0 |

| No, at risk | | | | | | | |
|---|---|---|---|---|---|---|---|
| Standard treatment arm | 204 | 127 | 76 | 49 | 31 | 17 | 6 |
| Study A | 608 | 374 | 234 | 130 | 66 | 22 | 10 |
| Study B | 272 | 174 | 128 | 86 | 58 | 31 | 11 |
| Study C | 171 | 105 | 83 | 73 | 57 | 31 | 8 |
| Study D | 561 | 348 | 253 | 184 | 129 | 91 | 44 |
| Study E | 421 | 226 | 137 | 79 | 32 | 10 | 0 |

**Fig. 9.2** Overall survival and relapse-free survival in over 3000 patients comparing standard 7 + 3 double induction followed by high-dose cytarabine consolidation with five alternative conventional induction and postremission strategies (Büchner et al. 2012)

and 5-year OS of 15% (Röllig et al. 2018c; Löwenberg et al. 2009).

The inclusion and exclusion criteria of clinical trials create a positive selection of patients who are fitter than the general population (Estey and Gale 2017; Estey et al. 2018). Therefore, it is important to look at registry data to get a more comprehensive picture (Röllig et al. 2019; Nagel et al. 2017; Juliusson et al. 2012).

### 9.3.4 Maintenance

Historically, the first approach to keep patients in remission was the prolonged application of classic cytostatic agents. Whereas neither 6-MP, MTX, BCG nor low-dose cytarabine with or without thioguanine did turn out successfully (Crowther et al. 1970; Carey et al. 1975; Cassileth et al. 1992), the combination of 6-thioguanine, cytarabine, and daunorubicin given in low doses sequentially over 3 years was equally effective as one cycle of high-dose cytarabine-based consolidation (Büchner et al. 2003). However, with regard to time, effort, and convenience, this maintenance approach has not been widely implemented. Randomized trials exploring alternative substances for maintenance such as interferon, IL-2 with or without histamine or androgens for maintenance showed an improvement in relapse-free survival (RFS) for IL-2 plus histamine and for androgens, but all failed to show a significant improvement in survival for the entire patient population (Pautas et al. 2010; Goldstone et al. 2001; Brune et al. 2006; Pigneux et al. 2018).

Recently, a small randomized trial using azacitidine as maintenance for patients >65 years in CR after intensive induction showed a significant improvement in RFS which did not translate into an OS benefit, potentially due to differences in relapse treatments in the two patient groups (Huls et al. 2019). In a similarly designed larger randomized trial, the orally available hypomethylating compound CC-486 was used versus placebo for maintenance in CR patients >=55 years with intermediate or adverse cytogenetic risk after intensive pre-treatment not eligible for allogeneic stem cell transplantation. CC-486 reduced the risk for relapse or death by 35% and for death by 31%, resulting in an OS prolongation of 9.9 months (HR: 0.69) (Wei et al. 2020). As relapses occurred later but to a similar extent in the CC-486 arm, the long-term remission rate was still similar between both patient groups, indicating a prolongation of survival by CC-486 maintenance, but not an increase in the proportion of cured patients.

As new compounds with a more specific mode of action are evaluated in the first-line treatment and enter clinical practice (see Chaps. 17–19), their continuous use beyond induction may become a new mode of maintenance with the option not only to prolong remission, but also to increase the rate of cure.

## 9.4 Novel Agents and Treatment Stratification for Induction

Cytogenetic and molecular methods revealed that AML patients share the same clinical features and findings, but that on the biological and cellular level, there is a wide heterogeneity (see Chap. 5). However, conventional cytoreductive agents such as cytarabine and daunorubicin do not target differences in genetic cellular configurations. Patients with high genetic risk showed an adverse disease course with standard therapy, no matter which conventional agents were used (see Sect. 9.3.3). Due to a lack of other effective drugs, a "one size fits all" approach has been common practice in AML treatment for decades, using the standard 7 + 3 or one of its variations for all newly diagnosed fit AML patients.

The development of novel agents targeting cellular pathways that may be essential for leukemogenesis has led to improvements in treatment outcomes, accompanied by differential responses in different genetic subgroups. The approval and subsequent availability of some of these agents have changed the treatment landscape and have led to a diversification of AML therapy.

### 9.4.1 Tyrosine-Kinase Inhibitors

The presence of an internal tandem duplication mutation (ITD) in the gene coding for the FLT3 tyrosine kinase can drive hematopoietic cells toward leukemia and lead to increased proliferation and resistance to apoptosis in myeloid blasts, corresponding to a high relapse rate and limited long-term survival (Mizuki et al. 2003; Thiede et al. 2002). It was hypothesized that small molecules inhibiting FLT3 signaling could improve the course of the disease (Larrosa-Garcia and Baer 2017). First-generation tyrosine-kinase inhibitors (TKI) target several cellular kinases and have limited single-agent activity.

The first randomized evidence for the efficacy of TKIs in combination with intensive chemotherapy came from sorafenib, which prolonged EFS and RFS, but not OS significantly in a younger patient population ≤60 years irrespective of the FLT3 mutational status (Röllig et al. 2015). In elderly patients, sorafenib led to increased toxicity that prevented a survival benefit (Serve et al. 2013).

The RATIFY trial evaluated midostaurin in combination with standard induction and consolidation chemotherapy and as maintenance for 12 months in a randomized placebo-controlled design. While the addition of midostaurin did not increase the CR rates, RFS and OS were significantly prolonged, with an increase in median OS from 26 to 75 months (HR: 0.78). These results led to the approval of midostaurin for the first-line treatment of FLT3-mutated AML in combination with standard chemotherapy (Stone et al. 2017). Although the value of midostaurin in maintenance was not clear based on the study design, the EMA approved the drug also for maintenance.

The second-generation TKIs are more specific for FLT3 and inhibit fewer additional kinases (Larrosa-Garcia and Baer 2017). Furthermore, agents, such as quizartinib, gilteritinib, and crenolanib, show significant single-agent activity. Quizartinib and gilteritinib have been shown to be more effective than standard salvage treatment in relapsed/refractory FLT3 mutated AML, and gilteritinib has been approved for single-agent use in this clinical setting (see Chaps. 11 and 12). Currently, all three agents are evaluated in combination with standard intensive treatment for newly diagnosed fit AML patients.

### 9.4.2 Monoclonal Antibodies

As CD33 can be found on blasts of almost all AML types (Ehninger et al. 2014), targeting

AML blasts with antibodies has been considered a promising treatment concept. Gemtuzumab ozogamicin (GO) is a humanized monoclonal CD33 antibody conjugated with the toxin calicheamicin. By binding to CD33 positive AML cells, the antibody–drug conjugate is internalized into the cell and broken down, releasing calicheamicin, which then binds to the DNA and causes apoptosis (Tsuchikama and An 2018). Several trials have shown proof of GO efficacy in relapsed and primary AML. For the combination of GO and standard intensive chemotherapy, meta-analyses of randomized trials have shown that (1) a low-dose fractionated administration results in the best tolerability, and (2) among AML subgroups, patients with favorable risk AML have the greatest benefit from GO in addition to standard therapy (Hills et al. 2014; Li et al. 2014). Results on the requirement of CD33 expression have been mixed (Walter et al. 2007; Khan et al. 2017); similarly, single-nucleotide polymorphisms (SNP) genotyping of large numbers of GO treatment patients disagree about its predictive ability (Lamba et al. 2017; Gale et al. 2018).

In the randomized open-label ALFA-0701 trial, GO was added to standard induction and consolidation treatment of newly diagnosed AML patients with mainly intermediate or adverse cytogenetic risk. The addition of GO led to a significant prolongation of event-free and relapse-free survival, whereas a benefit in OS did not reach statistical significance. Subgroup analyses revealed that the survival benefit was caused by patients with favorable or intermediate cytogenetics, whereas patients with adverse risk did not benefit from GO (Lambert et al. 2019). According to subgroup analyses, patients with $NPM1_{mut}$ and also FLT3-ITD showed a greater risk reduction by GO. A meta-analysis of five randomized trials identified the greatest survival benefit in patients with favorable risk (20% difference in 5-year OS), a smaller significant benefit in intermediate risk (6% difference in 5-year OS), and no benefit for adverse risk patients (Hills et al. 2014).

Based on the results of ALFA-0701, GO was approved by FDA and EMA for the treatment of newly diagnosed CD33 positive AML in combination with standard chemotherapy.

The effect of GO in addition to induction therapy with idarubicin, standard-dose cytarabine plus etoposide (ICE) in NPM1 positive AML patients, was assessed in the randomized open-label AML-SG 09-09 study. The use of GO was associated with a significant reduction in relapse risk, but the combination with ICE led to an increased early mortality rate in elderly patients, most likely due to the combination with etoposide and ATRA (Schlenk et al. 2019).

The impact of GO in postremission treatment is currently uncertain since there is no randomized evidence for a benefit in postremission (Burnett et al. 2011).

Several CD33 immunotherapy approaches are in clinical development. Also, CD123, CD70, and CD47 targets are in advanced clinical development and may become relevant for the first-line treatment in the future (see Chap. 19).

### 9.4.3 Liposomal Formulation of Cytarabine and Daunorubicin (CPX-351)

CPX-351 is a liposomal formulation of a fixed molar ratio (1:5) of daunorubicin and cytarabine. After cellular internalization, liposomes undergo degradation, releasing cytarabine and daunorubicin intracellularly to induce DNA damage resulting in cell death. In vitro studies demonstrated that the 1:5 ratio resulted in synergistic in vitro cytotoxicity in the majority of cancer cell lines evaluated (Krauss et al. 2019).

Study CLTR0310-301, a randomized, multicenter, open-label, active-controlled trial compared CPX-351 with a standard 7 + 3 combination of daunorubicin and cytarabine in 309 patients 60–75 years of age with newly diagnosed t-AML or AML-MRC. The results demonstrated higher remission rates (48% versus 33%), and an improvement in overall survival (HR: 0.69) by CPX-351 with an estimated median overall survival of 9.6 months compared with 5.9 months for the 7 + 3 control arm. The survival benefit was pronounced in patients who were able to proceed to allogeneic stem cell transplantation after receiving CPX-351 (HR: 0.46) compared with 7 + 3 induction (Lancet et al. 2018). Based on these results, CPX-351 was approved by FDA and EMA for newly diagnosed tAML or AML-MRC of all age groups.

## 9.5 Balancing Risks and Benefits in Postremission Treatment

Standard induction treatment without the addition of novel agents will bring around 60–80% of younger adults and 40–60% of older patients in complete morphologic remission, depending on prognostic factors, of which age and genetics are the most important (see Chap. 7). Still more than half of all intensively treated patients die from the disease (Dinmohamed et al. 2016), as relapse and subsequent treatment failure remain the biggest challenge in AML treatment (see Chaps. 11 and 12). As (1) the physical condition of patients in a relapsed situation after intensive first-line therapy may limit the option of salvage treatment, and (2) the relapsed disease is generally more difficult to treat, the primary goal of the first-line treatment is to prevent relapses. They will occur in almost 100% of CR patients if treatment is stopped after induction due to small quantities of residual leukemia cells (see Chap. 18).

In general, either dose intensive chemotherapy ("consolidation") or allogeneic stem cell transplantation (allo-SCT) will be used for postremission treatment. Whereas autologous transplantation can be considered as being part of the first option, the graft versus leukemia immune mechanisms after allogeneic SCT introduce a different antileukemic mode of action (see Chap. 13). Allogeneic lymphocytes and the resulting immune mechanisms are at the same time boon and bane of allo-SCT. Whereas the graft versus leukemia effect eliminates chemoresistant leukemic cells and reduces the relapse rate compared with chemo-consolidation, the delayed immune reconstitution after SCT and the organ damage of graft versus host disease reduce the quality of life and increase the number of patients dying in remission (nonrelapse mortality).

The best way to balance the risks and benefits of consolidation chemotherapy versus allo-SCT is to weigh up the estimated relapse risk and the expected transplant-related mortality. The latter can be assessed by the EBMT score integrating age, disease stage, donor type, donor–recipient gender combination, and time interval from diagnosis to transplantation (Gratwohl 2012). Additionally, information on comorbidities contribute to the assessment of post-transplant mortality (Sorror et al. 2008). If the risk of non-relapse mortality (NRM) exceeds the risk of relapse after allo-SCT, the use of chemo-consolidation should be favored according to the guidelines of the ELN AML working party (Cornelissen et al. 2012). In fit patients in first CR with a good matched and readily available donor, the preferred postremission option for patients with favorable genetics would be chemotherapy, whereas allo-SCT would be recommended for an adverse risk constellation. In an intermediate-risk patient, a more detailed and individualized assessment is necessary (see Chap. 13).

Patients with FLT3-ITD at a low ITD-WT allelic ratio (FLT3-ITD$^{low}$) and co-occurring NPM1 mutation (NPM1$_{mut}$) who have access to midostaurin represent a more complex scenario regarding relapse risk and postremission treatment decision. The low FLT3-ITD ratio, the NPM1 mutation, and midostaurin treatment reduce the relapse risk compared with other FLT3-ITD patients, who have a generally high risk of relapse compared with FLT3$_{wt}$ or FLT3-TKD and should be advised to undergo allo-SCT. If FLT3-ITD$^{low}$-NPNM1$_{mut}$ patients under midostaurin treatment are in hematologic CR and the level of minimal residual disease (MRD) is low as defined by NPM1$_{mut}$/ABL levels or Multicolor Flow Cytometry (MFC), the relapse risk can be considered low based on studies on disease kinetics in NPM1mut patients after the end of consolidation (Krönke et al. 2011; Shayegi et al. 2013). Therefore, these patients can be advised to continue conventional treatment plus midostaurin, whereas allo-SCT should be recommended to patients with relevant MRD (see Fig. 9.3).

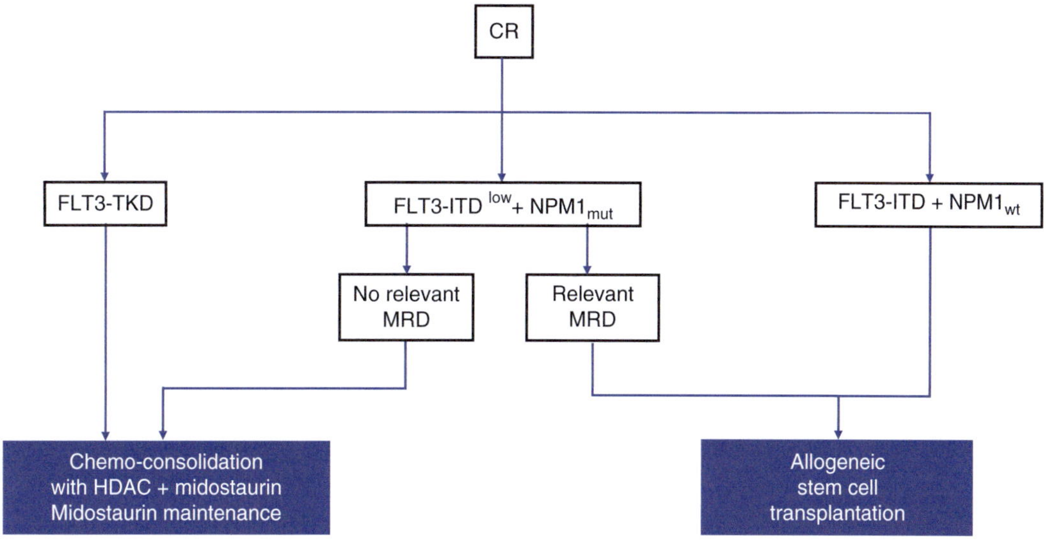


**Fig. 9.3** Decision tree for the modality of postremission treatment depending on FLT3, NPM1 mutational status, and NPM1 MRD

## 9.6 Treatment Stratification

Before discussing algorithms for treatment, the authors would like to emphasize the utmost importance of enrolling patients in clinical trials as the first priority whenever these are available. As clinical trials offer the standard of care as control treatment, patients are not put at risk of undertreatment. The development and availability of novel agents that may cause prolonged survival have been and will be only possible on the basis of clinical trials. The authors would therefore like to stress the necessity to reach out for clinical trials, ideally as part of an academic cooperative group and embedded in a general registry and biobanking infrastructure in order to continuously improve treatment options and outcomes for AML patients.

With midostaurin, GO and CPX-351 expanding the antineoplastic armamentarium by three agents with the potential for prolonged overall survival in certain subgroups of AML, the diagnostic workup at initial diagnosis is important not only for prognostication, but also for treatment stratification. As outlined in Sect. 9.2, the general prognosis of patients is not dependent on the time from diagnosis to treatment (TDT). Still, the turn-around time for genetic diagnosis should be as short as possible. In conclusion, the potential benefits of correct stratification seem to outweigh the risks of disease progression in clinically stable patients. High WBC counts do not automatically indicate an emergency as they can be managed by the use of hydroxyurea.

Patients with acute AML-related problems such as leukostasis syndrome (see Chap. 14), or disease-related coagulation disorders should start treatment immediately with 7 + 3 based standard induction. Patients presenting with leukocytosis without clinical signs of leukostasis should be treated with hydroxyurea to reduce the white blood cell (WBC) count until the start of intensive chemotherapy (Röllig and Ehninger 2015).

Based on the results of diagnostic tests, the treatment algorithms depicted in Fig. 9.4 can be recommended outside of clinical trials.

## 9.7 Open Questions and Future Perspectives

Although "standard" intensive treatment approaches have been around for several decades now, there are still open questions and issues, for which evidence is sparse and which may be worth clinical research. Many institutions aim for

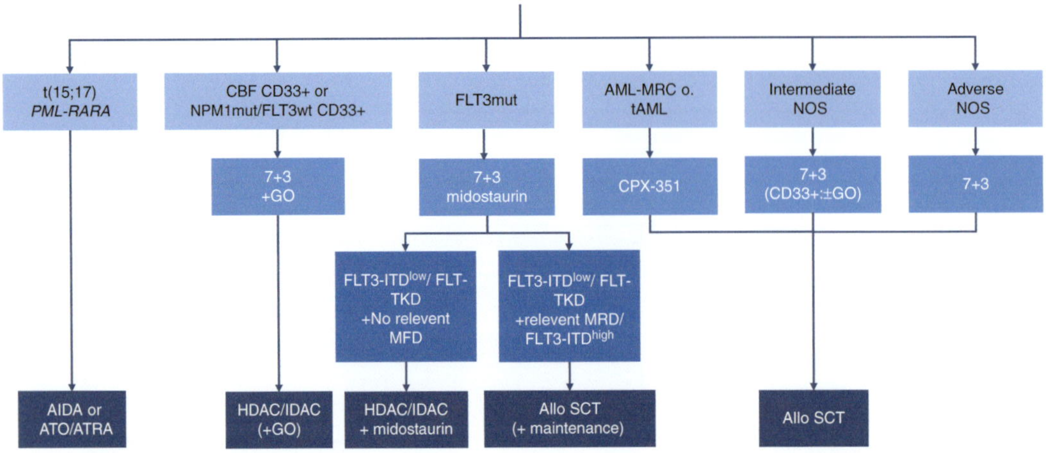


**Fig. 9.4** Genetically stratified first-line treatment for fit patients outside clinical trials

two induction cycles (double induction) in order to reduce the leukemic burden whereas others proceed to postremission treatment as soon as the blast count was reduced to <5% even after only one induction (Fernandez et al. 2009). Likewise, it is uncertain if the application of at least one cycle of high-dose cytarabine may be beneficial even for patients proceeding to allo-SCT or if allo-SCT should follow CR achievement directly. The dose and amount of cytarabine cycles in postremission treatment is the subject of an ongoing debate (Löwenberg 2013; Paul et al. 2020). Randomized trials will contribute to answering these questions, and new insights on the levels and behavior of measurable residual disease markers will help us optimizing the first-line treatment.

Standard intensive first-line treatment can cure a significant proportion of newly diagnosed patients. Due to advances in anti-infective prophylaxis and treatment and other supportive measures (see Chap. 16), the tolerability of intensive regimens has improved and early mortality is constantly going down (see Fig. 9.5) (Percival et al. 2015). Pilot studies suggest that it may be even feasible to complete a complete intensive induction course in an outpatient setting if patients are carefully selected and monitored on a daily basis (Mabrey et al. 2020). Although comprehensive and complex inpatient treatment is required for most patients, the cost of standard treatment is low in comparison with the prices of novel agents. Based on these considerations, intensive treatment will remain the backbone and reference of curative AML treatment for the time being.

Thanks to a promising pipeline of novel agents in advanced clinical development, treatment of AML will become not only more efficacious, more refined, individualized, and challenging, but also more expensive. We have seen that novel agents with limited single-agent activity can be successfully added to the standard cytoreductive treatment, but will they be able to replace standard approaches while still be curative? Will we maintain a less specific broad treatment backbone and add specific targeted agents, and how many conventional and novel agents can we combine at a tolerable level and with manageable toxicity? Finally, novel agents with low toxicity but high curative potential may blur the fit–unfit frontier and sever the connection fit = intensive = curative and unfit = nonintensive = palliative and replace it by "eligible for."

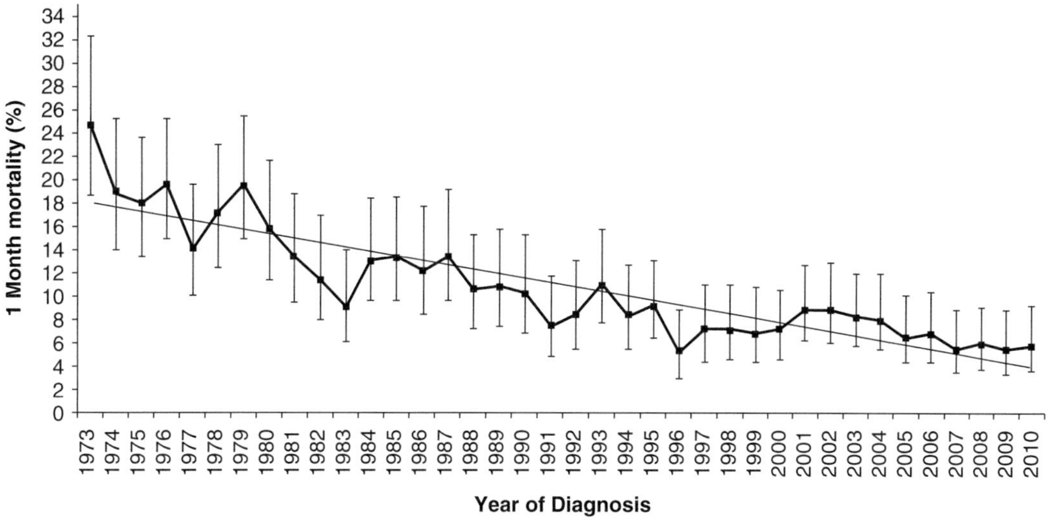


**Fig. 9.5** Decline in early mortality in AML treatment from the SEER database (Percival et al. 2015)

## References


Appelbaum FR, Gundacker H, Head DR, Slovak ML, Willman CL, Godwin JE et al (2006) Age and acute myeloid leukemia. Blood 107(9):3481–3485

Atallah E, Cortes J, O'Brien S, Pierce S, Rios MB, Estey E et al (2007) Establishment of baseline toxicity expectations with standard frontline chemotherapy in acute myelogenous leukemia. Blood 110:3547–3551

Bertoli S, Bérard E, Huguet F, Huynh A, Tavitian S, Vergez F et al (2013) Time from diagnosis to intensive chemotherapy initiation does not adversely impact the outcome of patients with acute myeloid leukemia. Blood 121(14):2618–2626

Boiron M, Jacquillat C, Weil M, Tanzer J, Levy D, Sultan C et al (1969) Daunorubicin in the treatment of acute myelocytic leukaemia. Lancet:330–333

Braess J, Amler S, Kreuzer K-A, Spiekermann K, Lindemann HW, Lengfelder E et al (2018) Sequential high-dose cytarabine and mitoxantrone (S-HAM) versus standard double induction in acute myeloid leukemia-a phase 3 study. Leukemia 32(12):2558–2571

Brune M, Castaigne S, Catalano J, Gehlsen K, Ho AD, Hofmann WK et al (2006) Improved leukemia-free survival after postconsolidation immunotherapy with histamine dihydrochloride and interleukin-2 in acute myeloid leukemia: results of a randomized phase 3 trial. Blood 108(1):88–96

Büchner T, Hiddemann W, Berdel WE, Wormann B, Schoch C, Fonatsch C et al (2003) 6-Thioguanine, cytarabine, and daunorubicin (TAD) and high-dose cytarabine and mitoxantrone (HAM) for induction, TAD for consolidation, and either prolonged maintenance by reduced monthly TAD or TAD-HAM-TAD and one course of intensive consolidation by seq. J Clin Oncol 21(24):4496–4504

Büchner T, Schlenk RF, Schaich M, Dohner K, Krahl R, Krauter J et al (2012) Acute myeloid leukemia (AML): different treatment strategies versus a common standard arm—combined prospective analysis by the German AML Intergroup. J Clin Oncol 30(29):3604–3610

Burnett AK, Hills RK, Milligan DW, Goldstone AH, Prentice AG, McMullin MF et al (2010a) Attempts to optimize induction and consolidation treatment in acute myeloid leukemia: results of the MRC AML12 trial. J Clin Oncol 28(4):586–595

Burnett AK, Hills RK, Green C, Jenkinson S, Koo K, Patel Y et al (2010b) The impact on outcome of the addition of all-trans retinoic acid to intensive chemotherapy in younger patients with nonacute promyelocytic acute myeloid leukemia: overall results and results in genotypic subgroups defined by mutations in NPM1, FLT3, and C. Blood 115(5):948–956

Burnett AK, Hills RK, Milligan D, Kjeldsen L, Kell J, Russell NH et al (2011) Identification of patients with acute myeloblastic leukemia who benefit from the addition of gemtuzumab ozogamicin: results of the MRC AML15 trial. J Clin Oncol 29(4):369–377

Burnett AK, Russell NH, Hills RK, Hunter AE, Kjeldsen L, Yin J et al (2013) Optimization of chemotherapy for younger patients with acute myeloid leukemia: results of the medical research council AML15 trial. J Clin Oncol 31(27):3360–3368

Burnett AK, Russell NH, Hills RK, Kell J, Cavenagh J, Kjeldsen L et al (2015) A randomized comparison of daunorubicin 90 mg/m2 vs 60 mg/m2 in AML induction: results from the UK NCRI AML17 trial in 1206 patients. Blood 125(25):3878–3885

Burnett AK, Russell NH, Hills RK (2016) Higher daunorubicin exposure benefits FLT3 mutated acute myeloid leukemia. Blood 128:449–452

Carey RW, Ribas-Mundo M, Ellison RR, Glidewell O, Lee ST, Cuttner J et al (1975) Comparative study of cytosine arabinoside therapy alone and combined with thioguanine, mercaptopurine, or daunorubicin in acute myelocytic leukemia. Cancer 36(5):1560–1566

Cassileth PA, Lynch E, Hines JD, Oken MM, Mazza JJ, Bennett JM et al (1992) Varying intensity of postremission therapy in acute myeloid leukemia. Blood 79(8):1924–1930

Cornelissen JJ, Gratwohl A, Schlenk RF, Sierra J, Bornhauser M, Juliusson G, et al (2012) The European LeukemiaNet AML Working Party consensus statement on allogeneic HSCT for patients with AML in remission: an integrated-risk adapted approach [Internet]. Nat Rev Clin Oncol 9:579–90. https://doi.org/10.1038/nrclinonc.2012.150

Cornelissen JJ, Versluis J, Passweg JR, van Putten WLJ, Manz MG, Maertens J et al (2015) Comparative therapeutic value of post-remission approaches in patients with acute myeloid leukemia aged 40-60 years. Leukemia 29(5):1041–1050

Crowther D, Bateman CJ, Vartan CP, Whitehouse JM, Malpas JS, Fairley GH et al (1970) Combination chemotherapy using L-asparaginase, daunorubicin, and cytosine arabinoside in adults with acute myelogenous leukaemia. Br Med J 4:513–517

Dillman RO, Davis RB, Green MR, Weiss RB, Gottlieb AJ, Caplan S et al (1991) A comparative study of two different doses of cytarabine for acute myeloid leukemia: a phase III trial of cancer and leukemia group B. Blood 78(10):2520–2526

Dinmohamed AG, Visser O, van Norden Y, Blijlevens NMA, Cornelissen JJ, Huls GA et al (2016) Treatment, trial participation and survival in adult acute myeloid leukemia: a population-based study in the Netherlands, 1989-2012. Leukemia 30(1):24–31

Ehninger A, Kramer M, Röllig C, Thiede C, Bornhäuser M, Von Bonin M et al (2014) Distribution and levels of cell surface expression of CD33 and CD123 in acute myeloid leukemia. Blood Cancer J 4:e218

Ellison RR, Holland JF, Weil M, Jacquillat C, Boiron J, Bernard J et al (1968) Arabinosyl cytosine: a useful agent in the treatment of acute leukemia in adults. Blood 32(4):507–523

Estey E, Gale RP (2017) Acute myeloid leukemia therapy and the chosen people. Leukemia 31:269–271

Estey EH, Thall PF, Pierce S, Cortes J, Beran M, Kantarjian H et al (1999) Randomized phase II study of fludarabine + cytosine arabinoside + idarubicin +/− all-trans retinoic acid +/− granulocyte colony-stimulating factor in poor prognosis newly diagnosed acute myeloid leukemia and myelodysplastic syndrome. Blood 93(8):2478–2484

Estey EH, Gale RP, Sekeres MA (2018) New drugs in AML: uses and abuses. Leukemia 32:1479–1481

Fairley GH (1971) The treatment of acute myeloblastic leukaemia. Br J Haematol 20(6):567–570

Fernandez HF, Sun Z, Yao X, Litzow MR, Luger SM, Paietta EM et al (2009) Anthracycline dose intensification in acute myeloid leukemia. N Engl J Med 361(13):1249–1259

Ferrara F, Barosi G, Venditti A, Angelucci E, Gobbi M, Pane F et al (2013) Consensus-based definition of unfitness to intensive and non-intensive chemotherapy in acute myeloid leukemia: a project of SIE, SIES and GITMO group on a new tool for therapy decision making. Leukemia 27(5):997–999

Gale RE, Popa T, Wright M, Khan N, Freeman SD, Burnett AK et al (2018) No evidence that CD33 splicing SNP impacts the response to GO in younger adults with AML treated on UK MRC/NCRI trials. Blood 131:468–471

Gardin C, Chevret S, Pautas C, Turlure P, Raffoux E, Thomas X et al (2013) Superior long-term outcome with idarubicin compared with high-dose daunorubicin in patients with acute myeloid leukemia age 50 years and older. J Clin Oncol 31:321–327

Goldstone AH, Burnett AK, Wheatley K, Smith AG, Michael Hutchinson R, Clark RE (2001) Attempts to improve treatment outcomes in acute myeloid leukemia (AML) in older patients: the results of the United Kingdom Medical Research Council AML11 trial. Blood 98(5):1302–1311

Gratwohl A (2012) The EBMT risk score. Bone Marrow Transplant 47(6):749–756

Hills RK, Castaigne S, Appelbaum FR, Delaunay J, Petersdorf S, Othus M et al (2014) Addition of gemtuzumab ozogamicin to induction chemotherapy in adult patients with acute myeloid leukaemia: a meta-analysis of individual patient data from randomised controlled trials. Lancet Oncol 15:986–996

Holowiecki J, Grosicki S, Giebel S, Robak T, Kyrcz-Krzemien S, Kuliczkowski K et al (2012) Cladribine, but not fludarabine, added to daunorubicin and cytarabine during induction prolongs survival of patients with acute myeloid leukemia: a multicenter, randomized phase III study. J Clin Oncol 30(20):2441–2448

Huls G, Chitu DA, Havelange V, Jongen-Lavrencic M, van de Loosdrecht AA, Biemond BJ et al (2019) Azacitidine maintenance after intensive chemotherapy improves DFS in older AML patients. Blood 133(13):1457–1464

Juliusson G, Lazarevic V, Horstedt AS, Hagberg O, Hoglund M (2012) Acute myeloid leukemia in the real world: why population-based registries are needed. Blood 119:3890–3899

Kern W, Estey EH (2006) High-dose cytosine arabinoside in the treatment of acute myeloid leukemia: review of three randomized trials. Cancer 107(1):116–124

Khan N, Hills RK, Virgo P, Couzens S, Clark N, Gilkes A, et al (2017) Expression of CD33 is a predictive factor for effect of gemtuzumab ozogamicin at different doses in adult acute myeloid leukaemia. Leukemia [Internet] 31(5):1059–68. https://doi.org/10.1038/leu.2016.309

Klepin HD, Geiger AM, Tooze JA, Kritchevsky SB, Williamson JD, Pardee TS et al (2013) Geriatric assessment predicts survival for older adults receiving

induction chemotherapy for acute myelogenous leukemia. Blood 121(21):4287–4294
Krauss AC, Gao X, Li L, Manning ML, Patel P, Fu W et al (2019) FDA approval summary: (Daunorubicin and Cytarabine) liposome for injection for the treatment of adults with high-risk acute myeloid leukemia. Clin Cancer Res 25(9):2685–2690
Krönke J, Schlenk RF, Jensen KO, Tschurtz F, Corbacioglu A, Gaidzik VI et al (2011) Monitoring of minimal residual disease in NPM1-mutated acute myeloid leukemia: a study from the German-Austrian acute myeloid leukemia study group. J Clin Oncol 29:2709–2716
Krug U, Röllig C, Koschmieder A, Heinecke A, Sauerland MC, Schaich M et al (2010) Complete remission and early death after intensive chemotherapy in patients aged 60 years or older with acute myeloid leukaemia: a web-based application for prediction of outcomes. Lancet 376(9757):2000–2008
Krug U, Berdel WE, Gale RP, Haferlach C, Schnittger S, Müller-Tidow C et al (2016) Increasing intensity of therapies assigned at diagnosis does not improve survival of adults with acute myeloid leukemia. Leukemia 30(6):1230–1236
Lancet et al J Clin Oncol 2018. https://pubmed.ncbi.nlm.nih.gov/30024784/
Lamba JK, Chauhan L, Shin M, Loken MR, Pollard JA, Wang YC et al (2017) CD33 splicing polymorphism determines gemtuzumab ozogamicin response in de novo acute myeloid leukemia: report from randomized phase III children's oncology group trial AAML0531. J Clin Oncol 35(23):674–2682
Lambert J, Pautas C, Terre C, Raffoux E, Turlure P, Caillot D et al (2019) Gemtuzumab ozogamicin for de novo acute myeloid leukemia: final efficacy and safety updates from the open-label, phase III ALFA-0701 trial. Haematologica 104(1):113–119
Larrosa-Garcia M, Baer MR (2017) FLT3 inhibitors in acute myeloid leukemia: current status and future directions. Mol Cancer Ther 16(6):991–1001
Lee JH, Kim H, Joo YD, Lee WS, Bae SH, Zang DY et al (2017) Prospective randomized comparison of idarubicin and high-dose daunorubicin in induction chemotherapy for newly diagnosed acute myeloid leukemia. J Clin Oncol 35(24):2754–2763
Li X, Xu SN, Qin DB, Tan Y, Gong Q, Chen JP (2014) Effect of adding gemtuzumab ozogamicin to induction chemotherapy for newly diagnosed acute myeloid leukemia: a meta-analysis of prospective randomized phase III trials. Ann Oncol 25:455–461
Löwenberg B (2013) Sense and nonsense of high-dose cytarabine for acute myeloid leukemia. Blood 121(1):26–28
Löwenberg B, Suciu S, Archimbaud E, Haak H, Stryckmans P, de Cataldo R et al (1998) Mitoxantrone versus daunorubicin in induction-consolidation chemotherapy—the value of low-dose cytarabine for maintenance of remission, and an assessment of prognostic factors in acute myeloid leukemia in the elderly: final report. European Organization. J Clin Oncol 16(3):872–881
Löwenberg B, Ossenkoppele GJ, van Putten W, Schouten HC, Graux C, Ferrant A et al (2009) High-dose daunorubicin in older patients with acute myeloid leukemia. N Engl J Med 361(13):1235–1248
Löwenberg B, Pabst T, Vellenga E, van Putten W, Schouten HC, Graux C et al (2011) Cytarabine dose for acute myeloid leukemia. N Engl J Med 364:1027–1036
Mabrey FL, Gardner KM, Shannon Dorcy K, Perdue A, Smith HA, Davis AM et al (2020) Outpatient intensive induction chemotherapy for acute myeloid leukemia and high-risk myelodysplastic syndrome. Blood Adv 4(4):611–616
Mandelli F, Vignetti M, Suciu S, Stasi R, Petti MC, Meloni G et al (2009) Daunorubicin versus mitoxantrone versus idarubicin as induction and consolidation chemotherapy for adults with acute myeloid leukemia: the EORTC and GIMEMA groups study AML-10. J Clin Oncol 27(32):5397–5403
Mayer RJ, Davis RB, Schiffer CA, Berg DT, Powell BL, Schulman P et al (1994) Intensive postremission chemotherapy in adults with acute myeloid leukemia. Cancer and Leukemia Group B. N Engl J Med 331:896–903
Michaelis LC (2018) Cytotoxic therapy in acute myeloid leukemia: not quite dead yet. Hematology 2018(1):51–62
Mizuki M, Schwäble J, Steur C, Choudhary C, Agrawal S, Sargin B et al (2003) Suppression of myeloid transcription factors and induction of STAT response genes by AML-specific Flt3 mutations. Blood 101(8):3164–3173
Nagel G, Weber D, Fromm E, Erhardt S, Lübbert M, Fiedler W et al (2017) Epidemiological, genetic, and clinical characterization by age of newly diagnosed acute myeloid leukemia based on an academic population-based registry study (AMLSG BiO). Ann Hematol 96(12):1993–2003
Niederwieser D, Hoffmann VS, Pfirrmann M, Al-Ali HK, Schwind S, Vucinic V, et al (2016) Comparison of treatment strategies in patients over 60 years with AML: final analysis of a prospective randomized German AML Intergroup Study. Blood [Internet]. 128(22):1066. https://doi.org/10.1182/blood.V128.22.1066.1066
Ossenkoppele G, Lowenberg B (2015) How I treat the older patient with acute myeloid leukemia. Blood 125(5):767–774
Paul S, Rausch CR, Jabbour EJ (2020) The face of remission induction. Br J Haematol 188(1):101–115
Pautas C, Merabet F, Thomas X, Raffoux E, Gardin C, Corm S et al (2010) Randomized study of intensified anthracycline doses for induction and recombinant interleukin-2 for maintenance in patients with acute myeloid leukemia age 50 to 70 years: results of the ALFA-9801 study. J Clin Oncol 28(5):808–814
Percival M-EM, Tao L, Medeiros BC, Clarke CA (2015) Improvements in the early death rate among 9380 patients with acute myeloid leukemia after

initial therapy: a SEER database analysis. Cancer 121(12):2004–2012

Pfirrmann M, Ehninger G, Thiede C, Bornhäuser M, Kramer M, Röllig C et al (2012) Prediction of post-remission survival in acute myeloid leukaemia: a post-hoc analysis of the AML96 trial. Lancet Oncol 13(2):207–214

Pigneux A, Bene MC, Salmi L-R, Dumas P-Y, Delaunay J, Bonmati C et al (2018) Improved survival by adding lomustine to conventional chemotherapy for elderly patients with AML without unfavorable cytogenetics: results of the LAM-SA 2007 FILO trial. J Clin Oncol 36(32):3203–3210

Pluta A, Robak T, Wrzesien-Kus A, Katarzyna BB, Sulek K, Wawrzyniak E et al (2017) Addition of cladribine to the standard induction treatment improves outcomes in a subset of elderly acute myeloid leukemia patients. Results of a randomized polish adult leukemia group (PALG) phase II trial. Am J Hematol 92(4):359–366

Rai KR, Holland JF, Glidewell OJ, Weinberg V, Brunner K, Obrecht JP et al (1981) Treatment of acute myelocytic leukemia: a study by cancer and leukemia group B. Blood 58(6):1203–1212

Röllig C, Ehninger G (2015) How I treat hyperleukocytosis in acute myeloid leukemia. Blood 125(21):3246–3252

Röllig C, Serve H, Huttmann A, Noppeney R, Muller-Tidow C, Krug U et al (2015) Addition of sorafenib versus placebo to standard therapy in patients aged 60 years or younger with newly diagnosed acute myeloid leukaemia (SORAML): a multicentre, phase 2, randomised controlled trial. Lancet Oncol 16(16):1691–1699

Röllig C, Kramer M, Gabrecht M, Hänel M, Herbst R, Kaiser U et al (2018a) Intermediate-dose cytarabine plus mitoxantrone versus standard-dose cytarabine plus daunorubicin for acute myeloid leukemia in elderly patients. Ann Oncol 29(4):973–978

Röllig C, Steffen B, Herbst R, Noppeney R, Racil Z, Schäfer-Eckart K et al (2018b) Randomized comparison of 90 mg versus 60 mg daunorubicin in 7+3 standard induction for newly diagnosed acute myeloid leukemia: results from the SAL-DaunoDouble trial. HemaSphere 2(S1):Abstract S861

Röllig C, Kramer M, Gabrecht M, Hänel M, Herbst R, Kaiser U et al (2018c) Intermediate-dose cytarabine plus mitoxantrone versus standard-dose cytarabine plus daunorubicin for acute myeloid leukemia in elderly patients. Ann Oncol 29:973–978

Röllig C, Kramer M, Schliemann C (2019) Time from diagnosis to treatment does not affect outcome in intensively treated patients with newly diagnosed acute myeloid leukemia. Annu Meet Am Soc Hematol 134(Suppl 1):Abstract 13

Röllig C, Beelen DW, Braess J, Greil R, Niederwieser D, Passweg JR, et al (n.d.) Onkopedia-Leitlinie Akute Myeloische Leukämie [Internet]. https://www.onkopedia.com/de/onkopedia/guidelines/akute-myeloische-leukaemie-aml

Schaich M, Röllig C, Soucek S, Kramer M, Thiede C, Mohr B et al (2011) Cytarabine dose of 36 g/m2 compared with 12 g/m2 within first consolidation in acute myeloid leukemia: results of patients enrolled onto the prospective randomized AML96 study. J Clin Oncol 29(19):2696–2702

Schaich M, Parmentier S, Kramer M, Illmer T, Stolzel F, Rollig C et al (2013) High-dose cytarabine consolidation with or without additional Amsacrine and Mitoxantrone in acute myeloid leukemia: results of the prospective randomized AML2003 trial. J Clin Oncol 31(17):2094–2102

Schlenk RF, Weber D, Herr W, Wulf G, Salih HR, Derigs HG et al (2019) Randomized phase-II trial evaluating induction therapy with idarubicin and etoposide plus sequential or concurrent azacitidine and maintenance therapy with azacitidine. Leukemia 33:1923–1933

Sekeres MA, Elson P, Kalaycio ME, Advani AS, Copelan EA, Faderl S et al (2009) Time from diagnosis to treatment initiation predicts survival in younger, but not older, acute myeloid leukemia patients. Blood 113:28–36

Serve H, Krug U, Wagner R, Sauerland MC, Heinecke A, Brunnberg U et al (2013) Sorafenib in combination with intensive chemotherapy in elderly patients with acute myeloid leukemia: results from a randomized, placebo-controlled trial. J Clin Oncol 31:3110–3118

Shayegi N, Kramer M, Bornhäuser M, Schaich M, Schetelig J, Platzbecker U et al (2013) The level of residual disease based on mutant NPM1 is an independent prognostic factor for relapse and survival in AML. Blood 122:83–92

Sorror M, Storer B, Sandmaier BM, Maloney DG, Chauncey TR, Langston A et al (2008) Hematopoietic cell transplantation-comorbidity index and Karnofsky performance status are independent predictors of morbidity and mortality after allogeneic nonmyeloablative hematopoietic cell transplantation. Cancer 112(9):1992–2001

Southam CM, Craver LF, Dargeon HW, Burchenal JH (1951) A study of the natural history of acute leukemia with special reference to the duration of the disease and the occurrence of remissions. Cancer 4:39–59

Stone RM, Mandrekar SJ, Sanford BL, Laumann K, Geyer S, Bloomfield CD et al (2017) Midostaurin plus chemotherapy for acute myeloid leukemia with a FLT3 mutation. N Engl J Med 377:454–464

Teuffel O, Leibundgut K, Lehrnbecher T, Alonzo TA, Beyene J, Sung L (2013) Anthracyclines during induction therapy in acute myeloid leukaemia: a systematic review and meta-analysis. Br J Haematol 161(2):192–203

Thiede C, Steudel C, Mohr B, Schaich M, Schakel U, Platzbecker U et al (2002) Analysis of FLT3-activating mutations in 979 patients with acute myelogenous leukemia: association with FAB subtypes and identification of subgroups with poor prognosis. Blood 99:4326–4335

Tsuchikama K, An Z (2018) Antibody-drug conjugates: recent advances in conjugation and linker chemistries. Protein Cell 9(1):33–46

Valcárcel D, Montesinos P, Sánchez-Ortega I, Brunet S, Esteve J, Martínez-Cuadrón D et al (2012) A scoring system to predict the risk of death during induction with anthracycline plus cytarabine-based chemotherapy in patients with de novo acute myeloid leukemia. Cancer 118(2):410–417

Vellenga E, van Putten W, Ossenkoppele GJ, Verdonck LF, Theobald M, Cornelissen JJ et al (2011) Autologous peripheral blood stem cell transplantation for acute myeloid leukemia. Blood 118(23):6037–6042

Walter RB, Gooley TA, Van Der Velden VHJ, Loken MR, Van Dongen JJM, Flowers DA et al (2007) CD33 expression and P-glycoprotein-mediated drug efflux inversely correlate and predict clinical outcome in patients with acute myeloid leukemia treated with gemtuzumab ozogamicin monotherapy. Blood 109(10):4168–4170

Walter RB, Othus M, Borthakur G, Ravandi F, Cortes JE, Pierce SA et al (2011) Prediction of early death after induction therapy for newly diagnosed acute myeloid leukemia with pretreatment risk scores: a novel paradigm for treatment assignment. J Clin Oncol 29(33):4417–4423

Wei AH, Döhner H, Pocock C, Montesinos P, Afanasyev B, Dombret H, et al (2020) Oral azacitidine maintenance therapy for acute myeloid leukemia in first remission. N Engl J Med 383(26):2526–2537

Wheatley K, Brookes CL, Howman AJ, Goldstone AH, Milligan DW, Prentice AG et al (2009) Prognostic factor analysis of the survival of elderly patients with AML in the MRC AML11 and LRF AML14 trials. Br J Haematol 145(5):598–605

Willemze R, Suciu S, Meloni G, Labar B, Marie JP, Halkes CJ et al (2014) High-dose cytarabine in induction treatment improves the outcome of adult patients younger than age 46 years with acute myeloid leukemia: results of the EORTC-GIMEMA AML-12 trial. J Clin Oncol 32:219–228

Yates JW, Wallace HJ Jr, Ellison RR, Holland JF (1973) Cytosine arabinoside (NSC-63878) and daunorubicin (NSC-83142) therapy in acute nonlymphocytic leukemia. Cancer Chemother Rep 57:485–488

# Treatment of Newly Diagnosed AML in Unfit Patients

# 10

Norbert Vey

## 10.1 Introduction

As demonstrated by large population-based studies (Menzin et al. 2002; Juliusson et al. 2009), the majority of older patients with acute myeloid leukemia (AML) are deemed ineligible for intensive chemotherapy (ICT; i.e., regimens based on the combination of anthracyclines and cytarabine), which is the standard of care for AML in children and young adults. In the Swedish registry (Juliusson et al. 2009), more than 90% of patients younger than 65 years received ICT as compared to 45% of those older than 65 years. Historically, unfit patients who were ineligible for intensive treatment approaches may have received only supportive care. Given that this population is projected to increase due to demographic changes and improved life expectancy, the improvement of their therapeutic options is of paramount importance. The recent development of low-intensity therapies over the past few years has thus provided an alternative to the typically binary choice between intensive treatment and no treatment at all.

The concepts of both low-intensity therapy and unfit patients have unclear definitions as they are often defined by default, that is, "low-intensity" automatically applies to any therapy that is not intensive induction/consolidation chemotherapy, while an "unfit" patient is any patient that cannot tolerate an intensive treatment. Patient outcomes result from the interactions of variables related to (1) the patient, (2) the disease, and (3) the treatment. From this perspective, the treatment of older unfit AML patients with low-intensity approaches is a losing battle fought with weak therapies (low-intensity having been synonymous with low-efficacy until recently) against resistant AML cells as reflected by the frequency of adverse cytogenetics and secondary AML (Vey 2013) in fragile patients with an increased risk of toxicity and treatment-related mortality. Fortunately, substantial progress has been made over the past decade with improvements in supportive care, identification of the most fragile patients, AML genetic-risk stratification, and new therapeutic approaches.

In this chapter, we will discuss the current definition of patient fitness and review treatment results for low-intensity approaches and their impact on the clinical management of AML. We will focus on low-dose cytarabine (LDAC) and and hypomethylating agents (HMA), which represent the current standard of care for unfit AML patients. We will also discuss the attempts made to improve these therapies with their combination to a variety of agents and the recent advent of more effective regimens based on the addition of venetoclax. Treatments based on therapies that target oncogenes, such as FLT3 or IDH1 and IDH2, are discussed in another chapter of this book.

N. Vey (✉)
Hematology Department, Institut Paoli-Calmettes, Aix-Marseille Université, CRCM, Marseille, France
e-mail: VEYN@ipc.unicancer.fr



C. Röllig, G. J. Ossenkoppele (eds.), *Acute Myeloid Leukemia*, Hematologic Malignancies, https://doi.org/10.1007/978-3-030-72676-8_10

## 10.2 Who Is Unfit?

To date, there is no clear and univocal answer to this question, though consensus criteria have emerged that now form the basis of current eligibility criteria for clinical trials dedicated to unfit AML patients. Attempts to formalize criteria by which unfitness can be defined have been based on retrospective studies. The goal of these studies was to identify variables that predict a poor outcome following ICT such as low response rate, high early mortality (30- to 60-day mortality rate), or poor overall survival. In most of these studies, the following were independently associated with a poor patient outcome: age > 75 years, performance status (PS) > 2, hematopoietic cell transplantation comorbidity index (HCT-CI) > 3, high white blood cell counts (WBCs), and unfavorable cytogenetics (Etienne et al. 2007; Malfuson et al. 2008; Kantarjian et al. 2010). Sorror et al. recently proposed a scoring system built on the basis of a large retrospective study's results from 1100 AML patients aged 20–89 years (Sorror et al. 2017). Comorbidities, including those already incorporated into the HCT-CI (Sorror et al. 2005), were evaluated. The addition of parameters such as hypoalbuminemia and thrombocytopenia, a high level of lactate dehydrogenase, age, and European LeukemiaNet (ELN) risk categories further improved the model. The proposed AML-composite model (AML-CM) allowed for the identification of four risk groups with one-year overall survival of 84%, 65%, 52%, and 21%. Concerning patients aged 65–75 years, the two intermediate categories were associated with the same one-year overall survival and could be merged. The three subsequent risk categories were associated with one-year overall survival of 86%, 50% and 23%. As proposed by the authors, the first group would benefit from an intensive approach while the third clearly would not. With 50% one-year overall survival, there is some uncertainty as to whether the intermediate group would benefit from intensive or low-intensity therapy and may represent the appropriate target population for randomized trials.

Three important limitations of the proposed definition criteria for unfitness should be noted. First, with the exception of a single study (Sorror et al. 2017), the criteria are derived from analyses of intensively treated patient populations. Second, PS changes and certain comorbidities may be confounded with potentially reversible leukemia-related complications such as anemia, infection, and hyperleukocytosis. It is therefore advisable to reassess patients after correcting complications such as these in order to avoid an overestimation of a patient's unfitness. The third limitation is linked to insufficient awareness of the multiple dimensions of frailty in older patients. These include physical function, polypharmacy, cognition, social support, and nutritional status (Loh and Klepin 2018). A comprehensive geriatric evaluation of older AML patients revealed that more than 30% had significant cognitive impairment. The Short Physical Performance Battery (SPPB) was able to identify patients at high risk of early mortality among patients with a performance status of 0 to 1 (Klepin et al. 2013).

As reflected by several recommendations for AML management in older patients, age, performance status, comorbidities, and disease features, as well as patient wishes and physician appraisals, are major determinants in the decision-making process (Ferrara et al. 2013; Dohner et al. 2017). The results of the British Medical Research Council (MRC) AML-14 trial (Wheatley et al. 2009) have highlighted the importance of physician assessments. Initially, this trial planned to randomize patients to intensive or nonintensive treatment, but only eight were randomized out of 1485 patients included in the trial. When examining the variables associated with treatment modality decisions in centers where both treatment types were available, the physician emerged as a significant independent factor, after PS and age, in multivariate analysis. In the large study by Sorror et al., 20% of all patients received low-intensity treatment but this varied from 4 to 33% among the five participating centers (Sorror et al. 2017). This variability was not explained by differences in patient characteristics, further illustrating the subjectivity in treatment choice even between highly specialized centers. Some may argue that an experienced physician's assessment may be as good as an imperfect scoring system; however, Bories et al. demonstrated that, besides their expertise, a physician's behavioral characteristics and in particular their individual attitudes toward risk and uncertainty have an impact on the decision-making process for older patients with AML (Bories et al. 2018). Thus, it is important to base treatment decisions on objective criteria and utilize stratification systems, such as the one proposed by Sorror et al. (Sorror et al. 2017), or simpler systems such as the one proposed by the Italian GIMEMA group, which used a consensus-based process to define unfitness according to the following criteria: age > 75 years, poor PS, and severe cardiac, pulmonary, renal, or other comorbidities (Ferrara et al. 2013).

## 10.3 Treatment with Low-Dose Cytarabine

### 10.3.1 Single-Agent LDAC

The efficacy of single-agent cytarabine has been known since the '60s (Lichtman 2013). Two randomized studies showed that overall survival was similar between older AML patients treated with single-agent low-dose cytarabine (LDAC) as compared to conventional induction chemotherapy (Lowenberg et al. 1989; Tilly et al. 1990). Yet in spite of its 50-year history, there is currently no established schedule and it remains unclear as to whether LDAC activity relates to cytotoxicity or to induction of differentiation. Following a large study conducted by the British Medical Research Council (MRC AML-14 trial), which compared LDAC to best supportive care (BSC) in older AML patients who were ineligible for ICT (Burnett et al. 2007), the use of a 20 mg twice daily for 10 days dose-schedule is currently widely used and serves as a control arm in the majority of recent trials. Their results indicated that LDAC produced a complete remission (CR) rate of 18% that translated into significantly prolonged overall survival as compared to BSC. Another important finding of this study was that the oldest patients derived the same benefit from LDAC as younger patients and that LDAC was ineffective in AML with adverse cytogenetics. Table 10.1 summarizes the results of seven clinical trials conducted on LDAC. A meta-analysis that included most of these trials revealed a pooled CR/CRi rate of 19% (95% CI [13%–27%]) and a pooled median overall survival of 5.4 (95% CI [4.4–6.7]) (Stone et al. 2019). The 60-day mortality rates, which reflect both efficacy and treatment toxicity, ranged from 18 to

**Table 10.1** Patient characteristics and outcomes for those treated with LDAC in recent multicenter prospective trials

| Study | No. of pts. | Median age | Adverse cytogenetics (%) | Median No. of cycles | CR (%) | 60-day mortality | Median OS (months) |
|---|---|---|---|---|---|---|---|
| AML14 (Burnett et al. 2007) | 103 | 74 | 17 | 2 | 18 | 29% | NR |
| AML AZA-001 (Dombret et al. 2015) | 158 | 75 | 34 | 4 | 26 | NR | 6.4 |
| DACO-016 (Kantarjian et al. 2012b) | 215 | 73 | 36 | 2[a] | 11.3 | 23% | 5.0 |
| Glasdegib-LDAC phase III trial (Cortes et al. 2018) | 44 | 75 | 43 | 2 | 5.3 | NR | 4.3 |
| Volasertib-LDAC phase II trial (Dohner et al. 2014) | 42 | 76 | 39 | 2 | 13 | 18% | 5.2 |
| Sapacitabine vs. LDAC (Burnett et al. 2015) | 73 | 75 | 17 | 3 | 28 | 23% | 5.9 |
| Lintuzumab-LDAC (Sekeres et al. 2013) | 104 | 70 | 48 | 3 | NR | NR | 5.1 |

*CR* complete response, *LDAC* low-dose cytarabine, *NR* not reported, *OS* overall survival, *Pts* patients
[a]LDAC dose schedule was 20 mg/m$^2$ once daily for 10 days in this study and 20 mg twice daily in all others

29% (Burnett et al. 2007; Kantarjian et al. 2012b; Dohner et al. 2014; Burnett et al. 2015). Median ages were consistent across trials (median age ranged from 73 to 76 years), while the proportion of patients with adverse cytogenetics varied widely from 17 to 48% (Burnett et al. 2007; Kantarjian et al. 2012b; Sekeres et al. 2013; Dohner et al. 2014; Burnett et al. 2015; Dombret et al. 2015; Cortes et al. 2018). Factors predicting LDAC response have not been formally evaluated but some trends can be observed. An age of greater than 75 years was significantly associated with decreased overall survival in a meta-analysis (Stone et al. 2019). The detrimental effect of adverse cytogenetics was reported in a pooled analysis of all patients treated with lintuzumab-LDAC or LDAC alone with a median overall survival of 4.5 months in the group with adverse cytogenetics as compared to 8.7 months in the other patients ($P = 0.002$) (Sekeres et al. 2013). A similar trend was observed in two other studies (Burnett et al. 2007; Dohner et al. 2014). A poor PS was also associated with a trend toward worse outcomes (Burnett et al. 2007). There was no clear difference in patient outcome according to the LDAC dose-schedule. In the DACO-016 trial (Kantarjian et al. 2012b), LDAC was given once daily with 20 mg/m$^2$/day as opposed to the other trials presented in Table 10.1, which used the MRC AML-14 schedule. The response rate was lower (11.3%) in the DACO-016 trial but the overall survival was similar to that of the other trials.

### 10.3.2 LDAC-Based Combination Regimens

Several attempts have been made to improve LDAC results with the addition of new drugs. The MRC developed a "Pick a Winner" program devised to screen for new active therapies, mainly in combination with LDAC and compared to LDAC alone following random allocation (Hills and Burnett 2011). Based on previous experience, the program operated under the hypothesis that the CR rate would be a reliable surrogate for survival. Four new LDAC combinations have been tested using the anti-CD33 antibody–drug conjugate gemtuzumab ozogamicin (Burnett et al. 2013), arsenic trioxide (Burnett et al. 2011), the farnesyltransferase inhibitor tipifarnib (Burnett et al. 2012), or the quinolone-derived intercalating agent vosaroxin (Dennis et al. 2015). There was no indication of any improvement in patient outcomes as compared to the LDAC alone arm. However, the gemtuzumab ozogamicin combination achieved a significantly better CR/CRi rate, but this did not translate into a survival improvement (Burnett et al. 2013). Similarly, volasertib, a small molecule inhibitor of Polo-like kinase I that induces cell cycle arrest and apoptosis, in combination with LDAC as compared to LDAC alone in a randomized phase II trial demonstrated enhanced overall response rates (31% vs. 13.3%, respectively) and a prolonged median overall survival (8 months vs. 5.2 months, respectively), but these results were not confirmed in a large phase III randomized trial (Dohner et al., European Hematology Association meeting 2016, Abstract S501).

Venetoclax has been evaluated in combination with LDA (Wei et al. 2019). Based on initial encouraging results, the VIALE-C study, a multicenter, randomized, phase 3 trial comparing Venetoclax-LDAC to LDAC alone has been conducted in adult patients with previously untreated de novo or secondary AML ineligible for intensive chemotherapy (Wei et al. 2020). 143 and 68 patients were randomized to venetoclax plus LDAC and LDAC alone, respectively. The study failed to meet its primary endpoint of improved OS with the addition of venetoclax to LDAC (7.2 vs. 4.1 months; HR = 0.75 [95% CI: 0.52, 1.07]; $P = 0.11$); however, an unplanned analysis with an additional 6 months of follow up showed a significantly superior median OS of 8.4 months for the venetoclax arm (HR 0.70; 95% CI 0.50–0.98; $P = 0.04$). The CR/CRi rates were 48% and 13% for the venetoclax plus LDAC arm and LDAC-alone arm, respectively. The combination of venetoclax plus LDAC was primarily associated with grade 3 to 4 hematologic adverse events.

Altogether, these results have indicated that while CR may be a prerequisite for survival improvement with LDAC, CR alone is insufficient and a superior CR rate does not guarantee a survival benefit. Although not reaching its primary endpoint, the VIALE-C trial showed that the combination of venetoclax with LDAC showed clinically meaningful outcome improvement.

Glasdegib is an oral smoothened (SMO) inhibitor recently approved by the FDA and EMEA for the treatment of AML in unfit patients in combination with LDAC. SMO is involved in the Hedghog pathway that has been shown to contribute to the maintenance and expansion of leukemic stem cells (Irvine and Copland 2012). The BRIGHT-1003 trial(Cortes et al. 2018) was a randomized open-label controlled phase 2 study that compared glasdegib-LDAC to LDAC in previously untreated elderly patients with AML or higher-risk MDS. Glasdegib (100 mg/day) was given orally on a continuous basis and LDAC (20 mg) was given subcutaneously twice daily for 10 days every 28 days. About 88 patients were allocated to the glasdegib/LDAC arm and 44 to the LDAC. About 124 patients had AML and 16 MDS. Half of them were older than 75 years. Thirty-two percent were classified in the adverse group of the ELN 2010 classification in the glasdegib/LDAC arm versus 42% in the LDAC arm. CR/CRi rate was significantly higher in the glasdegib/LDAC arm (17% vs. 2.3%, $P < 0.05$) and overall survival was significantly longer (8.8 months with glasdegib/LDAC vs. 4.9 months with LDAC, $P = 0.0004$). The most frequently reported AEs with glasdegib/LDAC were pneumonia, fatigue, dyspnea, hyponatremia, and sepsis. Although positive, this study showed poor results in terms of response and overall survival that are in the range of what has previously been reported with LDAC or HMA as single agents. In the absence of direct comparison with the other low-intensity regimens, the place of glasdegib/LDAC in the current AML treatment algorithm thus remains to be established.

## 10.4 Hypomethylating Agents

Epigenetic deregulation plays an important role in the pathogenesis of AML. Recurrent somatic mutations in key genes involved in the epigenetic machinery (DNMT3A, TET2, IDH1, IDH2, and ASXL1) are frequently observed in AML and preleukemic clones (Papaemmanuil et al. 2016). Therapies targeting DNA methyltransferases (DNMTs) have been investigated in MDS and AML. The hypomethylating agents, decitabine and azacitidine, are pyrimidine analogs acting as DNMT inhibitors. They induce global hypomethylation of cytosine residues at cytosine–guanine dinucleotide–rich gene promoters and distal enhancers critical for gene expression regulation (Glass et al. 2017). Both azacitidine and decitabine have been approved in the EU (but not in the US, although widely used off-label) for the frontline treatment of AML in older patients ineligible for ICT.

### 10.4.1 Azacitidine

The AZA AML-001 study compared the outcome of 488 patients aged 65 years and above with newly diagnosed AML who were randomly assigned to receive either azacitidine (75 mg/m$^2$/day subcutaneous injections for 7 days per cycle) or conventional care regimens (CCR, including LDAC, ICT, or BSC) (Dombret et al. 2015). Although it did not meet the primary endpoint, the study reported an improved median overall survival of 10.4 months with azacitidine versus 6.5 months with CCR ($P = 0.1$) that reached statistical significance in a prespecified analysis censoring patients that received AML treatment after discontinuing the study drug (stratified log-rank $P = 0.0190$). Interestingly, the overall CR/CRi rates were relatively low and not different between the azacitidine arm (27.8%) and the CCR (25.1%) arm.

### 10.4.2 Decitabine

Similarly, the DACO-016 phase III trial compared the efficacy of decitabine with treatment choice (TC, supportive care, or LDAC) in older patients with newly diagnosed AML and poor or intermediate-risk cytogenetics (Kantarjian et al. 2012b). About 485 patients were randomly assigned to receive decitabine 20 mg/m²/day intravenously for 5 days every 4 weeks or TC. The results demonstrated a nonsignificant increase in median OS with decitabine (7.7 months) versus TC (5.0 months; $P = 0.108$). An unplanned analysis with more events indicated the same median OS but a statistically significant difference ($P = 0.037$). The CR/CRi with incomplete platelet recovery (CRp) rate was 17.8% with decitabine versus 7.8% with TC. Alternative dose-schedules of decitabine have been developed including a 10-day schedule, which may be more effective than the 5-day schedule (Blum et al. 2010).

### 10.4.3 Guadecitabine

Guadecitabine is a hypomethylating dinucleotide of decitabine linked to guanosine. Guadecitabine is resistant to degradation by cytidine deaminase and has a prolonged half-life as compared to decitabine. An encouraging CR/CRi rate of 54% was reported in a randomized phase II trial conducted in treatment-naïve older AML patients treated with guadecitabine as 60 or 90 mg/m²/day for 5 days, (Kantarjian et al. 2017). However, the ASTRAL-1 study that compared guadecitabine to the standard of care (azacitidine, decitabine, or LDAC) in unfit AML patients demonstrated no significant difference in CR rates (19% vs. 17.4% in the guadecitabine vs. control arms, respectively) and overall survival (median of 7.1 vs. 8.4 months in the guadecitabine vs. control arms, respectively) (Fenaux et al. 2019).

### 10.4.4 Predictors of Response to HMAs

Older age (Kantarjian et al. 2012b), a poor performance status (Thepot et al. 2014; Pleyer et al. 2016), high WBC counts at diagnosis (Kantarjian et al. 2012b), and adverse cytogenetics (Bories et al. 2014; Pleyer et al. 2016) were associated with poorer response rates and/or survival. However, it is worth noting that the group with adverse cytogenetics had the greatest survival benefit from HMAs as compared to conventional care regimens in a subgroup analysis of the AZA AML-001 trial (Seymour et al. 2010). As expected, prior exposure to HMAs before AML transformation was associated with poor survival (median 7.8 months) in a retrospective study of 32 patients (Talati et al. 2020). The analysis of a large international retrospective series of older AML patients treated with azacitidine identified three covariates independently associated with overall survival: ECOG (0 vs. 1–2 vs. 3–4), WBC count before AZA onset ($\leq 10 \times 10^9$/L vs. $>10 \times 10^9$/L), and cytogenetics (normal vs. abnormal) (Ramos et al. 2015). The European ALMA (E-ALMA) scoring system was designed on the basis of these results. As shown in Table 10.2, the E-ALMA system adequately discriminates between three risk groups with different OS and may help with decision-making.

Several studies have suggested that gene mutations can impact prognosis; the TET2, DNMT3A, and NPM1 gene mutations were associated with higher response rates and survival after treatment with azacitidine (Itzykson et al. 2011; Metzeler et al. 2012; Craddock et al. 2017), and the TP53 gene mutation with improved response after treatment with a 10-day schedule of decitabine (Welch et al. 2016).

### 10.4.5 Real-World Data

As reflected by the opposing opinions of the US and European agencies, the interpretation of the

**Table 10.2** Distribution of risk categories, response rates, and overall survival by the European ALMA score (Ramos et al. 2015)

| Risk group | Score | *N* (%) | CR rate (%) | Median OS |
|---|---|---|---|---|
| Favorable | 0 | 44 (13.4) | 36.4 | 17.6 months |
| Intermediate | 1–2 | 237 (72) | 19.8 | 10.6 months |
| Poor | 3–4 | 48 (14.6) | 14.6 | 4.5 months |

*CR* complete remission, *N* number of patients, *OS* overall survival

results of the two pivotal studies is still a matter of debate (Kantarjian et al. 2012b; Dombret et al. 2015). However, HMAs are considered as the standard of treatment for older unfit AML patients as revealed by various recent treatment recommendations (Dohner et al. 2017; Tallman et al. 2019). Several studies have addressed the issue of the impact of HMAs in the real world and their results are summarized in Table 10.3. The majority of these studies focused on AML patients treated with azacitidine and in general the results of the AZA AML-001 trial (Dombret et al. 2015) were reproduced both in terms of response (CR/CRi rate between 17 and 23% vs. 28% for real-world studies versus AZA AML-001, respectively) and in terms of median overall survival (between 10 and 14 months vs. 10 months for real-world studies vs. AZA AML-001, respectively) (Bories et al. 2014; Pleyer et al. 2016; Talati et al. 2020).

In a comparison of 214 patients treated with azacitidine within the AZA AML-001 trial with 95 patients selected according to AZA AML-001 inclusion criteria (i.e., WBC < 30 G/L, marrow blasts >30%) in the Austrian registry, no difference in overall survival was observed between the trial and real-world groups (9.9 and 10.8 months, respectively; $P = 0.616$) (Pleyer et al. 2017). Interestingly, this was also true when compared to patients from the Austrian registry who did not fulfill the AZA AML-001 trial eligibility criteria.

### 10.4.6 Insights into the Mechanisms of Resistance to HMAs

Recent studies have investigated the mechanisms of HMA resistance. Although global hypomethylation is generally observed following treatment with HMAs, the correlation between methylation levels and response has not been consistently documented (Voso et al. 2014). A study of patients treated with decitabine for chronic myelomonocytic leukemia (CMML) demonstrated that the methylation of specific DNA sites rather than global methylation was associated with response (Merlevede et al. 2016). Interestingly, clinical responses were achieved without either decreasing the mutant allele burden or preventing the

**Table 10.3** Characteristics and outcomes of unfit patients treated with HMAs in multicenter prospective trials or in retrospective real-world studies for previously untreated AML

| Study | No. of pts. | HMA/Schedule | Median age | Median WBC | Adverse cytogenetics (%) | Median No. of cycles | CR/CRi (%)/Time to response | Median OS (months) |
|---|---|---|---|---|---|---|---|---|
| AML AZA-001 (Dombret et al. 2015) | 241 | AZA/EMEA | 75 | 3.1 | 35 | 6 | 28%/NR | 10.4 |
| DACO-016 (Kantarjian et al. 2012b) | 242 | DAC/20X5 | 73 | 3.1 | 36 | 4 | 28%/4.3 months | 7.7 |
| French ATU (Thepot et al. 2014) | 149 | AZA/EMEA and alternate | 74 | 3.2 | 40 | 5 | 33%/4.7 months | 4.7 |
| Toulouse (Bories et al. 2014) | 95 | AZA/EMEA and alternate | 76 | 2.3 | 45 | 6 | 19%/4.5 months | 11.3 |
| Italian registry (Bocchia et al. 2019) | 306 | DAC | 75 | NR | 30 | 5 | 23%/NR | 10 |
| Moffitt CC (Talati et al. 2020) | 255 | AZA and DAC | 76 | 3.3 | 31 | NR | 23%/NR | 14.4 |
| Austrian registry (Pleyer et al. 2016) | 139 | AZA/EMEA | 76 | NR | 31 | 3 | 17%/3 months | 12.9 |

*NR* not reported, *EMEA* EMEA approved dose schedule, i.e., 75 mg/m$^2$/day × 7 days, *alternate* alternate schedules, i.e., 75 mg/m$^2$/day days 1–5 and 8–9 or 50 mg/m$^2$/day × 7

emergence of new genetic alterations. In myelodysplastic syndromes (MDS), treatment with azacitidine was able to modify the subclonal distribution but founder clones were not eliminated (Unnikrishnan et al. 2017). In AML, the number of leukemic stem cells (LSC) as measured by lymphoid multipotential progenitor populations (LMPP) persistence was lower in responders to azacitidine but persisted in the majority and increased prior to relapse (Craddock et al. 2017). Altogether, these data confirmed that HMA clinical activity relies on epigenetic mechanisms and show that HMAs are unable to induce a clonal eradication. The persistence of LCS may explain why HMAs alone are unable to produce long-term disease-free survival, making combinations of HMAs with LCS-targeting drugs an attractive approach.

## 10.5 The Lessons of HMA Therapy: A Paradigm Shift

One striking observation on HMA therapies was the dissociation between response and survival, challenging the basis upon which the classical International Working Group (IWG) response criteria for AML were established (Cheson et al. 2003). Indeed, after conventional ICT the achievement of CR is associated with survival improvements, which is also true for relapsed AML (Vey et al. 1999) and for the oldest patients (Vey et al. 2004). However, in the AZA AML-001 study, the survival benefit of azacitidine was retained even after excluding the responders from the analysis (Dombret et al. 2015). Approximately 30% of patients without bone marrow response improved their cytopenia. This indicates that normal hematopoiesis could be restored in the absence of significant bone marrow blast reduction, which may partially explain the survival benefit. In the DACO-016 study, the achievement of transfusion independence was associated with a significant increase in survival (median overall survival of 9.8 months and 6.4 months for patients with and without hematologic improvement (HI), respectively; $P = 0.02$). In a posthoc analysis of the AZA AML-001 trial, Schuh et al. revealed that among patients who achieved a stable disease, those with HI with azacitidine had improved survival (median overall survival increase of 7.9 months), which was not the case for patients treated in the CCR arm (Schuh et al. 2017b). In the Austrian registry study (Pleyer et al. 2014), bone marrow response was not an independent predictor of survival, whereas HI was, suggesting that the disease's natural history may be modified by HMAs even in the absence of blast reduction. This is consistent with the epigenetic mechanisms and induction of differentiation. Comparable treatment effects have recently been observed with new therapies such as the IDH1 or 2 inhibitors ivosidenib and enasidenib, which also target epigenetic mechanisms and were shown to induce differentiation (Stein et al. 2020). Though HI is commonly used as a response criterion in MDS (Cheson et al. 2006) but not in AML (Dohner et al. 2017), it appears to be relevant for evaluating the effects of low-intensity therapies on AML and may be integrated into future AML response criteria (Bloomfield et al. 2018). This observation also has practical implications as it supports the recommendation to continue HMA therapy even in the absence of a response, so long as patients can tolerate the treatment and the disease does not progress (Estey 2013; Schuh et al. 2017a). In addition, registry data indicate that continuous treatment is more important than azacitidine dosage or dosing schedule regarding OS benefits, which is consistent with the transience of demethylation observed in HMA treatment (Thepot et al. 2014; Pleyer et al. 2014; Ramos et al. 2015).

## 10.6 HMA-Based Combination Regimens

Although the use of HMAs has led to significant improvements in the outcome of older unfit AML patients, results remain unsatisfactory with an overall median survival that does not exceed 1 year (see Table 10.3). Consequently, when this information is combined with the favorable tolerance profile of HMAs, they are regarded as attractive drugs for the design of novel combination regimens. Based on preclinical evidence demonstrating that the dual inhibition of epigenetic pathways via HMAs and histone deacetylase inhibitors (HDAC) leads to synergistic in vitro activity (Cameron et al. 1999), the combination of HMAs with HDAC has been extensively investigated. Regimens combining azacitidine or decitabine with a variety of HDAC, such as valproic acid, vorinostat, and entinostat, were studied in MDS and AML with disappointing clinical effects. This was possibly due to HDAC toxicity leading to early treatment interruption, not only of the HDAC but also of the HMAs, which may have counteracted the potential beneficial effects (Garcia-Manero et al. 2008; Griffiths and Gore 2013). Recently, encouraging results have been reported in a phase II study of pracinostat and azacitidine with a CR/CRi rate of 44% and a median overall survival of 19 months that need to be confirmed (Garcia-Manero et al. 2019). The antitumor immune response was positively affected by HMAs upregulating the expression of tumor antigens, HLA class-1, or co-stimulatory molecules, but this can be offset by the concomitant upregulation of inhibitory immune checkpoint molecules, which makes the combination of HMAs with immune checkpoints inhibitors appealing (Daver et al. 2018). Encouraging preliminary clinical results have been reported (Daver et al. 2017) but were not confirmed by the results of a randomized phase II study comparing durvalumab and azacitidine to azacitidine alone in previously untreated AML patients ineligible for ICT (Zeidan et al. 2019a). In many other instances, combination regimens have been developed empirically in the absence of biological rationale and were listed in Schuh's review article (Schuh et al. 2017a). Most of these attempts failed to improve patient overall survival as compared to HMA monotherapy, in spite of a substantial increase in the response rate. This underlines the importance of safety and tolerance issues in older fragile patient populations as illustrated by vadastuximab talirine (SGN-CD33A), an antibody–drug conjugate directed toward CD33 (Kung Sutherland et al. 2013). A phase I trial found that the combination of SGN-33A with AZA yielded responses in 70% of patients with the majority of them achieving MRD negativity (Fathi et al. 2018), but the phase III CASCADE trial comparing vadastuximab and HMAs to HMAs alone was put on hold due to excessive toxicity. In a study combining alternating courses of LDAC-cladribine and decitabine in 118 AML patients ineligible for ICT, Kadia et al. reported a CR/CRi rate of 68% and a median overall survival of 13.8 months, which compared favorably to decitabine alone (Kadia et al. 2018). It should be noted, however, that study patients had a median age of 69 years, a median ECOG performance status of 1, and 25% of them could receive transplantations. These characteristics correspond to those of older patients who are eligible for ICT (Pigneux et al. 2007; Lowenberg et al. 2009) rather than those of unfit patients (Kantarjian et al. 2012b; Dombret et al. 2015). This suggests that "intensified low-intensity" regimens may provide improved patient outcomes as compared to HMAs, but that not every unfit patient would be able to tolerate an increase in treatment intensity (Vey 2018).

Venetoclax in combination with azacitidine was evaluated versus azacitidine alone in the multicenter, randomized, phase 3 VIALE-A study (DiNardo et al. 2020). Eligible patients had newly diagnosed AML and were either aged ≥75 years or aged ≥18 years and considered ineligible for standard induction therapy based on the presence of prespecified comorbidities. The study included 286 patients in the venetoclax (VEN) plus azacitidine arm and 145 in the azacitidine plus placebo (PBO) arm. The addition of venetoclax to azacitidine was associated with improved OS (14.7 months in AZA + VEN vs. 9.6 mos in AZA + PBO (HR: 0.66, 95% CI: 0.52–0.85, $P < 0.001$)). CR + CRi rate was 66% and 28% in AZA + VEN and AZA + PBO respectively, $P < 0.001$). Venetoclax plus azacitidine was primarily associated with grade 3 and 4 hematologic adverse events and manageable gastrointestinal toxicity. The combination of venetoclax and HMA has been approved by the FDA in 2019. The confirmation of the efficacy of this regimen by the phase 3 VIALE-A trial makes it a new standard for the frontline therapy of elderly patients with AML unfit for intensive chemotherapy (Richard-Carpentier and DiNardo 2019).

## 10.7 LDAC Versus HMAs, Azacitidine Versus Decitabine: Did We Pick a Winner?

So far in randomized studies, HMAs have not demonstrated significantly superior survival to LDAC (Kantarjian et al. 2012b; Dombret et al. 2015). However, converging evidence suggests HMA superiority. As discussed above, overall results with LDAC are disappointing, with a median overall survival of less than 6 months in most studies. In addition, achieving CR with LDAC is generally restricted to patients with favorable or intermediate-risk cytogenetics, and survival benefits are mainly restricted to patients who achieve CR (Burnett et al. 2007). HMAs have also demonstrated several potential advantages over LDAC. First, HMAs produce higher HI rates as revealed by the AZA AML-001 study with a red blood cell (RBC) transfusion independence rate of 70% as compared to 17% in the control arm ($P = 0.03$) (Dombret et al. 2015) and this may translate into a survival benefit (Pleyer et al. 2014). Second, HMAs are effective in poor-risk genetic categories, such as inv(3) or TP53 mutations (Wanquet et al. 2015; Welch et al. 2016), with a statistically significant survival benefit in combination with azacitidine versus LDAC in the group with adverse cytogenetics (Döhner et al. 2014). Third, some real-world data provided additional evidence for the superiority of HMAs as compared to LDAC (Talati et al. 2020).

The comparison of azacitidine with ICT has not been directly addressed in comparative studies for the AZA AML-001 study. However, only 87 patients were randomized between azacitidine and ICT. The results showed a higher CR/CRi rate in the ICT arm (47% vs. 28% in the azacitidine arm) but a similar median overall survival (13.3 vs. 12.2 in the azacitidine arm, $P = 0.5$), yet given the small number of patients, no definitive conclusion could be drawn. Two single-institution retrospective studies that used propensity score-based analysis reported conflicting results with better overall survival for ICT versus azacitidine in one study (Bories et al. 2014) and the opposite in the other (Talati et al. 2020), where the proportions of patients treated with ICT were comparable (34% and 36.7%). Collectively, these results indicate that ICT yields higher CR rates as compared with azacitidine, but there is no clear evidence that this translates into better overall survival.

No prospective trial comparing azacitidine with decitabine has been reported as of yet. The available data are derived from indirect comparisons and retrospective studies in MDS and AML, suggesting that azacitidine is at least as effective as decitabine and may have a greater impact on overall survival (Kumar et al. 2010; Kantarjian et al. 2012b; Xie et al. 2015; Dombret et al. 2015). A recent large phase 3 trial compared guadecitabine to a control arm in which patients may receive azacitidine or decitabine based on physician choice. Respectively 171 and 167 patients were allocated to azacitidine or decitabine and they characteristics were well balanced. The composite CR rate (CR + CRi + CRp) was 22.2% vs. 25.1% and the median OS 8.7 vs. 8.2 (HR: 0.97; 95% CI: 0.77–1.23; Log-rank $P$ value: 0.81).

## 10.8 Other Low-Intensity Therapies

In the pre-HMA era, since no established therapy was available, it was possible to include unfit patients with previously untreated AML in early phase trials, which had the advantage of allowing the evaluation of new drugs in treatment-naïve patients instead of the usual heavily pretreated refractory/relapsed patient populations. Many new agents have been tested in this setting and scarce responses have been achieved with most of them (Stahl et al. 2017), though few have been tested in phase III trials. The farnesyltransferase inhibitor tipifarnib was not associated with improved patient outcomes as compared to BSC in a randomized study (Harousseau et al. 2009). More recently, the orally available nucleoside analog sapacitabine has been investigated in unfit AML patients based on initial reports showing a favorable tolerance profile and significant activity in this setting (Kantarjian et al. 2012a). In a phase III trial of the British MRC comparing single-agent sapacitabine and LDAC (Burnett et al. 2015), the CR rate with sapacitabine was 16% while the median overall survival was 4.7 months, and these were not superior to LDAC.

## 10.9 Conclusion

Low-intensity therapies represent a significant advance in the clinical management of older patients with AML. Over the past decade, a growing proportion of older patients were offered therapy as shown by population-based studies and registries (Medeiros et al. 2015; Nagel et al. 2017; Talati et al. 2020). In a study of Surveillance, Epidemiology, and End Results(SEER)-Medicare data from 14,089 older patients with AML residing in the US, the proportion of patients who did not receive active treatment decreased over time from 59.7% among patients diagnosed in 2001 to 42.8% among those diagnosed in 2013 (Zeidan et al. 2019b).

Azacitidine and decitabine are effective new forms of low-intensity therapy and may be superior to LDAC. In large cohorts from specialized centers, HMAs are used in approximately one-third of patients older than 65 years (Bories et al. 2014; Talati et al. 2020), while less than 10% of patients received LDAC, highlighting the growing importance of HMAs in the current AML therapeutic armory. Existing data from clinical trials or retrospective studies indicate a survival benefit as compared to LDAC, particularly in patients with unfavorable cytogenetics who represent 35–40% of patients in this age group. Whether HMAs are superior or equivalent to ICT has not been established. With the currently dynamic AML therapeutic landscape, it is unlikely and probably undesirable to perform such studies. The new and more effective venetoclax-based low-intensity regimens that are currently being developed will challenge conventional ICT and their validation is now a priority.

HMAs have also revealed that epigenetic therapies do not have the same clinical effects as conventional chemotherapy. Indeed, the dissociation between response and survival, the transience of demethylation, and the achievement of hematologic improvements in the absence of blast reduction imply that treatment should be continued until progression, even in the absence of bone marrow response. This also demonstrates that achieving CR should not be a primary goal of any clinical trials evaluating these therapies and that hematologic improvements may represent a meaningful clinical endpoint as it does in MDS.

The development of novel active low-intensity therapies for older AML patients has emphasized the need for objective and reproducible criteria to define "unfitness." Several simple stratification systems have been developed as well as more sophisticated geriatric tools, and their implementation in clinical practice should improve physicians' decisions.

With the recently reported results of venetoclax-HMA combination (DiNardo et al. 2020), a new standard has emerged that will probably have a significant impact on the outcome of elderly patients with AML. However, even if improved, the survival of these patients remains short and further improvements are warranted. This will rely on the ongoing development of several novel agents as described in another chapter of this book that could be added to the venetoclax-HMA backbone or be incorporated into sequential strategies. This underlines the importance of including elderly patients in clinical trials.

## References

Bloomfield CD, Estey E, Pleyer L, Schuh AC, Stein EM, Tallman MS, Wei A (2018) Time to repeal and replace response criteria for acute myeloid leukemia? Blood Rev 32:416–425. https://doi.org/10.1016/j.blre.2018.03.006

Blum W, Garzon R, Klisovic RB, Schwind S, Walker A, Geyer S, Liu S, Havelange V, Becker H, Schaaf L, Mickle J, Devine H, Kefauver C, Devine SM, Chan KK, Heerema NA, Bloomfield CD, Grever MR, Byrd JC, Villalona-Calero M, Croce CM, Marcucci G (2010) Clinical response and miR-29b predictive significance in older AML patients treated with a 10-day schedule of decitabine. Proc Natl Acad Sci U S A 107:7473–7478. https://doi.org/10.1073/pnas.1002650107

Bocchia M, Candoni A, Borlenghi E, Defina M, Filì C, Cattaneo C, Sammartano V, Fanin R, Sciumè M,

Sicuranza A, Imbergamo S, Riva M, Fracchiolla N, Latagliata R, Caizzi E, Mazziotta F, Alunni G, Di Bona E, Crugnola M, Rossi M, Consoli U, Fontanelli G, Greco G, Nadali G, Rotondo F, Todisco E, Bigazzi C, Capochiani E, Molteni A, Bernardi M, Fumagalli M, Rondoni M, Scappini B, Ermacora A, Simonetti F, Gottardi M, Lambertenghi Deliliers D, Michieli M, Basilico C, Galeone C, Pelucchi C, Rossi G (2019) Real-world experience with decitabine as a first-line treatment in 306 elderly acute myeloid leukaemia patients unfit for intensive chemotherapy. Hematol Oncol 37:447–455. https://doi.org/10.1002/hon.2663

Bories P, Bertoli S, Berard E, Laurent J, Duchayne E, Sarry A, Delabesse E, Beyne-Rauzy O, Huguet F, Recher C (2014) Intensive chemotherapy, azacitidine, or supportive care in older acute myeloid leukemia patients: an analysis from a regional healthcare network. Am J Hematol 89:E244–E252. https://doi.org/10.1002/ajh.23848

Bories P, Lamy S, Simand C, Bertoli S, Delpierre C, Malak S, Fornecker L, Moreau S, Recher C, Nebout A (2018) Physician uncertainty aversion impacts medical decision making for older patients with acute myeloid leukemia: results of a national survey. Haematologica 103:2040–2048. https://doi.org/10.3324/haematol.2018.192468

Burnett AK, Milligan D, Prentice AG, Goldstone AH, McMullin MF, Hills RK, Wheatley K (2007) A comparison of low-dose cytarabine and hydroxyurea with or without all-trans retinoic acid for acute myeloid leukemia and high-risk myelodysplastic syndrome in patients not considered fit for intensive treatment. Cancer 109:1114–1124. https://doi.org/10.1002/cncr.22496

Burnett AK, Hills RK, Hunter A, Milligan D, Kell J, Wheatley K, Yin J, McMullin MF, Cahalin P, Craig J, Bowen D, Russell N (2011) The addition of arsenic trioxide to low-dose Ara-C in older patients with AML does not improve outcome. Leukemia 25:1122–1127. https://doi.org/10.1038/leu.2011.59

Burnett AK, Russell NH, Culligan D, Cavanagh J, Kell J, Wheatley K, Virchis A, Hills RK, Milligan D, AML Working Group of the UK National Cancer Research Institute (2012) The addition of the farnesyl transferase inhibitor, tipifarnib, to low dose cytarabine does not improve outcome for older patients with AML. Br J Haematol 158:519–522. https://doi.org/10.1111/j.1365-2141.2012.09165.x

Burnett AK, Hills RK, Hunter AE, Milligan D, Kell WJ, Wheatley K, Yin J, McMullin MF, Dignum H, Bowen D, Russell NH, UK National Cancer Research Institute AML Working Group (2013) The addition of gemtuzumab ozogamicin to low-dose Ara-C improves remission rate but does not significantly prolong survival in older patients with acute myeloid leukaemia: results from the LRF AML14 and NCRI AML16 pick-a-winner comparison. Leukemia 27:75–81. https://doi.org/10.1038/leu.2012.229

Burnett AK, Russell N, Hills RK, Panoskaltsis N, Khwaja A, Hemmaway C, Cahalin P, Clark RE, Milligan D (2015) A randomised comparison of the novel nucleoside analogue sapacitabine with low-dose cytarabine in older patients with acute myeloid leukaemia. Leukemia 29:1312–1319. https://doi.org/10.1038/leu.2015.38

Cameron EE, Bachman KE, Myohanen S, Herman JG, Baylin SB (1999) Synergy of demethylation and histone deacetylase inhibition in the re-expression of genes silenced in cancer. Nat Genet 21:103–107. https://doi.org/10.1038/5047

Cheson BD, Bennett JM, Kopecky KJ, Buchner T, Willman CL, Estey EH, Schiffer CA, Doehner H, Tallman MS, Lister TA, Lo-Coco F, Willemze R, Biondi A, Hiddemann W, Larson RA, Lowenberg B, Sanz MA, Head DR, Ohno R, Bloomfield CD (2003) Revised recommendations of the international working group for diagnosis, standardization of response criteria, treatment outcomes, and reporting standards for therapeutic trials in acute myeloid leukemia. J Clin Oncol 21:4642–4649

Cheson BD, Greenberg PL, Bennett JM, Lowenberg B, Wijermans PW, Nimer SD, Pinto A, Beran M, de Witte TM, Stone RM, Mittelman M, Sanz GF, Gore SD, Schiffer CA, Kantarjian H (2006) Clinical application and proposal for modification of the international working group (IWG) response criteria in myelodysplasia. Blood 108:419–425

Cortes JE, Heidel FH, Hellmann A, Fiedler W, Smith BD, Robak T, Montesinos P, Pollyea DA, DesJardins P, Ottmann O, Ma WW, Shaik MN, Laird AD, Zeremski M, O'Connell A, Chan G, Heuser M (2018) Randomized comparison of low dose cytarabine with or without glasdegib in patients with newly diagnosed acute myeloid leukemia or high-risk myelodysplastic syndrome. Leukemia 33(2):379–389. https://doi.org/10.1038/s41375-018-0312-9

Craddock CF, Houlton AE, Quek LS, Ferguson P, Gbandi E, Roberts C, Metzner M, Garcia-Martin N, Kennedy A, Hamblin A, Raghavan M, Nagra S, Dudley L, Wheatley K, McMullin MF, Pillai SP, Kelly RJ, Siddique S, Dennis M, Cavenagh JD, Vyas P (2017) Outcome of Azacitidine therapy in acute myeloid leukemia is not improved by concurrent Vorinostat therapy but is predicted by a diagnostic molecular signature. Clin Cancer Res 23:6430–6440. https://doi.org/10.1158/1078-0432.CCR-17-1423

Daver N, Garcia-Manero G, Basu S, Cortes JE, Ravandi F, Jabbour EJ, Assi R, Brandt M, Pierce S, Gordon T, Pemmaraju N, Andreeff M, Ning J, Kornblau S, Kadia T, Flores W, Matthews J, DiNardo CD, Borthakur G, Konopleva M, Allison J, Sharma P, Kantarjian HM (2017) Nivolumab (Nivo) with Azacytidine (AZA) in patients (pts) with relapsed acute myeloid leukemia (AML) or frontline elderly AML. Blood 130:1345–1345

Daver N, Boddu P, Garcia-Manero G, Yadav SS, Sharma P, Allison J, Kantarjian H (2018) Hypomethylating agents in combination with immune checkpoint inhibitors in acute myeloid leukemia and myelodysplastic syndromes. Leukemia 32:1094–1105. https://doi.org/10.1038/s41375-018-0070-8

Dennis M, Russell N, Hills RK, Hemmaway C, Panoskaltsis N, McMullin M-F, Kjeldsen L, Dignum H, Thomas IF, Clark RE, Milligan D, Burnett AK (2015) Vosaroxin and vosaroxin plus low-dose Ara-C (LDAC) vs low-dose Ara-C alone in older patients with acute myeloid leukemia. Blood 125:2923–2932. https://doi.org/10.1182/blood-2014-10-608117

DiNardo CD, Jonas B, Pullarkat V, Thirman M, Garcia J, Wei A, Döhner H, Fenaux P, Recher C, Konopleva M, Fiedler W, Koller E, Havelange V, Schuh A, Esteve J, Wang J, Vrhovac R, Hajek R, Porkka K, Illes A, Wolach O, Olivieri A, Yamamoto K, Jang J, Juliusson G, Vorobyev V, Yeh SP, Ozcan M, Hong WJ, Zhou Y, Potluri J, Pratz K, Jonas B, Pullarkat V, Thirman M, Garcia J, Wei A, Döhner H, Fenaux P, Recher C, Konopleva M, Fiedler W, Koller E, Havelange V, Schuh A, Esteve J, Wang J, Vrhovac R, Hajek R, Porkka K, Pratz K (2020) A randomized, double-blind, placebo-controlled study of Venetoclax. https://library.ehaweb.org/eha/2020/eha25th/303390/courtney.dinardo.a.randomized.double-blind.placebo-controlled.study.of.html?f=menu%3D6%2Abrowseby%3D8%2Asortby%3D2%2Ace_id%3D1766%2Amarker%3D794. Accessed 9 Aug 2020

Dohner H, Lubbert M, Fiedler W, Fouillard L, Haaland A, Brandwein JM, Lepretre S, Reman O, Turlure P, Ottmann OG, Muller-Tidow C, Kramer A, Raffoux E, Dohner K, Schlenk RF, Voss F, Taube T, Fritsch H, Maertens J (2014) Randomized, phase 2 trial of low-dose cytarabine with or without volasertib in AML patients not suitable for induction therapy. Blood 124:1426–1433. https://doi.org/10.1182/blood-2014-03-560557

Döhner H, Seymour JF, Butrym A, Wierzbowska A, Selleslag D, Jang JH, Cavenagh JD, Kumar R, Schuh AC, Candoni A, Récher C, Sandhu I, Bernal del Castillo T, Al-Ali HK, Martinelli G, Falantes J, Stone RM, Minden MD, McIntyre H, Songer S, Lucy LM, Beach CL, Dombret H (2014) Overall survival in older patients with newly diagnosed acute myeloid leukemia (AML) with >30% bone marrow blasts treated with Azacitidine by cytogenetic risk status: results of the AZA-AML-001 study. Blood 124:621. https://doi.org/10.1182/blood.V124.21.621.621

Dohner H, Estey E, Grimwade D, Amadori S, Appelbaum FR, Buchner T, Dombret H, Ebert BL, Fenaux P, Larson RA, Levine RL, Lo-Coco F, Naoe T, Niederwieser D, Ossenkoppele GJ, Sanz M, Sierra J, Tallman MS, Tien HF, Wei AH, Lowenberg B, Bloomfield CD (2017) Diagnosis and management of AML in adults: 2017 ELN recommendations from an international expert panel. Blood 129(4):424–447. https://doi.org/10.1182/blood-2016-08-733196

Dombret H, Seymour JF, Butrym A, Wierzbowska A, Selleslag D, Jang JH, Kumar R, Cavenagh J, Schuh AC, Candoni A, Recher C, Sandhu I, Bernal del Castillo T, Al-Ali HK, Martinelli G, Falantes J, Noppeney R, Stone RM, Minden MD, McIntyre H, Songer S, Lucy LM, Beach CL, Dohner H (2015) International phase 3 study of azacitidine vs conventional care regimens in older patients with newly diagnosed AML with >30% blasts. Blood 126:291–299. https://doi.org/10.1182/blood-2015-01-621664

Estey EH (2013) Epigenetics in clinical practice: the examples of azacitidine and decitabine in myelodysplasia and acute myeloid leukemia. Leukemia 27:1803–1812. https://doi.org/10.1038/leu.2013.173

Etienne A, Esterni B, Charbonnier A, Mozziconacci MJ, Arnoulet C, Coso D, Puig B, Gastaut JA, Maraninchi D, Vey N (2007) Comorbidity is an independent predictor of complete remission in elderly patients receiving induction chemotherapy for acute myeloid leukemia. Cancer 109:1376–1383. https://doi.org/10.1002/cncr.22537

Fathi AT, Erba HP, Lancet JE, Stein EM, Ravandi F, Faderl S, Walter RB, Advani AS, DeAngelo DJ, Kovacsovics TJ, Jillella A, Bixby D, Levy MY, O'Meara MM, Ho PA, Voellinger J, Stein AS (2018) A phase 1 trial of vadastuximab talirine combined with hypomethylating agents in patients with CD33-positive AML. Blood 132:1125–1133. https://doi.org/10.1182/blood-2018-03-841171

Fenaux P, Gobbi M, Kropf PL, Mayer J, Roboz GJ, Döhner H, Krauter J, Döhner K, Robak T, Kantarjian H, Novak J, Jedrzejczak W, Thomas X, Ojeda-Uribe M, Miyazaki Y, Min YH, Yeh S-P, Brandwein J, Gercheva-Kyuchukova L, Demeter J, Griffiths E, Yee K, Azab M, Issa J-P (2019) Results of ASTRAL-1 study, a phase 3 randomized trial of guadecitabine (G) vs treatment choice (TC) in treatment NAÏVE acute myeloid leukemia (TN-AML) not eligible for intensive chemotherapy (IC). HemaSphere 3:394–395. https://doi.org/10.1097/01.HS9.0000561796.30124.a4

Ferrara F, Barosi G, Venditti A, Angelucci E, Gobbi M, Pane F, Tosi P, Zinzani P, Tura S (2013) Consensus-based definition of unfitness to intensive and non-intensive chemotherapy in acute myeloid leukemia: a project of SIE, SIES and GITMO group on a new tool for therapy decision making. Leukemia 27:997–999. https://doi.org/10.1038/leu.2012.303

Garcia-Manero G, Assouline S, Cortes J, Estrov Z, Kantarjian H, Yang H, Newsome WM, Miller WH, Rousseau C, Kalita A, Bonfils C, Dubay M, Patterson TA, Li Z, Besterman JM, Reid G, Laille E, Martell RE, Minden M (2008) Phase 1 study of the oral isotype specific histone deacetylase inhibitor MGCD0103 in leukemia. Blood 112:981–989

Garcia-Manero G, Abaza Y, Takahashi K, Medeiros BC, Arellano M, Khaled SK, Patnaik M, Odenike O, Sayar H, Tummala M, Patel P, Maness-Harris L, Stuart R, Traer E, Karamlou K, Yacoub A, Ghalie R, Giorgino R, Atallah E (2019) Pracinostat plus azacitidine in older patients with newly diagnosed acute myeloid leukemia: results of a phase 2 study. Blood Adv 3:508–518. https://doi.org/10.1182/bloodadvances.2018027409

Glass JL, Hassane D, Wouters BJ, Kunimoto H, Avellino R, Garrett-Bakelman FE, Guryanova OA, Bowman R, Redlich S, Intlekofer AM, Meydan C, Qin T, Fall M, Alonso A, Guzman ML, Valk PJM, Thompson CB, Levine R, Elemento O, Delwel R, Melnick A, Figueroa ME (2017) Epigenetic identity in AML depends on disruption of non-promoter regulatory elements and is affected by antagonistic effects of mutations in epigenetic modifiers. Cancer Discov 7:868–883. https://doi.org/10.1158/2159-8290.CD-16-1032

Griffiths EA, Gore SD (2013) Epigenetic therapies in MDS and AML. Adv Exp Med Biol 754:253–283. https://doi.org/10.1007/978-1-4419-9967-2_13

Harousseau JL, Martinelli G, Jedrzejczak WW, Brandwein JM, Bordessoule D, Masszi T, Ossenkoppele GJ, Alexeeva JA, Beutel G, Maertens J, Vidriales MB, Dombret H, Thomas X, Burnett AK, Robak T, Khuageva NK, Golenkov AK, Tothova E, Mollgard L, Park YC, Bessems A, De Porre P, Howes AJ (2009) A randomized phase 3 study of tipifarnib compared with best supportive care, including hydroxyurea, in the treatment of newly diagnosed acute myeloid leukemia in patients 70 years or older. Blood 114:1166–1173

Hills RK, Burnett AK (2011) Applicability of a "pick a winner" trial design to acute myeloid leukemia. Blood 118:2389–2394. https://doi.org/10.1182/blood-2011-02-337261

Irvine DA, Copland M (2012) Targeting hedgehog in hematologic malignancy. Blood 119:2196–2204. https://doi.org/10.1182/blood-2011-10-383752

Itzykson R, Kosmider O, Cluzeau T, Mansat-De Mas V, Dreyfus F, Beyne-Rauzy O, Quesnel B, Vey N, Gelsi-Boyer V, Raynaud S, Preudhomme C, Ades L, Fenaux P, Fontenay M (2011) Impact of TET2 mutations on response rate to azacitidine in myelodysplastic syndromes and low blast count acute myeloid leukemias. Leukemia 25:1147–1152. https://doi.org/10.1038/leu.2011.71

Juliusson G, Antunovic P, Derolf A, Lehmann S, Mollgard L, Stockelberg D, Tidefelt U, Wahlin A, Hoglund M (2009) Age and acute myeloid leukemia: real world data on decision to treat and outcomes from the Swedish acute leukemia registry. Blood 113:4179–4187. https://doi.org/10.1182/blood-2008-07-172007

Kadia TM, Cortes J, Ravandi F, Jabbour E, Konopleva M, Benton CB, Burger J, Sasaki K, Borthakur G, DiNardo CD, Pemmaraju N, Daver N, Ferrajoli A, Wang X, Patel K, Jorgensen JL, Wang S, O'Brien S, Pierce S, Tuttle C, Estrov Z, Verstovsek S, Garcia-Manero G, Kantarjian H (2018) Cladribine and low-dose cytarabine alternating with decitabine as front-line therapy for elderly patients with acute myeloid leukaemia: a phase 2 single-arm trial. Lancet Haematol 5:e411–e421. https://doi.org/10.1016/S2352-3026(18)30132-7

Kantarjian H, Ravandi F, O'Brien S, Cortes J, Faderl S, Garcia-Manero G, Jabbour E, Wierda W, Kadia T, Pierce S, Shan J, Keating M, Freireich EJ (2010) Intensive chemotherapy does not benefit most older patients (age 70 years or older) with acute myeloid leukemia. Blood 116:4422–4429. https://doi.org/10.1182/blood-2010-03-276485

Kantarjian H, Faderl S, Garcia-Manero G, Luger S, Venugopal P, Maness L, Wetzler M, Coutre S, Stock W, Claxton D, Goldberg SL, Arellano M, Strickland SA, Seiter K, Schiller G, Jabbour E, Chiao J, Plunkett W (2012a) Results of a randomized phase II study of oral sapacitabine in elderly patients with previously untreated or first relapsed acute myeloid leukemia. Lancet Oncol 13:1096–1104. https://doi.org/10.1016/S1470-2045(12)70436-9

Kantarjian HM, Thomas XG, Dmoszynska A, Wierzbowska A, Mazur G, Mayer J, Gau JP, Chou WC, Buckstein R, Cermak J, Kuo CY, Oriol A, Ravandi F, Faderl S, Delaunay J, Lysak D, Minden M, Arthur C (2012b) Multicenter, randomized, open-label, phase III trial of decitabine versus patient choice, with physician advice, of either supportive care or low-dose cytarabine for the treatment of older patients with newly diagnosed acute myeloid leukemia. J Clin Oncol 30:2670–2677. https://doi.org/10.1200/JCO.2011.38.9429

Kantarjian HM, Roboz GJ, Kropf PL, Yee KWL, O'Connell CL, Tibes R, Walsh KJ, Podoltsev NA, Griffiths EA, Jabbour E, Garcia-Manero G, Rizzieri D, Stock W, Savona MR, Rosenblat TL, Berdeja JG, Ravandi F, Rock EP, Hao Y, Azab M, Issa JJ (2017) Guadecitabine (SGI-110) in treatment-naive patients with acute myeloid leukaemia: phase 2 results from a multicentre, randomised, phase 1/2 trial. Lancet Oncol 18:1317–1326. https://doi.org/10.1016/S1470-2045(17)30576-4

Klepin HD, Geiger AM, Tooze JA, Kritchevsky SB, Williamson JD, Pardee TS, Ellis LR, Powell BL (2013) Geriatric assessment predicts survival for older adults receiving induction chemotherapy for acute myelogenous leukemia. Blood 121:4287–4294. https://doi.org/10.1182/blood-2012-12-471680

Kumar A, List AF, Hozo I, Komrokji R, Djulbegovic B (2010) Decitabine versus 5-azacitidine for the treatment of myelodysplastic syndrome: adjusted indirect meta-analysis. Haematologica 95:340–342; author reply 343–344. https://doi.org/10.3324/haematol.2009.017764

Kung Sutherland MS, Walter RB, Jeffrey SC, Burke PJ, Yu C, Kostner H, Stone I, Ryan MC, Sussman D, Lyon RP, Zeng W, Harrington KH, Klussman K, Westendorf L, Meyer D, Bernstein ID, Senter PD, Benjamin DR, Drachman JG, McEarchern JA (2013) SGN-CD33A: a novel CD33-targeting antibody-drug conjugate using a pyrrolobenzodiazepine dimer is active in models of drug-resistant AML. Blood 122:1455–1463. https://doi.org/10.1182/blood-2013-03-491506

Lichtman MA (2013) A historical perspective on the development of the cytarabine (7days) and daunorubicin (3days) treatment regimen for acute myelogenous leukemia: 2013 the 40th anniversary of 7+3. Blood Cells Mol Dis 50:119–130. https://doi.org/10.1016/j.bcmd.2012.10.005

Loh KP, Klepin HD (2018) Geriatric assessment in older patients with acute myeloid leukemia. Cancers 10:225. https://doi.org/10.3390/cancers10070225

Lowenberg B, Zittoun R, Kerkhofs H, Jehn U, Abels J, Debusscher L, Cauchie C, Peetermans M, Solbu G, Suciu S et al (1989) On the value of intensive remission-induction chemotherapy in elderly patients of 65+ years with acute myeloid leukemia: a randomized phase III study of the European Organization for Research and Treatment of Cancer Leukemia Group. J Clin Oncol 7:1268–1274

Lowenberg B, Ossenkoppele GJ, van Putten W, Schouten HC, Graux C, Ferrant A, Sonneveld P, Maertens J, Jongen-Lavrencic M, von Lilienfeld-Toal M, Biemond BJ, Vellenga E, van Marwijk KM, Verdonck LF, Beck J, Dohner H, Gratwohl A, Pabst T, Verhoef G (2009) High-dose daunorubicin in older patients with acute myeloid leukemia. N Engl J Med 361:1235–1248. https://doi.org/10.1056/NEJMoa0901409

Malfuson JV, Etienne A, Turlure P, de Revel T, Thomas X, Contentin N, Terre C, Rigaudeau S, Bordessoule D, Vey N, Gardin C, Dombret H (2008) Risk factors and decision criteria for intensive chemotherapy in older patients with acute myeloid leukemia. Haematologica 93:1806–1813. https://doi.org/10.3324/haematol.13309

Medeiros BC, Satram-Hoang S, Hurst D, Hoang KQ, Momin F, Reyes C (2015) Big data analysis of treatment patterns and outcomes among elderly acute myeloid leukemia patients in the United States. Ann Hematol 94:1127–1138. https://doi.org/10.1007/s00277-015-2351-x

Menzin J, Lang K, Earle CC, Kerney D, Mallick R (2002) The outcomes and costs of acute myeloid leukemia among the elderly. Arch Intern Med 162:1597–1603

Merlevede J, Droin N, Qin T, Meldi K, Yoshida K, Morabito M, Chautard E, Auboeuf D, Fenaux P, Braun T, Itzykson R, de Botton S, Quesnel B, Commes T, Jourdan E, Vainchenker W, Bernard O, Pata-Merci N, Solier S, Gayevskiy V, Dinger ME, Cowley MJ, Selimoglu-Buet D, Meyer V, Artiguenave F, Deleuze J-F, Preudhomme C, Stratton MR, Alexandrov LB, Padron E, Ogawa S, Koscielny S, Figueroa M, Solary E (2016) Mutation allele burden remains unchanged in chronic myelomonocytic leukaemia responding to hypomethylating agents. Nat Commun 7:10767. https://doi.org/10.1038/ncomms10767

Metzeler KH, Walker A, Geyer S, Garzon R, Klisovic RB, Bloomfield CD, Blum W, Marcucci G (2012) DNMT3A mutations and response to the hypomethylating agent decitabine in acute myeloid leukemia. Leukemia 26:1106–1107. https://doi.org/10.1038/leu.2011.342

Nagel G, Weber D, Fromm E, Erhardt S, Lübbert M, Fiedler W, Kindler T, Krauter J, Brossart P, Kündgen A, Salih HR, Westermann J, Wulf G, Hertenstein B, Wattad M, Götze K, Kraemer D, Heinicke T, Girschikofsky M, Derigs HG, Horst HA, Rudolph C, Heuser M, Göhring G, Teleanu V, Bullinger L, Thol F, Gaidzik VI, Paschka P, Döhner K, Ganser A, Döhner H, Schlenk RF, German-Austrian AML Study Group (AMLSG) (2017) Epidemiological, genetic, and clinical characterization by age of newly diagnosed acute myeloid leukemia based on an academic population-based registry study (AMLSG BiO). Ann Hematol 96:1993–2003. https://doi.org/10.1007/s00277-017-3150-3

Papaemmanuil E, Gerstung M, Bullinger L, Gaidzik VI, Paschka P, Roberts ND, Potter NE, Heuser M, Thol F, Bolli N, Gundem G, Van Loo P, Martincorena I, Ganly P, Mudie L, McLaren S, O'Meara S, Raine K, Jones DR, Teague JW, Butler AP, Greaves MF, Ganser A, Dohner K, Schlenk RF, Dohner H, Campbell PJ (2016) Genomic classification and prognosis in acute myeloid leukemia. N Engl J Med 374:2209–2221. https://doi.org/10.1056/NEJMoa1516192

Pigneux A, Perreau V, Jourdan E, Vey N, Dastugue N, Huguet F, Sotto J-J, Salmi LR, Ifrah N, Reiffers J (2007) Adding lomustine to idarubicin and cytarabine for induction chemotherapy in older patients with acute myeloid leukemia: the BGMT 95 trial results. Haematologica 92:1327–1334. https://doi.org/10.3324/haematol.11068

Pleyer L, Burgstaller S, Girschikofsky M, Linkesch W, Stauder R, Pfeilstocker M, Schreder M, Tinchon C, Sliwa T, Lang A, Sperr WR, Krippl P, Geissler D, Voskova D, Schlick K, Thaler J, Machherndl-Spandl S, Theiler G, Eckmullner O, Greil R (2014) Azacitidine in 302 patients with WHO-defined acute myeloid leukemia: results from the Austrian Azacitidine registry of the AGMT-Study Group. Ann Hematol 93:1825–1838. https://doi.org/10.1007/s00277-014-2126-9

Pleyer L, Burgstaller S, Stauder R, Girschikofsky M, Sill H, Schlick K, Thaler J, Halter B, Machherndl-Spandl S, Zebisch A, Pichler A, Pfeilstöcker M, Autzinger E M, Lang A, Geissler K, Voskova D, Geissler D, Sperr WR, Hojas S, Rogulj IM, Andel J, Greil R (2016) Azacitidine front-line in 339 patients with myelodysplastic syndromes and acute myeloid leukaemia: comparison of French-American-British and World Health Organization classifications. J Hematol Oncol 9:39. https://doi.org/10.1186/s13045-016-0263-4

Pleyer L, Döhner H, Dombret H, Seymour JF, Schuh AC, Beach CL, Swern AS, Burgstaller S, Stauder R, Girschikofsky M, Sill H, Schlick K, Thaler J, Halter B, Machherndl Spandl S, Zebisch A, Pichler A, Pfeilstöcker M, Autzinger EM, Lang A, Geissler K, Voskova D, Sperr WR, Hojas S, Rogulj IM, Andel J, Greil R (2017) Azacitidine for front-line therapy of patients with AML: reproducible efficacy established by direct comparison of international phase 3 trial data with registry data from the Austrian Azacitidine registry of the AGMT Study Group. Int J Mol Sci 18:415. https://doi.org/10.3390/ijms18020415

Ramos F, Thépot S, Pleyer L, Maurillo L, Itzykson R, Bargay J, Stauder R, Venditti A, Seegers V, Martínez-Robles V, Burgstaller S, Récher C, Debén G, Gaidano G, Gardin C, Musto P, Greil R, Sánchez-Guijo F, Fenaux P, European ALMA Investigators (2015) Azacitidine frontline therapy for unfit acute myeloid leukemia patients: clinical use and outcome prediction. Leuk Res 39:296–306. https://doi.org/10.1016/j.leukres.2014.12.013

Richard-Carpentier G, DiNardo CD (2019) Venetoclax for the treatment of newly diagnosed acute myeloid leukemia in patients who are ineligible for intensive chemotherapy. Therap Adv Hematol 10:2040620719882822. https://doi.org/10.1177/2040620719882822

Schuh AC, Döhner H, Pleyer L, Seymour JF, Fenaux P, Dombret H (2017a) Azacitidine in adult patients with acute myeloid leukemia. Crit Rev Oncol Hematol 116:159–177. https://doi.org/10.1016/j.critrevonc.2017.05.010

Schuh AC, Döhner H, Seymour JF, Turlure P, Junghanss C, MacWhannell A, Tu N, Songer S, Beach CL, Dombret H (2017b) Stable disease with hematologic improvement is clinically meaningful for older patients with acute myeloid leukemia (AML) treated with Azacitidine. Leuk Res S1:S68–S69. https://doi.org/10.1016/S0145-2126(17)30222-9

Sekeres MA, Lancet JE, Wood BL, Grove LE, Sandalic L, Sievers EL, Jurcic JG (2013) Randomized, phase IIb study of low-dose cytarabine and lintuzumab versus low-dose cytarabine and placebo in older adults with untreated acute myeloid leukemia. Haematologica 98:119–128. https://doi.org/10.3324/haematol.2012.066613

Seymour JF, Fenaux P, Silverman LR, Mufti GJ, Hellstrom-Lindberg E, Santini V, List AF, Gore SD, Backstrom J, McKenzie D, Beach CL (2010) Effects of azacitidine compared with conventional care regimens in elderly (>/= 75 years) patients with higher-risk myelodysplastic syndromes. Crit Rev Oncol Hematol 76:218–227. https://doi.org/10.1016/j.critrevonc.2010.04.005

Sorror ML, Maris MB, Storb R, Baron F, Sandmaier BM, Maloney DG, Storer B (2005) Hematopoietic cell transplantation (HCT)-specific comorbidity index: a new tool for risk assessment before allogeneic HCT. Blood 106:2912–2919. https://doi.org/10.1182/blood-2005-05-2004

Sorror ML, Storer BE, Fathi AT, Gerds AT, Medeiros BC, Shami P, Brunner AM, Sekeres MA, Mukherjee S, Pena E, Elsawy M, Wardyn S, Whitten J, Moore R, Becker PS, McCune JS, Appelbaum FR, Estey EH (2017) Development and validation of a novel acute myeloid leukemia-composite model to estimate risks of mortality. JAMA Oncol 3:1675–1682. https://doi.org/10.1001/jamaoncol.2017.2714

Stahl M, Lu BY, Kim TK, Zeidan AM (2017) Novel therapies for acute myeloid leukemia: are we finally breaking the deadlock? Target Oncol 12:413–447. https://doi.org/10.1007/s11523-017-0503-8

Stein EM, DiNardo CD, Pollyea DA, Schuh AC (2020) Response kinetics and clinical benefits of nonintensive AML therapies in the absence of morphologic response. Clin Lymphoma Myeloma Leuk 20(2):e66–e75. https://doi.org/10.1016/j.clml.2019.11.017

Stone A, Zukerman T, Flaishon L, Yakar RB, Rowe JM (2019) Efficacy outcomes in the treatment of older or medically unfit patients with acute myeloid leukaemia: a systematic review and meta-analysis. Leuk Res 82:36–42. https://doi.org/10.1016/j.leukres.2019.05.007

Talati C, Dhulipala VC, Extermann MT, Ali NA, Kim J, Komrokji R, Sweet K, Kuykendall A, Sehovic M, Reljic T, Djulbegovic B, Lancet JE (2020) Comparisons of commonly used front-line regimens on survival outcomes in patients aged 70 years and older with acute myeloid leukemia. Haematologica 105:398–406. https://doi.org/10.3324/haematol.2018.208637

Tallman MS, Wang ES, Altman JK, Appelbaum FR, Bhatt VR, Bixby D, Coutre SE, De Lima M, Fathi AT, Fiorella M, Foran JM, Hall AC, Jacoby M, Lancet J, TW LB, Mannis G, Marcucci G, Martin MG, Mims A, O'Donnell MR, Olin R, Peker D, Perl A, Pollyea DA, Pratz K, Prebet T, Ravandi F, Shami PJ, Stone RM, Strickland SA, Wieduwilt M, Gregory KM, Hammond L, Ogba N (2019) Acute myeloid leukemia, version 3.2019, NCCN clinical practice guidelines in oncology. J Natl Comp Cancer Netw 17:721–749. https://doi.org/10.6004/jnccn.2019.0028

Thepot S, Itzykson R, Seegers V, Recher C, Raffoux E, Quesnel B, Delaunay J, Cluzeau T, Marfaing Koka A, Stamatoullas A, Chaury MP, Dartigeas C, Cheze S, Banos A, Morel P, Plantier I, Taksin AL, Marolleau JP, Pautas C, Thomas X, Isnard F, Beve B, Chait Y, Guerci A, Vey N, Dreyfus F, Ades L, Ifrah N, Dombret H, Fenaux P, Gardin C (2014) Azacitidine in untreated acute myeloid leukemia: a report on 149 patients. Am J Hematol 89:410–416. https://doi.org/10.1002/ajh.23654

Tilly H, Castaigne S, Bordessoule D, Casassus P, Le Prise PY, Tertian G, Desablens B, Henry-Amar M, Degos L (1990) Low-dose cytarabine versus intensive chemotherapy in the treatment of acute nonlymphocytic leukemia in the elderly. J Clin Oncol 8:272–279

Unnikrishnan A, Papaemmanuil E, Beck D, Deshpande NP, Verma A, Kumari A, Woll PS, Richards LA, Knezevic K, Chandrakanthan V, Thoms JAI, Tursky ML, Huang Y, Ali Z, Olivier J, Galbraith S, Kulasekararaj AG, Tobiasson M, Karimi M, Pellagatti A, Wilson SR, Lindeman R, Young B, Ramakrishna R, Arthur C, Stark R, Crispin P, Curnow J, Warburton P, Roncolato F, Boultwood J, Lynch K, Jacobsen SEW, Mufti GJ, Hellstrom-Lindberg E, Wilkins MR, MacKenzie KL, Wong JWH, Campbell PJ, Pimanda JE (2017) Integrative genomics identifies the molecular basis of resistance to Azacitidine therapy in myelodysplastic syndromes. Cell Rep 20:572–585. https://doi.org/10.1016/j.celrep.2017.06.067

Vey N (2013) Targeting age-related changes in the biology of acute myeloid leukemia: is the patient seeing the progress? Interdiscip Top Gerontol 38:73–84. https://doi.org/10.1159/000343623

Vey N (2018) Blurring lines between treatment intensity and patient fitness in elderly people with AML. Lancet Haematol 5:e383–e384. https://doi.org/10.1016/S2352-3026(18)30136-4

Vey N, Keating M, Giles F, Cortes J, Beran M, Estey E (1999) Effect of complete remission on survival in patients with acute myelogenous leukemia receiving first salvage therapy. Blood 93:3149–3150

Vey N, Coso D, Bardou V-J, Stoppa A-M, Braud A-C, Bouabdallah R, Sainty D, Mozziconacci M-J, Lafage M, Damaj G, Blaise D, Gastaut J-A, Maraninchi D (2004) The benefit of induction chemotherapy in patients age > or = 75 years. Cancer 101:325–331. https://doi.org/10.1002/cncr.20353

Voso MT, Santini V, Fabiani E, Fianchi L, Criscuolo M, Falconi G, Guidi F, Hohaus S, Leone G (2014) Why methylation is not a marker predictive of response to hypomethylating agents. Haematologica 99:613–619. https://doi.org/10.3324/haematol.2013.099549

Wanquet A, Prebet T, Berthon C, Sebert M, Roux C, Kulasekararaj A, Micol JB, Esterni B, Itzykson R, Thepot S, Recher C, Delaunay J, Dreyfus F, Mufti G, Fenaux P, Vey N (2015) Azacitidine treatment for patients with myelodysplastic syndrome and acute myeloid leukemia with chromosome 3q abnormalities. Am J Hematol 90:859–863. https://doi.org/10.1002/ajh.24099

Wei AH, Strickland SA, Hou JZ, Fiedler W, Lin TL, Walter RB, Enjeti A, Tiong IS, Savona M, Lee S, Chyla B, Popovic R, Salem AH, Agarwal S, Xu T, Fakouhi KM, Humerickhouse R, Hong WJ, Hayslip J, Roboz GJ (2019) Venetoclax combined with low-dose cytarabine for previously untreated patients with acute myeloid leukemia: results from a phase Ib/II study. J Clin Oncol 37:1277–1284. https://doi.org/10.1200/JCO.18.01600

Wei AH, Montesinos P, Ivanov V, DiNardo CD, Novak J, Laribi K, Kim I, Stevens DA, Fiedler W, Pagoni M, Samoilova O, Hu Y, Anagnostopoulos A, Bergeron J, Hou J-Z, Murthy V, Yamauchi T, McDonald A, Chyla B, Gopalakrishnan S, Jiang Q, Mendes W, Hayslip J, Panayiotidis P (2020) Venetoclax plus LDAC for newly diagnosed AML ineligible for intensive chemotherapy: a phase 3 randomized placebo-controlled trial. Blood 135:2137–2145. https://doi.org/10.1182/blood.2020004856

Welch JS, Petti AA, Miller CA, Fronick CC, O'Laughlin M, Fulton RS, Wilson RK, Baty JD, Duncavage EJ, Tandon B, Lee YS, Wartman LD, Uy GL, Ghobadi A, Tomasson MH, Pusic I, Romee R, Fehniger TA, Stockerl-Goldstein KE, Vij R, Oh ST, Abboud CN, Cashen AF, Schroeder MA, Jacoby MA, Heath SE, Luber K, Janke MR, Hantel A, Khan N, Sukhanova MJ, Knoebel RW, Stock W, Graubert TA, Walter MJ, Westervelt P, Link DC, DiPersio JF, Ley TJ (2016) TP53 and Decitabine in acute myeloid leukemia and myelodysplastic syndromes. N Engl J Med 375:2023–2036. https://doi.org/10.1056/NEJMoa1605949

Wheatley K, Brookes CL, Howman AJ, Goldstone AH, Milligan DW, Prentice AG, Moorman AV, Burnett AK (2009) Prognostic factor analysis of the survival of elderly patients with AML in the MRC AML11 and LRF AML14 trials. Br J Haematol 145:598–605. https://doi.org/10.1111/j.1365-2141.2009.07663.x

Xie M, Jiang Q, Xie Y (2015) Comparison between decitabine and azacitidine for the treatment of myelodysplastic syndrome: a meta-analysis with 1392 participants. Clin Lymphoma Myeloma Leuk 15:22–28. https://doi.org/10.1016/j.clml.2014.04.010

Zeidan AM, Cavenagh J, Voso MT, Taussig D, Tormo M, Boss I, Copeland WB, Gray VE, Previtali A, O'Connor T, Rose S, Beach CL, Silverman LR (2019a) Efficacy and safety of Azacitidine (AZA) in combination with the anti-PD-L1 Durvalumab (durva) for the front-line treatment of older patients (pts) with acute myeloid leukemia (AML) who are unfit for intensive chemotherapy (IC) and pts with higher-risk myelodysplastic syndromes (HR-MDS): results from a large, international, randomized phase 2 study. Blood 134:829. https://doi.org/10.1182/blood-2019-122896

Zeidan AM, Podoltsev NA, Wang X, Bewersdorf JP, Shallis RM, Huntington SF, Gore SD, Davidoff AJ, Ma X, Wang R (2019b) Temporal patterns and predictors of receiving no active treatment among older patients with acute myeloid leukemia in the United States: a population-level analysis. Cancer 125:4241–4251. https://doi.org/10.1002/cncr.32439

# Treatment of Relapsed and Refractory AML: Intensive Approach in Fit Patients

# 11

Sonia Jaramillo and Richard F. Schlenk

## 11.1 Introduction

Acute myeloid leukemia (AML) is a genetically heterogeneous disorder (Papaemmanuil et al. 2016) with an incidence of 3 to 4 per 100,000 per year and a median age at diagnosis ranging from 65 to 71 years (Nagel et al. 2017; Juliusson et al. 2012; Dinmohamed et al. 2016). It is characterized by the accumulation of somatically acquired genetic changes in hematopoietic progenitor cells that alter normal mechanisms of self-renewal, proliferation, and differentiation. Importantly, this accumulation of genetic changes may also occur at treatment failure in relapsed or refractory AML (Ding et al. 2012). Therefore, repeated molecular and cytogenetic analysis is necessary at first diagnosis, at relapse, and after treatment failure (Döhner et al. 2017). Outcome is influenced by various factors of which age and genetic profile of the disease are the most important (Papaemmanuil et al. 2016; Döhner et al. 2017).

S. Jaramillo
Department of Hematology and Oncology, University of Heidelberg, Heidelberg, Germany

R. F. Schlenk (✉)
Department of Hematology and Oncology, University of Heidelberg, Heidelberg, Germany

NCT-Trial Center, German Cancer Research Center and Heidelberg University Hospital, Heidelberg, Germany
e-mail: richard.schlenk@nct-heidelberg.de

After initiation of intensive treatment, failure to respond to intensive induction chemotherapy is another major unfavorable prognostic factor (Döhner et al. 2017; Thol et al. 2015). However, the definition of induction failure varies widely with regard to the time point of assessment and the intensity of the administered treatment. It can be assessed and defined either (1) early day 15 or 16 of first induction therapy during aplasia with persistence of a significant blast population (Kern et al. 2003), (2) at blood count recovery after induction therapy between day 21 and day 35 with <50% reduction of blast percentage and a blast percentage above 25% (Schlenk et al. 2003), or (3) in cases of partial response after first induction therapy persistence of >5% blasts in the bone marrow after a second induction therapy (Döhner et al. 2017). In addition, some investigators require the application of high dose cytarabine-containing regimens during induction therapy to define refractory AML (Ravandi et al. 2010). Thus, it's no wonder that the proportion of induction failure varies broadly from 10 to 40% due to different definitions (Döhner et al. 2017; Thol et al. 2015; Ravandi et al. 2010; Wattad et al. 2017; Ferguson et al. 2016). In addition, the definition of refractory disease have changed considerably over time and will vary in the future concerning the availability of molecularly targeted therapy in an individual patient (Table 11.1) in clinical practice, but even more important within clinical trials.



C. Röllig, G. J. Ossenkoppele (eds.), *Acute Myeloid Leukemia*, Hematologic Malignancies,
https://doi.org/10.1007/978-3-030-72676-8_11

**Table 11.1** Definitions used for induction failure or primary refractory AML over time

| | |
|---|---|
| No CR or CRi after two courses of intensive induction cycles, excluding patients with death in aplasia or due to indeterminate cause | Döhner et al. (2017) |
| Less than a 50% reduction in blast numbers with >15% residual blasts after one cycle of induction chemotherapy | Ferguson et al. (2016) |
| >15% blasts in the bone marrow, 2 weeks after the completion of the cycle | Wheatley et al. (1999) |
| Persistent leukemic blasts in either the peripheral blood or the bone marrow in a patient alive 7 days or more following treatment | Cheson et al. (2003) |
| < 50% blast percentage reduction following one course of intensive chemotherapy (Ravandi et al. 2010) | Schlenk et al. (2003) |
| Persistence of a significant leukemic blasts 7 days or more following high-dose cytarabine therapy | National Comprehensive Cancer Network (2016) |

*CR* complete remission, *CRi* CR with incomplete hematologic recovery
Modified from Montesinos et al. (Megías-Vericat et al. 2018)

Once a first complete remission (CR) is achieved, approximately half of the younger (≤60 years) patients and about 80–90% of the older patients still relapse despite intensive consolidation therapy and the majority of relapsed patients succumb to their disease (Döhner et al. 2017; Dombret and Gardin 2016; Heuser et al. 2020).

In both clinical situations, refractory and relapsed (r/r)-AML, the prognosis is dismal despite intensive treatment approaches, including allogeneic hematopoietic cell transplantation (allo-HCT). In two individual patient data (IPD) meta-analyses, outcome data in refractory and relapsed patients were very similar in intensively treated patients with a 2-year survival of 29% (95% Confidence Interval [CI], 26–33%) and 27% (95% CI, 25–30%), respectively (Wattad et al. 2017; Wheatley et al. 1999). Outcome data for patients treated non-intensively with low-dose cytarabine or hypomethylating agents and best supportive care are very dismal with a median and 2-year survival of 3.1 and 1.6 months as well as 0% and 4% (95% CI, 2–8%), respectively (Wattad et al. 2017; Schlenk et al. 2017). Overall, these figures clearly illustrate that new treatment strategies are urgently needed. The better understanding of the molecular complexity and biology of AML has led to a large spectrum of new treatment approaches ranging from new and modified cytotoxic drugs (e.g., CPX-351 (Lancet et al. 2018)), to targeted approaches (e.g., FLT3-inhibitors in *FLT3*-mutated (Stone et al. 2017; Perl et al. 2019) and IDH-inhibitors in *IDH*-mutated AML (Stein et al. 2017, 2019; DiNardo et al. 2018)). After years of stagnancy in drug approval for AML, new drugs are approved in frontline therapy and also for relapsed/refractory patients. However, in the relapsed/refractory setting, several attempts have failed (Ravandi et al. 2015; Roboz et al. 2014) in recent years, illustrating the difficulty of compound and treatment strategy development in this patient population. In the following section, we focus on prognostic and predictive factors, treatment approaches, and on statistical considerations for future clinical trials in r/r-AML.

## 11.2 Prognostic and Predictive Factors

Prognostic and predictive markers (Ballman 2015) are important in clinical practice since risks and benefits of specific therapeutic interventions have to be carefully assessed, presented, and discussed with the patient. Especially, predictive markers are indispensable in this context since they indicate whether a given treatment intervention is specifically effective in clinically or molecularly defined subgroups (Ballman 2015). The framework of prognostic markers for survival in relapsed AML was based on a pivotal HOVON IPD meta-analysis in 667 younger adults (15–60 years) which revealed a longer relapse-free interval after first complete remission (CR1), presence of a core-binding-factor AML at diagnosis, lower age at relapse, and no previous stem-cell transplantation during first-line therapy as factors associated with more favorable prognosis (Breems et al. 2005). The Spanish study group (PETHEMA) published a prognostic score for r/r-AML for survival integrating the before-mentioned factors and the molecular marker *FLT3*-ITD (Bergua et al. 2016). More recently, the German–Austrian AMLSG study group published two separate models based on extended Cox regression analysis including allo-HCT as time-dependent co-variable for r/r-AML. Beyond the before-mentioned factors, three molecular markers entered the models for r/r-AML, *FLT3*-ITD in both models, and mutated *IDH1* in refractory and biallelic *CEBPA* mutations in relapsed AML (Wattad et al. 2017; Schlenk et al. 2017). In addition, the possibility to perform an allo-HCT was a strong favorable marker in both models underlining the curative impact of this treatment strategy. In particular, allo-HCT seems to be most effective, if chronic Graft versus Host Disease (GvHD) is present (Ram et al. 2019). Table 11.2 summarizes prognostic markers in r/r-AML identified in patient populations treated with intensive chemotherapy and allo-HCT. Thus, the effects of molecularly targeted therapies are not reflected.

Most published prognostic models based on large individual patient data (IPD) meta-analyses do not take into account clonal evolution but use the pretreatment karyotype and molecular profile instead (Wattad et al. 2017; Schlenk et al. 2017; Breems et al. 2005; Bergua et al. 2016). In one smaller study of 144 patients with relapsed AML Shimizu et al. claimed that clonal evolution detected with conventional cytogenetic analysis is an unfavorable factor for survival (Shimizu et al. 2018). This study demonstrated that the assessment of cytogenetics and probably also of molecular markers (Krönke et al. 2013) at the time of relapse is essential not only for prognostication but also to identify druggable targets.

**Table 11.2** Prognostic markers in r/r-AML

| | |
|---|---|
| *Favorable markers* | |
| Longer relapse-free interval | Schlenk et al. (2017), Breems et al. (2005), Chevallier et al. (2011) |
| Core binding factor AML [t(8;21) or inv(16)] | Schlenk et al. (2017), Breems et al. (2005), Bergua et al. (2016) |
| Lower age at relapse | Breems et al. (2005) |
| No previous stem-cell transplantation | Breems et al. (2005), Bergua et al. (2016) |
| Double mutant *CEBPA* | Schlenk et al. (2017) |
| Allo-HCT to treat r/r-AML | Wattad et al. (2017), Schlenk et al. (2017) |
| *Unfavorable marker* | |
| *FLT3*-ITD | Wattad et al. (2017), Schlenk et al. (2017), Bergua et al. (2016) |
| Mutated-*IDH1* (only in refractory AML) | Wattad et al. (2017) |
| High-risk cytogenetics | Wattad et al. (2017), Schlenk et al. (2017), Bergua et al. (2016), Ram et al. (2019) |

*CEBPA* CCAAT/enhancer-binding protein alpha, *FLT3*-ITD FMS-related tyrosine kinase 3-internal tandem duplication, *IDH1* isocitrate dehydrogenase-1

## 11.3 Intensive Salvage Chemotherapy

In patients with r/r-AML intensive combination chemotherapy including high-dose cytarabine is frequently used, whereby no specific salvage regimen has emerged as standard (Döhner et al. 2017). Using combination chemotherapy the rates of CR/CRi were reported nearly similar with 36% and 36.8% in refractory and relapsed AML (Wattad et al. 2017; Schlenk et al. 2017). Higher rates were consistently reported in regimens combining gemtuzumab ozogamicin (GO), an antibody drug (calicheamicin) conjugate targeting CD33, with intermediate to high-dose cytarabine plus an anthracycline or an anthracedione (Paubelle et al. 2017; Hütter-Krönke et al. 2016; Debureaux et al. 2020). Of note, treatment with the salvage regimen GO-A-HAM (Hütter-Krönke et al. 2016) was associated with an excellent CR rate of 50% and was a significant favorable factor in a logistic regression model predicting the probability of achievement of a CR/CRi after salvage therapy (Wattad et al. 2017). In a double-blinded randomized phase-III study on vosaroxin versus placebo in combination with intermediate-dose cytarabine in r/r-AML, CR rates were significantly superior in patients randomized into the experimental arm with vosaroxin plus cytarabine. But only a trend ($p = 0.06$) toward better survival was achieved in the whole study population, whereas a significant benefit was present in the subgroup of older (age ≥ 60 years) patients (Ravandi et al. 2015). In addition, adverse events grade 3–5 were significantly more frequent in the experimental arm of the study including stomatitis, sepsis, and bacteraemia (Ravandi et al. 2015). On the background of these data, approval of vosaroxin was not granted in Europe and the United States. In a phase-II study, combination chemotherapy including either fludarabine or cladribine was reported similarly active with a CR rate of roughly 60% (Bao et al. 2018). However, based on the background of the international randomized phase-III study comparing elacytarabine with physician's choice, no difference between the comparators (FLAG/FLAG-Ida, MEC, HiDAC, hypomethylating agents, low-dose cytarabine) within the doctors' choice standard treatment arm showed superiority compared with the other options (Roboz et al. 2014). Therefore, the good results of the before-mentioned recently published phase-II study are probably not due to true superiority rather than selection bias. A recent comparison of MEC and high-dose cytarabine plus mitoxantrone (HAM) revealed similar response rates but significantly less toxicity with HAM (Christian et al. 2020). Although the results seem to support the use of HAM, this was not a randomized comparison. These examples clearly demonstrate that future studies should rely less on single-arm phase-II studies without adequate controls but on either randomized or adapted phase-II approaches including matched controls, which are discussed in the last part of the chapter.

## 11.4 Timing of Allogeneic Hematopoietic Cell Transplantation

In physically fit patients, the combined strategy of intensive salvage therapy to induce remission or blast count reduction followed by subsequent allo-HCT is mentioned as one option in reviews (Döhner et al. 2015) and guidelines (Döhner et al. 2017). However, long-term survival rates remain limited because of the common failure to achieve the necessary response and other factors that limit this approach for a large majority of patients. Therefore, an alternative approach for patients with r/r-AML is a short course of chemotherapy such as fludarabine, cytarabine, and amsacrine immediately prior to reduced intensity conditioning and allo-HCT (Döhner et al. 2017). However, the question of which strategy is preferable in an individual patient cannot be answered so far; a randomized trial addressing this question is active (NCT02461537). In a retrospective cohort study, Holtic et al. showed comparable outcome results of patients transplanted in first or second complete remission as well as primary induction failure, whereas patients who failed response to intensive salvage chemotherapy had inferior outcome (Holtick et al. 2016). Comparable results came from the IPD meta-analysis in patients with induction failure (Wattad et al. 2017). Allo-HCT without prior salvage chemotherapy ($n = 87$) and allo-HCT in CR after salvage chemotherapy ($n = 193$) resulted in comparable survival outcome and both strategies were significantly superior compared to allo-HCT performed after failure of salvage chemotherapy (Wattad et al. 2017). Results from a logistic regression model with the endpoint overall response to salvage therapy in the same work based on $n = 761$ patients suggested that patients with older age, unfavorable cytogenetics, and high WBC were not candidates for intensive salvage therapy due to the expected very low response probability. Especially, these patients may qualify for allo-HCT without prior salvage chemotherapy (Wattad et al. 2017). Similarly, in relapsed patients, prediction of response to salvage therapy may help to select the best treatment strategy (Schlenk et al. 2017). Based again on a logistic regression model including $n = 907$ patients, high CR/CRi rates were achieved in patients with biallelic *CEBPA* mutations, core-binding-factor AML, and a CR-duration >18 months whereas patients exhibiting adverse cytogenetics or a *FLT3*-ITD had a low probability to respond to salvage therapy and may again qualify for allo-HCT without prior salvage chemotherapy (Schlenk et al. 2017) (Table 11.3).

**Table 11.3** Useful factors for decision-making (in the absence of targeted approaches). Direct allogeneic HCT versus intensive salvage therapy followed by allogeneic HCT

| | |
|---|---|
| Direct allogeneic HCT | |
| Older age | Wattad et al. (2017) |
| High-risk cytogenetics | Wattad et al. (2017), Schlenk et al. (2017) |
| Intensive salvage therapy followed by allogeneic HCT | |
| Double mutant *CEBPA* | Schlenk et al. (2017) |
| Core-binding-factor AML [t(8;21) or inv(16)] | Schlenk et al. (2017) |

*CEBPA* CCAAT/enhancer-binding protein alpha

## 11.5 Targeted Approaches

### 11.5.1 IDH-Inhibitors

Mutations in *IDH1* and *IDH2* are detected in about 8% and 12% of patients with AML, respectively (Papaemmanuil et al. 2016). Treatment in r/r-AML patients with IDH2 inhibitor enasidenib showed promising activity as single agent in r/r-AML patients with mutated *IDH2* (Stein et al. 2019), CR rate of single agent enasidenib was 19.6% and overall response rate 38.8% with no difference between relapsed and refractory patients (Stein et al. 2019). Furthermore, response and survival were comparable among patients with *IDH2*-R140 or *IDH2*-R172 mutations. The most common grade 3 or 4 treatment-related adverse events were hyperbilirubinemia (10%), thrombocytopenia (7%), and differentiation syndrome (6%) in 345 treated patients. The recommended dose for further clinical development was reported with 100 mg enasidenib daily (Stein et al. 2017). With this dose, survival was longest in patients achieving a CR (median survival 22.9 months, $n = 42$), whereas the benefit was limited in those patients achieving a non-CR response (median survival 10.6 months) (Stein et al. 2019). Comparable outcome has been reported in r/r-AML from a trial with ivosidenib single agent 500 mg once daily, an IDH1 inhibitor (DiNardo et al. 2018). Complete remission was achieved in 21.6% and the overall response rate was 41.6%. In particular, patients achieving a CR had excellent overall survival with an 18-month survival rate of 50.1%. Estimates of median overall survival were 9.3 months among patients who had a response other than complete remission or complete remission with partial hematologic recovery and 3.9 months among patients who did not have a response (DiNardo et al. 2018). Although both IDH inhibitors provide a major step forward in r/r-AML, still only a minority of patients achieve a CR with single agent treatment and experience an enormous survival benefit. Both inhibitors are evaluated in numerous clinical trials in newly diagnosed as well as r/r-AML, as single agent but even more important in combination with chemotherapy.

### 11.5.2 FLT3-Inhibitors

*FLT3* mutations are accounting for one third of AML cases in intensively treated populations (Papaemmanuil et al. 2016), whereas results from a population-based registry study indicate an incidence of 23% with decreasing incidence rates with increasing age (Nagel et al. 2017). Activating *FLT3* mutations comprise internal tandem duplication (ITD) and point mutations most frequently at residue D835 affecting the tyrosine kinase domain (TKD) (Daver et al. 2019). Several FLT3 inhibitors are in clinical development including the type-I inhibitors midostaurin, sunitinib, lestaurtinib, crenolanib, and gilteritinib as well as the type-II inhibitors sorafenib, quizartinib, and ponatenib (Daver et al. 2019). Apart from the approval of midostaurin in newly diagnosed AML exhibiting activating *FLT3* mutations (Stone et al. 2017), data from randomized studies in r/r-AML are available for gilteritinib (Perl et al. 2019) and quizartinib (Cortes et al. 2019). Gilteritinib is an oral FLT3/AXL inhibitor which has been evaluated in a single agent phase-I/II study (Perl et al. 2016). Gilteritinib was well tolerated at a dose of 300 mg QD, and responses were seen in particular in AML with *FLT3*-ITD. In the subsequent randomized trial (ADMIRAL), 247 patients with r/r-AML exhibiting an activating *FLT3* mutation were randomly assigned to gilteritinib single agent and 124 to salvage chemotherapy (Perl et al. 2019). Overall (0.64; 95% confidence interval

[CI], 0.49–0.83; $p < 0.001$) and event-free survival (hazard ratio for treatment failure or death, 0.79; 95% CI, 0.58–1.09) were better in patients randomized to gilteritinib; a CR with full or partial hematologic recovery was achieved in 34.0% in the gilteritinib arm and in only 15.3% in the chemotherapy arm. The most common adverse events of grade 3 or higher in the gilteritinib arm were febrile neutropenia (45.9%), anemia (40.7%), and thrombocytopenia (22.8%). Based on these results gilteritinib was approved in the United States and the EU.

Another large randomized trial (QuANTUM-R) was conducted in patients with *FLT3*-ITD positive AML with single-agent quizartinib, an oral, highly potent and selective type II FLT3 inhibitor. In contrast to the ADMIRAL trial, the randomized QuANTUM-R trial included high-risk patients with duration of first complete remission of ≤6 months and only AML with *FLT3*-ITD. In total 367 patients were enrolled, of whom 245 were randomly allocated to quizartinib and 122 to chemotherapy. Overall survival was significantly longer for quizartinib compared to chemotherapy (hazard ratio 0.76 [95% CI 0.58–0.98; $p = 0.02$]). The most frequent treatment-related serious adverse events were febrile neutropenia (7%) sepsis or septic shock (5%), QT prolongation (2%), and nausea (2%) in the quizartinib arm. Although the QuANTUM-R study was positive, neither FDA nor EMA approved Quizartinib in r/r-AML.

Of note, the survival curves in both trials showed a beneficial effect of the FLT3 inhibitor to prolong overall survival. However, beyond 24 months, the outcome was dismal and similar in both, the FLT3-inhibitor as well as in the chemotherapy arms. This was seen despite a much higher percentage of patients proceeding to an allogeneic HCT in the FLT3-inhibitor arms and clearly indicates development of secondary resistance.

## 11.6 Statistical Considerations for Future Clinical Trials

Inclusion of patients with r/r-AML into clinical trials should be the first priority in the care of r/r-AML patients. Although randomized controlled trials are the gold standard to show superiority of a new treatment strategy compared to the current standard, this principle comes to its limits when no standard can be defined as in r/r-AML. This raises the question, how clinical evidence can be strengthened in early clinical trials to better inform on the decision to move forward or suspend a new treatment approach in clinical development.

One possibility would be to engage already in an early stage of clinical development on randomized instead of single-arm phase Ib/II studies (Rubinstein et al. 2009). In an attempt to keep sample size at this stage of development in a manageable scale, Rubinstein et al. recommended for phase-II randomized trials to select one-sided type-I (alpha) and type-II (beta) error rates relatively large with up to 20% each thus inducing considerable risk of false conclusions. By introducing a standard arm within the randomized approach, the external validity of trial results is increased. However, in a very heterogeneous disease such as AML (Papaemmanuil et al. 2016), a balanced distribution of prognostic and predictive factors will hardly be achieved even in a randomized approach due to small sample sizes (Gan et al. 2010). Further reservations against randomized phase II trials in this setting have been pointed out recently (Gan et al. 2010). On the other side, however, single-arm designs are criticized due to the intrinsic need to rely on the comparison of historical data. Therefore, the question arises why not use controls from existing large datasets (Wattad et al. 2017; Schlenk et al. 2017; Gerstung et al. 2017) for benchmarking. One solution is to combine a threshold-crossing (Eichler et al. 2016) phase-II/III approach with drawing matched controls from available datasets. Matching may be based on significant factors of prognostic models (Wattad et al. 2017; Schlenk et al. 2017) as described above enriched by additional important genetic and clinical factors. This approach (Edelmann et al. 2020) is used already in a trial (EudraCT No.: 2017-005158-12) in r/r-AML evaluating the efficacy of bortezomib to restore EZH2 levels (Göllner et al. 2017). Furthermore, the Q-HAM study

(Clinicaltrials.gov: NCT03989713, EudraCT No.:2018-002675-17) evaluating the combination of chemotherapy with quizartinib in r/r-AML also integrates matched controls to increase external validity (Krisam et al. n.d.).

## References


Ballman KV (2015) Biomarker: predictive or prognostic? J Clin Oncol 33(33):3968–3971

Bao Y, Zhao J, Li ZZ (2018) Comparison of clinical remission and survival between CLAG and FLAG induction chemotherapy in patients with refractory or relapsed acute myeloid leukemia: a prospective cohort study. Clin Transl Oncol 20(7):870–880

Bergua JM, Montesinos P, Martinez-Cuadrón D et al (2016) A prognostic model for survival after salvage treatment with FLAG-Ida +/− gemtuzumab-ozogamicine in adult patients with refractory/relapsed acute myeloid leukaemia. Br J Haematol 174(5):700–710

Breems DA, Van Putten WL, Huijgens PC et al (2005) Prognostic index for adult patients with acute myeloid leukemia in first relapse. J Clin Oncol 23:1969–1978

Cheson BD, Bennett JM, Kopecky KJ et al (2003) Revised recommendations of the international working group for diagnosis, standardization of response criteria, treatment outcomes, and reporting standards for therapeutic trials in acute myeloid leukemia. J Clin Oncol 21(24):4642–4649

Chevallier P, Labopin M, Turlure P et al (2011) Anew leukemia prognostic scoring system for refractory/relapsed adult acute myelogeneous leukaemia patients: a GOELAMS study. Leukemia 25(6):939–944

Christian S, Arain S, Patel P et al (2020) A multi-institutional comparison of mitoxantrone, etoposide, and cytarabine (MEC) versus high-dose cytarabine and mitoxantrone (Ara-C couplets) therapy for patients with relapsed or refractory acute myeloid leukemia. Am J Hematol 95(8):937–943. Epub ahead of print. https://doi.org/10.1002/ajh.25838

Cortes JE, Khaled S, Martinelli G et al (2019) Quizartinib versus salvage chemotherapy in relapsed or refractory FLT3-ITD acute myeloid leukaemia (QuANTUM-R): a multicentre, randomised, controlled, open-label, phase 3 trial. Lancet Oncol 20(7):984–997

Daver N, Schlenk RF, Russell NH, Levis MJ (2019) Targeting FLT3 mutations in AML: review of current knowledge and evidence. Leukemia 33(2):299–312

Debureaux PE, Labopin M, Mamez AC et al (2020) Fractionated gemtuzumabozogamicin in association with high dose chemotherapy: a bridge to allogeneic stem cell transplantation in refractory and relapsed acute myeloid leukemia. Bone Marrow Transplant 55:452–460

DiNardo CD, Stein EM, de Botton S et al (2018) Durable remissions with Ivosidenib in IDH1-mutated relapsed or refractory AML. N Engl J Med 378(25):2386–2398

Ding L, Ley TJ, Larson DE (2012) Clonal evolution in relapsed acute myeloid leukaemia revealed by whole-genome sequencing. Nature 481(7382):506–510

Dinmohamed AG, Visser O, van Norden Y et al (2016) Treatment, trial participation and survival in adult acute myeloid leukemia: a population-based study in the Netherlands, 1989-2012. Leukemia 30(1):24–31

Döhner H, Weisdorf DJ, Bloomfield CD. Acute myeloid leukemia. N Engl J Med. 2015;373(12):1136–52

Döhner H, Estey E, Grimwade D et al (2017) Diagnosis and management of AML in adults: 2017 ELN recommendations from an international expert panel. Blood 129(4):424–447

Dombret H, Gardin C (2016) An update of current treatments for adult acute myeloid leukemia. Blood 127(1):53–61

Edelmann D, Habermehl C, Schlenk RF, Benner A (2020) Adjusting Simon's optimal two-stage design for heterogeneous populations based on stratification or using historical controls. Biom J 62(2):311–329

Eichler HG, Bloechl-Daum B, Bauer P et al (2016) "Threshold-crossing": a useful way to establish the counterfactual in clinical trials? Clin Pharmacol Ther 100(6):699–712

Ferguson P, Hills RK, Grech A et al (2016) An operational definition of primary refractory acute myeloid leukemia allowing early identification of patients who may benefit from allogeneic stem cell transplantation. Haematologica 101:1351–1358

Gan HK, Grothey A, Pond GR et al (2010) Randomized phase II trials: inevitable or inadvisable? J Clin Oncol 28(15):2641–2647

Gerstung M, Papaemmanuil E, Martincorena I et al (2017) Precision oncology for acute myeloid leukemia using a knowledge bank approach. Nat Genet 49(3):332–340

Göllner S, Oellerich T, Agrawal-Singh S et al (2017) Loss of the histone methyltransferase EZH2 induces resistance to multiple drugs in acute myeloid leukemia. Nat Med 23(1):69–78

Heuser M, Ofran Y, Boissel N et al (2020) Acute myeloid leukaemia in adult patients: ESMO clinical practice guidelines for diagnosis, treatment and follow-up. Ann Oncol 31(6):697–712

Holtick U, Shimabukuro-Vornhagen A, Chakupurakal G et al (2016) FLAMSA reduced-intensity conditioning is equally effective in AML patients with primary induction failure as well as in first or second complete remission. Eur J Haematol 96(5):475–482

Hütter-Krönke ML, Benner A, Döhner K et al (2016) Salvage therapy with high-dose cytarabine and mitoxantrone in combination with all-trans retinoic acid and gemtuzum abozogamicin in acute myeloid leukemia refractory to first induction therapy. Haematologica 101(7):839–845

Juliusson G, Lazarevic V, Hörstedt AS, et al, Swedish Acute Leukemia Registry Group (2012) Acute

myeloid leukemia in the real world: why population-based registries are needed. Blood 119(17):3890–3899
Kern W, Haferlach T, Schoch C et al (2003) Early blast clearance by remission induction therapy is a major independent prognostic factor for both achievement of complete remission and long-term outcome in acute myeloid leukemia: data from the German AML Cooperative Group (AMLCG) 1992 trial. Blood 101(1):64–70
Krisam J, Weber D, Schlenk RF, Kieser M (n.d.) Enhancing single-arm phase II trials by inclusion of matched control patients—the matched-threshold-crossing (MTC) design. Submitted
Krönke J, Bullinger L, Teleanu V et al (2013) Clonal evolution in relapsed NPM1-mutated acute myeloid leukemia. Blood 122(1):100–108
Lancet JE, Uy GL, Cortes JE, Newell LF et al (2018) CPX-351 (cytarabine and daunorubicin) liposome for injection versus conventional Cytarabine plus Daunorubicin in older patients with newly diagnosed secondary acute myeloid leukemia. J Clin Oncol 36(26):2684–2692
Megías-Vericat JE, Martínez-Cuadrón D, Sanz MÁ, Montesinos P (2018) Salvage regimens using conventional chemotherapy agents for relapsed/refractory adult AML patients: a systematic literature review. Ann Hematol 97(7):1115–1153
Nagel G, Weber D, Fromm E et al (2017) Epidemiological, genetic and clinical characterization of newly diagnosed acute myeloid leukemia based on an academic population-based registry study (AMLSG BiO). Ann Hematol 96(12):1993–2003
National Comprehensive Cancer Network (NCCN) Guidelines: acute myeloid leukemia. 2016
Papaemmanuil E, Gerstung M, Bullinger L et al (2016) Genomic classification and prognosis in acute myeloid leukemia. N Engl J Med 374(23):2209–2221
Paubelle E, Ducastelle-Leprêtre S, Labussière-Wallet H et al (2017) Fractionated gemtuzumabozogamicin combined with intermediate-dose cytarabine and daunorubicin as salvage therapy in very high-risk AML patients: a bridge to reduced intensity conditioning transplant? Ann Hematol 96(3):363–371
Perl AE, Altman JK, Cortes JE et al (2016) Final results of the Chrysalis trial: a first-in-human phase 1/2 dose-escalation, dose-expansion study of Gilteritinib (ASP2215) in patients with relapsed/refractory acute myeloid leukemia (R/R AML). Blood 128:1069
Perl AE, Martinelli G, Cortes JE et al (2019) Gilteritinib or chemotherapy for relapsed or refractory FLT3-mutated AML. N Engl J Med 381(18):1728–1740
Ram R, Scheid C, Amit O et al (2019) Sequential therapy for patients with primary refractory acute myeloid leukemia: a historical prospective analysis of the German and Israeli experience. Haematologica 104(9):1798–1803
Ravandi F, Cortes J, Faderl S, O'Brien S, Garcia-Manero G, Verstovsek S et al (2010) Characteristics and outcome of patients with acute myeloid leukemia refractory to 1 cycle of high-dose cytarabine-based induction chemotherapy. Blood 116:5818–5823
Ravandi F, Ritchie EK, Sayar H et al (2015) Vosaroxin plus cytarabine versus placebo plus cytarabine in patients with first relapsed or refractory acute myeloid leukaemia (VALOR): a randomised, controlled, double-blind, multinational, phase 3 study. Lancet Oncol 16(9):1025–1036
Roboz GJ, Rosenblat T, Arellano M et al (2014) International randomized phase III study of elacytarabine versus investigator choice in patients with relapsed/refractory acute myeloid leukemia. J Clin Oncol 32(18):1919–1926
Rubinstein L, Crowley J, Ivy P et al (2009) Randomized phase II designs. Clin Cancer Res 15(6):1883–1890
Schlenk RF, Benner A, Hartmann F et al (2003) Risk-adapted postremission therapy in acute myeloid leukemia: results of the German multicenter AML HD93 treatment trial. Leukemia 17(8):1521–1528
Schlenk RF, Frech P, Weber D et al (2017) Impact of pretreatment characteristics and salvage strategy on outcome in patients with relapsed acute myeloid leukemia. Leukemia 31(5):1217–1220
Shimizu H, Yokohama A, Ishizaki T et al (2018) Clonal evolution detected with conventional cytogenetic analysis is a potent prognostic factor in adult patients with relapsed AML. Hematol Oncol 36(1):252–257
Stein EM, DiNardo CD, Pollyea DA et al (2017) Enasidenib in mutant IDH2 relapsed or refractory acute myeloid leukemia. Blood 130(6):722–731
Stein EM, DiNardo CD, Fathi AT et al (2019) Molecular remission and response patterns in patients with mutant-IDH2 acute myeloid leukemia treated with enasidenib. Blood 133(7):676–687
Stone RM, Mandrekar S, Sanford LB et al (2017) Midostaurin plus chemotherapy for acute myeloid leukemia with a FLT3 mutation. N Engl J Med 377(5):454–464
Thol F, Schlenk RF, Heuser M, Ganser A (2015) How I treat refractory and early relapsed acute myeloid leukemia. Blood 126(3):319–327
Wattad M, Weber D, Döhner K et al (2017) Impact of salvage regimens on response and overall survival in acute myeloid leukemia with induction failure. Leukemia 31(6):1306–1313. https://doi.org/10.1038/leu.2017.23
Wheatley K, Burnett AK, Goldstone AH et al (1999) A simple, robust, validated and highly predictive index for the determination of risk-directed therapy in acute myeloid leukaemia derived from the MRC AML 10 trial. United Kingdom Medical Research Council's Adult and Childhood Leukaemia Working Parties. Br J Haematol 107(1):69–79

# 12 Treatment of Relapsed and Refractory AML: Non-intensive Approach in Unfit Patients

Christian Récher

## 12.1 Introduction

Acute myeloid leukemia (AML) patients unable to achieve a complete response (CR) with standard induction therapy (refractory AML) or whose disease relapses after achieving remission are likely to die from their disease (Thol et al. 2015). The treatment of relapsed or refractory (R/R) AML in patients who are candidate for intensive chemotherapy consists in reducing the leukemia burden, with the aim to achieve complete remission (CR), CR with incomplete hematologic recovery (CRi), or to significantly reduce the percentage of bone marrow blasts before performing an allogeneic stem cell transplantation, which is currently the treatment with the highest probability of cure. Even with this high intensity strategy, the outcome remains poor with, across the board, less than 50% CR/CRi and a median survival of 6 months. The prognosis is even more dismal in patients not selected and thus deemed unfit for intensive chemotherapy in this setting. In these unfit patients, the main objective of treatment is to limit both disease progression and treatment-related toxicity on an outpatient basis to keep a meaningful quality of life. To this, non-intensive approaches are generally proposed including hypomethylating agents, low dose cytarabine, or single agent gemtuzumab ozogamicin (Megias-Vericat et al. 2018). Response rates are generally lower than 30% and median overall survival rarely exceeds 3–6 months (Roboz et al. 2014). More recently, owing to the considerable progress in understanding the molecular basis of AML and subsequent drug development, new important therapeutic options including small molecules inhibitors have been approved in R/R AML patients (Wei and Tiong 2017; Papaemmanuil et al. 2016a; Dohner et al. 2015). These targeted therapies are particularly relevant in unfit patients because, besides efficacy, their safety profiles are completely different and much more acceptable as compared to intensive chemotherapy. Moreover, they open the way to design new drug combinations by adding targeted therapies to low intensity therapy such as hypomethylating agents or by combining the targeted molecules.

## 12.2 How to Define Unfit Patients in the Relapse/Refractory Setting?

Although a large amount of literature addressed the issue of how to define fit versus unfit patients for intensive therapeutic strategies at diagnosis of

C. Récher (✉)
CHU Toulouse, IUCT-Oncopole, University of Toulouse 3, Toulouse, France
e-mail: recher.christian@iuct-oncopole.fr


C. Röllig, G. J. Ossenkoppele (eds.), *Acute Myeloid Leukemia*, Hematologic Malignancies,
https://doi.org/10.1007/978-3-030-72676-8_12

AML, data in the R/R setting remain very scarce, if any (Podoltsev et al. 2017). However, similar to first-line therapy, both patients and disease characteristics are routinely taken into account to help defining patients unfit for intensive therapeutic strategies including older age, performance status, comorbidities according to scoring systems such as HCT-IC, as well as poor disease characteristics such as adverse cytogenetic or molecular risks. In older patients, geriatric assessments may also help for clinical decision-making (Klepin et al. 2020; Molga et al. 2020). Moreover, sequelae from toxicity of previous treatments, patient's willingness, and/or physician attitude that may differ from diagnosis in the R/R setting where the chances for cure are so weak are also important points to consider. For example, relapses after allogeneic stem cell transplantation are particularly challenging because AML cells emerging at relapse are per se chemo- and immune-resistant while comorbidities and immunosuppression induced by the procedure weaken the capacities to well tolerate salvage treatments (Bejanyan et al. 2015).

The German–Austrian AML Study Group has recently analyzed the distribution of treatments at time of refractory disease or relapse in a large cohort of 3324 patients treated by first-line intensive chemotherapy within 5 different multicenter trials (Wattad et al. 2017; Schlenk et al. 2017). Out of 1025 patients who had refractory disease after induction chemotherapy, 875 patients (85%) received intensive salvage regimens whereas 150 patients (15%) received non-intensive or palliative treatment. Median overall survival of these latter was 3.1 months. As compared to patients who received an intensive salvage regimen, patients selected for non-intensive treatment were older (68 vs. 55 years), had more often secondary AML (20% vs. 7.9%), poor performance status (ECOG performance status 2–3, 25.7% vs. 12%), and differences in few gene mutations (*FLT3*-ITD, *DNMT3A*, and *IDH2*) (Wattad et al. 2017). In the same cohort, out of 2170 patients who achieved a first CR, 1307 patients relapsed. Median duration of CR1 was 274.5 days. Of these 1307 relapsed patients, 1120 patients (86%, median age, 53.6 years) received different salvage regimens in which non-intensive treatment such as hypomethylating agents and low-dose cytarabine represented only 5.5% of patients, whereas 187 patients (14%) (median age, 60.5 years) received palliative care only. Median and 24-month survival of patients who received salvage therapy and those who had palliative care were 7.9 months and 27.3%, and 1.6 months and 3.7%, respectively (Schlenk et al. 2017).

In two recent phase III trials assessing FLT3 inhibitors in R/R AML patients with *FLT3* mutations, 24–40% of patients were preselected by investigators for low intensity regimen (Perl et al. 2019a; Cortes et al. 2019a). A recent study from a real-world AML database on 896 patients treated by intensive induction chemotherapy showed that 64% of refractory and 59% of relapsed patients did not receive intensive salvage and were treated by low intensity regimen or supportive care (Bertoli et al. 2019). Thus, it is estimated that, after first-line intensive treatment, 20–40% of R/R AML (and probably more in real world) are generally not selected for further intensive salvage regimen and referred for low-intensity regimen or nothing.

Age, comorbidities, performance status, and disease characteristics are the main factors to stratify treatments of R/R AML (i.e., fitness vs. unfitness for intensive salvage and transplantation). Although exceptionally primary refractory to induction, approximately 30–40% of patients with favorable cytogenetic or molecular features (i.e., core binding factor (CBF)-AML, *NPM1*, *CEBPA* biallelic mutations) relapse. Intensive salvage chemotherapy induces more than 60% of second CR in these subgroups and long-term survival can be achieved (Rollig et al. 2015; Hospital et al. 2014; Burnett et al. 2013). Therefore, these patients should not be referred to low-intensity regimens for salvage. In addition, one way to define patients not candidate for intensive strategies and thus to be referred to low-intensity regimen is to estimate their prognosis according to a score established with intensive approaches. A study in 667 relapsed younger adults of the HOVON study group showed a longer relapse-free interval after CR1, presence of a CBF-AML at diagnosis, lower age at relapse, and no previous stem-cell transplantation during first-line therapy as factors associated with more favorable prognosis (Breems et al. 2005). Refractory patients were not included in this study. With these four factors three prognostic groups could be identified. According to this score, patients of the unfavorable group represented 67% of the cohort, had a low second CR rate (34%) and poor overall survival (16% at 1 year and 4% at 5 years, respectively). Another score for R/R AML has been proposed by the FILO study group (formerly GOELAMS) in a series of patients who had received intensive chemotherapy plus gemtuzumab ozogamicin as salvage treatment (Chevallier et al. 2010). Disease status (relapse <12 months including refractory patients), *FLT3*-ITD mutation, and high-risk cytogenetics were the strongest adverse prognostic factors and were used to generate a simple scoring system in which patients with 2 or 3 factors (31% of the cohort) had a 2-year OS of 12%. A similar score in patients treated by FLAG-Ida (+/−GO) was proposed by the PETHEMA study group (Bergua et al. 2016). Based on these scoring systems that share similar factors, patients "unfit" for intensive salvage regimen, belonging to the unfavorable groups, can be selected to offer them low-intensity treatments.

It should be noted that these prognosis scoring systems were mainly based on younger patients and did not integrate patient or disease characteristics at the time of relapse or refractory disease, particular performance status, or clonal evolution that may strongly impact outcome (Shimizu et al. 2018). Indeed, acquisition of additional cytogenetic abnormalities at first relapse is an adverse risk factor for both response to salvage treatment and overall survival independent from age, duration of CR1, and cytogenetic risk. Evaluation of clonal evolution assessed at the cytogenetic and molecular levels at the time of R/R is mandatory to better select patients for salvage therapies (see below).

Defining R/R patients as fit or unfit for intensive approaches remains challenging and more complex than this simple dichotomy (Table 12.1). Simplest situations are unfortunately the rarest: patients with a favorable risk disease and a fit condition are easily referred to intensive chemotherapy and conversely, patients with adverse risk cytogenetics and worse performance status or comorbidities are referred to non-intensive approach. In between, a caseby-case analysis is needed to weight benefit and risk of each option. In addition, the advent of new molecules, as discussed below, completely challenges the current therapeutic landscape by offering more effective and less toxic treatment options giving hope that non-intensive approaches will no longer be synonymous of palliative care.

## 12.3 Treatment Options in Unfit R/R AML Patients

Therapeutic possibilities and their objectives should be discussed with patients and their families even more carefully than at time of diagnosis.

**Table 12.1** Disease and patient characteristics to consider for defining treatments in R/R AML

| | Disease[a] | Patients[a] | Treatment[b] |
|---|---|---|---|
| Fitness for intensive salvage regimen | CBF/*CEBPA*$^{dm}$/*NPM1*$^{mut}$/*FLT3*$^{wt}$<br>No clonal evolution<br>Duration of CR1 > 12 months | Age < 65–70 years<br>PS < 2<br>No comorbidity<br>No allo-SCT in CR1 | Intensive chemotherapy<br>Targeted therapies |
| Unfitness for intensive salvage regimen | High-risk cytogenetics<br>TP53 mutation<br>Clonal evolution<br>Duration of CR1 ≤ 12 months | Age > 65–70 years<br>PS ≥ 2<br>Comorbidities<br>Allo-SCT in CR1 | Non intensive treatment<br>Targeted therapies |

[a]Prognostic scoring systems, comorbidities scores, and geriatric assessment may help for clinical decision-making (Klepin et al. 2020; Molga et al. 2020; Breems et al. 2005; Chevallier et al. 2010; Bergua et al. 2016; Sorror et al. 2017)
[b]Combinations of high- or low-intensity chemotherapy and targeted agents or monoclonal antibodies may be proposed in clinical trials

Indeed, the clinical picture at R/R setting is often very different owing to the toxicities of previous treatments including bone marrow transplantation, clonal evolution of the disease, and psychological experience of first-line treatment. Treatment options need to be weighed against each other by taking into account this very complex picture. Additional molecular screen is mandatory since targetable mutations could emerge at R/R through clonal evolution and sometimes, these targets present at diagnosis may be lost. Given the poor results of available therapies, enrolment in clinical trials is strongly recommended. Here, we will review therapies that are currently available and novel emerging therapies.

### 12.3.1 Standard Non-intensive Approaches

#### 12.3.1.1 Hypomethylating Agents

Hypomethylating agents (HMA) including azacitidine or decitabine are widely used as frontline treatment in older AML patients judged unfit for intensive chemotherapy because of comorbidities, age, or disease risk factors such as unfavorable cytogenetics (Dombret et al. 2015). These agents are also often used in R/R AML although neither evaluated in prospective clinical trials nor approved in this indication. Azacitidine and decitabine provide an acceptable compromise between efficacy, tolerability, and quality of life in this setting. HMA activity in R/R AML has been recently reported in an international multicenter retrospective study including 290 refractory and 365 relapsed patients (Stahl et al. 2018). Median age at diagnosis was 65 years. HMA induced 11% CR and 5.3% CR with incomplete count recovery (CRi; 5.3%) whereas 8.5% obtained hematologic improvement with no difference between refractory or relapsed patients. Thirty-day mortality was relatively low (6.4%). Although the global median OS was poor (6.7 months), CR/CRi patients had a median OS of 25.3 and 14.6 months, respectively. Interestingly, patients whose best response was hematological improvement or stable disease had a median OS of 11.7 months or 10.4 months, significantly better than those who had progressive disease, a finding that is similar to first-line setting (Bories et al. 2014). Presence of ≤5% circulating blasts and decitabine used in a 10-day schedule were associated with better response rates, whereas the presence of >5% circulating blasts and >20% bone marrow blasts were associated with decreased OS in multivariate analyses indicating that only patients with low proliferative disease may benefit from HMA. It is also noteworthy that a substantial number of patients (28%) received a second drug in combination azacitidine or decitabine suggesting that HMA may represent a valuable therapeutic platform, both in term of safety and efficacy, on which novel drugs could be added in clinical trials to improve outcome. So far, HMA likely represent the more interesting low-intensity treatment in R/R AML outside clinical trials.

#### 12.3.1.2 Low Dose Cytarabine

Low dose cytarabine is also an option that is proposed so far as control arm in recent phase 3 trials for unfit R/R AML patients although prospective trials in these setting have not been conducted (Perl et al. 2019a; Cortes et al. 2019a). This treatment may control disease with lower toxicity compared to intensive chemotherapy and CR had been anecdotally reported in selected patients (Sarkozy et al. 2013; Jensen et al. 1994). More recent controlled studies reported virtually no CR and a median OS of 3.7 months making this treatment considered a palliative option (Roboz et al. 2014; Cortes et al. 2019a). However, combined with old or novel drugs such as BCL-2 or Hedgehog pathway inhibitors, higher response rate may be achieved and should be assessed prospectively (Bewersdorf et al. 2020; Cortes et al. 2019b; Wei et al. 2019).

### 12.3.2 Targeted Therapies

#### 12.3.2.1 IDH1 Inhibitors

Somatic mutations of isocitrate dehydrogenase 1 (*IDH1*$^{R132}$) genes are found in 6–10% of AML (Bullinger et al. 2017). *IDH1*$^{R132}$ mutations are most frequent in cytogenetically normal AML and significantly associated with *NPM1* and DNMT3A mutations (Duchmann et al. 2019). Their prognostic impact is not clearly defined and may depend on mutational context (Patel et al. 2012; Paschka et al. 2010; Abbas et al. 2010). *IDH1*$^{R132}$ mutations induce a neomorphic enzyme that overproduces the 2-hydroxyglutarate oncometabolite which can inhibit many cellular processes and alter epigenetics and myeloid differentiation (Montalban-Bravo and DiNardo 2018). Moreover, these mutations are early events in leukemogenesis, which persist at relapse and thus, have emerged as promising therapeutic targets.

Ivosidenib, an oral, targeted, small-molecule inhibitor of mutant IDH1, has been evaluated as a single agent in a phase 1 dose-escalation and dose-expansion study in *IDH1*-mutated AML (DiNardo et al. 2018a). Patients were included if they had relapsed after stem cell transplantation, were refractory to induction or reinduction chemotherapy, had early relapse within 12 months after initial therapy, or second or later relapse, thus representing a very high-risk population in which unfit patients were likely well represented although fitness to intensive chemotherapy was not included in study criteria. It should be noted that the molecular landscape of AML with *IDH1* mutations observed in R/R patients under chemotherapy selection pressure differs from diagnosis with increased frequency of *SRSF2*, *ASXL1*, *RUNX1*, *NRAS*, and *TP53* co-occurring mutations (Duchmann et al. 2019; DiNardo et al. 2018a). The frequency of treatment-related adverse events of grade >2 was low, mainly prolongation of the QT interval, leukocytosis, and differentiation syndrome which are manageable with appropriate interventions including supportive care, hydroxyurea and corticosteroids (DiNardo and Wei 2020). Among the 125 patients of the primary efficacy population, the rate of CR or CR with partial hematologic recovery (CRh) was 30.4% with 21.8% CR whereas CRi was 11.7%. Moreover, mutation clearance was observed in 21% of responding patients demonstrating that deep response may be achieved in some patients. The median duration of response was 9.3 months in CR patients. Median overall survival was 8.8 months. Based on these promising results, ivosidenib has been recently approved by the Food and Drug Administration (FDA).

Mechanisms of resistance to ivosidenib have been recently described in patients who have progressed under treatment or who have relapsed after a response (Choe et al. 2019). Receptor tyrosine kinase (RTK) pathway mutations (excluding JAK2 mutations) and mutations in the individual genes *NRAS* and *PTPN11* are significantly associated with lack of response to ivosidenib. Of note, clonal or subclonal mIDH1 had similar CR/CRh rates. Interestingly, emerging mutations in patients who relapsed or progressed under ivosidenib were *IDH* or non-*IDH* related. Indeed, mutations in a second site of *IDH1* (associated with in vitro resistance to ivosidenib) or emergence of *IDH2*$^{R140}$ clones were detected in 23% of resistant patients whereas potentially actionable mutations in genes such as *FLT3*, *NRAS*, or *KRAS* were also identified indicating that molecular rescreening is important at each stage of the disease.

Preliminary results of ivosidenib combined with azacitidine as in treatment naive patients showed a complete response rate of 70% suggesting that R/R AML patients may also benefit from this combination by limiting the emergence of mutant resistant clones (Dinardo et al. 2019).

Olutasidenib (FT-2102) is the second oral selective inhibitor of mutant IDH1 currently in early phase clinical trial. Preliminary results showed similar efficacy to that of ivosidenib (Watts et al. 2019).

#### 12.3.2.2 IDH2 Inhibitors

Somatic mutations of *IDH2* gene, either *IDH2*$^{R140}$ or *IDH2*$^{R172}$, occur in 5–15% and 1–4% of AML, respectively (Bullinger et al. 2017). Similar to IDH1, *IDH2* mutations are frequently, but not exclusively, found in cytogenetically normal AML and induce 2-HG overproduction (Ward et al. 2010; Figueroa et al. 2010). However, despite a common mechanism of action, both mutations differ regarding co-occurring mutational events and outcome. At diagnosis, *IDH2*$^{R140}$

mutations are associated with *NPM1* and *DNMT3A* mutations whereas in the relapse/refractory setting, mutations in *SRSF2*, *DNMT3A*, *RUNX1*, *ASXL1*, *NRAS*, and *BCOR* genes emerge as the most frequent co-mutations (Bullinger et al. 2017; Amatangelo et al. 2017; Papaemmanuil et al. 2016b). Contrasting with *IDH2*$^{R140}$, *IDH2*$^{R172}$ mutations are mutually exclusive with *NPM1* and other class-defining mutations whereas it is frequently co-mutated with DNMT3A and BCOR (Duchmann et al. 2019). Therefore, AML with *IDH2*$^{R172}$ has been recognized as a defined subgroup of the AML genomic classification (Papaemmanuil et al. 2016b).

Enasidenib, an oral, targeted, small-molecule inhibitor of mutant IDH2, has been evaluated as a single agent in a phase 1 dose-escalation and dose-expansion study in mutant *IDH2*R/R AML patients and subsequently approved by the FDA (Stein 2018). A low frequency of treatment-related adverse events of grade 3 or higher was reported, mainly indirect hyperbilirubinemia (off-target effect related to UGT1A1 inhibition), leukocytosis, and differentiation syndrome (Amatangelo et al. 2017; Fathi et al. 2018). The overall response rate was 40.3% including 19.3% CR and 6.8% CRi. Median overall survival was 9.3 months and reaches 19.7 months in CR patients. Similar to ivosidenib, some interesting points need to be considered upon enasidenib treatment which induces responses through cell differentiation (Amatangelo et al. 2017). Interestingly, the variant allele frequency of IDH2 mutant, which measure mutational burden, was not associated with response and CRs were observed in patients with subclonal IDH2 mutations. Also, whereas in some CR patients, *IDH2* mutation clearance was achieved, *IDH2* mutational burden did not decrease in all responding patients during treatment, possibly due to the maturation of leukemic blasts into functional neutrophils carrying the mutation. Moreover, suppression of 2-HG induced by enasidenib did not predict response, as strong reduction of 2-HG levels was observed both in responders and non-responders. Last, mechanisms of resistance may involve the emergence of second-site IDH2 mutations, IDH2-mutant subclones with neomorphic mutations in *IDH1*, co-occurring mutations in NRAS, and other MAPK pathway effectors or complex clonal evolution (Amatangelo et al. 2017; Intlekofer et al. 2018; Quek et al. 2018).

A recent randomized phase 2 trial of azacitidine versus azacitidine plus enasidenib in newly diagnosed AML patients unfit for intensive chemotherapy showed a significant higher CR rate with the combination compared to azacitidine alone (53% vs. 12%) indicating that this treatment could be also a relevant option in R/R patients (DiNardo et al. 2019b).

#### 12.3.2.3 FLT3 Inhibitors

Mutations in the *FLT3* gene are among the most common mutations in AML occurring in up to 30% of patients (Papaemmanuil et al. 2016a). Two distinct activating *FLT3* mutations are described: internal tandem duplications (ITD) in the juxta membrane domain and point mutations in the tyrosine kinase domain (TKD). *FLT3* mutations are associated with an aggressive disease course especially *FLT3*-ITD which predicts early relapse and poor prognosis. Through clonal selection under chemotherapy, a higher mutant allelic burden is frequently observed at relapse indicating that AML cells have become more addicted to FLT3 signaling. This is an important point because at least in preclinical setting, FLT3-mutant allelic burden and clinical status (i.e., diagnosis vs. relapse samples) are predictive of response to FLT3inhibitors in AML (Pratz et al. 2010). Furthermore, as described above, *FLT3*-ITD is an independent poor prognostic factor in R/R AML.

Two randomized phase 3 trials with second generation FLT3 inhibitors, namely quizartinib and gilteritinib, have been recently conducted in R/R AML patients with *FLT3* mutations (gilteritinib) or *FLT3*-ITD only mutations (quizartinib) (Perl et al. 2019a; Cortes et al. 2019a). In both studies, the targeted molecule used as single agent was superior to standard treatment with high or low intensity chemotherapy in improving both response and overall survival.

Quizartinib, an oral, highly potent, and selective inhibitor of FLT3-ITD without activity against *FLT3*-TKD mutations, has been the first tyrosine kinase inhibitor to be compared in a randomized phase 3 trials to standard salvage therapy (Cortes et al. 2019a). In this phase 3 QUANTUM-R study, R/R AML patients with *FLT3*-ITD mutations and a first CR duration of less than 6 months were randomized between 30–60 mg/day quizartinib and a standard salvage chemotherapy regimen selected among MEC, FLAG-ida, or low dose cytarabine prior to randomization. The rate of composite CR (CRc) which included CR, Cri, and CRp was significantly higher with quizartinib than standard of care (48.2 vs. 27%). Of note, quizartinib induced very few true CRs (4%), most responses being CRi due to its myelosuppressive effect, an adverse effect already described in early phase trials and likely related to the inhibitory spectrum of quizartinib which includes cKIT (Cortes et al. 2018). Median time to first CRc was 4.9 weeks and median duration of CRc was 12.1 weeks. Median overall survival was longer for quizartinib than for standard of care (6.2 vs. 4.7 months). Main adverse event upon quizartinib treatment are QTc prolongation (3% grade 3), myelosuppression, and differentiation syndrome (Sexauer et al. 2012). Although QUANTUM-R was the first positive trial in the field, quizartinib was not approved by FDA and European Medicines Agency. Quizartinib resistance has been studied through single cell analysis showing highly complex mechanisms related to clonal heterogeneity (Smith et al. 2017).

Gilteritinib is an oral, small molecule inhibitor, highly selective of FLT3 with activity against both *FLT3*-ITD and -TKD mutations and only weak activity against cKIT (Lee et al. 2017; Mori et al. 2017). The spectrum of this molecule also extends to other tyrosine kinases such as AXL, which has been implicated in resistance to chemotherapy and FLT3 inhibitors (Ben-Batalla et al. 2013; Dumas et al. 2019). In the pivotal phase 3 ADMIRAL study, AML patients with R/R FLT3 mutated AML were randomized between 120 mg/day gilteritinib or salvage chemotherapy which included high or low intensity regimen defined by physicians prior to randomization (Perl et al. 2019a). Gilteritinib induced higher CR/CRh and CR rates (34.0% vs. 15.3% and 21.1% vs. 10.5%, respectively), enabled more patients to receive an allogeneic stem cell transplantation, and significantly improved overall survival as compared with standard salvage regimen (median OS, 9.3 vs. 5.6 months). Adverse events were more frequent in the standard chemotherapy arm with the exception of liver transaminase elevations. QTc prolongation, differentiation syndrome, and lipase elevation are very rare events upon gilteritinib treatment (<5%), whereas posterior reversible encephalopathy syndrome has been exceptionally reported (DiNardo and Wei 2020; McMahon et al. 2019a). Based on these results, gilteritinib was approved in North America, Europe, and Japan for the treatment of patients with R/R FLT3 mutated AML. Off-target activating mutations in genes of the *RAS/MAPK* pathway have been identified as a key mechanism of resistance to gilteritinib and confirmed in patients of the ADMIRAL trial who relapsed on gilteritinib treatment in whom in-target *FLT3*-F691L mutations were also detected (Smith et al. 2019; McMahon et al. 2019b).

As stated above, patients relapsing after allogeneic stem cell transplantation cumulate chemo and immune resistance, frailty, and comorbidities rendering them unfit for intensive salvage. Interestingly, sorafenib, a multikinase inhibitor with potent activity against FLT3, has demonstrated clinical activity in *FLT3*-ITD patients relapsing after transplantation (Metzelder et al. 2012). A subsequent comprehensive preclinical study elegantly demonstrated that sorafenib (and other FLT3 inhibitors) increased IL-15 production by *FLT3*-ITD leukemic cells leading to potentiation of allogeneic CD8+ T cell response and disease eradication in preclinical models (Mathew et al. 2018).

#### 12.3.2.4 Gemtuzumab Ozogamicin

Gemtuzumab ozogamicin (GO) is an anti-CD33 antibody drug conjugate carrying calicheamicin, a DNA damaging toxin. GO was first approved in 2000 on a 9 $mg/m^2$ dosing regimen in R/R AML patients (Larson RA Cancer 2005) but subsequently withdrawn due to preliminary results of a phase 3 randomized trial which demonstrated increased early deaths and lack of clinical benefit in patients treated by GO+ intensive chemotherapy (Larson et al. 2005; Baron and Wang 2018). GO single agent has been recently reapproved by the FDA in older patients with $CD33^{+}$R/R AML based on a phase 2 uncontrolled trial testing fractionated doses of GO (3 mg/$m^2$ on days 1, 4 and 7) in 57 patients in first relapse (Taksin et al. 2007). Overall response (CR + CRp) rate was 33% with 26% CR and 7% CRi. Median relapse-free and overall survival was 11 and 8.4 months, respectively. Main toxicity was myelosuppression while no veno-occlusive disease occurred. In this study, most patients achieving response received high dose cytarabine as consolidation indicating that this patient population very likely included fit patients. Nevertheless, since extra-hematological toxicity seems relatively low with this schedule, GO could be an option both as single agent in unfit patients, especially those with intermediate or favorable genetic risk, or in combination with small molecules inhibitors.

#### 12.3.2.5 APR-246

AML patients with *TP53* mutations are among the poorest responders to intensive chemotherapy (Hunter and Sallman 2019). Less than 50% of them achieved CR after intensive chemotherapy, most patients relapse even after allogeneic stem cell transplantation, and are referred to low intensity regimen. Although hypomethylating agents are popular in this subgroup (relative to the dismal results of chemotherapy), response rate and overall survival remain very poor (Welch et al. 2016; Bally et al. 2014).

APR-246 is the first-in-class small molecule that selectively targets *TP53 mutated* cancer cells through protein stabilization and structural reconfirmation and reactivates its cell cycle arrest and pro-apoptotic activities (Perdrix et al. 2017). In patients with *TP53* mutated myelodysplastic syndrome or AML, APR-246 combined with azacitidine induced CR rates of 53% and 56% in 2 ongoing phase 2 trials representing the first hope for relevant therapeutic improvement in this subgroup (Sallman et al. 2019; Cluzeau et al. 2019).

#### 12.3.2.6 Venetoclax

The anti-apoptotic B-cell lymphoma 2 (BCL-2) protein is overexpressed AML, especially in leukemic stem cells that are supposed to be responsible for chemoresistance and relapse (Lagadinou et al. 2013).

Venetoclax, an oral, selective, small-molecule inhibitor of BCL-2, has been recently approved in combination with hypomethylating agents as first-line therapy in AML patients who are ineligible to receive standard induction therapy on the basis of high response rates and promising response duration in a phase 1b/2 trial (DiNardo et al. 2018b, 2019c). These results have been recently confirmed in the VIALE-A phase 3 trial which demonstrated the superiority of azacitidine plus venetoclax over azacitidine plus placebo in terms of complete response rate, duration of response, and overall survival (DiNardo C, 25th congress of the European Hematology Association, abstract: LB2601,2020). Venetoclax combined with low dose cytarabine was also superior to low dose cytarabine in the VIALE-C phase 3 trial (Wei et al. 2020). In R/R patients, venetoclax has shown modest single-agent clinical activity, with 19% of overall response in a phase 2 trial (Konopleva et al. 2016). Retrospective real-world data from small series of R/R patients treated by combination of venetoclax and hypomethylating agents reported a CR rate of 5–30%, which is much less than response rates observed in first line (DiNardo et al. 2018c; Aldoss et al. 2018). However, combination with other small molecules inhibitors such as FLT3 or MDM2 inhibitors appears promising in R/R patients (Perl et al. 2019b; Daver et al. 2019).

## 12.4 Conclusion

Only 5% of quizartinib treated patients in the QUANTUM-R trial were >75 years and 11% had an ECOG performance status of 2. These data were not reported in the ADMIRAL trial. In the IDH1/2 trials, median age was 68–70 y and 19–20% of patients had a performance status of 2. Thus, the real impact of these new drugs in

AML patients with poor performance status, older age, or multiple comorbidities deserves further studies. Nevertheless, IDH and FLT3 inhibitors are likely appropriate drugs for unfit R/R AML patients since their safety profile are neglectable in comparison to the huge amount of toxicities induced by intensive salvage regimen. Beside specific side effects (QTc, differentiation syndrome, liver abnormalities) that are manageable, most adverse events reported with these inhibitors are mainly related to disease burden, and once response is achieved, tolerability and compliance are optimal. Yet, although overall response rate and disease control are of value, CR rates remain lower to 50% and a lot has to be done to further improve anti-leukemic activity. Obviously, the logical way to achieve this goal will be combination therapies. First results of HMA plus IDH1 or IDH2 inhibitors in first line are encouraging. Combinations (even triple) with targeted agents are also under study and will be hopefully the subject of future review in this topic.

## References


Abbas S, Lugthart S, Kavelaars FG, Schelen A, Koenders JE, Zeilemaker A, van Putten WJ, Rijneveld AW, Lowenberg B, Valk PJ (2010) Acquired mutations in the genes encoding IDH1 and IDH2 both are recurrent aberrations in acute myeloid leukemia: prevalence and prognostic value. Blood 116:2122–2126

Aldoss I, Yang D, Aribi A, Ali H, Sandhu K, Al Malki MM, Mei M, Salhotra A, Khaled S, Nakamura R, Snyder D, O'Donnell M, Stein AS, Forman SJ, Marcucci G, Pullarkat V (2018) Efficacy of the combination of venetoclax and hypomethylating agents in relapsed/refractory acute myeloid leukemia. Haematologica 103:e404–e407

Amatangelo MD, Quek L, Shih A, Stein EM, Roshal M, David MD, Marteyn B, Farnoud NR, de Botton S, Bernard OA, Wu B, Yen KE, Tallman MS, Papaemmanuil E, Penard-Lacronique V, Thakurta A, Vyas P, Levine RL (2017) Enasidenib induces acute myeloid leukemia cell differentiation to promote clinical response. Blood 130:732–741

Bally C, Ades L, Renneville A, Sebert M, Eclache V, Preudhomme C, Mozziconacci MJ, de The H, Lehmann-Che J, Fenaux P (2014) Prognostic value of TP53 gene mutations in myelodysplastic syndromes and acute myeloid leukemia treated with azacitidine. Leuk Res 38:751–755

Baron J, Wang ES (2018) Gemtuzumab ozogamicin for the treatment of acute myeloid leukemia. Expert Rev Clin Pharmacol 11:549–559

Bejanyan N, Weisdorf DJ, Logan BR, Wang HL, Devine SM, de Lima M, Bunjes DW, Zhang MJ (2015) Survival of patients with acute myeloid leukemia relapsing after allogeneic hematopoietic cell transplantation: a center for international blood and marrow transplant research study. Biol Blood Marrow Transplant 21:454–459

Ben-Batalla I, Schultze A, Wroblewski M, Erdmann R, Heuser M, Waizenegger JS, Riecken K, Binder M, Schewe D, Sawall S, Witzke V, Cubas-Cordova M, Janning M, Wellbrock J, Fehse B, Hagel C, Krauter J, Ganser A, Lorens JB, Fiedler W, Carmeliet P, Pantel K, Bokemeyer C, Loges S (2013) Axl, a prognostic and therapeutic target in acute myeloid leukemia mediates paracrine crosstalk of leukemia cells with bone marrow stroma. Blood 122:2443–2452

Bergua JM, Montesinos P, Martinez-Cuadron D, Fernandez-Abellan P, Serrano J, Sayas MJ, Prieto-Fernandez J, Garcia R, Garcia-Huerta AJ, Barrios M, Benavente C, Perez-Encinas M, Simiele A, Rodriguez-Macias G, Herrera-Puente P, Rodriguez-Veiga R, Martinez-Sanchez MP, Amador-Barciela ML, Riaza-Grau R, Sanz MA, group P (2016) A prognostic model for survival after salvage treatment with FLAG-Ida +/− gemtuzumab-ozogamicine in adult patients with refractory/relapsed acute myeloid leukaemia. Br J Haematol 174:700–710

Bertoli S, Tavitian S, Berard E, Gadaud N, Luquet I, Huynh A, Sarry A, Huguet F, Recher C (2019) Outcome of relapsed or refractory acute myeloid leukemia treated with intensive salvage chemotherapy in real life in comparison to intermediate dose cytarabine in phase 3 studies. Leuk Lymphoma 60(1):238–241

Bewersdorf JP, Giri S, Wang R, Williams RT, Tallman MS, Zeidan AM, Stahl M (2020) Venetoclax as monotherapy and in combination with hypomethylating agents or low dose cytarabine in relapsed and treatment refractory acute myeloid leukemia: a systematic review and meta-analysis. Haematologica 105(11):2659–2663

Bories P, Bertoli S, Berard E, Laurent J, Duchayne E, Sarry A, Delabesse E, Beyne-Rauzy O, Huguet F, Recher C (2014) Intensive chemotherapy, azacitidine, or supportive care in older acute myeloid leukemia patients: an analysis from a regional healthcare network. Am J Hematol 89:E244–E252

Breems DA, Van Putten WL, Huijgens PC, Ossenkoppele GJ, Verhoef GE, Verdonck LF, Vellenga E, De Greef GE, Jacky E, Van der Lelie J, Boogaerts MA, Lowenberg B (2005) Prognostic index for adult patients with acute myeloid leukemia in first relapse. J Clin Oncol 23:1969–1978

Bullinger L, Dohner K, Dohner H (2017) Genomics of acute myeloid leukemia diagnosis and pathways. J Clin Oncol 35:934–946

Burnett AK, Goldstone A, Hills RK, Milligan D, Prentice A, Yin J, Wheatley K, Hunter A, Russell N (2013)

Curability of patients with acute myeloid leukemia who did not undergo transplantation in first remission. J Clin Oncol 31:1293–1301

Chevallier P, Prebet T, Pigneux A, Hunault M, Delaunay J, Perry F, Lode L, Richebourg S, Blanchet O, Vey N, Ifrah N, Milpied N, Blaise D, Harousseau JL, Mohty M (2010) Influence of NPM1 and FLT3-ITD status on outcome in relapsed/refractory AML patients receiving salvage therapy including gemtuzumab ozogamicin. Leukemia 24:467–469

Choe S, Wang H, DiNardo CD, Stein EM, De Botton S, Fathi AT, Tallman MS, Kantarjian HM, Stone RM, Quek L, Konteatis Z, Dang L, Zhang V, Liu H, Attar EC, Wu B (2019) Molecular mechanisms mediating relapse following ivosidenib monotherapy in patients with IDH1-mutant relapsed or refractory acute myeloid leukemia. Blood 134:545

Cluzeau T, Sebert M, Rahmé R, Cuzzubbo S, Walter-petrich A, Lehmann-che J, Peterlin P, Beve B, Attalah H, Chermat F, Miekoutima E, Beyne-Rauzy O, Recher C, Stamatoullas A, Willems L, Raffoux E, Berthon C, Quesnel B, Carpentier A, Sallman DA, Chevret S, Ades L, Fenaux P (2019) APR-246 combined with azacitidine (AZA) in TP53 mutated myelodysplastic syndrome (MDS) and acute myeloid leukemia (AML). A phase 2 study by the Groupe Francophone Des Myélodysplasies (GFM). Blood 134:677

Cortes J, Perl AE, Dohner H, Kantarjian H, Martinelli G, Kovacsovics T, Rousselot P, Steffen B, Dombret H, Estey E, Strickland S, Altman JK, Baldus CD, Burnett A, Kramer A, Russell N, Shah NP, Smith CC, Wang ES, Ifrah N, Gammon G, Trone D, Lazzaretto D, Levis M (2018) Quizartinib, an FLT3 inhibitor, as monotherapy in patients with relapsed or refractory acute myeloid leukaemia: an open-label, multicentre, single-arm, phase 2 trial. Lancet Oncol 19:889–903

Cortes JE, Khaled S, Martinelli G, Perl AE, Ganguly S, Russell N, Kramer A, Dombret H, Hogge D, Jonas BA, Leung AY, Mehta P, Montesinos P, Radsak M, Sica S, Arunachalam M, Holmes M, Kobayashi K, Namuyinga R, Ge N, Yver A, Zhang Y, Levis MJ (*2019a*) Quizartinib versus salvage chemotherapy in relapsed or refractory FLT3-ITD acute myeloid leukaemia (QuANTUM-R): a multicentre, randomised, controlled, open-label, phase 3 trial. Lancet Oncol 20:984–997

Cortes JE, Heidel FH, Hellmann A, Fiedler W, Smith BD, Robak T, Montesinos P, Pollyea DA, DesJardins P, Ottmann O, Ma WW, Shaik MN, Laird AD, Zeremski M, O'Connell A, Chan G, Heuser M (*2019b*) Randomized comparison of low dose cytarabine with or without glasdegib in patients with newly diagnosed acute myeloid leukemia or high-risk myelodysplastic syndrome. Leukemia 33:379–389

Daver NG, Garcia JS, Jonas BA, Kelly KR, Assouline S, Brandwein JM, Fenaux P, Olin RL, Martinelli G, Paolini S, Pigneux A, Pollyea DA, Powell BL, Roboz GJ, Tafuri A, Vey N, Visani G, Yee KWL, Dail M, Green C, Kirschbrown WP, Hong W-J, Ott MG, Onishi M, Wang J, Konopleva MY, Andreeff M (2019) Updated results from the venetoclax (Ven) in combination with idasanutlin (Idasa) arm of a phase 1b trial in elderly patients (Pts) with relapsed or refractory (R/R) AML ineligible for cytotoxic chemotherapy. Blood 134:229

DiNardo CD, Wei AH (2020) How I treat acute myeloid leukemia in the era of new drugs. Blood 135:85–96

DiNardo CD, Stein EM, de Botton S, Roboz GJ, Altman JK, Mims AS, Swords R, Collins RH, Mannis GN, Pollyea DA, Donnellan W, Fathi AT, Pigneux A, Erba HP, Prince GT, Stein AS, Uy GL, Foran JM, Traer E, Stuart RK, Arellano ML, Slack JL, Sekeres MA, Willekens C, Choe S, Wang H, Zhang V, Yen KE, Kapsalis SM, Yang H, Dai D, Fan B, Goldwasser M, Liu H, Agresta S, Wu B, Attar EC, Tallman MS, Stone RM, Kantarjian HM (*2018a*) Durable remissions with ivosidenib in IDH1-mutated relapsed or refractory AML. N Engl J Med 378:2386–2398

DiNardo CD, Pratz KW, Letai A, Jonas BA, Wei AH, Thirman M, Arellano M, Frattini MG, Kantarjian H, Popovic R, Chyla B, Xu T, Dunbar M, Agarwal SK, Humerickhouse R, Mabry M, Potluri J, Konopleva M, Pollyea DA (*2018b*) Safety and preliminary efficacy of venetoclax with decitabine or azacitidine in elderly patients with previously untreated acute myeloid leukaemia: a non-randomised, open-label, phase 1b study. Lancet Oncol 19:216–228

DiNardo CD, Rausch CR, Benton C, Kadia T, Jain N, Pemmaraju N, Daver N, Covert W, Marx KR, Mace M, Jabbour E, Cortes J, Garcia-Manero G, Ravandi F, Bhalla KN, Kantarjian H, Konopleva M (*2018c*) Clinical experience with the BCL2-inhibitor venetoclax in combination therapy for relapsed and refractory acute myeloid leukemia and related myeloid malignancies. Am J Hematol 93:401–407

Dinardo CD, Stein AS, Stein EM, Fathi AT, Frankfurt O, Schuh AC, Martinelli G, Patel PA, Raffoux E, Tan P, Zeidan AM, Botton SD, Kantarjian HM, Stone RM, Lam DH, Gong J, Zhang V, Winkler T, Wu B, Vyas P (*2019*) Mutant IDH1 inhibitor ivosidenib (IVO; AG-120) in combination with azacitidine (AZA) for newly diagnosed acute myeloid leukemia (ND AML). J Clin Oncol 37:7011

DiNardo CD, Schuh AC, Stein EM, Fernandez PM, Wei A, De Botton S, Zeidan AM, Fathi AT, Quek L, Kantarjian HM, Frattini MG, Lersch F, Gong J, Franovic A, MacBeth K, Vyas P, Döhner H (*2019b*) Enasidenib plus azacitidine significantly improves complete remission and overall response compared with azacitidine alone in patients with newly diagnosed acute myeloid leukemia (AML) with isocitrate dehydrogenase 2 (IDH2) mutations: interim phase II results from an ongoing, randomized study. Blood 134:643

DiNardo CD, Pratz K, Pullarkat V, Jonas BA, Arellano M, Becker PS, Frankfurt O, Konopleva M, Wei AH, Kantarjian HM, Xu T, Hong WJ, Chyla B, Potluri J, Pollyea DA, Letai A (*2019c*) Venetoclax combined with decitabine or azacitidine in treatment-naive, elderly patients with acute myeloid leukemia. Blood 133:7–17

Dohner H, Weisdorf DJ, Bloomfield CD (2015) Acute myeloid leukemia. N Engl J Med 373:1136–1152

Dombret H, Seymour JF, Butrym A, Wierzbowska A, Selleslag D, Jang JH, Kumar R, Cavenagh J, Schuh AC, Candoni A, Recher C, Sandhu I, Bernal del Castillo T, Al-Ali HK, Martinelli G, Falantes J, Noppeney R, Stone RM, Minden MD, McIntyre H, Songer S, Lucy LM, Beach CL, Dohner H (2015) International phase 3 study of azacitidine vs conventional care regimens in older patients with newly diagnosed AML with >30% blasts. Blood 126:291–299

Duchmann M, Micol J-B, Duployez N, Raffoux E, Thomas X, Marolleau J-P, Braun T, Ades L, Chantepie S, Lemasle E, Berthon C, Malfuson JV, Pautas C, Lambert J, Boissel N, Celli-Lebras K, Caillot D, Turlure P, Vey N, Pigneux A, Recher C, Terré C, Gardin C, Itzykson R, Preudhomme C, Dombret H, De Botton S (2019) Prognostic significance of concurrent gene mutations in intensively treated patients with IDH1/2 mutated AML. Blood 134:1416

Dumas PY, Naudin C, Martin-Lanneree S, Izac B, Casetti L, Mansier O, Rousseau B, Artus A, Dufossee M, Giese A, Dubus P, Pigneux A, Praloran V, Bidet A, Villacreces A, Guitart A, Milpied N, Kosmider O, Vigon I, Desplat V, Dusanter-Fourt I, Pasquet JM (2019) Hematopoietic niche drives FLT3-ITD acute myeloid leukemia resistance to quizartinib via STAT5-and hypoxia-dependent upregulation of AXL. Haematologica 104:2017–2027

Fathi AT, DiNardo CD, Kline I, Kenvin L, Gupta I, Attar EC, Stein EM, de Botton S, Investigators ACS (2018) Differentiation syndrome associated with Enasidenib, a selective inhibitor of mutant Isocitrate dehydrogenase 2: analysis of a phase 1/2 study. JAMA Oncol 4:1106–1110

Figueroa ME, Abdel-Wahab O, Lu C, Ward PS, Patel J, Shih A, Li Y, Bhagwat N, Vasanthakumar A, Fernandez HF, Tallman MS, Sun Z, Wolniak K, Peeters JK, Liu W, Choe SE, Fantin VR, Paietta E, Lowenberg B, Licht JD, Godley LA, Delwel R, Valk PJ, Thompson CB, Levine RL, Melnick A (2010) Leukemic IDH1 and IDH2 mutations result in a hypermethylation phenotype, disrupt TET2 function, and impair hematopoietic differentiation. Cancer Cell 18:553–567

Hospital MA, Prebet T, Bertoli S, Thomas X, Tavernier E, Braun T, Pautas C, Perrot A, Lioure B, Rousselot P, Tamburini J, Cluzeau T, Konopacki J, Randriamalala E, Berthon C, Gourin MP, Recher C, Cahn JY, Ifrah N, Dombret H, Boissel N (2014) Core-binding factor acute myeloid leukemia in first relapse: a retrospective study from the French AML Intergroup. Blood 124:1312–1319

Hunter AM, Sallman DA (2019) Current status and new treatment approaches in TP53 mutated AML. Best Pract Res Clin Haematol 32:134–144

Intlekofer AM, Shih AH, Wang B, Nazir A, Rustenburg AS, Albanese SK, Patel M, Famulare C, Correa FM, Takemoto N, Durani V, Liu H, Taylor J, Farnoud N, Papaemmanuil E, Cross JR, Tallman MS, Arcila ME, Roshal M, Petsko GA, Wu B, Choe S, Konteatis ZD, Biller SA, Chodera JD, Thompson CB, Levine RL, Stein EM (2018) Acquired resistance to IDH inhibition through trans or cis dimer-interface mutations. Nature 559:125–129

Jensen MK, Johansen P, Stentoft J, Jensen MK (1994) Salvage therapy with low-dose cytosine arabinoside in refractory or relapsed acute non-lymphocytic leukaemia: a report on 25 patients. Eur J Haematol 52:236–239

Klepin HD, Ritchie E, Major-Elechi B, Le-Rademacher J, Seisler D, Storrick L, Sanford BL, Marcucci G, Zhao W, Geyer SA, Ballman KV, Powell BL, Baer MR, Stock W, Cohen HJ, Stone RM, Larson RA, Uy GL (2020) Geriatric assessment among older adults receiving intensive therapy for acute myeloid leukemia: report of CALGB 361006 (Alliance). J Geriatr Oncol 11:107–113

Konopleva M, Pollyea DA, Potluri J, Chyla B, Hogdal L, Busman T, McKeegan E, Salem AH, Zhu M, Ricker JL, Blum W, DiNardo CD, Kadia T, Dunbar M, Kirby R, Falotico N, Leverson J, Humerickhouse R, Mabry M, Stone R, Kantarjian H, Letai A (2016) Efficacy and biological correlates of response in a phase II study of venetoclax monotherapy in patients with acute myelogenous leukemia. Cancer Discov 6:1106–1117

Lagadinou ED, Sach A, Callahan K, Rossi RM, Neering SJ, Minhajuddin M, Ashton JM, Pei S, Grose V, O'Dwyer KM, Liesveld JL, Brookes PS, Becker MW, Jordan CT (2013) BCL-2 inhibition targets oxidative phosphorylation and selectively eradicates quiescent human leukemia stem cells. Cell Stem Cell 12:329–341

Larson RA, Sievers EL, Stadtmauer EA, Lowenberg B, Estey EH, Dombret H, Theobald M, Voliotis D, Bennett JM, Richie M, Leopold LH, Berger MS, Sherman ML, Loken MR, van Dongen JJ, Bernstein ID, Appelbaum FR (2005) Final report of the efficacy and safety of gemtuzumab ozogamicin (Mylotarg) in patients with CD33-positive acute myeloid leukemia in first recurrence. Cancer 104:1442–1452

Lee LY, Hernandez D, Rajkhowa T, Smith SC, Raman JR, Nguyen B, Small D, Levis M (2017) Preclinical studies of gilteritinib, a next-generation FLT3 inhibitor. Blood 129:257–260

Mathew NR, Baumgartner F, Braun L, O'Sullivan D, Thomas S et al (2018) Sorafenib promotes graft-versus-leukemia activity in mice and humans through IL-15 production in FLT3-ITD-mutant leukemia cells. Nat Med 24:282–291

McMahon CM, Canaani J, Rea B, Sargent RL, Qualtieri JN, Watt CD, Morrissette JJD, Carroll M, Perl AE (*2019a*) Gilteritinib induces differentiation in relapsed and refractory FLT3-mutated acute myeloid leukemia. Blood Adv 3:1581–1585

McMahon CM, Ferng T, Canaani J, Wang ES, Morrissette JJD, Eastburn DJ, Pellegrino M, Durruthy-Durruthy R, Watt CD, Asthana S, Lasater EA, DeFilippis R, Peretz CAC, McGary LHF, Deihimi S, Logan AC,

Luger SM, Shah NP, Carroll M, Smith CC, Perl AE (*2019b*) Clonal selection with RAS pathway activation mediates secondary clinical resistance to selective FLT3 inhibition in acute myeloid leukemia. Cancer Discov 9:1050–1063

Megias-Vericat JE, Martinez-Cuadron D, Sanz MA, Montesinos P (2018) Salvage regimens using conventional chemotherapy agents for relapsed/refractory adult AML patients: a systematic literature review. Ann Hematol 97:1115–1153

Metzelder SK, Schroeder T, Finck A, Scholl S, Fey M, Gotze K, Linn YC, Kroger M, Reiter A, Salih HR, Heinicke T, Stuhlmann R, Muller L, Giagounidis A, Meyer RG, Brugger W, Vohringer M, Dreger P, Mori M, Basara N, Schafer-Eckart K, Schultheis B, Baldus C, Neubauer A, Burchert A (2012) High activity of sorafenib in FLT3-ITD-positive acute myeloid leukemia synergizes with allo-immune effects to induce sustained responses. Leukemia 26:2353–2359

Molga A, Wall M, Chhetri R, Wee LY, Singhal D, Edwards S, Singhal N, Ross D, To LB, Caughey G, Shakib S, Germing U, To T, Hiwase D (2020) Comprehensive geriatric assessment predicts azacitidine treatment duration and survival in older patients with myelodysplastic syndromes. J Geriatr Oncol 11:114–120

Montalban-Bravo G, DiNardo CD (2018) The role of IDH mutations in acute myeloid leukemia. Future Oncol 14:979–993

Mori M, Kaneko N, Ueno Y, Yamada M, Tanaka R, Saito R, Shimada I, Mori K, Kuromitsu S (2017) Gilteritinib, a FLT3/AXL inhibitor, shows antileukemic activity in mouse models of FLT3 mutated acute myeloid leukemia. Invest New Drugs 35:556–565

Papaemmanuil E, Dohner H, Campbell PJ (*2016a*) Genomic classification in acute myeloid leukemia. N Engl J Med 375:900–901

Papaemmanuil E, Gerstung M, Bullinger L, Gaidzik VI, Paschka P, Roberts ND, Potter NE, Heuser M, Thol F, Bolli N, Gundem G, Van Loo P, Martincorena I, Ganly P, Mudie L, McLaren S, O'Meara S, Raine K, Jones DR, Teague JW, Butler AP, Greaves MF, Ganser A, Dohner K, Schlenk RF, Dohner H, Campbell PJ (*2016b*) Genomic classification and prognosis in acute myeloid leukemia. N Engl J Med 374:2209–2221

Paschka P, Schlenk RF, Gaidzik VI, Habdank M, Kronke J, Bullinger L, Spath D, Kayser S, Zucknick M, Gotze K, Horst HA, Germing U, Dohner H, Dohner K (2010) IDH1 and IDH2 mutations are frequent genetic alterations in acute myeloid leukemia and confer adverse prognosis in cytogenetically normal acute myeloid leukemia with NPM1 mutation without FLT3 internal tandem duplication. J Clin Oncol 28:3636–3643

Patel JP, Gonen M, Figueroa ME, Fernandez H, Sun Z, Racevskis J, Van Vlierberghe P, Dolgalev I, Thomas S, Aminova O, Huberman K, Cheng J, Viale A, Socci ND, Heguy A, Cherry A, Vance G, Higgins RR, Ketterling RP, Gallagher RE, Litzow M, van den Brink MR, Lazarus HM, Rowe JM, Luger S, Ferrando A, Paietta E, Tallman MS, Melnick A, Abdel-Wahab O, Levine RL (2012) Prognostic relevance of integrated genetic profiling in acute myeloid leukemia. N Engl J Med 366:1079–1089

Perdrix A, Najem A, Saussez S, Awada A, Journe F, Ghanem G, Krayem M (2017) PRIMA-1 and PRIMA-1(Met) (APR-246): from mutant/wild type p53 reactivation to unexpected mechanisms underlying their potent anti-tumor effect in combinatorial therapies. Cancers 9:172

Perl AE, Martinelli G, Cortes JE, Neubauer A, Berman E, Paolini S, Montesinos P, Baer MR, Larson RA, Ustun C, Fabbiano F, Erba HP, Di Stasi A, Stuart R, Olin R, Kasner M, Ciceri F, Chou WC, Podoltsev N, Recher C, Yokoyama H, Hosono N, Yoon SS, Lee JH, Pardee T, Fathi AT, Liu C, Hasabou N, Liu X, Bahceci E, Levis MJ (*2019a*) Gilteritinib or chemotherapy for relapsed or refractory FLT3-mutated AML. N Engl J Med 381:1728–1740

Perl AE, Daver NG, Pratz KW, Maly J, Hong W-J, Bahceci E, Tong B, Tian T, Dilley K (*2019b*) Venetoclax in combination with gilteritinib in patients with relapsed/refractory acute myeloid leukemia: a phase 1b study. Blood 134:3910

Podoltsev NA, Stahl M, Zeidan AM, Gore SD (2017) Selecting initial treatment of acute myeloid leukaemia in older adults. Blood Rev 31:43–62

Pratz KW, Sato T, Murphy KM, Stine A, Rajkhowa T, Levis M (2010) FLT3-mutant allelic burden and clinical status are predictive of response to FLT3 inhibitors in AML. Blood 115:1425–1432

Quek L, David MD, Kennedy A, Metzner M, Amatangelo M, Shih A, Stoilova B, Quivoron C, Heiblig M, Willekens C, Saada V, Alsafadi S, Vijayabaskar MS, Peniket A, Bernard OA, Agresta S, Yen K, MacBeth K, Stein E, Vassiliou GS, Levine R, De Botton S, Thakurta A, Penard-Lacronique V, Vyas P (2018) Clonal heterogeneity of acute myeloid leukemia treated with the IDH2 inhibitor enasidenib. Nat Med 24:1167–1177

Roboz GJ, Rosenblat T, Arellano M, Gobbi M, Altman JK, Montesinos P, O'Connell C, Solomon SR, Pigneux A, Vey N, Hills R, Jacobsen TF, Gianella-Borradori A, Foss O, Vetrhusand S, Giles FJ (2014) International randomized phase III study of elacytarabine versus investigator choice in patients with relapsed/refractory acute myeloid leukemia. J Clin Oncol 32:1919–1926

Rollig C, Bornhauser M, Kramer M, Thiede C, Ho AD, Kramer A, Schafer-Eckart K, Wandt H, Hanel M, Einsele H, Aulitzky WE, Schmitz N, Berdel WE, Stelljes M, Muller-Tidow C, Krug U, Platzbecker U, Wermke M, Baldus CD, Krause SW, Stolzel F, von Bonin M, Schaich M, Serve H, Schetelig J, Ehninger G (2015) Allogeneic stem-cell transplantation in patients with NPM1-mutated acute myeloid leukemia: results from a prospective donor versus no-donor analysis of patients after upfront HLA typing within the SAL-AML 2003 trial. J Clin Oncol 33:403–410

Sallman DA, DeZern AE, Garcia-Manero G, Steensma DP, Roboz GJ, Sekeres MA, Cluzeau T, Sweet KL, McLemore AF, McGraw K, Puskas J, Zhang L, Yao J, Mo Q, Nardelli L, Al Ali N, Padron E, Korbel G,

Attar EC, Kantarjian HM, Lancet JE, Fenaux P, List AF, Komrokji RS (2019) Phase 2 results of APR-246 and azacitidine (AZA) in patients with TP53 mutant myelodysplastic syndromes (MDS) and oligoblastic acute myeloid leukemia (AML). Blood 134:676

Sarkozy C, Gardin C, Gachard N, Merabet F, Turlure P, Malfuson JV, Pautas C, Micol JB, Thomas X, Quesnel B, Celli-Lebras K, Preudhomme C, Terre C, Fenaux P, Chevret S, Castaigne S, Dombret H (2013) Outcome of older patients with acute myeloid leukemia in first relapse. Am J Hematol 88:758–764

Schlenk RF, Frech P, Weber D, Brossart P, Horst HA, Kraemer D, Held G, Ringhoffer M, Burchardt A, Kobbe G, Gotze K, Nachbaur D, Fischer T, Lubbert M, Salih HR, Salwender H, Wulf G, Koller E, Wattad M, Fiedler W, Kremers S, Kirchen H, Hertenstein B, Paschka P, Gaidzik VI, Teleanu V, Heuser M, Thol F, Dohner K, Krauter J, Ganser A, Dohner H, the German-Austrian A. (2017) Impact of pretreatment characteristics and salvage strategy on outcome in patients with relapsed acute myeloid leukemia. Leukemia 31:1217–1220

Sexauer A, Perl A, Yang X, Borowitz M, Gocke C, Rajkhowa T, Thiede C, Frattini M, Nybakken GE, Pratz K, Karp J, Smith BD, Levis M (2012) Terminal myeloid differentiation in vivo is induced by FLT3 inhibition in FLT3/ITD AML. Blood 120:4205–4214

Shimizu H, Yokohama A, Ishizaki T, Hatsumi N, Takada S, Saitoh T, Sakura T, Nojima Y, Handa H (2018) Clonal evolution detected with conventional cytogenetic analysis is a potent prognostic factor in adult patients with relapsed AML. Hematol Oncol 36:252–257

Smith CC, Paguirigan A, Jeschke GR, Lin KC, Massi E, Tarver T, Chin CS, Asthana S, Olshen A, Travers KJ, Wang S, Levis MJ, Perl AE, Radich JP, Shah NP (2017) Heterogeneous resistance to quizartinib in acute myeloid leukemia revealed by single-cell analysis. Blood 130:48–58

Smith CC, Levis MJ, Perl AE, Martinelli G, Neubauer A, Berman E, Montesinos P, Baer MR, Larson RA, Chou W-C, Yokoyama H, Recher C, Yoon S-S, Hill JE, Rosales M, Bahceci E (2019) Emerging mutations at relapse in patients with FLT3-mutated relapsed/refractory acute myeloid leukemia who received gilteritinib therapy in the phase 3 admiral trial. Blood 134:14

Sorror ML, Storer BE, Fathi AT, Gerds AT, Medeiros BC, Shami P, Brunner AM, Sekeres MA, Mukherjee S, Pena E, Elsawy M, Wardyn S, Whitten J, Moore R, Becker PS, McCune JS, Appelbaum FR, Estey EH (2017) Development and validation of a novel acute myeloid leukemia-composite model to estimate risks of mortality. JAMA Oncol 3:1675–1682

Stahl M, DeVeaux M, Montesinos P, Itzykson R, Ritchie EK, Sekeres MA, Barnard JD, Podoltsev NA, Brunner AM, Komrokji RS, Bhatt VR, Al-Kali A, Cluzeau T, Santini V, Fathi AT, Roboz GJ, Fenaux P, Litzow MR, Perreault S, Kim TK, Prebet T, Vey N, Verma V, Germing U, Bergua JM, Serrano J, Gore SD, Zeidan AM (2018) Hypomethylating agents in relapsed and refractory AML: outcomes and their predictors in a large international patient cohort. Blood Adv 2:923–932

Stein EM (2018) Enasidenib, a targeted inhibitor of mutant IDH2 proteins for treatment of relapsed or refractory acute myeloid leukemia. Future Oncol 14:23–40

Taksin AL, Legrand O, Raffoux E, de Revel T, Thomas X, Contentin N, Bouabdallah R, Pautas C, Turlure P, Reman O, Gardin C, Varet B, de Botton S, Pousset F, Farhat H, Chevret S, Dombret H, Castaigne S (2007) High efficacy and safety profile of fractionated doses of mylotarg as induction therapy in patients with relapsed acute myeloblastic leukemia: a prospective study of the ALFA Group. Leukemia 21:66–71

Thol F, Schlenk RF, Heuser M, Ganser A (2015) How I treat refractory and early relapsed acute myeloid leukemia. Blood 126:319–327

Ward PS, Patel J, Wise DR, Abdel-Wahab O, Bennett BD, Coller HA, Cross JR, Fantin VR, Hedvat CV, Perl AE, Rabinowitz JD, Carroll M, Su SM, Sharp KA, Levine RL, Thompson CB (2010) The common feature of leukemia-associated IDH1 and IDH2 mutations is a neomorphic enzyme activity converting alpha-ketoglutarate to 2-hydroxyglutarate. Cancer Cell 17:225–234

Wattad M, Weber D, Dohner K, Krauter J, Gaidzik VI, Paschka P, Heuser M, Thol F, Kindler T, Lubbert M, Salih HR, Kundgen A, Horst HA, Brossart P, Gotze K, Nachbaur D, Kohne CH, Ringhoffer M, Wulf G, Held G, Salwender H, Benner A, Ganser A, Dohner H, Schlenk RF (2017) Impact of salvage regimens on response and overall survival in acute myeloid leukemia with induction failure. Leukemia 31:1306–1313

Watts JM, Baer MR, Yang J, Prebet T, Lee S, Schiller GJ, Dinner S, Pigneux A, Montesinos P, Wang ES, Seiter K, Wei AH, De Botton S, Arnan Sangerman M, Donnellan WB, Jonas BA, Ferrell PB Jr, Dao K-H, Kelly P, Sweeney J, Forsyth S, Guichard S, Brevard J, Henrick P, Mohamed H, Cortes JE (2019) Olutasidenib (FT 2102), an IDH1m inhibitor as a single agent or in combination with azacitidine, induces deep clinical responses with mutation clearance in patients with acute myeloid leukemia treated in a phase 1 dose escalation and expansion study. Blood 134:231

Wei AH, Tiong IS (2017) Midostaurin, enasidenib, CPX-351, gemtuzumab ozogamicin, and venetoclax bring new hope to AML. Blood 130:2469–2474

Wei AH, Strickland SA Jr, Hou JZ, Fiedler W, Lin TL, Walter RB, Enjeti A, Tiong IS, Savona M, Lee S, Chyla B, Popovic R, Salem AH, Agarwal S, Xu T, Fakouhi KM, Humerickhouse R, Hong WJ, Hayslip J, Roboz GJ (2019) Venetoclax combined with low-dose cytarabine for previously untreated patients with acute myeloid leukemia: results from a phase Ib/II study. J Clin Oncol 37:1277–1284

Wei AH, Montesinos P, Ivanov V, DiNardo CD, Novak J, Laribi K, Kim I, Stevens DA, Fiedler W, Pagoni M, Samoilova O, Hu Y, Anagnostopoulos A, Bergeron J, Hou JZ, Murthy V, Yamauchi T, McDonald A, Chyla B, Gopalakrishnan S, Jiang Q, Mendes W, Hayslip J, Panayiotidis P (2020) Venetoclax plus LDAC for newly diagnosed AML ineligible for intensive chemotherapy: a phase 3 randomized placebo-controlled trial. Blood 135:2137–2145

Welch JS, Petti AA, Miller CA, Fronick CC, O'Laughlin M, Fulton RS, Wilson RK, Baty JD, Duncavage EJ, Tandon B, Lee YS, Wartman LD, Uy GL, Ghobadi A, Tomasson MH, Pusic I, Romee R, Fehniger TA, Stockerl-Goldstein KE, Vij R, Oh ST, Abboud CN, Cashen AF, Schroeder MA, Jacoby MA, Heath SE, Luber K, Janke MR, Hantel A, Khan N, Sukhanova MJ, Knoebel RW, Stock W, Graubert TA, Walter MJ, Westervelt P, Link DC, DiPersio JF, Ley TJ (2016) TP53 and decitabine in acute myeloid leukemia and myelodysplastic syndromes. N Engl J Med 375:2023–2036

# Allogeneic Hematopoietic Cell Transplantation

13

Martin Bornhäuser

## 13.1 Introduction

Recent statistics of the European Group for Blood and Marrow Transplantation (EBMT) suggest that AML is by far the No. 1 indication for allogeneic HCT in Europe. https://www.ebmt.org/registry/transplant-activity-survey/ 22.07.2020 (Fig. 13.1).

The most important point is to check the availability of potential allogeneic HCT donors as possible after the diagnosis of AML in patients with an acceptable performance status. This will ensure that timely transplant procedure can be planned in case of intermediate or high-risk profile. In patients with favorable risk profile, persistence, or reoccurrence of measurable residual disease may also be an indication for a donor search. Results of HLA typing of patients and potential donors should be available as late as 2–3 weeks after the first induction cycle had been started. This will ensure to plan allogeneic HCT in the first 20–30% of patients who are refractory to first induction therapy. As time from diagnosis or relapse to transplant remains an important confounder of outcome, timely donor identification of potential donors is key for successful therapy.

M. Bornhäuser (✉)
Med. Klinik und Poliklinik I, Universitätsklinikum Carl Gustav Carus, Dresden, Germany
e-mail: Martin.bornhaeuser@ukdd.de

### 13.1.1 Principles of Allogeneic Hematopoietic Cell Transplantation

Allogeneic HCT is clearly offering the highest chance of long-term cure in patients with high-risk AML. In intermediate-risk disease, patient, and donor-specific factors have to be integrated to weigh the individual risk of transplant-related mortality against the disease-specific risks (Cornelissen et al. 2012). Several models are offered with the EBMT risk score and the Sorror score being the most well-established systems allowing assessment of transplant-specific parameters and comorbidities (Gratwohl 2012; Elsawy and Sorror 2016). Besides the antileukemic activity of conditioning therapy, the eradication of leukemic cells is mainly achieved by the allogeneic immune effects of the graft (Graft-versus-Leukemia Reaction, GvL). The most relevant effector cells in this context are CD8+ cytotoxic T cells and CD4 helper cells. Apart from major histocompatibility antigens (HLA), minor HLA but also leukemia-associated antigens may act as target antigen for GvL effects.

The profound allogeneic immune effects result in a significantly lower incidence of relapse compared to any other postremission therapy (Cornelissen et al. 2007). As alloimmunity also leads to life-threatening Graft-versus-Host disease (GvHD), several efforts have been undertaken to reduce the risk for GvHD by T cell



C. Röllig, G. J. Ossenkoppele (eds.), *Acute Myeloid Leukemia*, Hematologic Malignancies,
https://doi.org/10.1007/978-3-030-72676-8_13

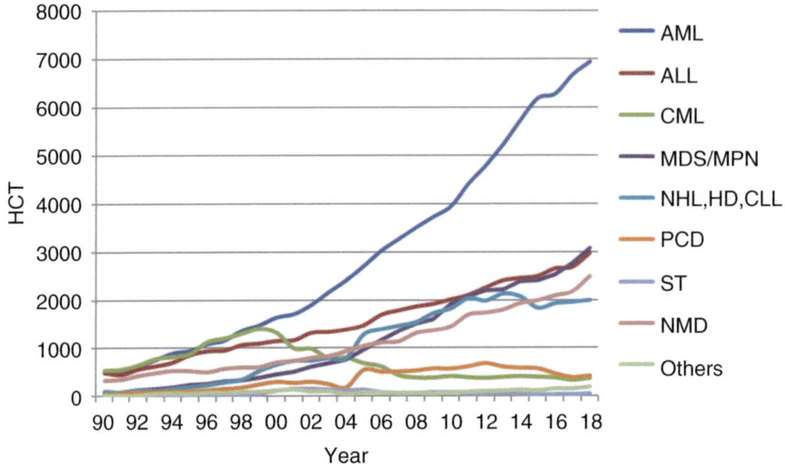


**Fig. 13.1** Number of allogeneic HCT procedures per indication performed in Europe between 1990 and 2018. *MDS* Myelodysplastic syndrome, *AML* acute myeloid leukemia, *ALL* acute lymphoblastiuc leukemia, *CML* chronic myeloid leukemia, *MPN* myeloproliferative neoplasm, *NHL* Non-Hoddgkin's disease, *HD* Hodgkins lymphoma, *CLL* chronic lymphocytic leukemia, PCD plasma cell dyscrasia, *ST* solid tumor, *NMD* non-malignant disease

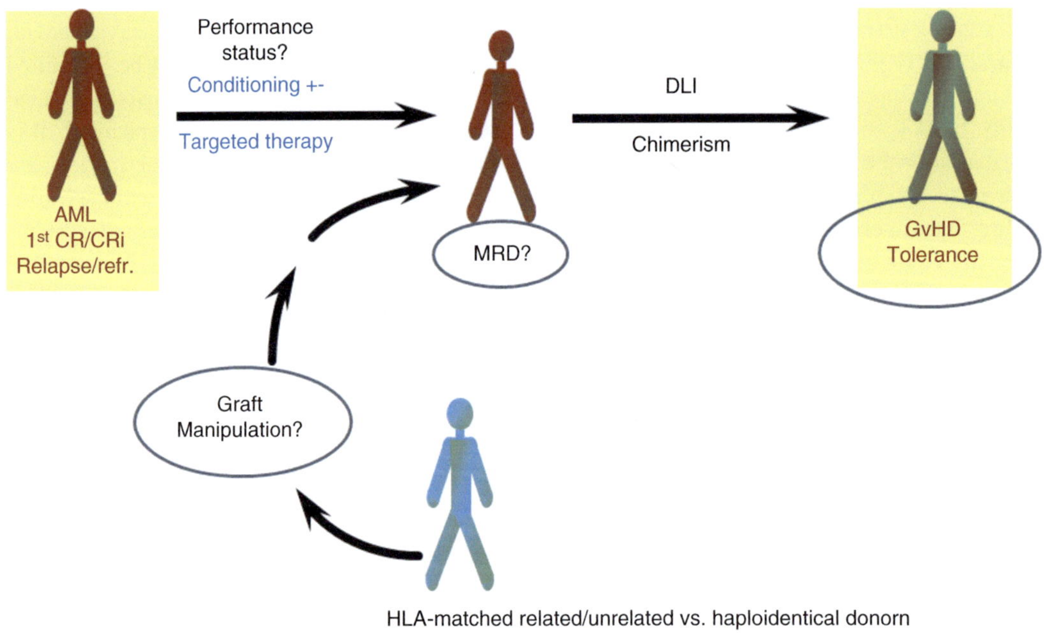


**Fig. 13.2** Principle of allogeneic HCT. *MRD* measurable residual disease, *CR* complete remission, *CRi* complete remission with inclomplete platelet recovery, *refr.* refractory, *DLI* donor lymphocyte infusion, *HLA* human leukocyte antigen, *GvHD* graft-versus-host disease

depletion either in vitro in the graft or by the infusion of T cell-depleting agents (e.g., antithymocyte globulin (ATG), MabCampath). In patients with measurable residual disease or mixed chimerism after transplantation, the infusion of donor lymphocytes (DLI) may be an appropriate intervention to avoid hematologic relapse. Ideally, immunologic tolerance between donor and recipient may occur later after HCT allowing the cessation of pharmacologic immunosuppression.

The overall concept of allogeneic HCT is depicted in Fig. 13.2.

### 13.1.2 Indications for Allogeneic HCT

In general, the indication for allogeneic HCT in AML patients has to balance the risk of non-relapse mortality with that of disease recurrence using conventional postremission therapy (Cornelissen et al. 2012). Outweighing these risk and benefits is valid for all recipients of allogeneic HCT but may become specifically difficult to assess in older patients with AML and comorbidities with impaired residual organ function. Still, it may be worthwhile to reevaulate a patient after having responded to induction therapy when performance status may have improved. As the available donor is a critical determinant of transplantation-associated risk assessment, the availability of information on this parameter needs to be acquired as soon as possible after initial diagnosis.

Whereas two most widely used scoring system, the Hematopoietic Cell Transplantation Comorbidity Index (http://hctci.org), focuses on non-hematologic organ function, the Pretransplant Assessment of Mortality (PAM; http://pamscore.org) Score includes information on AML subcategory, donor type, and cytomegalovirus (CMV) serostatus of both patient and donor. In this regard, the PAM score is similar to the EBMT risk score (https://hematol.ch/scorecalc/stem-cell-transplantation/ebmt) but may be more useful for the many patients within the age category of >65 years. In general, allogeneic HCT should be recommended if the expected survival benefit exceeds 15%.

Incorporating AML disease-risk and transplant-associated risk may lead to the following weighting algorithms (Table 13.1, adapted and edited from Cornelissen et al. (2012):

Besides objective parameters, the patients and his/her family's expectations have to be integrated in the overall concept. Additional factors here might be the intolerance of consolidation therapy and protracted cytopenia with no signs of recovery. In order to plan and prepare allogeneic HCT the following aspects have to be taken into account:

- Choice of the ideal donor/graft source
- Preparative regimen allowing for cytoreduction and elimination of residual disease
- Serotherapy and immunosuppression to overcome HLA barriers and to reduce the risk for severe Graft-versus-Host Disease (GvHD)
- Social/psychological wishes of patients and family members

### 13.1.3 Donor Selection and Graft Source

Although the recommendations on donor selection are based on large retrospective data, the algorithms in which available siblings are initially HLA-typed with the patient have remained

**Table 13.1** Indication for allogeneic HCT in AML according to an integrated risk scoring

| Stage of disease | MRD after induction or during cons | Risk of relapse | EBMT score | HCT-CI | Donor |
|---|---|---|---|---|---|
| CR 1 intermediate | Neg. | 50% | ≤2 | ≤2 | MSD, 10/10 or 9/10 permissive DBP1 |
| | Pos. | >60% | ≤3 | ≤3 | MSD, UD 10/10 or 9/10 or Haplo |
| CR 1 adverse | Neg./pos. | • 80% | ≤3–4 | ≤3–4 | MSD, UD 10/10 or 9/10 or Haplo |
| CR 2 | – | • >70% | ≤4 | ≤4 | MSD, UD 10/10 or 9/10 or Haplo |
| Primary refractory | – | • >90% | ≤5 | ≤5 | MSD, UD 10/10 or 9/10 or Haplo |

*CR1* 1. First complete remission, *MSD* matched sibling donor, *UD* unrelated donor, *cons.* consolidation, *neg.* negative, *pos.* positive, *haplo* haploidentical

[a]Non-acute promyelocytic leukemia (APL)

stable. In many patients without an eligible donor or in older in patients in whom siblings may be medically ineligible, an early initiation of an unrelated donor search is key. Given the many available donors in international registries, 70–80% of patients should find a suitable match within 4–6 weeks. According to the most recent National Marrow Donor Program (NMDP) guidelines, patients and donors should be typed at high-resolution level for HLA-A, B, C, DRB1, and in case of unrelated donor selection, DBP1 should be included in order to identify potentially permissive mismatches (Dehn et al. 2019). As DBP1 is a relevant target antigen for Graft-versus-Leukemia reactions, acceptance of a non-permissive mismatch may be an acceptable option in patients with adverse risk or relapsed disease. Current prospective registry trials have been initiated in order to confirm the relevance and feasibility of prospective DBP1 matching.

Finally, patients with a clear indication for allogeneic HCT are candidates for haploidentical transplantation. In this case children, and parents for younger patients, and extended family members may be suitable donors and should be asked for HLA-typing when no 9/10 matched unrelated donor can be identified. This algorithm allows identifying a donor for >95% of patients within 3–4 weeks from initial diagnosis.

Prospective and retrospective data do not suggest that the use of G-CSF mobilized blood is significantly superior to transplantation of bone marrow. Most centers prefer G-CSF mobilized peripheral blood in patients with AML to enhance the speed of engraftment and to mediate more profound allogeneic GvL effects coming with an increased risk of chronic GvHD. The use of cord blood from sibling and unrelated donors is an option as alternative graft source. Give the differences in donor availability, cord blood has become a standard source for allogeneic HCT in the United States and in southern Europe but is virtually not used in northern Europe.

### 13.1.4 Preparative Regimen

In patients with AML, conditioning intensity has still to be considered as important component of the overall cytoreductive treatment concept. Most recently, a randomized trial has suggested that the risk of relapse increases significantly when lower doses of alkylating agents are applied in AML and MDS (Scott et al. 2017). Therefore, younger patients (<40 years) with no comorbidities should receive standard intensity regimens based on 12.8 mg/kg intravenous busulfan (Bu) or total-body irradiation (TBI, 10–12 Gy). Whether Bu or TBI should be combined with cyclophosphamide (Cy) or fludarabine (Flu) has also been addressed in randomized trials of smaller size. Currently, the use of Flu/Bu with ablative doses of Bu seems to be the most widely adopted protocol with preserved antileukemic activity but better tolerability. Along these lines, the combination of 8 Gy TBI combined with Flu was associated with lower non-relapse mortality, preserved relapse-free survival, and convincing long-term results in patients with AML in first CR (Fasslrinner et al. 2018). With the advent of postgrafting Cy as effective prophylaxis of GvHD, the use of Flu before transplantation gains additional rationale (Fig. 13.3).

The Flu/Bu regimen can be safely applied until the age of 60. Above this age category, the use of Treosulfan (Treo) at 3 × 10 g/sqm combined with Flu has been shown to have superior outcomes when combined with 50% of the ablative Bu dose and Flu (Beelen et al. 2020). This has led to the licensure of Treo as conditioning therapy. Further potential combination partners for Flu in reduced-intensity protocols (RIC) can be melphalan at 100–140 mg/sqm or cyclophosphamide (e.g., 2 × 40–60 mg/kg). Minimal conditioning with Flu and 2 Gy TBI or Cy is feasible but is associated with a high incidence of relapse in patients with AML (Gyurkocza et al. 2010).

In patients with refractory AML or relapse in whom a suitable donor is in sight and can be approached within weeks may benefit from a so called "sequential" conditioning therapy (Fig. 13.4). Compared to conventional conditioning, sequential regimens, with FLAMSA-RIC as a prototypic example integrate intermediate dose cytarabine with amsacrine or anthracyclines shortly followed by a RIC regimen based on busulfan or lower doses of TBI (Heinicke et al. 2018).

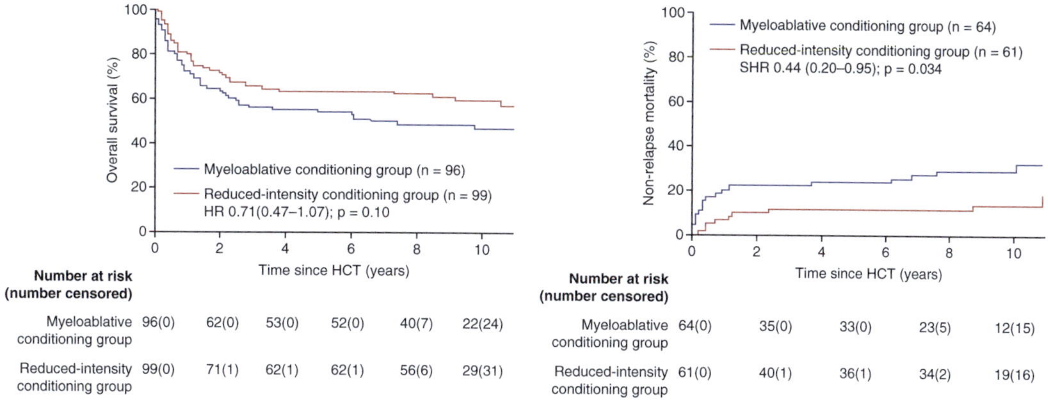


**Fig. 13.3** 10 year follow-up of a randomized trial of 12 Gy TBI/Cy and Flu/8 Gy TBI showing a significantly lower non-relapse mortality for RIC (right panel) in patients with AML in first CR (Fasslrinner et al. 2018)

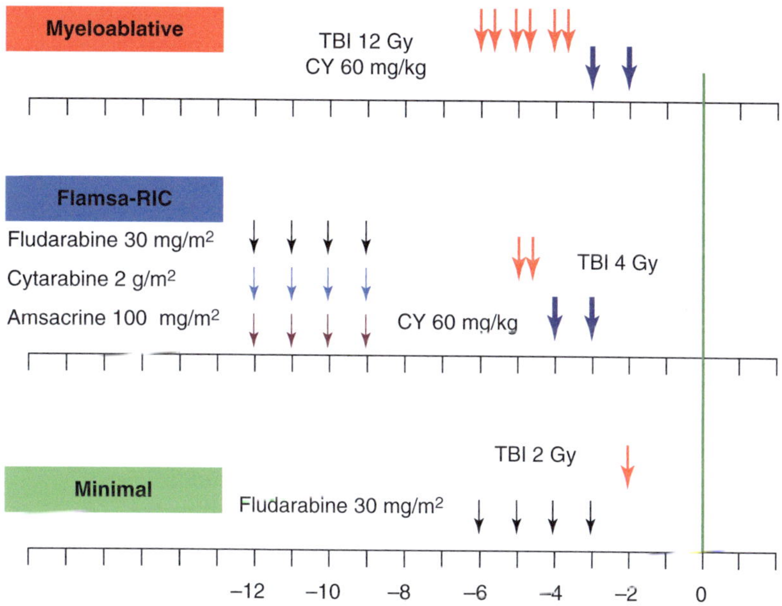


**Fig. 13.4** Comparison of conventional myeloablative, sequential (FLAMSA-RIC), and minimal conditioning. *TBI* total-body irradiation, *Cy* cyclophosphamide, *RIC* reduced-intensity conditioning (Courtesy of Gesine Bug, University Hospital Frankfurt)

### 13.1.5 GvHD Prophylaxis

Besides relapse of leukemia, GvHD is the major reason for treatment failure after allogeneic HCT. The disease is categorized according to onset and severity in an acute and a chronic subtype. While acute GvHD occurs in the first months after HCT and may affect skin, liver, and gut, chronic GvHD is a systemic disease mimicking autoimmune diseases like sclerodermia and vasculitis. Steroid refractory acute GvHD is a life-threatening complication, chronic GvHD is associated with relevant morbidity and a dramatic decrease of quality of life.

Since the introduction of calcineurin inhibitors (CNIs) in the 1980s of the last century, cyclosporine and later tacrolimus have been established as the core component of most prophylactic regimens. They are typically combined with methotrexate on days 1, 3, 6, and 11 or with Mycophenolate mofetil (MMF), although MMF has never been established as equivalent. Serotherapy with Antithymocyte globulin (ATG) or the anti-CD52 antibody MabCampath is used in patients receiving grafts from unrelated or mismatched donors. ATG has shown to significantly reduce the incidence of acute and chronic GvHD (Finke et al. 2009). Patients may also receive mTOR inhibitors (e.g., sirolimus or everolimus) in combination with tacrolimus or MMF (Rodriguez et al. 2010). A more recent development is the use of high-dose Cy on days 3 and 4 after allogeneic HCT (PTCy) followed by CNI ± MMF with the aim of preferentially targeting alloreactive T cells. This strategy has been shown to be superior in preventing chronic GvHD in a randomized trial (De Jong et al. 2019).

Finally, T cell depletion from the graft is the most efficient way of reducing the risk of relapse but has repeatedly been associated with an increased risk of relapse and graft failure (Pasquini et al. 2012). The results of randomized trials comparing CD34+ selection with pharmacologic regimens have to be awaited.

Table 13.2 summarizes the most widely used pharamcologic regimens applied as prophylaxis for GvHD.

The risk for acute and secondary chronic GvHD is determined by the following factors:

- HLA match
- Female donor for male patients
- Patient and donor age
- Graft source (Peripheral blood associated with more chronic GvHD)
- Graft manipulation (in vivo/in vitro T cell depletion)
- GvHD prophylaxis
- Intestinal dysbiosis

Until now, pre-transplant cellular assays have not been established as predictive biomarkers for the risk of GvHD. Post-transplant biomarkers in serum and urine have been validated to predict for the occurrence of acute GvHD albeit no controlled trial has indicated so far, that early intervention can change the outcome of these high-risk patients (Major-Monfried et al. 2018; Kaiser et al. 2004). Until now, optimized HLA matching and efficient prophylactic regimens are the mainstay for the successful outcome of allogeneic HCT.

### 13.1.6 Therapy of GvHD

Therapy of acute GvHD is based on steroids (prednisolone equivalents of 1–2 mg/kg) whenever grade II disease is diagnosed. Two-thirds of patients require escalation of immunosuppres-

**Table 13.2** Pharmacologic regimens for GvHD prophylaxis

| Regimen | Mode of application | Remarks |
|---|---|---|
| Cyclosporine A (CsA) + Methotrexate (Mtx) | CsA from day −1<br>Mtx 10 mg/m$^2$ day 1, 3, 6, 11 | Target trough levels need to be controlled<br>Rescue with calcium folinate accodting to local standard |
| Tacrolimus (FK506) + Mtx | Tacrolimus from day −1<br>Mtx s.o. | Target trough levels. Folinate s.o. |
| CsA or Tacrolimus + Mycophenolate mofetil (MMF) | CsA/Tacrolimus from day −3 or −1<br>MMF 2–3 × 15 mg/kg from day 0 | Most frequently after RIC or minimal conditioning |
| Tacrolimus + Sirolimus or Everolimus | Tacrolimus from day −3<br>Sirolimus from day −3 | Needs drug monitoring. Cave: Sinusoidal obstruction syndrome |
| Antithymocyte globulin (ATG) | Grafalon (Neovi) 3 × 10–20 mg/kg, Thymoglobulin (Sanofi) 3 × 1.0–1.5 mg/kg from day −3 bis −1 | Doses of different preparations. Acute side effects require premedication and monitoring |
| Post Grafting Cyclophosphamide (PTCy) | 50 mg/kg on days +3 and +4 | Requires hydration and MESNA |
| Sirolimus + MMF | Sirolimus from day −3<br>MMF from day 0 | Limited clinical experience |
| MabCampath | 20–100 mg over 3–4 days | Requires regular chimerism analyses and DLI in 50–60% of patients |

sion including higher doses of steroids and targeted therapies with ruxolitinib being the only compound tested in randomized trial with signs of superior activity (Zeiser et al. 2020). Further second line therapies may include pentostatin, anti-TNFalpha antibodies, Mycophenolate mofetil (MMF), Tocilizumab, Vedolizumab, Alemtuzumab, ATG, and extracorporeal photopheresis (ECP). Cell-based therapies with Mesenchymal Stromal Cells (MSC) have shown promising results especially in children with acute GvHD (Hashmi et al. 2016). As mentioned above, patients with steroid refractory acute GvHD have dismal prognosis despite advances in therapy and supportive care.

Chronic GvHD is also treated with steroids again followed by second line immunosuppressants with ibrutinib being the only licensed compound in the United States for this indication so far. Second line therapies include ECP, rituximab, MMF, mTOR inhibitors, methotrexate, and low-dose interleukin-2.

### 13.1.7 Supportive Care

All patients after allogeneic HCT need to be regularly screened for the occurrence of opportunistic infections. This includes monitoring of CMV and other herpesviridae via PCR testing and the application of antifungal and antiviral prophylactic medication. Patients receiving steroids for GvHD therapy should receive prophylaxis with mold-active antifungals (e.g., posaconazole). In addition, cotrimoxazole should be applied to prevent pneumocystis jiroveci infection. For further details, dedicated reviews are recommended (Ullmann et al. 2016).

## 13.2 Results of Allogeneic HCT

### 13.2.1 AML in First CR

In the last two decades several cooperative AML study groups have tried to compare the efficacy of allogeneic HCT with conventional consolidation therapy based on an intent-to-treat analysis based on the availability of a HLA matched sibling donor (Cornelissen et al. 2007; Ho et al. 2016). Despite this effort of "biological randomisation" the bias associated with such a comparison could hardly be ruled out. Still, the use of allogeneic HCT was shown to be superior in patients with high-risk disease until the age of 60 and in patients with intermediate risk up to the age of 40. This risk-based approach could be confirmed in two large meta-analyses which could include 4 and 21 prospectively treated cohorts included between 1982 and 2002 (Koreth et al. 2009; Yanada et al. 2005). Once again, only patients with intermediate and high-risk disease having a risk of relapse of over 35% seemed to benefit from allogeneic HCT in first CR. Patients with low-risk AML had no survival advantage after allogeneic HCT due to the increased risk of transplant-related mortality of 15–35%. Recent analyses suggest that NRM has again decreased about 5–10% in the last 10 years due to improvements in supportive care and donor selection (McDonald et al. 2020).

Allogeneic HCT performed in first CR improves the 5-year overall survival of patients with high-risk and intermediate-risk disease by 10% to about 31% and 52%, respectively. Subgroup analyses suggest that patients below the age of 35 had the highest relative benefit.

In high-risk patients defined by cytogenetics, blast reduction, or molecular features, prospective trials have even investigated upfront allogeneic HCT without awaiting results of induction therapy (Stolzel et al. 2013). Although such a strategy clearly increased the proportion of high-risk patients undergoing transplantation, it could not demonstrate a clear advantage over applying allogeneic HCT in a conventional fashion after induction therapy (Schetelig et al. 2015).

### 13.2.2 Relapsed AML

Patients with relapsed AML may have a chance of 50–60% of achieving a second CR with reinduction chemotherapy. Subsequent allogeneic HCT can lead to 5-year survival probabilities of 30–50%. The subsequent risk-factors for failure have been identified by Breems et al. (Breems et al. 2005).

- <18 months between first CR and relapse
- Intermediate or high-risk cytogenetics
- Age > 35 years
- Previous autologous (or allogeneic) HCT

In case of slowly proliferating disease or when relapse is detected early by monitoring of measurable residual disease (MRD) and a donor had already been identified, allogeneic HCT may be performed immediately without reinduction chemotherapy.

### 13.2.3 Primary or Secondary Refractory Disease

About 20–30% of patients with AML either have primary refractory disease or experience relapse within 6 months after induction therapy. In both cases, allogeneic HCT needs to be scheduled for these patients as early as possible although some of these patients are difficult to prepare for the procedure. The challenge in these cases is a rapid identification of the potential donor and a bridging strategy until transplantation can be performed. If no matched sibling or unrelated donor can be identified within the first weeks, these patients may benefit from haploidentical HCT. Whether it is advantageous to aggressively strive for the induction of remission with a regimen based on high-dose cytarabine or whether it should be enough to control disease dynamics and plan a sequential conditioning therapy.

According to an analysis of the Center for International Blood and Marrow Transplant Research (CIBMTR) 34% of all patients with AML undergoing allogeneic HCT were not in remission by the time of transplantation. The probability of survival for these 1.673 patients was 19% after standard intensive conditioning therapy. Major reasons for death were progressive disease (42%), followed by infection (15%) and organ failure (12%) (Duval et al. 2009).

To assess the potential benefit of allogeneic HCT in patients being not in CR, a predictive model was developed incorporating five easily accessible parameters:

- Duration of remission <6 months
- Unfavorable cytogenetics
- Blasts in peripheral blood
- Karnofsky Index <90%
- Alternative donor (No HLA-matched sibling)

Patients with <3 risk factors had a 3 years probability of survival of 15–42%. In case of ≥3 risk factors, a conventional transplant procedure seems to offer no real curative potential. In such cases, other transplantation strategies or treatment within a clinical trial should be offered.

In a retrospective analysis of the European Group for Blood and Marrow Transplantation (EBMT) performed in refractory cases, the application of more than two induction chemotherapy cycles turned out to be the most prominent negative prognostic factor again arguing for a rapid decision making and therapeutic intervention in these cases (Craddock et al. 2011). Interestingly, the intensity of conditioning therapy was irrelevant in this high-risk population.

In the last 15 years, the development of "so called" sequential conditioning regimens (see Sect. 13.1.4) was tested in several non-controlled clinical trials. In European centers, the FLAMSA-RIC and similar protocols have been shown to be effective in high-risk patients with and acceptable toxicity profile (Schmid et al. 2006). Recent modifications have made this approach feasible also for older patient applying a non–TBI-based approach (Sheth et al. 2019).

The first clinical trials comparing sequential conditioning with standard intensity or RIC have completed recruitment and will report results very soon. Anyhow, having the results of HLA-typing available as soon as possible in patients with AML receiving intensive induction therapy can be recommended in any case.

Having seen a similar outcome of allogeneic HCT in recipients of grafts from sibling and intelligently matched unrelated donors, several study groups have started recommending allogeneic HCT from an unrelated donor immediately in first CR in patients with ELN high-risk disease having no sibling donor. Currently, prospective clinical trials are under way to demonstrate the non-inferiority of haploidentical versus 9/10 matched unrelated donor HCT (HAMLET trial, NCT03275636).

## 13.3 Monitoring Measurable Residual Disease

### 13.3.1 Rationale and Technology

It has become clear, that in most patients, conditioning therapy will not eradicate the leukemic clone completely and that many patients require additional immunologic effects (GvL) to achieve durable remission and cure. Similar to other hematologic diseases, residual leukemic cells can be detected with different methods before and after allogeneic HCT. Whereas marrow morphology and cytogenetics have a limited sensitivity, multiparameter flow cytometry (MFC) and real-time quantitative polymerase chain reaction (qPCR), and newer technologies offer sensitive tools allowing MRD detection at levels as low as 10e-6. The prognostic role of residual MRD by MFC and molecular technologies by the time of conditioning therapy and after allogeneic HCT has been clearly demonstrated (Shayegi et al. 2013; Getta et al. 2016). Molecular methods may comprise chimerism analyses with a set of adequate STR markers and potentially including a sensitive SRY assay in sex-mismatched settings. Performing chimerism analyses in enriched progenitor cells significantly increases the sensitivity and predictive value of chimerism as MRD parameter (Thiede et al. 2001). Ideally, leukemia-specific aberrations like NPM-1, MLL, or CBF fusions may be amplified with quantitative PCR assays. Recently, next-generation sequencing (NGS) has been introduced into MRD monitoring with first data suggesting prognostic relevance of persistent NGS-based disease detection in the first months after HCT (Thol et al. 2018). Whereas most molecular genetic assays can be standardized and tested in a multicentric fashion, MFC is rather investigator-dependent and difficult to standardize within a multicentric setting.

### 13.3.2 Prophylactic and Pre-emptive Interventions

The detection of persistent or increasing levels of MRD in the first 3 months after allogeneic HCT should prompt increased attention in the treating physician. The MRD signals may trigger a more rapid tapering of immunosuppression and/or subsequent infusion of increasing doses of donor lymphocyte infusions (DLI). Prophylactic DLI have been applied in the context of sequential conditioning regimens and may be especially indicated in patients having received in vivo T cell depletion with MabCampath or ATG (Schmid et al. 2007). If patients are early after HCT or still have signs of acute or chronic GvHD, taper of immunosuppression of DLI is not feasible and alternative pharmacologic interventions can be discussed. The feasibility of applying 5-azacytidine in patients with MRD with or without DLI has been demonstrated within a prospective clinical trial (Platzbecker et al. 2018). Although long-term efficacy was only observed in a minor proportion of patients, the approach has been shown to be non-toxic and may be combined with novel pharmacologic approaches including BCL2-antagonism or immunotherapy. In patients with FLT3-mutated AML, disease dynamics may be too fast to apply pre-emptive interventions. In these cases, prophylactic application of sorafenib was associated with a significant improvement in event-free survival (Burchert et al. 2020). Future interventions may include IDH1/2 inhibition, bispecific antibodies, or CAR T cells within clinical trials. In summary, MRD monitoring before and after allogeneic HCT and subsequent prophylactic and/or pre-emptive interventions have become standard in patients with AML undergoing allogeneic HCT. Still, the relative contribution of each strategy needs to be assessed within prospective controlled trials.

## References

Beelen DW, Trenschel R, Stelljes M, Groth C, Masszi T, Reményi P, et al (2020) Treosulfan or busulfan plus fludarabine as conditioning treatment before allogeneic haemopoietic stem cell transplantation for older patients with acute myeloid leukaemia or myelodysplastic syndrome (MC-FludT.14/L): a randomised, non-inferiority, phase 3. Lancet Haematol [Internet]. 7(1):e28–e39. https://linkinghub.elsevier.com/retrieve/pii/S2352302619301577

Breems DA, Van Putten WLJ, Huijgens PC, Ossenkoppele GJ, Verhoef GEG, Verdonck LF et al (2005) Prognostic index for adult patients with acute myeloid leukemia in first relapse. J Clin Oncol 23(9):1969–1978

Burchert A, Bug G, Fritz LV, Finke J, Stelljes M, Röllig C et al (2020) Sorafenib maintenance after allogeneic hematopoietic stem cell transplantation for acute myeloid leukemia with FLT3-internal tandem duplication mutation (SORMAIN). J Clin Oncol 38(26): 2993–3002. https://doi.org/10.1200/JCO.19.03345

Cornelissen JJ, van Putten WLJ, Verdonck LF, Theobald M, Jacky E, Daenen SMG, et al (2007) Results of a HOVON/SAKK donor versus no-donor analysis of myeloablative HLA-identical sibling stem cell transplantation in first remission acute myeloid leukemia in young and middle-aged adults: benefits for whom? Blood [Internet]. 109(9):3658–66. https://ashpublications.org/blood/article/109/9/3658/23619/Results-of-a-HOVONSAKK-donor-versus-nodonor

Cornelissen JJ, Gratwohl A, Schlenk RF, Sierra J, Bornhauser M, Juliusson G et al (2012) The European LeukemiaNet AML working party consensus statement on allogeneic HSCT for patients with AML in remission: an integrated-risk adapted approach. Nat Rev Clin Oncol 9(10):579–590

Craddock C, Labopin M, Pillai S, Finke J, Bunjes D, Greinix H et al (2011) Factors predicting outcome after unrelated donor stem cell transplantation in primary refractory acute myeloid leukaemia. Leukemia 25(5):808–813

De Jong CN, Meijer E, Bakunina K, Nur E, van Marwijk Kooij M, de Groot MR, et al (2019) Post-transplantation cyclophosphamide after allogeneic hematopoietic stem cell transplantation: results of the prospective randomized HOVON-96 trial in recipients of matched related and unrelated donors. Blood [Internet]. 134(Suppl_1):1. https://doi.org/10.1182/blood-2019-124659

Dehn J, Spellman S, Hurley CK, Shaw BE, Barker JN, Burns LJ et al (2019) Selection of unrelated donors and cord blood units for hematopoietic cell transplantation: guidelines from the NMDP/CIBMTR. Blood 134(12):924–934

Duval M, He W, Klein JP, Tallman MS, DiPersio JF, Bunjes DW et al (2009) Allogeneic hematopoietic cell transplantation can cure some patients with acute leukemia in relapse or primary induction failure: a CIBMTR study. Blood 114(22):528

Elsawy M, Sorror ML (2016) Up-to-date tools for risk assessment before allogeneic hematopoietic cell transplantation. Bone Marrow Transplant [Internet]. 51(10):1283–300. http://www.nature.com/articles/bmt2016141

Fasslrinner F, Schetelig J, Burchert A, Kramer M, Trenschel R, Hegenbart U, et al (2018) Long-term efficacy of reduced-intensity versus myeloablative conditioning before allogeneic haemopoietic cell transplantation in patients with acute myeloid leukaemia in first complete remission: retrospective follow-up of an open-label, randomised phase . Lancet Haematol [Internet] 5(4):e161–e169. http://www.ncbi.nlm.nih.gov/pubmed/29550384

Finke J, Bethge WA, Schmoor C, Ottinger HD, Stelljes M, Zander AR et al (2009) Standard graft-versus-host disease prophylaxis with or without anti-T-cell globulin in haematopoietic cell transplantation from matched unrelated donors: a randomised, open-label, multicentre phase 3 trial. Lancet Oncol 10(9):855–864

Getta BM, Devlin S, Maloy MA, Mohanty A, Arcila M, Tallman MS, et al (2016) Multicolor flow cytometry and multi-gene next generation sequencing are complimentary and highly predictive for relapse in acute myeloid leukemia following allogeneic hematopoietic stem cell transplant. Blood [Internet]. 128(22):834. https://ashpublications.org/blood/article/128/22/834/99294/Multicolor-Flow-Cytometry-and-MultiGene-Next

Gratwohl A (2012) The EBMT risk score. Bone Marrow Transplant [Internet]. 47(6):749–56. http://www.nature.com/articles/bmt2011110

Gyurkocza B, Storb R, Storer BE, Chauncey TR, Lange T, Shizuru JA, et al (2010) Nonmyeloablative allogeneic hematopoietic cell transplantation in patients with acute myeloid leukemia. J Clin Oncol [Internet] 28(17):2859–67. http://ascopubs.org/doi/10.1200/JCO.2009.27.1460

Hashmi S, Ahmed M, Murad MH, Litzow MR, Adams RH, Ball LM et al (2016) Survival after mesenchymal stromal cell therapy in steroid-refractory acute graft-versus-host disease: systematic review and meta-analysis. Lancet Haematol 3(1):e45–e52

Heinicke T, Labopin M, Schmid C, Polge E, Socié G, Blaise D, et al (2018) Reduced relapse incidence with FLAMSA–RIC compared with Busulfan/Fludarabine for acute myelogenous leukemia patients in first or second complete remission: a study from the acute leukemia working party of the European Society for blood and marrow transplantation. Biol Blood Marrow Transplant [Internet] 24(11):2224–32. https://linkinghub.elsevier.com/retrieve/pii/S108387911830394X

Ho AD, Schetelig J, Bochtler T, Schaich M, Schafer-Eckart K, Hanel M et al (2016) Allogeneic stem cell transplantation improves survival in patients with acute myeloid leukemia characterized by a high allelic ratio of mutant FLT3-ITD. Biol Blood Marrow Transplant 22(3):462–469

Kaiser T, Kamal H, Rank A, Kolb H-J, Holler E, Ganser A, et al (2004) Proteomics applied to the clinical follow-up of patients after allogeneic hematopoietic stem cell transplantation. Blood [Internet]. 104(2):340–9. https://ashpublications.org/blood/article/104/2/340/18325/Proteomics-applied-to-the-clinical-followup-of

Koreth J, Schlenk R, Kopecky KJ, Honda S, Sierra J, Djulbegovic BJ, et al (2009) Allogeneic stem cell transplantation for acute myeloid leukemia in first complete remission. JAMA [Internet]. 301(22):2349. http://jama.jamanetwork.com/article.aspx?doi=10.1001/jama.2009.813

Major-Monfried H, Renteria AS, Pawarode A, Reddy P, Ayuk F, Holler E, et al (2018) MAGIC biomarkers predict long-term outcomes for steroid-resistant acute GVHD. Blood [Internet]. 131(25):2846–55. https://ashpublications.org/blood/article/131/25/2846/37158/MAGIC-biomarkers-predict-longterm-outcomes-for

McDonald GB, Sandmaier BM, Mielcarek M, Sorror M, Pergam SA, Cheng GS et al (2020) Survival, nonrelapse mortality, and relapse-related mortality after allogeneic hematopoietic cell transplantation: comparing 2003–2007 versus 2013–2017 cohorts. Ann Intern Med 172(4):229–239

Pasquini MC, Devine S, Mendizabal A, Baden LR, Wingard JR, Lazarus HM et al (2012) Comparative outcomes of donor graft CD34+ selection and immune suppressive therapy as graft-versus-host disease prophylaxis for patients with acute myeloid leukemia in complete remission undergoing HLA-matched sibling allogeneic hematopoietic cell transpl. J Clin Oncol 30(26):3194–3201

Platzbecker U, Middeke JM, Sockel K, Herbst R, Wolf D, Baldus CD, et al (2018) Measurable residual disease-guided treatment with azacitidine to prevent haematological relapse in patients with myelodysplastic syndrome and acute myeloid leukaemia (RELAZA2): an open-label, multicentre, phase 2 trial. Lancet Oncol [Internet] 19(12):1668–79. https://linkinghub.elsevier.com/retrieve/pii/S1470204518305801

Rodriguez R, Nakamura R, Palmer JM, Parker P, Shayani S, Nademanee A et al (2010) A phase II pilot study of tacrolimus/sirolimus GVHD prophylaxis for sibling donor hematopoietic stem cell transplantation using 3 conditioning regimens. Blood 115(5):1098–1105

Schetelig J, Schaich M, Schafer-Eckart K, Hanel M, Aulitzky WE, Einsele H et al (2015) Hematopoietic cell transplantation in patients with intermediate and high-risk AML: results from the randomized study alliance leukemia (SAL) AML 2003 trial. Leukemia 29(5):1060–1068

Schmid, C, Schleuning, M, Schwerdtfeger R et al (2006) Long-term survival in refractory acute myeloid leukemia after sequential treatment with chemotherapy and reduced-intensity conditioning for allogeneic stem cell transplantation. Blood [Internet]. 108(3):1092–9. http://www.bloodjournal.org/cgi/doi/10.1182/blood-2005-10-4165

Schmid C, Labopin M, Nagler A, Bornhäuser M, Finke J, Fassas A et al (2007) Donor lymphocyte infusion in the treatment of first hematological relapse after allogeneic stem-cell transplantation in adults with acute myeloid leukemia: a retrospective risk factors analysis and comparison with other strategies by the EBMT acute leukem. J Clin Oncol 25(31):4938–4945

Scott BL, Pasquini MC, Logan BR, Wu J, Devine SM, Porter DL, et al (2017) Myeloablative versus reduced-intensity hematopoietic cell transplantation for acute myeloid leukemia and myelodysplastic syndromes. J Clin Oncol [Internet]. 35(11):1154–61. http://ascopubs.org/doi/10.1200/JCO.2016.70.7091

Shayegi N, Kramer M, Bornhauser M, Schaich M, Schetelig J, Platzbecker U et al (2013) The level of residual disease based on mutant NPM1 is an independent prognostic factor for relapse and survival in AML. Blood 122(1):83–92

Sheth V, Labopin M, Canaani J, Volin L, Brecht A, Ganser A, et al (2019) Comparison of FLAMSA-based reduced intensity conditioning with treosulfan/fludarabine conditioning for patients with acute myeloid leukemia: an ALWP/EBMT analysis. Bone Marrow Transplant [Internet] 54(4):531–9. http://www.nature.com/articles/s41409-018-0288-0

Stolzel F, Platzbecker U, Mohr B, Rollig C, Middeke JM, Thiede C et al (2013) Early intervention with allogeneic hematopoietic cell transplantation during chemotherapy-induced aplasia in patients with high-risk acute myeloid leukemia. Leukemia 27:2068–2072

Thiede C, Bornhauser M, Oelschlagel U, Brendel C, Leo R, Daxberger H et al (2001) Sequential monitoring of chimerism and detection of minimal residual disease after allogeneic blood stem cell transplantation (BSCT) using multiplex PCR amplification of short tandem repeat-markers. Leukemia 15(2):293–302

Thol F, Gabdoulline R, Liebich A, Klement P, Schiller J, Kandziora C, et al (2018) Measurable residual disease monitoring by NGS before allogeneic hematopoietic cell transplantation in AML. Blood [Internet]. 132(16):1703–13. https://www.ncbi.nlm.nih.gov/pubmed/30190321

Ullmann AJ, Schmidt-Hieber M, Bertz H, Heinz WJ, Kiehl M, Krüger W et al (2016) Infectious diseases in allogeneic haematopoietic stem cell transplantation: prevention and prophylaxis strategy guidelines 2016. Ann Hematol 95(9):1435–1455

Yanada M, Matsuo K, Emi N, Naoe T (2005) Efficacy of allogeneic hematopoietic stem cell transplantation depends on cytogenetic risk for acute myeloid leukemia in first disease remission: a metaanalysis. Cancer 103(8):1652–1658

Zeiser R, von Bubnoff N, Butler J, Mohty M, Niederwieser D, Or R et al (2020) Ruxolitinib for glucocorticoid-refractory acute graft-versus-host disease. N Engl J Med 383:500–502

# Special Clinical Scenarios: Hyperleukocytosis

# 14

Gesine Bug and Halvard Bonig

## 14.1 Definition and Epidemiology

Acute myeloid leukemia (AML) patients will present with hyperleukocytosis in approximately 10–20% of cases irrespective of age (Porcu et al. 2000; de Jonge et al. 2011; Creutzig et al. 1987). Technically hyperleukocytosis is a laboratory abnormality which may be entirely asymptomatic or associated with leukostasis, a medical emergency (Porcu et al. 2000; Rollig and Ehninger 2015). The term hyperleukocytosis is most often used for peripheral white blood cell (WBC) counts in excess of $100 \times 10^9$/L. As signs and symptoms of hyperleukocytosis may also occur at lower WBC numbers, some centers accept a cut-off of $50 \times 10^9$/L or even $30 \times 10^9$/L WBC (Stahl et al. 2018; Tien et al. 2018).

Hyperleukocytosis reflects rapid disease kinetics and thus is more common in conjunction with other high-risk features such as FLT3-ITD with increasing FLT3-ITD/FLT3 ratios correlating with significantly higher WBC counts (Gale et al. 2008). Hyperleukocytosis is also more commonly seen in myelomonocytic or monoblastic AML, APL micrygranular variant (AML M3v), and AML with 11q23 rearrangements or CBFB/MYH11 fusion protein (Porcu et al. 2000; Cuttner et al. 1980). The prognosis of AML with hyperleukocytosis is poor, but whether this is a reflection of the underlying biology of the leukemia or of the hyperleukocytosis itself (in other words, whether hyperleukocytosis is an additional, independent prognostic factor) has been debated controversially (Porcu et al. 2000; Marbello et al. 2008; Cornelissen and Blaise 2016). This is compounded by differences between various risk scores in considering elevated WBC as a risk factor. For example, the HOVON-SAKK consortium includes a higher WBC count as an independent prognostic factor for poor outcome in t(8;21) or RUNX1-RUNX1T1 (AML1-ETO) positive and cytogenetically normal AML with $20 \times 10^9$/L and $100 \times 10^9$/L as the cut-off, respectively, irrespective of clinical manifestations of hyperleukocytosis (Cornelissen and Blaise 2016).

The principles of management of AML with hyperleukocytosis in adults and children do not differ and will be discussed together. While the fundamentals of supportive care in hyperleukocytosis are universally accepted, the issue of how to best reduce the high leukocyte count in which patient is a matter of controversial debate and

G. Bug (✉)
Department of Medicine 2, Goethe University, Frankfurt/Main, Germany
e-mail: Gesine.Bug@kgu.de

H. Bonig
Institute for Transfusion Medicine and Immunohematology, Goethe University, Frankfurt/Main, Germany

German Red Cross Blood Service Baden-Württemberg-Hessen, Frankfurt/Main, Germany

Division of Hematology, Department of Medicine, University of Washington, Seattle, WA, USA


C. Röllig, G. J. Ossenkoppele (eds.), *Acute Myeloid Leukemia*, Hematologic Malignancies,
https://doi.org/10.1007/978-3-030-72676-8_14

suffers from a paucity of robust clinical trial data. Understanding the pathophysiological underpinnings of hyperleukocytosis as well as the strengths and weaknesses of the different treatment approaches will assist in making clinical management decisions and are the focus of this review.

## 14.2 Clinical Features and Pathophysiology of Hyperleukocytosis

Approximately one-third of patients with hyperleukocytosis will present with serious clinical manifestations that constitute a medical emergency. This is commonly attributed to leukostasis, a phenomenon in which the excess of large leukemic blasts impairs the blood flow in the capillary systems. This explains why the principal target organs of leukostasis are kidneys, lung, and brain, but heart and eyes may also be affected. Hyperleukocytosis is also indicative of large tumor load and may predispose for TLS and its sequelae. All possible signs and symptoms should be meticulously queried and assessed as to not be overlooked in the face of emergency management. The diagnosis of symptomatic hyperleukocytosis may be clinically challenging due to the coexistence of numerous medical problems that are either associated with the leukemia or may be due to an underlying medical condition. Therefore, signs and symptoms of acute renal failure, dyspnea with arterial oxygen desaturation, dizziness, confusion, somnolence, delirium, impaired vision, angina, or electrocardiographic (ECG) abnormalities should be considered as possible manifestations of leukostasis and distinguished from those attributable to, for example, sepsis, hypotension, pneumonia, coronary artery disease, and cerebral hemorrhage, to name just a few. It should be noted that CNS leukostasis is often accompanied by disseminated small hemorrhagic lesions and may occasionally be associated with catastrophic cerebral hemorrhage. In general, patients with hyperleukocytosis carry a higher risk for organ failure, and early death rates primarily due to cerebral hemorrhage or pulmonary leukostasis approach 20–30% (Creutzig et al. 1987; Walter et al. 2011; Oberoi et al. 2014; Chang et al. 2007; Dutcher et al. 1987; Bunin and Pui 1985).

## 14.3 Treatment and Clinical Management

Symptomatic hyperleukocytosis is far more common in AML than in acute lymphoblastic leukemia (ALL) or chronic myeloid leukemia (except for blast crisis) and requires immediate intervention to reverse organ failure and correct the disturbance in electrolytes, acid base disorders, and coagulation. It is widely accepted that in addition to aggressive and immediate supportive measures this entails rapid cytoreduction. Supportive therapy generally includes hyperhydration with careful fluid balancing, anti-gout medication (uric acid oxidase) and correction of electrolytes and acid-base status. Oxygen by nasal prongs should be given when saturation on room air is insufficient. The large numbers of spontaneously disintegrating leukemia cells in the blood stream can be misinterpreted by automatic hemocytometers as platelets, thus overestimating true platelet counts. In patients displaying clinical signs of thrombocytopenia, a microscopic (manual) platelet count should be ordered. The indication for platelet transfusions can be made independently of the leukocyte count and should be instructed by platelet counts and coagulation studies. For rheological reasons clinicians will typically defer RBC transfusions. If tolerated by the patient, hemoglobin as low as 60 g/L can temporarily be accepted until leukocyte counts have been relevantly lowered.

In contrast, the optimal approach to cytoreduction is controversial and not well supported by evidence from clinical trials. It most likely requires a degree of individualization based on the leading clinical presentation and the overall aim of AML treatment (curative or palliative). Essentially the choices include mild cytoreductive therapy with either hydroxyurea or cytarabine as "pre-phase," leukocyte-depleting apheresis, immediate intensive induction chemotherapy, or some combination of these options. We will discuss therapeutic strategies to manage symptomatic hyperleukocytosis on the basis of two patient cases, which represent two very different clinical scenarios.

### 14.3.1 Patient 1

A 71-year-old patient with a long-standing diagnosis of CMML-1 had been followed on a watch and wait basis for >3 years. Four weeks after the last routine visit, he presented in our emergency unit with a reduced performance score with fever, myalgia, and dyspnea; his arterial oxygen saturation was 79%. He was diagnosed with secondary AML complicated by symptomatic hyperleukocytosis with a WBC of $90 \times 10^9/L$, hemoglobin 93 g/L, platelet count $89 \times 10^9/L$, LDH 7050 U/L, and 17% blasts, 25% monocytes, and a pathologic left shift in the hemogram. The patient initially opted for palliative therapy and was put on hydroxyurea, broad spectrum antibiotics, and supportive care but changed his mind and agreed to mechanical ventilation when his pulmonary situation progressively deteriorated in spite of efficient cytoreduction to a WBC count of $8 \times 10^9/L$ and LDH of 2062 U/L. The computed tomography (CT) scan of the lung showed bilateral pulmonary infiltrates corresponding to an acute respiratory distress syndrome (ARDS), suggesting pulmonary leukostasis. As aggressive diagnostic procedures including bronchoalveolar lavage did not identify any pathogen, induction therapy with 7 + 3 was started and cytarabine administered for 3 days, resulting in rapid recovery of pulmonary function and extubation of the patient. Induction therapy was halted due to hyperbilirubinemia. The clinical situation was still improving when the patient refused further treatment and was discharged to receive best supportive treatment. He died 6 weeks later from his AML.

This case demonstrates that leukemic pulmonary infiltration and leukostasis may occur in spite of an efficiently lowered peripheral WBC count. Overlap between hyperleukocytosis and leukostasis is only partial (Porcu et al. 2000). Neither can a certain leukocyte count be tagged with a certain risk for leukostasis, nor can definitively "safe" leukocyte counts be defined. In other words, the majority of patients with hyperleukocytosis are clinically asymptomatic with respect to symptoms of leukostasis, as well as leukostasis can occur at leukocyte counts significantly below $100 \times 10^9/L$ and can persist long after the peripheral blood leukocyte count has been reduced with appropriate measures.

## 14.4 Chemotherapy

Aiming for an immediate start of intensive induction therapy (7 + 3) is crucial even, or all the more, if WBC counts are high as according to a systematic review hydroxyurea or low-dose chemotherapy do not ameliorate the early death rate (Oberoi et al. 2014; Dohner et al. 2017). Cytarabine (e.g., 100–200 mg/m$^2$ per day as continuous infusion) seems more efficient than hydroxyurea in treating signs and symptoms of leukostasis. However, if intensive induction chemotherapy cannot be started immediately due to patient-related factors or logistic reasons, we still rely on high doses of hydroxyurea (up to 6 g per day in 2–3 doses) as a bridge to definitive antileukemic treatment. Hydroxyurea may also be considered for elderly patients with hyperleukocytosis prior to treatment with a hypomethylating agent with or without venetoclax as such patients have not been included in the pivotal clinical trials and hence safety and efficacy data are not available (Kantarjian et al. 2012; Dombret et al. 2015; DiNardo et al. 2019).

### 14.4.1 Patient 2

A 63-year-old patient complained of progressive fatigue, weakness, and dyspnea upon mild exertion over the last 3 weeks, when a blood sample was taken in preparation for an unrelated orthopedic intervention and hyperleukocytosis was noticed. Upon admission to our hospital, the patient was in stable clinical condition despite high fever and partial pulmonary insufficiency ($pO_2$ 52 mmHg, $pCO_2$ 28 mmHg, arterial oxygen saturation 90%). Laboratory assessment showed a WBC of 332 × $10^9$/L, hemoglobin of 88 g/L, a platelet count of 85 × $10^9$/L, LDH of 1394 U/L, and acute kidney failure (creatinine 2.6 mg/dL). The patient was started on hydroxyurea and therapeutic leukapheresis was performed on two consecutive days which reduced leukocytes by 50% and 36%, respectively, for a total of 1.7 × $10^{12}$ leukocytes in the two apheresis products, at the end of which the peripheral blood WBC count was 85 × $10^9$/L. In spite of aggressive supportive care including rasburicase, he developed a sudden increase in LDH to 7000 U/L associated with symptomatic TLS with hyperuricemia (14 mg/dL), hyperkalemia (4.9 mmol/L), hyperphosphatemia (14.5 mg/dL), and hypocalcemia (free calcium 1.0 mmol/L) and renal failure with anuria requiring two sessions of dialysis. The first RBC transfusion was administered at a hemoglobin of 59 g/L on the fourth day. Bone marrow aspiration revealed an AML NOS with monocytic differentiation and expression of KMT2A-PTD. Induction with cytarabine and daunorubicin (7 + 3) was started when renal function had recovered 10 days after admission. The patient achieved a complete remission and after one cycle of consolidation chemotherapy proceeded to allogeneic stem cell transplantation in molecular remission which is currently ongoing 8 months after diagnosis.

This second case suggests that immediate leukapheresis may be a reasonable option in case of severe TLS with life-threatening laboratory and clinical symptoms to achieve rapid and gentle cytoreduction without overburdening critical organs. In contrast to TLS, leukostasis is not primarily a quantitative problem and thus possibly less responsive to leukapheresis: Leukocrits sufficiently high to cause meaningful rheological disturbance (i.e., hyperviscosity) are rarely observed, and the typically very low hematocrit of newly diagnosed AML patients further counteracts such effects (Porcu et al. 2000). Indeed, a significant body of data was put forth implicating endothelial dysfunction in response to mediators secreted by blasts as well as in response to adhesive interactions with the large and rigid blasts with their activated and sometimes overexpressed adhesion molecule repertoire. According to these data, there is no good correlation between leukostasis and WBC count, a notion that is supported by our first case report. Leukocytes form thrombotic plugs in small vessels but also extravasate and cause peri-vascular infiltrates (Porcu et al. 2000; Rollig and Ehninger 2015). Bertoli et al. report the short-term use of dexamethasone concurrent to induction chemotherapy, the rationale being the down-regulation of leukocyte adhesion molecules and inflammatory response genes by steroids. The authors conclude that this was associated with favorable outcomes (Bertoli et al. 2018), but use of corticosteroids has not become clinical practice. While some candidate cytokines have been identified as presumptive culprits in the pathogenesis of leukostasis (Porcu et al. 2000, 2002; Rollig and Ehninger 2015), treatment with anti-functional anti-cytokine antibodies has not been attempted.

## 14.5 Is There a Role for Therapeutic Apheresis? Evidence from Clinical Case Series

The concept of physically removing a large number of AML blasts from the circulation to rapidly "debulk" the tumor appears compelling and has been practiced ever since continuous-flow apheresis devices became available. In CML, the disease which triggered the advent of apheresis, leukodepleting apheresis was a very useful therapeutic addition before the advent of allogeneic stem cell transplantation (Bloom et al. 1979). By contrast, the evidence supporting therapeutic leukapheresis for hyperleukocytosis in AML is quite weak, 2B for leukapheresis for symptomatic ("therapeutic" apheresis) and 2C for leukapheresis for asymptomatic leukocytosis ("prophylactic" apheresis) >100 × $10^9$/L (Padmanabhan et al. 2019). Definition of the role of leukapheresis has not been helped by the differences in defining what could be construed to count as "success."

Technically, a well-performed leukapheresis will process approximately two total volumes of blood (TBV), thereby removing a trillion or more blasts and transiently lower the leukocyte count by more than 50% (Bloom et al. 1979; Pham and Schwartz 2015; Ganzel et al. 2012; Schulz et al. 2013; Porcu et al. 1997). Such a procedure could be considered successful from the laboratory perspective if it is achieved without harming the patient, but effective cytoreduction does not necessarily translate into clinical benefit. It is worth remembering that only a minority of blasts is circulating at any one time point and redistribution of blasts will quickly negate any short-term impact on WBC unless complemented by other approaches. Thus, in patient 2 over the course of the second apheresis, that is, within less than 2 hours during which 600 billion cells were removed, more than 300 billion more cells entered the blood stream from extravascular sites. Case 2 further illustrates that a profound reduction of the number of circulating blasts alone may not translate into clinically meaningful improvement, while case 1 reminds us that leukostasis, although more frequently associated with hyperleukocytosis, is not primarily a matter of cell count. Instead, it underscores the current understanding of leukostasis as an event involving activated adhesion molecules and endothelial dysfunction (see above). Supporting this notion is the observation that similar and even higher WBC counts in newly diagnosed ALL are rarely, if ever, associated with leukostasis so the hyperleukocytosis in ALL of at least $400 \times 10^9/L$ does not constitute an indication for leukodepletion by apheresis (Padmanabhan et al. 2019).

To date, no prospective, let alone randomized studies have been performed to address the value of leukapheresis on patient outcome (Padmanabhan et al. 2019). Conceptually, the procedure could at best be expected to reduce early, hyperleukocytosis-associated mortality, but whether this actually is achieved remains contentious with some authors (Giles et al. 2001; Bug et al. 2007; Nan et al. 2017) arguing in favor, several more (Oberoi et al. 2014; Porcu et al. 2002; Pastore et al. 2014; Malkan and Ozcebe 2017; Korkmaz 2018; Abla et al. 2016; Choi et al. 2018) explicitly failing to identify clinical benefit, yet others (Haase et al. 2009; Inaba et al. 2008) avoiding judgment of its efficacy. Irrespective of its effect on short-term mortality, available analyses agree that therapeutic leukapheresis has no bearing on long-term outcomes and the largest body of data summarized in a comprehensive review and meta-analysis discourages its practice due to a lack of effect on mortality (Oberoi et al. 2014).

This conclusion does not fully align with clinical experience which suggests that a technically successful leukapheresis may meaningfully contribute to early management in a subset of patients by resulting in symptomatic improvement and accordingly clinical practice only partly reflects this negative view (Stahl et al. 2018). Most retrospective studies have examined only small numbers of patients, were heterogeneous in terms of patient characteristics (e.g., WBC, RBC, platelet count, degree of coagulopathy, cardiovascular and performance status, indication for leukapheresis), and had an inherent bias for or against leukapheresis. Another temporal bias may be attributable to improvements in leukapheresis technology, better supportive care, and introduction of new treatment options.

## 14.6 Conclusions

An authoritative review of best-practice approaches to hyperleukocytosis in AML was recently published (Rollig and Ehninger 2015). In agreement therewith we summarize that symptomatic hyperleukocytosis, that is, hyperleukocytosis with leukostasis, is a medical emergency which besides supportive therapy requires forceful leukoreduction. Leukapheresis can be considered but should neither replace nor delay definitive chemotherapy.

There is no rationale for leukapheresis in patients with asymptomatic hyperleukocytosis irrespective of WBC counts; a diagnosis of acute promyelocytic leukemia (FAB M3) is a contraindication to therapeutic leukapheresis due to the disease-inherent risk of disseminated intravascular coagulopathy (Padmanabhan et al. 2019). Specifically does leukapheresis not seem to reduce the risk of tumor lysis syndrome and coagulopathy during induction, likely because compared to the total blast volume in bone marrow the number in blood is comparatively small. Even with best medical care, the prognosis of AML with hyperleukocytosis is guarded.

## References


Abla O, Angelini P, Di Giuseppe G, Kanani MF, Lau W, Hitzler J et al (2016) Early complications of hyperleukocytosis and leukapheresis in childhood acute leukemias. J Pediatr Hematol Oncol 38(2):111–117

Bertoli S, Picard M, Berard E, Griessinger E, Larrue C, Mouchel PL et al (2018) Dexamethasone in hyperleukocytic acute myeloid leukemia. Haematologica 103(6):988–998

Bloom R, Da Silva AMT, Bracey A (1979) Reversible respiratory failure due to intravascular leukostasis in chronic myelogenous leukemia. Relationship of oxygen transfer to leukocyte count. Am J Med 67(4):679–683

Bug G, Anargyrou K, Tonn T, Bialleck H, Seifried E, Hoelzer D et al (2007) Impact of leukapheresis on early death rate in adult acute myeloid leukemia presenting with hyperleukocytosis. Transfusion 47(10):1843–1850

Bunin NJ, Pui CH (1985) Differing complications of hyperleukocytosis in children with acute lymphoblastic or acute nonlymphoblastic leukemia. J Clin Oncol 3(12):1590–1595

Chang MC, Chen TY, Tang JL, Lan YJ, Chao TY, Chiu CF et al (2007) Leukapheresis and cranial irradiation in patients with hyperleukocytic acute myeloid leukemia: no impact on early mortality and intracranial hemorrhage. Am J Hematol 82(11):976–980

Choi MH, Choe YH, Park Y, Nah H, Kim S, Jeong SH et al (2018) The effect of therapeutic leukapheresis on early complications and outcomes in patients with acute leukemia and hyperleukocytosis: a propensity score-matched study. Transfusion 58(1):208–216

Cornelissen JJ, Blaise D (2016) Hematopoietic stem cell transplantation for patients with AML in first complete remission. Blood 127(1):62–70

Creutzig U, Ritter J, Budde M, Sutor A, Schellong G (1987) Early deaths due to hemorrhage and leukostasis in childhood acute myelogenous leukemia. Associations with hyperleukocytosis and acute monocytic leukemia. Cancer 60(12):3071–3079

Cuttner J, Conjalka MS, Reilly M, Goldberg J, Reisman A, Meyer RJ et al (1980) Association of monocytic leukemia in patients with extreme leukocytosis. Am J Med 69(4):555–558

de Jonge HJ, Valk PJ, de Bont ES, Schuringa JJ, Ossenkoppele G, Vellenga E et al (2011) Prognostic impact of white blood cell count in intermediate risk acute myeloid leukemia: relevance of mutated NPM1 and FLT3-ITD. Haematologica 96(9):1310–1317

DiNardo CD, Pratz K, Pullarkat V, Jonas BA, Arellano M, Becker PS et al (2019) Venetoclax combined with decitabine or azacitidine in treatment-naive, elderly patients with acute myeloid leukemia. Blood 133(1):7–17

Dohner H, Estey E, Grimwade D, Amadori S, Appelbaum FR, Buchner T et al (2017) Diagnosis and management of AML in adults: 2017 ELN recommendations from an international expert panel. Blood 129(4):424–447

Dombret H, Seymour JF, Butrym A, Wierzbowska A, Selleslag D, Jang JH et al (2015) International phase 3 study of azacitidine vs conventional care regimens in older patients with newly diagnosed AML with >30% blasts. Blood 126(3):291–299

Dutcher JP, Schiffer CA, Wiernik PH (1987) Hyperleukocytosis in adult acute nonlymphocytic leukemia: impact on remission rate and duration, and survival. J Clin Oncol 5(9):1364–1372

Gale RE, Green C, Allen C, Mead AJ, Burnett AK, Hills RK et al (2008) The impact of FLT3 internal tandem duplication mutant level, number, size, and interaction with NPM1 mutations in a large cohort of young adult patients with acute myeloid leukemia. Blood 111(5):2776–2784

Ganzel C, Becker J, Mintz PD, Lazarus HM, Rowe JM (2012) Hyperleukocytosis, leukostasis and leukapheresis: practice management. Blood Rev 26(3):117–122

Giles FJ, Shen Y, Kantarjian HM, Korbling MJ, O'Brien S, Anderlini P et al (2001) Leukapheresis reduces early mortality in patients with acute myeloid leukemia with high white cell counts but does not improve long- term survival. Leuk Lymphoma 42(1–2):67–73

Haase R, Merkel N, Diwan O, Elsner K, Kramm CM (2009) Leukapheresis and exchange transfusion in children with acute leukemia and hyperleukocytosis. A single center experience. Klin Padiatr 221(6):374–378

Inaba H, Fan Y, Pounds S, Geiger TL, Rubnitz JE, Ribeiro RC et al (2008) Clinical and biologic features and treatment outcome of children with newly diagnosed acute myeloid leukemia and hyperleukocytosis. Cancer 113(3):522–529

Kantarjian HM, Thomas XG, Dmoszynska A, Wierzbowska A, Mazur G, Mayer J et al (2012) Multicenter, randomized, open-label, phase III trial of decitabine versus patient choice, with physician advice, of either supportive care or low-dose cytarabine for the treatment of older patients with newly diagnosed acute myeloid leukemia. J Clin Oncol 30(21):2670–2677

Korkmaz S (2018) The management of hyperleukocytosis in 2017: do we still need leukapheresis? Transfus Apher Sci 57(1):4–7

Malkan UY, Ozcebe OI (2017) Leukapheresis do not improve early death rates in acute myeloid leukemia patients with hyperleukocytosis. Transfus Apher Sci 56(6):880–882

Marbello L, Ricci F, Nosari AM, Turrini M, Nador G, Nichelatti M et al (2008) Outcome of hyperleukocytic adult acute myeloid leukaemia: a single-center retrospective study and review of literature. Leuk Res 32(8):1221–1227

Nan X, Qin Q, Gentille C, Ensor J, Leveque C, Pingali SR et al (2017) Leukapheresis reduces 4-week mortality in acute myeloid leukemia patients with hyperleukocytosis—a retrospective study from a tertiary center. Leuk Lymphoma 58(9):1–11

Oberoi S, Lehrnbecher T, Phillips B, Hitzler J, Ethier MC, Beyene J et al (2014) Leukapheresis and low-dose chemotherapy do not reduce early mortality in acute myeloid leukemia hyperleukocytosis: a systematic review and meta-analysis. Leuk Res 38(4):460–468

Padmanabhan A, Connelly-Smith L, Aqui N, Balogun RA, Klingel R, Meyer E et al (2019) Guidelines on the use of therapeutic apheresis in clinical practice—evidence-based approach from the Writing Committee of the American Society for Apheresis: the eighth special issue. J Clin Apher 34(3):171–354

Pastore F, Pastore A, Wittmann G, Hiddemann W, Spiekermann K (2014) The role of therapeutic leukapheresis in hyperleukocytotic AML. PLoS One 9(4):e95062

Pham HP, Schwartz J (2015) How we approach a patient with symptoms of leukostasis requiring emergent leukocytapheresis. Transfusion 55(10):2306–2311; quiz 5

Porcu P, Danielson CF, Orazi A, Heerema NA, Gabig TG, McCarthy LJ (1997) Therapeutic leukapheresis in hyperleucocytic leukaemias: lack of correlation between degree of cytoreduction and early mortality rate. Br J Haematol 98(2):433–436

Porcu P, Cripe LD, Ng EW, Bhatia S, Danielson CM, Orazi A et al (2000) Hyperleukocytic leukemias and leukostasis: a review of pathophysiology, clinical presentation and management. Leuk Lymphoma 39(1–2):1–18

Porcu P, Farag S, Marcucci G, Cataland SR, Kennedy MS, Bissell M (2002) Leukocytoreduction for acute leukemia. Ther Apher 6(1):15–23

Rollig C, Ehninger G (2015) How I treat hyperleukocytosis in acute myeloid leukemia. Blood 125(21):3246–3252

Schulz M, Bug G, Bialleck H, Serve H, Seifried E, Bonig H (2013) Leucodepletion for hyperleucocytosis—first report on a novel technology featuring electronic interphase management. Vox Sang 105(1):47–53

Stahl M, Pine A, Hendrickson JE, Litzow MR, Luger SM, Stone RM et al (2018) Beliefs and practice patterns in hyperleukocytosis management in acute myeloid leukemia: a large U.S. web-based survey(.). Leuk Lymphoma 59(11):2723–2726

Tien FM, Hou HA, Tsai CH, Tang JL, Chen CY, Kuo YY et al (2018) Hyperleukocytosis is associated with distinct genetic alterations and is an independent poor-risk factor in de novo acute myeloid leukemia patients. Eur J Haematol 101(1):86–94

Walter RB, Othus M, Borthakur G, Ravandi F, Cortes JE, Pierce SA et al (2011) Prediction of early death after induction therapy for newly diagnosed acute myeloid leukemia with pretreatment risk scores: a novel paradigm for treatment assignment. J Clin Oncol 29(33):4417–4423

# 15 Special Clinical Scenarios: Extramedullary Disease

Friedrich Stölzel

*The difficulty in interpreting chloroma, in assigning to it its proper role within the categories of leukemia, arises from the fact that it belongs to that group of borderland cases which lies between genuine neoplasms and leukemias.*

*Heinrich Lehndorff, *1877 Vienna—†1965 New York*

## 15.1 Definition of Extramedullary AML

Extramedullary AML (syn. myeloid sarcoma, granulocytic sarcoma, myeloblastoma, or chloroma, the latter often being used synonymously with leukemia cutis) is defined as infiltration of extramedullary sites by AML blasts effacing tissue architecture of the tissue in which it is found (Vardiman et al. 2009). Importantly, any site of the body can be affected. Central nervous system (CNS) involvement of AML, that is, leukemic infiltration into the CSF per se does not fulfill the criteria for extramedullary AML (EM AML) and is therefore often delineated separately. Extramedullary AML is defined as a distinct AML entity in the WHO classification where it is referenced as "myeloid sarcoma" (Arber et al. 2016). Extramedullary manifestations may occur also in acute lymphoblastic leukemia (ALL), chronic lymphocytic leukemia (CLL), chronic myeloid leukemia (CML), and myelodysplastic syndromes/myeloproliferative neoplasms (MDS/MPN) whereas in the latter this may indicate the transformation into AML.

F. Stölzel (✉)
Medizinische Klinik und Poliklinik I, University Hospital Carl Gustav Carus Dresden, Technische Universität Dresden, Dresden, Germany
e-mail: friedrich.stoelzel@ukdd.de

## 15.2 Prevalence and Sites

In AML, the appearance of extramedullary leukemic infiltration has historically been correlated to appear in patients with certain balanced translocations such as t(8;21) and inv(16), flow-cytometric positivity of AML cells for CD56, cytomorphological features of M2-, M4-, or M5-FAB subtypes, patient age, and high WBC counts at diagnosis (Byrd et al. 1995; Byrd and Weiss 1994). However, it is now well acknowledged that EM AML can occur in any AML subtype and at every location of the body (Bakst et al. 2011; Ohanian et al. 2013; Stolzel et al. 2020), Fig. 15.1. Interestingly, apart from close proximity to neuralgic structures such as afferent nerves, EM AML manifestations seem to present rather indolent at presentation (Stolzel et al. 2011). Since screening for EM AML has recently not yet been performed on a regular basis in the



C. Röllig, G. J. Ossenkoppele (eds.), *Acute Myeloid Leukemia*, Hematologic Malignancies,
https://doi.org/10.1007/978-3-030-72676-8_15

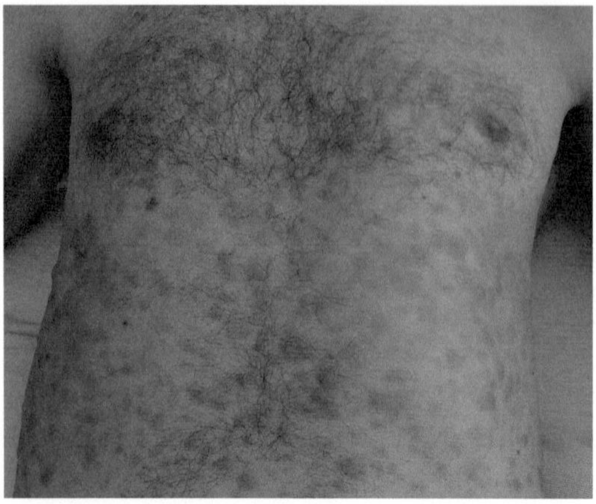

**Fig. 15.1** EM AML of the skin confirmed after histologic confirmation of a punch biopsy in a patient with EM AML at initial diagnosis concurrently with classical AML in the bone marrow

initial workup of AML patients, available data and analyses of prevalence or clinical relevance are skewed (Dohner et al. 2005; Ganzel et al. 2016). This skewing is caused by (a) a reporting of EM AML that is diagnosed as per clinical examination only since routine imaging studies are not performed, for example, with a dominance of EM AML of the skin as a "tip of the iceberg" phenomenon, by (b) a reporting of clinical diagnosed EM AML not having undergone biopsy as the "most likely" diagnosis although the simultaneous diagnosis of two distinct but unrelated neoplasms may occur or the co-appearance of, for example, an infectious complication of the skin that may be misdiagnosed as EM AML, and (c) confounding due to certain phenomena associated with AML such as gum hyperplasia or splenomegaly with EM AML, respectively. In rare occurrences, AML may present with the clinical picture of a Sweet syndrome (acute febrile neutrophilic dermatosis) which in this case fulfills diagnostic criteria (von den Driesch 1994) and reflects malignancy-associated Sweet syndrome, respectively (Cohen et al. 1988).

EM AML prevalence historically ranged from as low as 2.5–9.1% (Bakst et al. 2011; Avni and Koren-Michowitz 2011). However, these data are derived from either autopsy studies, naturally selecting for patients succumbing of AML with a supposedly advanced disease which might increase the prevalence for EM AML or from analyses reporting clinically detected EM AML and therefore reporting lower prevalences. The only prospective study assessing the prevalence of EM AML applying $^{18}$FDG-PET/CT imaging (delineated in detail in the following chapter) at diagnosis demonstrated a prevalence of 17% for newly diagnosed AML patients and a higher prevalence of 22% when also including patients with the diagnosis of relapse (Stolzel et al. 2020). The prevalence of EM AML at relapse after allogeneic hematopoietic stem cell transplantation (HCT) is generally thought to be higher than at initial diagnosis or at relapse after chemotherapy—furthermore, it has been observed frequently that patients with extramedullary manifestations at diagnosis experience extramedullary manifestations at relapse, too. This would suggest that the tropism for EM sites might be in part disease intrinsic (Stolzel et al. 2012; Vago 2019).

CNS involvement in AML is a rare manifestation as compared to, for example, CNS involvement in patients with acute lymphoblastic leukemia (ALL). The largest analysis from three prospective multicenter clinical trials found a low prevalence of 0.6% at diagnosis of AML and 2.9% at diagnosis of relapsed AML (Alakel et al. 2017).

## 15.3 Histology, Cytogenetic, and Molecular Markers

For diagnostic examination, either core-needle biopsy or surgical excision of the tumor should be performed. Morphologically EM AML exhibits myeloid cell infiltration that resembles the AML features found in the patient's bone marrow or peripheral blood. However, in infrequent occasions, EM AML is diagnosed in the absence of AML in the bone marrow or peripheral blood—in these cases AML the extramedullary site always precedes the systemic occurrence in the hematopoietic system. Primary EM AML is often misdiagnosed with lymphoma, specifically diffuse large cell B-cell lymphoma (DLBCL)—

therefore, integration of cytogenetic and molecular analyses techniques (see below) must be employed (Meis et al. 1986; Yamauchi and Yasuda 2002). The infiltration of extramedullary sites is described to be either diffuse or in a single-filing pattern usually with a high- to very-high KI-67/MIBI index. Cytochemical stains usually include AML-specific markers, respectively, while vice versa B- and T-lineage specific markers should be tested to exclude above-mentioned differential diagnoses.

Cytogenetic abnormalities are frequently detected in extramedullary tumor tissue of AML patients and can be performed either by conventional fluorescence in situ hybridization (FISH), array comparative genomic hybridization (array CGH) or chromosomal microarrays (CMA) (Deeb et al. 2005; Mirza et al. 2014; Pileri et al. 2007). Since concordance of cytogenetic abnormalities of bone marrow and EM AML sites is common, the finding of these abnormalities will either confirm those found in the bone marrow or, in case of isolated EM AML occurrence will help to reveal the risk status by unraveling the prognostic nature of the disease. The prevalence of certain cytogenetic abnormalities in EM AML is conflicting since available data still mostly rely on clinical manifestations of EM AML or are derived from retrospective analyses of prospective trials or registry data for whom the occurrence of EM AML reporting was not mandatory. In general, every genetic abnormality in AML can also be detected in EM AML. However, inversion of chromosome 16 (*CBFB-MYH11*) seems to have a predominance of occurrence in EM AML manifestation in the intestines (Pileri et al. 2007; Alvarez et al. 2011; Tsimberidou et al. 2008; Xavier et al. 2003; Zhang et al. 2010). In large series of AML patients with CNS manifestation reported, the co-occurrence of other extramedullary sites, the diagnosis of complex aberrant karyotypes, abnormalities of chromosome 11, inversion of chromosome 16, and *FLT3*-ITD mutations were observed, respectively (Alakel et al. 2017; Cheng et al. 2015; Shihadeh et al. 2012). In patients with acute promyelocytic leukemia (APL) carrying the characteristic t(15;17), an extramedullary disease most often occurs as CNS manifestation and most often during relapsed disease (Montesinos et al. 2009; Vega-Ruiz et al. 2009).

The genomic landscape of EM AML with regard to mutations is as heterogeneous as AML itself (see Chap. 5). While many studies have been able to identify the same mutations found in the bone marrow and peripheral blood of AML patients, some reports described a predominance of *NPM1* and *FLT3* mutations in EM AML while others couldn't confirm these findings but indicated a high frequency of RAS-pathway mutations, respectively (Ansari-Lari et al. 2004; Caraffini et al. 2018; Falini et al. 2007; Fernandez et al. 2019; Kashofer et al. 2018; Li et al. 2015).

In conclusion, EM AML carries frequently known genetic abnormalities regularly found in AML patients' bone marrow or peripheral blood. In isolated EM AML (without any evidence for the occurrence of AML in the bone marrow or peripheral blood) or when the diagnosis of EM AML is in doubt (e.g., when the dignity and the affiliation of a tumor occurring simultaneously to the diagnosis of AML cannot be specified clinically), chromosomal analyses and mutational screening can (a) help to ascertain the diagnosis of EM AML, (b) help to rule out another co-occurring malignancy, and (c) establish the genetic risk-factors and druggable lesions in isolated EM AML.

## 15.4 Imaging

Apart from EM AML occurring in the skin (i.e., leukemia cutis, although this term is not restricted to AML since this also occurs in CML, ALL, or CLL, respectively) or EM AML causing painful or function-degrading symptoms, EM AML is often clinically not observed causing a tip-of-the-iceberg phenomenon with regard to its prevalence. Reports have been published using computed tomography (CT) scans (Fig. 15.2), magnetic resonance imaging (MRI), and very early 67-Gallium scans for detection of EM AML (Larson et al. 1972; Pui et al. 1994). However, single patient reports as well as small patient series demonstrated repetitively that 18-fluoro-

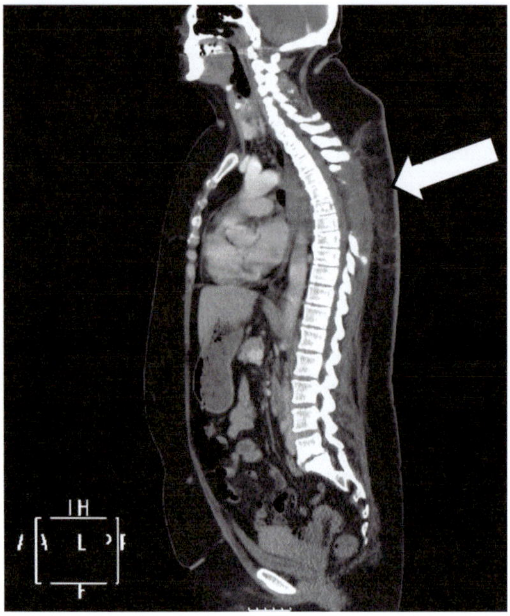

**Fig. 15.2** Sagittal CT-scan of a patient with EM AML of the soft tissue, destroying bone, and infiltrating the myelon (arrow) causing paraplegia of both lower extremities at initial diagnosis. In this patient, the correct diagnosis was made after molecular analyses revealed the existence of an *NPM1* mutation after conventional histological analyses remained inconclusive

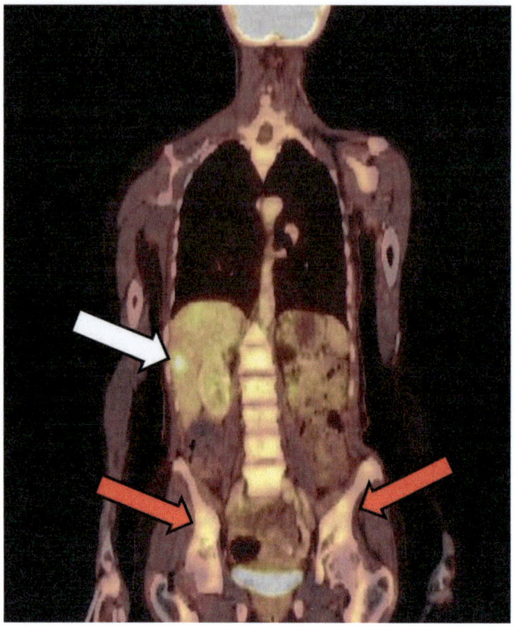

**Fig. 15.3** Pre-therapeutic coronal $^{18}$FDG-PET/CT (fused multiplanar reconstruction, MPR) of a patient with histologically confirmed EM AML of the liver (white arrow) and heterogeneous AML infiltration in the pelvic bone (red arrows) as compared to rather homogeneous AML infiltration of the vertebrae

deoxy-glucose ($^{18}$FDG) positron emission tomography (PET) combined with CT scans are a very useful tool to detect EM AML (Stolzel et al. 2011; Karlin et al. 2006; Kuenzle et al. 2002; Mantzarides et al. 2008; Ueda et al. 2010), Fig. 15.3. In the largest pilot study, $^{18}$FDG-PET/CT was able to detect the histologically proven EM AML sites in 90% of the patients and furthermore, unravel additional EM AML sites in 60% of the patients, respectively (Stolzel et al. 2011). The only prospectively performed study to assess the frequency of EM AML in AML patients was the PETAML trial that found a combined prevalence of EM AML of 22% utilizing $^{18}$FDG-PET/CT in a total of 93 consecutive patients (Stolzel et al. 2020). Moreover, in these 21 patients who had EM AML as per $^{18}$FDG-PET/CT, a total of 65 lesions suggestive for EM AML (range 1–12) with a median SUVmax of 6.1 (range 2.1–51.4) were detected. This study demonstrated a sensitivity and specificity of 77% and 97% for $^{18}$FDG-PET/CT in detecting EM AML in patients with AML, respectively. Interestingly, in six out of ten patients with histologically confirmed EM AML, still active EM AML as per $^{18}$FDG-PET/CT was detected on follow up during remission assessment (Stolzel et al. 2020).

Because of its broad availability that also most often occurs in institutions diagnosing and treating AML, $^{18}$FDG-PET/CT is considered as the diagnostic modality of choice when screening an AML patient for EM AML (Bakst et al. 2011; Stolzel et al. 2020; O'Donnell et al. 2017; Solh et al. 2016).

Patients with CNS manifestation (leukemic meningitis or focal EM AML of the CNS) of AML need to undergo either cranial CT or MRI scanning to exclude the possibility of increased intracranial pressure and for detection of focal EM AML in order to perform a lumbar puncture (LP) for diagnostic as well as therapeutic purposes. In this scenario, MRI (with contrast) is preferentially used because of the combined informative character of yielding information on the focal disease, leptomeningeal enhancement, and intracranial pressure albeit its time-consuming nature that might not always be appropriate, for example, in patients with imminent risk of seizure or hemorrhage.

## 15.5 Approach to AML Patients with Extramedullary Disease

In patients with isolated EM AML without bone marrow or peripheral blood involvement, an excisional tissue biopsy is necessary and superior to, for example, fine needle aspirate or punch biopsy. Albeit the latter might be the clinical compromise of choice when tumor excision cannot be performed in a timely manner or when other factors as, for example, hemorrhage or neutropenic sepsis are impeding a total excision. The work up is similar to analyses of the bone marrow and peripheral blood and includes morphologic examination, flow cytometry as well as cytogenetic and molecular studies, as recommended in the guidelines from the College of American Pathologists and the American Society of Hematology (Arber et al. 2017). In patients with AML detected in the bone marrow and peripheral blood, the workup using EM AML tissue samples may primarily focus on confirming the diagnosis (Arber et al. 2017). However, it should be noted that there exist patients (especially since more and more elderly AML patients undergo curative treatment approaches) who present with other in parallel diagnosed malignant tumors, a scenario that might alter the treatment approach and prognosis of a patient. Therefore, when in doubt whether a tumor in parallel to the diagnosis reflects the co-occurrence of EM AML or not, a tissue biopsy should be obtained to confirm or preclude the diagnosis. With regard to the implementation of imaging procedures please see "Imaging" as depicted above.

## 15.6 Treatment and Prognosis

The recent clinical perception of EM AML was that EM AML reflects a more aggressive form of the disease that was, for example, reflected by guidelines including EM AML in a high-risk category rendering patients with EM AML as candidates for allogeneic hematopoietic stem cell transplantation (HCT), respectively (Cornelissen et al. 2012).

On the contrary, a recent retrospective analysis of 11 ECOG-ACRIN-lead prospective clinical trials based on clinical data from a large number of AML patients revealed a high proportion of patients with EM AML (23.7%) but could not identify EM AML as an independent prognostic factor (Ganzel et al. 2016). However, since this analysis was based on (a) clinical diagnosis only (i.e., no screening for EM AML) and (b) also allocated AML patients into the EM AML category based on symptoms such as splenomegaly or gingival hyperplasia that does not strictly fulfill EM AML WHO criteria, and therefore (c) reported skewed data, the results of this analysis must be interpreted with caution. Another retrospective analysis from the ECOG-ACRIN 1900 trial revealed that in patients with EM AML or without EM AML complete response (CR) rates or DFS did not differ. EM AML was also not associated with a significantly inferior OS. Albeit, this trial randomized AML patients to standard dose 60 mg/m$^2$/day as part of induction chemotherapy versus 90 mg/m$^2$/day that resulted in an improved OS for those patients with EM AML receiving 90 mg/m$^2$/day as compared to those with EM AML receiving 60 mg/m$^2$/day with a median OS of 2.1 years versus 1.4 years, respectively (Fernandez et al. 2019). However, these overall survival differences were not statistically significant in the multivariate analysis of this retrospectively performed subgroup analysis.

Isolated diagnosis of myeloid sarcoma (i.e., EM AML), for example, based on a biopsy from suspicious tissue of a tumor always precedes the systemic, classical manifestation of AML; however, the time lag from isolated EM AML to classical AML may vary from weeks to even years. Therefore, the diagnosis of isolated myeloid sarcoma should be considered synonymous with AML (Vardiman et al. 2009). The same scenario occurs in patients with the occurrence of myeloid sarcoma during a CR (as per bone marrow and peripheral blood) of AML—this situation is synonymous with relapsed AML and an isolated manifestation of EM AML precedes systemic, classical AML in weeks or months.

Patients with isolated EM AML and EM AML in conjunction with marrow AML should be treated according to their age, their fitness, and adapted to their cytogenetic-, and molecular genetic risk profile either with the goal of remission induction or thereafter consolidating therapy. There exists no evidence supporting a beneficiary use of prophylactic intrathecal chemotherapy in patients with skin EM AML at diagnosis. Which consolidation therapy is applied should be based on the individual risk factors of the patient's AML and patient-related factors (including HCT donor status) itself. In patients in whom a curative therapeutic approach cannot be claimed and no clinical trials are available (or favored), local treatment options such as radiotherapy (RT) or surgery should be considered. The latter should only be considered as debulking therapy (and sometimes in combination with the need for a diagnostic biopsy) in patients, for example, with an imminent threat to irreversible organ dysfunction as, for example, compression of the myelon or peripheral nerves. RT should be preferred over surgery (if available in a timely manner) since doses of, for example, 24 Gy in 12 fractions offer a high rate of disease control with manageable side effects in most cases, respectively. However, local long-term disease control is low despite the achievement of intermittent local remission (Bakst et al. 2012; Bakst and Yahalom 2011). The short- and long-term effects of RT in combination with other palliative treatment options like hypomethylating agents (HMAs), Bcl-2 inhibitors like, for example, venetoclax, or *FLT3*-ITD inhibitors like, for example, gilteritinib are currently unknown.

In patients in whom RT is used as adjuvant therapy to induction chemotherapy due to necessary swift symptom relief or vital structure decompression, RT in the above-mentioned ranges does not preclude the use of total body irradiation (TBI) as part of conditioning regimen prior to allogeneic hematopoietic stem cell transplantation (Bakst et al. 2011). In case (a) RT was applied prior to chemotherapy or (b) conditioning therapy is applied after RT (in conjunction with induction chemotherapy), cutaneous radiation recall phenomena are seldom observed.

Patients with isolated EM AML or EM AML in conjunction with marrow AML as relapse after conventional chemotherapy should undergo reinduction chemotherapy and be referred to receive an allogeneic HCT, in case a curative approach for the patient is applicable.

Patients with isolated EM AML relapse after allogeneic HCT are observed more frequently than at relapse after conventional chemotherapy (Shimizu et al. 2013; Solh et al. 2012; Yoshihara et al. 2012; Ge et al. 2014; Harris et al. 2013; Shem-Tov et al. 2017), Fig. 15.4. This might be again an observation bias since follow-up care for patients after allogeneic HCT is more concise and well-structured since these patients received the therapeutic approach not only with the high-

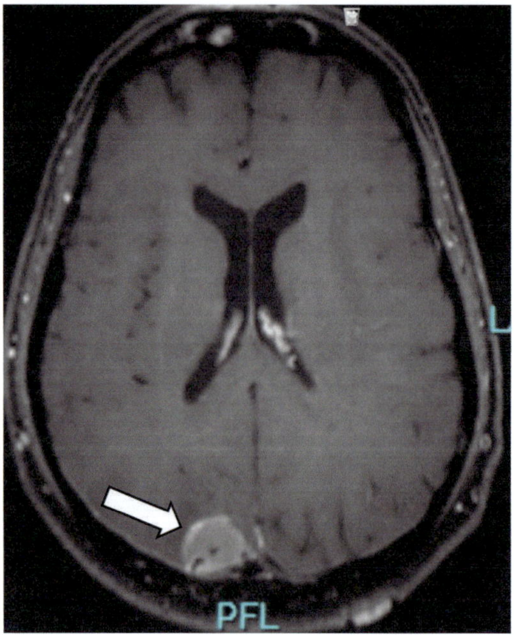


**Fig. 15.4** Axial cranial MRI of an AML patient with an *FLT3*-ITD who underwent haploidentical allogeneic HCT. The patient presented with diplopia 2.5 years after allogeneic HCT when subsequently this MRI was obtained—after neurosurgical removal, histological diagnosis of extramedullary relapse of AML, local radiotherapy, three cycles with intrathecal chemotherapy with dexamethasone and cytarabine, and administration of gilteritinib was initiated

est potential for curation but also with the highest frequency of potential treatment-related morbidities. However, from an immunological point of view, AML cells evading to sanctuary sites of the body in order to persist and expand at levels of reduced immunologic surveillance with lower numbers of patrolling donor T- and NK-cells seem reasonable (Stolzel et al. 2012; Vago 2019). Furthermore, EM AML relapses after allo-HCT occurs later than bone marrow relapse and was shown to have either a better prognosis or the same prognosis as a patient with isolated marrow relapse (Shimizu et al. 2013; Harris et al. 2013; Shem-Tov et al. 2017). Patients with isolated EM AML relapse and patients with EM AML and marrow AML after allogeneic HCT should be evaluated for several treatment options—whether a patient can be scheduled for potentially curative reinduction chemotherapy, HMA in combination with donor-lymphocyte infusion (DLI) or other targeted therapies, for example, gilteritinib and then subsequent retransplantation depending on the fitness of the patient, time lapse from first allogenic HCT to relapse, and the donor status for a second allogeneic HCT, of course. Again, reinduction therapy can be obtained in any modality with local treatment where RT would be the preferred therapy of choice. Combinatory effects of above-mentioned substances (HMAs, venetoclax, gilteritinib, and amongst others) or other frequently applied TKIs such as sorafenib or IDH1/2 inhibitors, or checkpoint-inhibitors (Davids et al. 2016), or targeting CD33 (Ando et al. 2010; Owonikoko et al. 2007; Piccaluga et al. 2004) together with RT and underlying graft-versus-leukemia (GvL) effects are possible on an individual basis but prospective data are missing. For patients with isolated CNS manifestation of AML, intrathecal injection of chemotherapy with a dual (dexamethasone and cytarabine) or a triple combination (dexamethasone, cytarabine, and methotrexate) are feasible whereas intrathecal application of DLI has been reported only once in the literature in three patients as a *coup de main*, respectively (Neumann et al. 2011). Ideally, however, all patients with EM AML should be included in clinical AML trials whenever possible.

**Citation** From Heinrich Lehndorff (1910), free translation by Clarence King (1934).

## References


Alakel N, Stolzel F, Mohr B, Kramer M, Oelschlagel U, Rollig C et al (2017) Symptomatic central nervous system involvement in adult patients with acute myeloid leukemia. Cancer Manag Res 9:97–102

Alvarez P, Navascues CA, Ordieres C, Pipa M, Vega IF, Granero P et al (2011) Granulocytic sarcoma of the small bowel, greater omentum and peritoneum associated with a CBFbeta/MYH11 fusion and inv(16) (p13q22): a case report. Int Arch Med 4(1):3

Ando T, Mitani N, Matsunaga K, Nakazora T, Gondo T, Yujiri T et al (2010) Gemtuzumab ozogamicin therapy for isolated extramedullary AML relapse after allogeneic hematopoietic stem-cell transplantation. Tohoku J Exp Med 220(2):121–126

Ansari-Lari MA, Yang CF, Tinawi-Aljundi R, Cooper L, Long P, Allan RH et al (2004) FLT3 mutations in myeloid sarcoma. Br J Haematol 126(6):785–791

Arber DA, Orazi A, Hasserjian R, Thiele J, Borowitz MJ, Le Beau MM et al (2016) The 2016 revision to the World Health Organization classification of myeloid neoplasms and acute leukemia. Blood 127(20):2391–2405

Arber DA, Borowitz MJ, Cessna M, Etzell J, Foucar K, Hasserjian RP et al (2017) Initial diagnostic workup of acute leukemia: guideline from the College of American Pathologists and the American Society of Hematology. Arch Pathol Lab Med 141(10):1342–1393

Avni B, Koren-Michowitz M (2011) Myeloid sarcoma: current approach and therapeutic options. Ther Adv Hematol 2(5):309–316

Bakst R, Yahalom J (2011) Radiation therapy for leukemia cutis. Pract Radiat Oncol 1(3):182–187

Bakst RL, Tallman MS, Douer D, Yahalom J (2011) How I treat extramedullary acute myeloid leukemia. Blood 118(14):3785–3793

Bakst R, Wolden S, Yahalom J (2012) Radiation therapy for chloroma (granulocytic sarcoma). Int J Radiat Oncol Biol Phys 82(5):1816–1822

Byrd JC, Weiss RB (1994) Recurrent granulocytic sarcoma. An unusual variation of acute myelogenous leukemia associated with 8;21 chromosomal translocation and blast expression of the neural cell adhesion molecule. Cancer 73(8):2107–2112

Byrd JC, Edenfield WJ, Shields DJ, Dawson NA (1995) Extramedullary myeloid cell tumors in acute nonlymphocytic leukemia: a clinical review. J Clin Oncol 13(7):1800–1816

Caraffini V, Perfler B, Berg JL, Uhl B, Schauer S, Kashofer K et al (2018) Loss of RKIP is a frequent event in myeloid sarcoma and promotes leukemic tissue infiltration. Blood 131(7):826–830

Cheng CL, Li CC, Hou HA, Fang WQ, Chang CH, Lin CT et al (2015) Risk factors and clinical outcomes of acute myeloid leukaemia with central nervous system involvement in adults. BMC Cancer 15:344

Cohen PR, Talpaz M, Kurzrock R (1988) Malignancy-associated Sweet's syndrome: review of the world literature. J Clin Oncol 6(12):1887–1897

Cornelissen JJ, Gratwohl A, Schlenk RF, Sierra J, Bornhauser M, Juliusson G et al (2012) The European LeukemiaNet AML working party consensus statement on allogeneic HSCT for patients with AML in remission: an integrated-risk adapted approach. Nat Rev Clin Oncol 9(10):579–590

Davids MS, Kim HT, Bachireddy P, Costello C, Liguori R, Savell A et al (2016) Ipilimumab for patients with relapse after allogeneic transplantation. N Engl J Med 375(2):143–153

Deeb G, Baer MR, Gaile DP, Sait SN, Barcos M, Wetzler M et al (2005) Genomic profiling of myeloid sarcoma by array comparative genomic hybridization. Genes Chromosomes Cancer 44(4):373–383

Dohner K, Schlenk RF, Habdank M, Scholl C, Rucker FG, Corbacioglu A et al (2005) Mutant nucleophosmin (NPM1) predicts favorable prognosis in younger adults with acute myeloid leukemia and normal cytogenetics: interaction with other gene mutations. Blood 106(12):3740–3746

Falini B, Lenze D, Hasserjian R, Coupland S, Jaehne D, Soupir C et al (2007) Cytoplasmic mutated nucleophosmin (NPM) defines the molecular status of a significant fraction of myeloid sarcomas. Leukemia 21(7):1566–1570

Fernandez HF, Sun Z, Litzow MR, Luger SM, Paietta E, Racevskis J et al (2019) Extramedullary acute myeloid leukemia presenting in young adults demonstrates sensitivity to high-dose anthracycline: a subset analysis from ECOG-ACRIN 1900. Haematologica 104(4):e147–ee50

Ganzel C, Manola J, Douer D, Rowe JM, Fernandez HF, Paietta EM et al (2016) Extramedullary disease in adult acute myeloid leukemia is common but lacks independent significance: analysis of patients in ECOG-ACRIN Cancer Research Group Trials, 1980-2008. J Clin Oncol 34(29):3544–3553

Ge L, Ye F, Mao X, Chen J, Sun A, Zhu X et al (2014) Extramedullary relapse of acute leukemia after allogeneic hematopoietic stem cell transplantation: different characteristics between acute myelogenous leukemia and acute lymphoblastic leukemia. Biol Blood Marrow Transplant 20(7):1040–1047

Harris AC, Kitko CL, Couriel DR, Braun TM, Choi SW, Magenau J et al (2013) Extramedullary relapse of acute myeloid leukemia following allogeneic hematopoietic stem cell transplantation: incidence, risk factors and outcomes. Haematologica 98(2):179–184

Karlin L, Itti E, Pautas C, Rachid M, Bories D, Cordonnier C et al (2006) PET-imaging as a useful tool for early detection of the relapse site in the management of primary myeloid sarcoma. Haematologica 91(12 Suppl):ECR54

Kashofer K, Gornicec M, Lind K, Caraffini V, Schauer S, Beham-Schmid C et al (2018) Detection of prognostically relevant mutations and translocations in myeloid sarcoma by next generation sequencing. Leuk Lymphoma 59(2):501–504

King C (1934) A case of chloroma with orbital involvement locally benefited by X-ray therapy. Trans Am Ophthalmol Soc 32:340–353

Kuenzle K, Taverna C, Steinert HC (2002) Detection of extramedullary infiltrates in acute myelogenous leukemia with whole-body positron emission tomography and 2-deoxy-2-[18F]-fluoro-D-glucose. Mol Imaging Biol 4(2):179–183

Larson SM, Graff KS, Tretner IH, Zager RF, Henderson EA, Johnston GS (1972) Positive gallium 677 photoscan in myeloblastoma. JAMA 222(3):321–323

Lehndorff (1910) Ergebnisse der inneren Medizin und Kinderheilkunde, p 221

Li Z, Stolzel F, Onel K, Sukhanova M, Mirza MK, Yap KL et al (2015) Next-generation sequencing reveals clinically actionable molecular markers in myeloid sarcoma. Leukemia 29(10):2113–2116

Mantzarides M, Bonardel G, Fagot T, Gontier E, Soret M, Revel TD et al (2008) Granulocytic sarcomas evaluated with F-18-fluorodeoxyglucose PET. Clin Nucl Med 33(2):115–117

Meis JM, Butler JJ, Osborne BM, Manning JT (1986) Granulocytic sarcoma in nonleukemic patients. Cancer 58(12):2697–2709

Mirza MK, Sukhanova M, Stolzel F, Onel K, Larson RA, Stock W et al (2014) Genomic aberrations in myeloid sarcoma without blood or bone marrow involvement: characterization of formalin-fixed paraffin-embedded samples by chromosomal microarrays. Leuk Res 38(9):1091–1096

Montesinos P, Diaz-Mediavilla J, Deben G, Prates V, Tormo M, Rubio V et al (2009) Central nervous system involvement at first relapse in patients with acute promyelocytic leukemia treated with all-trans retinoic acid and anthracycline monochemotherapy without intrathecal prophylaxis. Haematologica 94(9):1242–1249

Neumann M, Blau IW, Burmeister T, Tietze-Buerger C, Blau O, Gerbitz A et al (2011) Intrathecal application of donor lymphocytes in leukemic meningeosis after allogeneic stem cell transplantation. Ann Hematol 90(8):911–916

O'Donnell MR, Tallman MS, Abboud CN, Altman JK, Appelbaum FR, Arber DA et al (2017) Acute myeloid leukemia, version 3.2017, NCCN clinical practice guidelines in oncology. J Natl Compr Cancer Netw 15(7):926–957

Ohanian M, Faderl S, Ravandi F, Pemmaraju N, Garcia-Manero G, Cortes J et al (2013) Is acute myeloid leukemia a liquid tumor? Int J Cancer 133(3): 534–543

Owonikoko T, Agha M, Balassanian R, Smith R, Raptis A (2007) Gemtuzumab therapy for isolated extramed-

ullary AML relapse following allogeneic stem-cell transplant. Nat Clin Pract Oncol 4(8):491–495
Piccaluga PP, Martinelli G, Rondoni M, Malagola M, Gaitani S, Isidori A et al (2004) Gemtuzumab ozogamicin for relapsed and refractory acute myeloid leukemia and myeloid sarcomas. Leuk Lymphoma 45(9):1791–1795
Pileri SA, Ascani S, Cox MC, Campidelli C, Bacci F, Piccioli M et al (2007) Myeloid sarcoma: clinicopathologic, phenotypic and cytogenetic analysis of 92 adult patients. Leukemia 21(2):340–350
Pui MH, Fletcher BD, Langston JW (1994) Granulocytic sarcoma in childhood leukemia: imaging features. Radiology 190(3):698–702
Shem-Tov N, Saraceni F, Danylesko I, Shouval R, Yerushalmi R, Nagler A et al (2017) Isolated extramedullary relapse of acute leukemia after allogeneic stem cell transplantation: different kinetics and better prognosis than systemic relapse. Biol Blood Marrow Transplant 23(7):1087–1094
Shihadeh F, Reed V, Faderl S, Medeiros LJ, Mazloom A, Hadziahmetovic M et al (2012) Cytogenetic profile of patients with acute myeloid leukemia and central nervous system disease. Cancer 118(1):112–117
Shimizu H, Saitoh T, Hatsumi N, Takada S, Handa H, Jimbo T et al (2013) Prevalence of extramedullary relapses is higher after allogeneic stem cell transplantation than after chemotherapy in adult patients with acute myeloid leukemia. Leuk Res 37(11): 1477–1481
Solh M, DeFor TE, Weisdorf DJ, Kaufman DS (2012) Extramedullary relapse of acute myelogenous leukemia after allogeneic hematopoietic stem cell transplantation: better prognosis than systemic relapse. Biol Blood Marrow Transplant 18(1):106–112
Solh M, Solomon S, Morris L, Holland K, Bashey A (2016) Extramedullary acute myelogenous leukemia. Blood Rev 30(5):333–339
Stolzel F, Rollig C, Radke J, Mohr B, Platzbecker U, Bornhauser M et al (2011) (1)(8)F-FDG-PET/CT for detection of extramedullary acute myeloid leukemia. Haematologica 96(10):1552–1556
Stolzel F, Hackmann K, Kuithan F, Mohr B, Fussel M, Oelschlagel U et al (2012) Clonal evolution including partial loss of human leukocyte antigen genes favoring extramedullary acute myeloid leukemia relapse after matched related allogeneic hematopoietic stem cell transplantation. Transplantation 93(7):744–749
Stolzel F, Luer T, Lock S, Parmentier S, Kuithan F, Kramer M et al (2020) The prevalence of extramedullary acute myeloid leukemia detected by 18FDG-PET/CT: final results from the prospective PETAML trial. Haematologica 105(6):1552–1558
Tsimberidou AM, Kantarjian HM, Wen S, Keating MJ, O'Brien S, Brandt M et al (2008) Myeloid sarcoma is associated with superior event-free survival and overall survival compared with acute myeloid leukemia. Cancer 113(6):1370–1378
Ueda K, Ichikawa M, Takahashi M, Momose T, Ohtomo K, Kurokawa M (2010) FDG-PET is effective in the detection of granulocytic sarcoma in patients with myeloid malignancy. Leuk Res 34(9):1239–1241
Vago L (2019) Clonal evolution and immune evasion in posttransplantation relapses. Hematology Am Soc Hematol Educ Program 2019(1):610–616
Vardiman JW, Thiele J, Arber DA, Brunning RD, Borowitz MJ, Porwit A et al (2009) The 2008 revision of the World Health Organization (WHO) classification of myeloid neoplasms and acute leukemia: rationale and important changes. Blood 114(5):937–951
Vega-Ruiz A, Faderl S, Estrov Z, Pierce S, Cortes J, Kantarjian H et al (2009) Incidence of extramedullary disease in patients with acute promyelocytic leukemia: a single-institution experience. Int J Hematol 89(4):489–496
von den Driesch P (1994) Sweet's syndrome (acute febrile neutrophilic dermatosis). J Am Acad Dermatol 31(4):535–556; quiz 57–60
Xavier SG, Fagundes EM, Hassan R, Bacchi C, Conchon M, Tabak DG et al (2003) Granulocytic sarcoma of the small intestine with CBFbeta/MYH11 fusion gene: report of an aleukaemic case and review of the literature. Leuk Res 27(11):1063–1066
Yamauchi K, Yasuda M (2002) Comparison in treatments of nonleukemic granulocytic sarcoma: report of two cases and a review of 72 cases in the literature. Cancer 94(6):1739–1746
Yoshihara S, Ando T, Ogawa H (2012) Extramedullary relapse of acute myeloid leukemia after allogeneic hematopoietic stem cell transplantation: an easily overlooked but significant pattern of relapse. Biol Blood Marrow Transplant 18(12):1800–1807
Zhang XH, Zhang R, Li Y (2010) Granulocytic sarcoma of abdomen in acute myeloid leukemia patient with inv(16) and t(6;17) abnormal chromosome: case report and review of literature. Leuk Res 34(7):958–961

# Special Clinical Scenarios: Infectious Complications and Prophylaxis

16

Rosanne Sprute and Oliver A. Cornely

## 16.1 Introduction

Patients with acute myeloid leukemia, in particular when undergoing remission induction and consolidation chemotherapy, are particularly susceptible to severe infections. Immunocompromise may precede the diagnosis of leukemia for weeks, and antineoplastic treatment will aggravate immunosuppression. Insufficient myelopoiesis leads to neutropenia and additional humoral or cell-mediated immunosuppression. Chemotherapy treatments further deplete the number of neutrophils. Additionally, the iatrogenic disruption of skin barriers and loss of mucosal integrity increase the risk of infections with colonizing pathogens.

The duration and extent of neutropenia correlate with the risk to acquire infections. AML patients undergoing induction and consolidation therapy are generally considered to be at high risk due to the expected long episodes of neutropenia. The spectrum and complexity of infections in these patients are profound. Bacteria are mainly causative, but invasive fungal infections and virus reactivations also have a high incidence in AML patients and contribute significantly to morbidity and mortality. Additionally, infections have the potential to delay or compromise the continuation of antineoplastic therapy.

On the basis of the attenuated immune response, AML patients often do not show a strong inflammatory reaction and serious infections can occur with minimal signs and symptoms. The earliest and often the only clinical sign of infection may be an increased temperature ≥38 °C, which led to this particular definition of fever. It must be kept in mind when using analgesics (NSAR, metamizole, and acetaminophen) or steroids (Freifeld et al. 2011; Heinz et al. 2017) that may mask fever.

A fast diagnostic work-up of fever of unknown origin (FUO) in AML patients is essential, but in many patients, no site of infection or causative pathogen can be identified (Freifeld et al. 2011; Neumann et al. 2013). However, substantially better outcomes can be expected in neutropenic patients receiving prompt evidence-based empirical anti-infective therapy at the onset of fever. Infections can disseminate rapidly in patients with neutropenia, underscoring the importance of early therapy to avoid progression to life-threatening sepsis. Thus, after obtaining blood cultures, empiric therapy with broad-spectrum antibiotics should be initiated promptly in all febrile neutropenic patients, including those receiving antimicrobial prophylaxis.

R. Sprute · O. A. Cornely (✉)
Department I of Internal Medicine, Excellence Center for Medical Mycology (ECMM), University of Cologne, Faculty of Medicine and University Hospital Cologne, Cologne, Germany

University of Cologne, Faculty of Medicine and University Hospital Cologne, Chair Translational Research, Cologne Excellence Cluster on Cellular Stress Responses in Aging-Associated Diseases (CECAD), Cologne, Germany
e-mail: oliver.cornely@uk-koeln.de



C. Röllig, G. J. Ossenkoppele (eds.), *Acute Myeloid Leukemia*, Hematologic Malignancies,
https://doi.org/10.1007/978-3-030-72676-8_16

## 16.2 Definitions

**Neutropenia:** The definition of neutropenia varies in the literature. In line with recent guidelines, a neutrophil count <500/μL or <1000/μL with an expected decline to <500/μL within the next 48 h defines neutropenia (Freifeld et al. 2011; Heinz et al. 2017). Patients with a count <100/μL are considered to be at an even higher risk of infection.

**Fever:** Fever in neutropenic patients is typically defined as a single oral temperature measurement of ≥38.3 °C or a temperature of ≥38.0 °C sustained over 1 h. Noninfectious causes of a febrile reaction such as drug-induced fever, malignancy-associated cytokine release, or a transfusion of blood products should be ruled out to regard the symptom as a sign of infection.

### 16.2.1 First Fever in an Episode of Neutropenia

#### 16.2.1.1 Initial Assessment

To identify a possible site of infection, thorough knowledge of patient history and clinical examination is essential. Particular attention must be paid to the skin, oropharyngeal mucosa, indwelling catheters and devices, lungs, paranasal sinuses, and perianal region. Vital parameters should be frequently monitored in patients with febrile neutropenia.

Laboratory tests include a complete blood cell count including full white blood cell count with differential and platelet count, electrolytes, serum concentrations of creatinine and blood urea nitrogen, and total bilirubin, as well as serum activities of hepatic transaminase enzymes (Freifeld et al. 2011). Lactate, a blood gas analysis, and coagulation assays contribute to identify patients in need of intensive care early (Heinz et al. 2017).

Prior to the initiation of antibiotic therapy, a minimum of two separate pairs of blood cultures should be drawn by venipuncture and (if present) from the central venous catheter (CVC). Differential time to positivity (DTTP) >120 min indicates a CVC-related infection and CVC removal is usually necessary (Hentrich et al. 2014). If clinical signs or symptoms indicate a focus of infection, further cultures must be taken as appropriate, for example, urine, stool, sputum, or oral swabs. Of note, urinary tract infections in neutropenic patients often do not cause localized symptoms such as dysuria. A urine sample obtained prior initiation of antibiotic treatment increases the overall yield of relevant pathogens but must not delay empiric treatment.

In case of lower respiratory tract symptoms, a chest CT scan is indicated. A chest X-ray has lower sensitivity and specificity and is outdated. Other imaging procedures are indicated according to clinical signs or symptoms. For example, symptoms of sinusitis should prompt a CT scan of the paranasal sinuses, while abdominal complaints give the reason for abdominal ultrasound (Heinz et al. 2017).

## 16.3 Empirical First-Line Therapy

Current standard microbiological techniques do not allow to identify the causative pathogen and its susceptibility pattern earlier than within 24–48 h. Nevertheless, prompt initiation of empiric therapy is paramount until the results of pathogen identification and susceptibility testing are available to guide a more targeted approach. Patients with febrile neutropenia must receive their empirical antibiotic therapy urgently after the onset of fever to minimize the risk of life-threatening infection. Treatment initiation within 2 h is generally accepted, but the faster the better.

For empiric antibiotic therapy, the local epidemiology and local resistance patterns from individual institutions should always be considered before deciding on an antibacterial regimen. High-risk patients require a hospital-based therapy with a first-line broad-spectrum antibacterial agent. It should comprise activity against *Pseudomonas aeruginosa* and other gram-negative pathogens (Enterobacteria such as *Escherichia coli* and *Klebsiella spp.*) as well as gram-positives, predominantly *Staphylococcus aureus* and α-hemolytic streptococci (Heinz et al. 2017). In up to a third of patients, bacteremia with one of these pathogens will be diagnosed. Anaerobes are rare causes of infection and therefore do not need to be considered in first-line empirical therapy.

Several therapeutic choices are available. Monotherapy with cefepime, ceftazidime, a carbapenem (imipenem or meropenem), or piperacillin/tazobactam is generally appropriate as first-line therapy. Actually, multidrug combinations are not more effective (Freifeld et al. 2011; Heinz et al. 2017). Several studies tried to assess evidence for the superior efficacy of combination antibiotic regimes but a significant clinical benefit could not be reached (Bliziotis et al. 2005; Vardakas et al. 2005). This may be different in settings and regions of pronounced antimicrobial resistance.

Penicillin allergy is the most frequently reported drug allergy and most patients who believe to have had a weak reaction to penicillin never had a proper diagnosis of allergy, and will likely tolerate cephalosporins and carbapenems. Many hospitals provide a management pathway including skin testing and test dosing. However, patients with a history of immediate-type hypersensitivity reactions such as urticaria or bronchospasm should receive an alternative empiric combination regimen without beta-lactams or carbapenems, for example aztreonam plus vancomycin or ciprofloxacin plus clindamycin (Freifeld et al. 2011). Given the drastic reduction in therapeutic options, allergy must be ruled out before the next chemotherapy.

## 16.4 Re-evaluation of the First-Line Therapy

During empiric treatment, a daily reassessment of treatment response is mandatory. When an infection focus is identified or a causative pathogen has been isolated, the initial antibiotic regime may be adjusted based on susceptibility assay results.

The role of baseline screening for multi-resistant pathogens is still being defined. Screening of newly or re-admitted patients should be considered. In patients at risk for infections with multidrug-resistant bacteria (colonization, previous infection, or high rates of endemicity in the hospital), a modification to the initial therapy may be considered. For methicillin-resistant *Staphylococcus aureus* (MRSA), early addition of vancomycin or teicoplanin is indicated. For extended-spectrum β-lactamases (ESBL)-producing gram-negatives, the use of carbapenem is appropriate. Although vancomycin-resistant enterococci (VRE) colonization increases a patient's risk of developing VRE infections, the addition of linezolid to empirical first-line treatment has not shown a significant benefit and is not recommended in current guidelines.

## 16.5 Duration of Empirical Antimicrobial Therapy After Defervescence

The duration of therapy depends on the type of infection, the pathogen isolated, and the persistence of or recovery from neutropenia. In persistently neutropenic patients without identified focus nor pathogen but with a stable defervescence, empiric therapy can be discontinued a few days after all signs and symptoms of infection are resolved. In afebrile patients with no signs of infection and a good hematopoietic recovery, the empirical antibiotic therapy can be discontinued after 2 days (Heinz et al. 2017).

### 16.5.1 Second-Line Treatment

In patients with persisting fever for more than 96 h, with a second episode of fever in the neutropenic phase, or with signs of infectious disease progression, a complete physical examination must be repeated once more, blood cultures should be drawn and other diagnostic tests performed as guided by symptoms. The antibiotic spectrum should be reviewed and a change of the empiric antimicrobial treatment regimen considered. Independent of the presence of respiratory symptoms, a multi-slice pulmonary CT scan is recommended after 96 h of persistent or recurrent fever despite adequate therapy (Heinz et al.

2017). If a second febrile episode in the same neutropenic period begins, a CT scan should be done within hours.

## 16.6 Empirical Antifungal Treatment

AML patients are at high risk of invasive fungal infections. Fungi are mostly identified in patients with prolonged neutropenia and persistent or recurrent fever receiving empirical antibiotic therapy, rather than initially occurring in the early phases of neutropenia (Freifeld et al. 2011; Heinz et al. 2017).

Yeasts (primarily *Candida* species) are ubiquitous colonizers of human mucosal surfaces and can cause superficial infections such as stomatitis. Additionally, the breakdown of the mucosal integrity facilitates the translocation of yeasts to the bloodstream. Molds, such as *Aspergillus* species or emerging Mucorales, mainly cause pulmonary manifestations and sinusitis with substantial mortality in immunocompromised hosts (Cornely et al. 2019).

Serial monitoring for serum galactomannan levels can be used to guide antifungal therapy in high risk patients (Maertens et al. 2004). Of note, several confounders complicate the interpretation of test results, and sensitivity and specificity are generally lower in patients with hematologic malignancies (Pfeiffer et al. 2006). β-D-Glucan testing can detect many fungal pathogens, including *Candida* and *Aspergillus* species. The test has high sensitivity, but detects β-D-glucan of various sources apart from invasive fungal infection (Freifeld et al. 2011; Heinz et al. 2017).

A mold-active empirical antifungal therapy is recommended after 4–7 days in persistently febrile patients or if fever relapses despite adequate antibiotic therapy. The choice of antifungal depends on the use of antifungal prophylaxis and the suspected fungal infection. The echinocandin caspofungin and the polyene liposomal amphotericin B are empirical therapy options in neutropenic patients without prior antifungal prophylaxis and with fever persisting for ≥96 h (Walsh et al. 2004).

## 16.7 Empirical Antiviral Treatment

### 16.7.1 Herpes Viruses

Viruses that trigger fever in patients with AML often belong to the herpes virus family. These viral diseases are typically not newly acquired but mostly occur as reactivation of latent infections with herpes simplex virus (HSV) or varicella zoster virus (VZV). Epstein–Barr virus and cytomegalovirus mainly have importance in the setting of allogenic stem cell transplantation (Sandherr et al. 2015).

Empiric antiviral therapy is not indicated in the management of febrile neutropenic patients. Antiviral treatment for HSV or VZV is only recommended if there is active viral disease detected by clinical and laboratory examination. Most viral infections during neutropenia are due to HSV. However, typical lesions of grouped vesicles often do not occur, making the diagnosis of HSV-related mucositis more difficult. It requires proof of viral replication by molecular methods.

### 16.7.2 Respiratory Viruses

The risk of viral infections of the respiratory tract is notably increased in patients with neutropenia. Testing for respiratory viruses (influenza, parainfluenza, respiratory syncytial virus, SARS-CoV-2, etc.) and chest imaging are indicated for patients with respiratory complaints, including upper respiratory symptoms such as cough or rhinitis (Sandherr et al. 2015). Proven infections with the influenza virus should be treated with neuraminidase inhibitors. Empirical treatment of influenza-like symptoms is only recommended in outbreak situations or after exposure (Freifeld et al. 2011). For recommendations on vaccination, please see Sect. 16.7.3.1.4.3.

### 16.7.3 Hepatitis B Virus

Please see Sect. 16.7.3.1.4.2

#### 16.7.3.1 Prophylaxis

Despite prompt administration of empirical antibiotic therapy, infections in neutropenic cancer patients are still the leading cause for nonrelapse mortality (Neumann et al. 2013; Bucaneve et al. 2005; Cometta et al. 2003). To reduce infection rates and complications during neutropenia, prophylaxis may be considered in patients anticipated to have severe and long-lasting neutropenia. This risk is generally present in patients receiving induction and consolidation treatment for AML.

##### Antibacterial Prophylaxis

The routine use of antibacterial prophylaxis in patients with cancer and neutropenia is controversially discussed. Studies have demonstrated that antibacterial prophylaxis can reduce febrile events, and the number of documented infections is well-tolerated and cost-effective. The strongest evidence has been for prophylaxis with fluoroquinolones (Bucaneve et al. 2005).

On the other hand, trials have failed to convincingly demonstrate a survival benefit associated with antibacterial prophylaxis. A number of randomized clinical trials have suggested that prophylaxis with fluoroquinolones may have a survival advantage but could not demonstrate a significant, but only a numerical reduction in mortality rates (Bucaneve et al. 2005; Cullen et al. 2005).

Furthermore, prophylaxis can lead to drug-related adverse effects such as antibiotic-associated diarrhea and the promotion of antibiotic-resistant pathogens. A recent history of antibiotic exposure increases the risk of infections due to bacterial pathogens resistant to the antibiotic used (Ruhnke et al. 2014).

Additionally, fluoroquinolone prophylaxis in a patient strictly precludes the subsequent use of fluoroquinolones for initial empirical therapy in febrile neutropenic patients (Freifeld et al. 2011; Neumann et al. 2013). This drastically reduces the treatment options, particularly in settings of resistant pathogens or β-lactam-allergic patients.

Thus, the benefit of reduced febrile episode rates during neutropenia must be weighed against the lack of convincing evidence for a statistically robust reduction of mortality. Combined with concerns regarding drug-related adverse events and the promotion of resistance, this strengthens the arguments against routine use of antibacterial prophylaxis in AML patients.

##### Antifungal Prophylaxis

For patients who experience prolonged neutropenia, prophylaxis against invasive mold and *Candida* infections is considered beneficial. In patients with acute leukemia, antifungal prophylaxis is associated with significant reductions in invasive fungal infection rates and all-cause mortality (Robenshtok et al. 2007; Cornely et al. 2007).

The risk of an invasive fungal infection rises for patients with prolonged neutropenia for more than 7 days. Prophylaxis should be performed with posaconazole during remission induction chemotherapy for AML (Cornely et al. 2007). The delayed-release tablet formulation of posaconazole is usually well-tolerated, provides predictable absorption and should be favored over oral suspension if feasible. A loading dose of 2 × 300 mg on the first day should be given, followed by a maintenance dose of 300 mg daily from the second day (Mellinghoff et al. 2018; Cornely et al. 2016). Prophylaxis may be started several days before the expected onset of neutropenia.

Of note, posaconazole is an inhibitor of CYP3A4 and drug interactions need to be considered, for example, with midostaurin (reduction of midostaurin dose by 50%, monitoring) or venetoclax (reduction of venetoclax dose by 75%) (Gallogly et al. 2017; Agarwal et al. 2017). Anyhow, routine therapeutic drug monitoring during posaconazole prophylaxis with the tablet formulation is not recommended (Cornely et al. 2016). If posaconazole is contraindicated, screening for serum galactomannan three times per week is an option for the early diagnosis of invasive fungal infection (Maertens et al. 2001).

##### Pneumocystis jirovecii Pneumonia Prophylaxis

Pneumocystis jirovecii plays a special role as a yeast-like fungus with a history of misdetermination as a protozoan parasite. It can cause potentially life-threatening infections in immunocompromised individuals.

Prophylaxis with TMP-SMX is highly effective in preventing Pneumocystis jirovecii pneumonia (PCP) and associated with a decrease in mortality in patients with neoplastic disease. This has particularly been demonstrated in patients with acute lymphatic leukemia (Sepkowitz 1992). For AML patients, solid data on the actual risk for PCP and the benefit of prophylaxis are sparse (Pagano et al. 2002). As PCP is seldom seen in AML patients, prophylaxis should only be considered during intensive treatment regimens that place patients at particular risk.

Given these conditions, TMP-SMX is considered the first-line agent for prophylaxis. An administration of 960 mg three times per week is recommended for the period of treatment-induced immunosuppression.

Alternative drugs for prophylaxis are less well studied for hematological patients. Regimes that may be used in case of intolerance are oral atovaquone (1500 mg/day), oral dapsone (100 mg/day), or aerosolized pentamidine (300 mg every 4 weeks) (Neumann et al. 2013).

### Antiviral Prophylaxis

#### HSV and VZV

As mentioned above, most viral infections during neutropenia are due to HSV and VZV. Opinions differ on prophylaxis of virus reactivation: some authors recommend antiviral prophylaxis with acyclovir or valacyclovir for patients who are seropositive for HSV and are undergoing leukemia induction therapy (Freifeld et al. 2011). However, no significant effect of antiviral prophylaxis with acyclovir on the reduction of febrile days, the rate of bloodstream infections, and other opportunistic infections or mortality could be proven in several studies (Sandherr et al. 2015; Bergmann et al. 1997; Yahav et al. 2009). Due to this sparse evidence, antiviral prophylaxis in patients with AML undergoing induction or consolidation therapy is not a standard. Hematopoietic stem cell transplant (HCT) recipients who are seropositive for HSV and/or VZV should receive oral antiviral prophylaxis following transplant. Prophylaxis should be continued for up to 30 days after allogenic HCT for HSV and for up to 1 year for VZV (Ullmann et al. 2016).

#### Hepatitis B Virus

Reactivation of hepatitis B virus (HBV) infections is common in AML patients with a history of hepatitis B. Thus, HBV screening is recommended in AML patients (HBs antigen and anti-HBc) and if positive, prophylactic lamivudine (HBV-DNA < 2000 IU/mL), entecavir, or nucleotide analogs as tenofovir (HBV-DNA > 2000 IU/mL) are recommended to prevent reactivation (Cometta et al. 2003). Most data on effectiveness exist for lamivudine but entecavir and tenofovir have higher antiviral potency and are therefore recommended in patients with a high viral load. In the case of HBsAg negativity and anti-HBc negativity, immunization should be considered.

Randomized trials investigating the optimal duration of prophylaxis do not exist, but reactivations have been described even after the end of antineoplastic therapy. Thus, recent guidelines recommend to continue antiviral prophylaxis for 6–12 months after the completion of antineoplastic therapy (Sandherr et al. 2015).

After allogenic HCT, anti-HBc positive patients should be regularly monitored for HBV DNA and preemptive antiviral treatment should be initiated in case of viral load. Treatment should be continued until at least 6 months after the cessation of immunosuppression (Ullmann et al. 2016).

#### Influenza Virus

Seasonal influenza vaccination with an inactivated vaccine is recommended for all patients with AML regardless of antineoplastic therapy. The best timing for a good serological response is not established, but recent guidelines recommend an immunization between chemotherapy cycles. The second administration of influenza vaccine can be reasonable to enhance seroconversion (Rousseau et al. 2012). In addition, vaccination of all family members, health-care workers, and other close contacts is of particular importance to reduce the risk of infection (Freifeld et al. 2011; Sandherr et al. 2015).

Cytomegalovirus

Patients after allogenic HCT are at particularly high risk for cytomegalovirus (CMV) disease. CMV causes multiorgan disease both early (<100 days) and late (>100 days) after HCT and remains one of the most important pathogens for transplant-associated complications. All CMV-seronegative recipients ideally should receive a CMV-seronegative donor graft. CMV-seropositive patients have a poorer outcome than seronegative patients. To prevent transmission via transfusions in CMV-seronegative recipients, blood products from seronegative donors or leucocyte-depleted blood products should be used (Ullmann et al. 2016; Ljungman et al. 2019).

Prophylaxis of infection or early preemptive intervention, for example, with ganciclovir, foscarnet or letermovir, remains the foundations of effective CMV infection management for seropositive patients (Ljungman et al. 2019; Marty et al. 2017). The early initiation of antiviral preemptive treatment based on weekly quantitative PCR monitoring for at least 100 days after transplant is recommended over prophylaxis treatment (Ljungman et al. 2019).

### Myeloid Growth Factor for Infection Prophylaxis

Granulocyte colony stimulating factor (G-CSF) and granulocyte/macrophage colony stimulating factor (GM-CSF) are used to promote the production of leukocytes and can prevent infectious complications.

The preemptive use of hematopoietic growth factors has been shown to reduce the duration of treatment-induced neutropenia, the incidence of neutropenic fever, and the infection-related and all-cause mortality (Walsh et al. 2004; Mehta et al. 2015; Kuderer et al. 2007). CSF prophylaxis may be considered particularly in the elderly or for patients with additional risk factors. If indicated, CSFs should be started at the end of the chemotherapy cycle. For the treatment of established fever, CSFs are not generally recommended (Freifeld et al. 2011; Heinz et al. 2017; Vehreschild et al. 2014).

## References


Agarwal SK, DiNardo CD, Potluri J, Dunbar M, Kantarjian HM, Humerickhouse RA et al (2017) Management of Venetoclax-Posaconazole Interaction in acute myeloid leukemia patients: evaluation of dose adjustments. Clin Ther 39(2):359–367

Bergmann OJ, Mogensen SC, Ellermann-Eriksen S, Ellegaard J (1997) Acyclovir prophylaxis and fever during remission-induction therapy of patients with acute myeloid leukemia: a randomized, double-blind, placebo-controlled trial. J Clin Oncol 15(6):2269–2274

Bliziotis IA, Michalopoulos A, Kasiakou SK, Samonis G, Christodoulou C, Chrysanthopoulou S et al (2005) Ciprofloxacin vs an aminoglycoside in combination with a beta-lactam for the treatment of febrile neutropenia: a meta-analysis of randomized controlled trials. Mayo Clin Proc 80(9):1146–1156

Bucaneve G, Micozzi A, Menichetti F, Martino P, Dionisi MS, Martinelli G et al (2005) Levofloxacin to prevent bacterial infection in patients with cancer and neutropenia. N Engl J Med 353(10):977–987

Cometta A, Kern WV, De Bock R, Paesmans M, Vandenbergh M, Crokaert F et al (2003) Vancomycin versus placebo for treating persistent fever in patients with neutropenic cancer receiving piperacillin-tazobactam monotherapy. Clin Infect Dis 37(3):382–389

Cornely OA, Maertens J, Winston DJ, Perfect J, Ullmann AJ, Walsh TJ et al (2007) Posaconazole vs. fluconazole or itraconazole prophylaxis in patients with neutropenia. N Engl J Med 356(4):348–359

Cornely OA, Duarte RF, Haider S, Chandrasekar P, Helfgott D, Jimenez JL et al (2016) Phase 3 pharmacokinetics and safety study of a posaconazole tablet formulation in patients at risk for invasive fungal disease. J Antimicrob Chemother 71(3):718–726

Cornely OA, Alastruey-Izquierdo A, Arenz D, Chen SCA, Dannaoui E, Hochhegger B et al (2019) Global guideline for the diagnosis and management of mucormycosis: an initiative of the European Confederation of Medical Mycology in cooperation with the Mycoses Study Group Education and Research Consortium. Lancet Infect Dis 19(12):e405–e421

Cullen M, Steven N, Billingham L, Gaunt C, Hastings M, Simmonds P et al (2005) Antibacterial prophylaxis after chemotherapy for solid tumors and lymphomas. N Engl J Med 353(10):988–998

Freifeld AG, Bow EJ, Sepkowitz KA, Boeckh MJ, Ito JI, Mullen CA et al (2011) Clinical practice guideline for the use of antimicrobial agents in neutropenic patients with cancer: 2010 update by the Infectious Diseases Society of America. Clin Infect Dis 52(4):e56–e93

Gallogly MM, Lazarus HM, Cooper BW (2017) Midostaurin: a novel therapeutic agent for patients with FLT3-mutated acute myeloid leukemia and systemic mastocytosis. Ther Adv Hematol 8(9):245–261

Heinz WJ, Buchheidt D, Christopeit M, von Lilienfeld-Toal M, Cornely OA, Einsele H et al (2017) Diagnosis and empirical treatment of fever of unknown origin (FUO) in adult neutropenic patients: guidelines of the infectious diseases working party (AGIHO) of the German Society of Hematology and Medical Oncology (DGHO). Ann Hematol 96(11):1775–1792

Hentrich M, Schalk E, Schmidt-Hieber M, Chaberny I, Mousset S, Buchheidt D et al (2014) Central venous catheter-related infections in hematology and oncology: 2012 updated guidelines on diagnosis, management and prevention by the infectious diseases working party of the German Society of Hematology and Medical Oncology. Ann Oncol 25(5):936–947

Kuderer NM, Dale DC, Crawford J, Lyman GH (2007) Impact of primary prophylaxis with granulocyte colony-stimulating factor on febrile neutropenia and mortality in adult cancer patients receiving chemotherapy: a systematic review. J Clin Oncol 25(21):3158–3167

Ljungman P, de la Camara R, Robin C, Crocchiolo R, Einsele H, Hill JA et al (2019) Guidelines for the management of cytomegalovirus infection in patients with haematological malignancies and after stem cell transplantation from the 2017 European conference on infections in leukaemia (ECIL 7). Lancet Infect Dis 19(8):e260–e272

Maertens J, Verhaegen J, Lagrou K, Van Eldere J, Boogaerts M (2001) Screening for circulating galactomannan as a noninvasive diagnostic tool for invasive aspergillosis in prolonged neutropenic patients and stem cell transplantation recipients: a prospective validation. Blood 97(6):1604–1610

Maertens J, Theunissen K, Verbeken E, Lagrou K, Verhaegen J, Boogaerts M et al (2004) Prospective clinical evaluation of lower cut-offs for galactomannan detection in adult neutropenic cancer patients and haematological stem cell transplant recipients. Br J Haematol 126(6):852–860

Marty FM, Ljungman P, Chemaly RF, Maertens J, Dadwal SS, Duarte RF et al (2017) Letermovir prophylaxis for cytomegalovirus in hematopoietic-cell transplantation. N Engl J Med 377(25):2433–2444

Mehta HM, Malandra M, Corey SJ (2015) G-CSF and GM-CSF in neutropenia. J Immunol 195(4):1341–1349

Mellinghoff SC, Panse J, Alakel N, Behre G, Buchheidt D, Christopeit M et al (2018) Primary prophylaxis of invasive fungal infections in patients with haematological malignancies: 2017 update of the recommendations of the infectious diseases working party (AGIHO) of the German Society for Haematology and Medical Oncology (DGHO). Ann Hematol 97(2):197–207

Neumann S, Krause SW, Maschmeyer G, Schiel X, von Lilienfeld-Toal M, Infectious Diseases Working Party et al (2013) Primary prophylaxis of bacterial infections and Pneumocystis jirovecii pneumonia in patients with hematological malignancies and solid tumors: guidelines of the infectious diseases working party (AGIHO) of the German Society of Hematology and Oncology (DGHO). Ann Hematol 92(4):433–442

Pagano L, Fianchi L, Mele L, Girmenia C, Offidani M, Ricci P et al (2002) Pneumocystis carinii pneumonia in patients with malignant haematological diseases: 10 years' experience of infection in GIMEMA centres. Br J Haematol 117(2):379–386

Pfeiffer CD, Fine JP, Safdar N (2006) Diagnosis of invasive aspergillosis using a galactomannan assay: a meta-analysis. Clin Infect Dis 42(10):1417–1427

Robenshtok E, Gafter-Gvili A, Goldberg E, Weinberger M, Yeshurun M, Leibovici L et al (2007) Antifungal prophylaxis in cancer patients after chemotherapy or hematopoietic stem-cell transplantation: systematic review and meta-analysis. J Clin Oncol 25(34):5471–5489

Rousseau B, Loulergue P, Mir O, Krivine A, Kotti S, Viel E et al (2012) Immunogenicity and safety of the influenza A H1N1v 2009 vaccine in cancer patients treated with cytotoxic chemotherapy and/or targeted therapy: the VACANCE study. Ann Oncol 23(2):450–457

Ruhnke M, Arnold R, Gastmeier P (2014) Infection control issues in patients with haematological malignancies in the era of multidrug-resistant bacteria. Lancet Oncol 15(13):e606–e619

Sandherr M, Hentrich M, von Lilienfeld-Toal M, Massenkeil G, Neumann S, Penack O et al (2015) Antiviral prophylaxis in patients with solid tumours and haematological malignancies—update of the guidelines of the infectious diseases working party (AGIHO) of the German Society for Hematology and Medical Oncology (DGHO). Ann Hematol 94(9):1441–1450

Sepkowitz KA (1992) Pneumocystis carinii pneumonia among patients with neoplastic disease. Semin Respir Infect 7(2):114–121

Ullmann AJ, Schmidt-Hieber M, Bertz H, Heinz WJ, Kiehl M, Krüger W et al (2016) Infectious diseases in allogeneic haematopoietic stem cell transplantation: prevention and prophylaxis strategy guidelines 2016. Ann Hematol 95(9):1435–1455

Vardakas KZ, Samonis G, Chrysanthopoulou SA, Bliziotis IA, Falagas ME (2005) Role of glycopeptides as part of initial empirical treatment of febrile neutropenic patients: a meta-analysis of randomised controlled trials. Lancet Infect Dis 5(7):431–439

Vehreschild JJ, Bohme A, Cornely OA, Kahl C, Karthaus M, Kreuzer KA et al (2014) Prophylaxis of infectious complications with colony-stimulating factors in adult cancer patients undergoing chemotherapy-evidence-based guidelines from the infectious diseases working party AGIHO of the German Society for Haematology and Medical Oncology (DGHO). Ann Oncol 25(9):1709–1718

Walsh TJ, Teppler H, Donowitz GR, Maertens JA, Baden LR, Dmoszynska A et al (2004) Caspofungin versus liposomal amphotericin B for empirical antifungal therapy in patients with persistent fever and neutropenia. N Engl J Med 351(14):1391–1402

Yahav D, Gafter-Gvili A, Muchtar E, Skalsky K, Kariv G, Yeshurun M et al (2009) Antiviral prophylaxis in haematological patients: systematic review and meta-analysis. Eur J Cancer 45(18):3131–3148

# 17 Future Developments: Novel Agents

Chong Chyn Chua and Andrew H. Wei

## 17.1 Introduction

For patients with acute myeloid leukaemia (AML), the European Union (EU) has approved midostaurin (Stone et al. 2017), gemtuzumab ozogamicin (Castaigne et al. 2012) CPX-351(Lancet et al. 2018), gilteritinib (Perl et al. 2019b) and most recently glasdegib (DAURISMO; Pfizer Inc.). Most of these therapies are covered in detail in other chapters of this book. This paper will focus on new, non-immune-based therapies which have potential to make a clinical impact for patients with AML in the near future. These include venetoclax (VENCLEXTA; AbbVie Inc.), enasidenib (IDHIFA; Celgene Corp.), ivosidenib (TIBSOVO; Agios Pharmaceutical Inc.) and glasdegib (DAURISMO; Pfizer Inc.). We will also highlight a number of other non-immunologic novel agents that have medium-term potential for regulatory approval in AML.

Advancement of scientific research and genomic technologies over the last decade has drastically improved our understanding of AML pathogenesis, contributing to development of targeted therapeutic agents designed to target putative molecular drivers of AML. The resulting changes in the treatment landscape have resulted in a complex therapeutic environment in the United States with 8 anti-leukaemic drugs added to the treatment arsenal between 28 April 2017 and 28 November 2018. These include midostaurin, CPX-351, gemtuzumab ozogamicin, venetoclax, glasdegib, ivosidenib, enasidenib and gilteritinib. To date, five of these drugs have been approved by the European Medicines Agency (EMA) (Table 17.1). In many other parts of the world, midostaurin is the only recently approved new AML therapy. Consequently, what is considered 'standard of care' now differs substantially depending on which geographic jurisdiction the patient is diagnosed in.

With the advent of these new treatment options, the management of AML has rapidly evolved from a 'one size fits all' approach, to one where it is now imperative to acquire relevant molecular information both at diagnosis and at each relapse timepoint to ensure that the optimal treatment option is identified and tailored for each patient. In reality, however, the molecular architecture of AML is characteristically polyclonal and highly likely to evolve resistance to therapeutic pressure, as has been observed with inhibitors of IDH (Quek et al. 2018), FLT3 (McMahon et al. 2019b) and BCL-2 (DiNardo et al. 2020a). As a result, despite incremental improvements in disease outcomes with several new therapies, disease relapse remains a dominant

C. C. Chua · A. H. Wei (✉)
Department of Haematology, The Alfred Hospital, Melbourne, VIC, Australia

Australian Centre for Blood Diseases, Monash University, Melbourne, VIC, Australia
e-mail: a.wei@alfred.org.au



C. Röllig, G. J. Ossenkoppele (eds.), *Acute Myeloid Leukemia*, Hematologic Malignancies,
https://doi.org/10.1007/978-3-030-72676-8_17

**Table 17.1** Recent regulatory approved drugs for AML

| Indication | Drug | Mechanism of action | Regulatory approval | Resistance mechanisms | Predictors of sensitivity |
|---|---|---|---|---|---|
| *FLT3 mutant AML* | | | | | |
| Newly diagnosed | Midostaurin (RYDAPT, Novartis) | Type 2 inhibitor with multiple kinase targets | • EMA: 20 September 2017<br>• FDA: 28 April 2017<br>• In combination with standard cytarabine and daunorubicin induction and cytarabine consolidation | • Off-target: Upregulation of MCL-1 | • Effective in FLT3-ITD and FLT3-TKD |
| Relapsed refractory | Gilteritinib (XOSPATA, Astellas) | Type 1 FLT3 and AXL inhibitor | • EMA: 8 November 2019<br>• FDA: 28 November 2018<br>• Monotherapy | • On-target: FLT3 gatekeeper F691L mutation<br>• Off-target: RAS/MAPK pathway signalling mutations; clonal evolution | • Effective in FLT3-ITD and FLT3-TKD |
| *IDH2 mutant AML* | | | | | |
| Relapsed refractory | Enasidenib (IDHIFA, Celgene) | IDH2 inhibitor | • EMA: not approved<br>• FDA: 1 August 2017<br>• Monotherapy | • On-target: second-site mutations, IDH1 mutations<br>• Off-target: FLT3 (ITD and TKD), Receptor tyrosine kinase pathway mutations especially NRAS | • Similar response rates in IDH2 R140 or R172 mutant cases |
| *IDH1 mutant AML* | | | | | |
| Newly diagnosed or relapsed refractory | Ivosidenib (TIBSOVO, Agios) | IDH1 inhibitor | • EMA: not approved<br>• FDA: 20 July 2018 (RR); 2 May 2019 (Newly diagnosed)<br>• Monotherapy | • On-target: second-site mutations, IDH2 mutations<br>• Off-target: Receptor tyrosine kinase pathway mutations | • IDH1 mutations |
| *Unfit/elderly patients (age ≥ 75 years, or comorbidities that preclude intensive chemotherapy)* | | | | | |
| Newly diagnosed | Venetoclax (VENCLEXTA, Abbvie/ Genentech) | Selective BCL-2 inhibitor, induces cell apoptosis | • EMA: not approved<br>• FDA: 21 November 2018<br>• In combination with either hypomethylating agents or low-dose cytarabine | • On-target: BCL-2 binding site mutation (described only in chronic lymphocytic leukaemia at venetoclax failure)<br>• Off-target: Upregulation of other BH3 apoptosis pathways (MCL-1, BCL-xL); receptor tyrosine kinase pathway mutations (especially *FLT3*-ITD), *TP53* mutations | • NPM1, IDH2, IDH1 |

| | | | | | |
|---|---|---|---|---|---|
| Newly diagnosed | Glasdegib (DAURISMO, Pfizer) | Hedghog signalling pathway inhibitor | • EMA: 26 June 2020<br>• FDA: 21 November 2018<br>• In combination with low-dose cytarabine | • Requires further studies | • Requires further studies |
| *Fit patients with AML-MRC or t-AML* | | | | | |
| Newly diagnosed | CPX-351 (VYXEOS, Jazz Pharmaceuticals) | Liposomal formulation of cytarabine and daunorubicin at fixed 5:1 molar ratio | • EMA: 23 August 2018<br>• FDA: 3 August 2017<br>• Monotherapy | • On-target: N/A<br>• Off-target: *TP53* mutations | • AML-MRC or t-AML |
| *CD33 positive AML* | | | | | |
| Newly diagnosed or relapsed refractory | Gemtuzumab ozogamicin (MYLOTARG, Pfizer) | Anti-CD33 monoclonal antibody conjugated to calicheamicin | • EMA: 4 May 2018<br>• FDA: 1 September 2017<br>• May be used in combination with cytarabine and daunorubicin chemotherapy for newly diagnosed AML | • Adverse risk cytogenetics (associated with lower CD33 expression) | • Favourable risk cytogenetics |

cause of treatment failure, which mitigates the magnitude of overall survival (OS) gained with new drugs in the context of randomised studies with OS as the primary endpoint. Treatment failure may be either primary or adaptive in nature and related to on- or off-target resistance mechanisms, depending on the type of therapeutic pressure exerted by an individual agent.

The key challenge moving forward will be to devise effective combination treatment strategies able to overcome dynamic mechanisms of resistance, as well as identifying the optimal sequencing of therapies that will deliver the best long-term outcomes for patients with AML. This chapter will focus on emerging therapies that have potential to be approved by the EMA in the next few years. The discussion of immune-based and recently approved EMA therapies will be the subject of other chapters in this book. This chapter will be structured to discuss new drugs directed at improving AML outcomes for patients who are: (1) older or unfit for intensive chemotherapy, (2) relapsed or refractory to prior therapy, (3) in first remission and not eligible for allogeneic stem cell transplantation or (4) harbouring adverse risk *TP53* mutant AML.

## 17.2 New Therapies Aimed at Improving Outcomes for Older Patients with AML

### 17.2.1 Progress and Challenges in Targeting BCL-2

Venetoclax, a selective, potent, orally bioavailable small-molecule BCL-2 inhibitor has emerged as a promising therapy for frontline treatment of elderly AML. The BCL-2 family of proteins consists of pro- and anti-apoptotic proteins that tightly regulate mitochondrial outer membrane permealisation (MOMP), which when perturbed, may commit the cell to death by apoptosis (Czabotar et al. 2014). There are three classes of BCL-2 family proteins including (1) pro-survival proteins (e.g. BCL-2, BCL-xL, MCL-1), or (2) pro-apoptotic BCL-2 homology 3 (BH3) only proteins (e.g. BIM, BID, BAD, Puma) or (3) multidomain pro-apoptotic proteins (e.g. BAX, BAK, BOK) (Czabotar et al. 2014). Preclinical studies have demonstrated that some AML cells with expression of BCL-2 are particularly primed for cell death, owing to pre-bound BIM that is released upon venetoclax binding to BCL-2 (Konopleva and Letai 2018; Konopleva et al. 2006). AML blasts, however, also frequently express other related pro-survival BCL-2 family proteins, such as BCL-xL, MCL-1 and BFL1, thereby limiting the activity of single agent venetoclax, which had only modest activity in the phase 2 monotherapy clinical trial conducted predominantly in relapsed and refractory (R/R) patients with AML (Konopleva et al. 2016). Venetoclax at a dose of 800 mg daily was used in patients with R/R ($n$ = 30) or treatment naïve AML ($n$ = 2) (Konopleva et al. 2016). The overall response rate was 19% (6% complete remission [CR], 13% CR with incomplete count recovery [CRi]). Notably, 4 out of 6 patients who achieved CR had *IDH1/2* mutations, suggesting potential venetoclax sensitivity in this subgroup of patients. This prompted two parallel phase 1/2 trials to explore the activity of venetoclax in older patients with AML ineligible for intensive chemotherapy in the frontline setting in combination with either low-dose ara-C (LDAC) or the hypomethylating agents (HMA) azacitidine and decitabine (DiNardo et al. 2018a; Wei et al. 2017).

#### 17.2.1.1 Venetoclax in Combination with LDAC

The phase 2 study combined venetoclax at 600 mg daily (recommended phase 2 dose [RP2D]) in 28-day cycles with LDAC at 20 mg/m$^2$/day administered subcutaneously (SC) on days 1 to 10 (Wei et al. 2019b). The median age of enrolled patients was 74 years (range: 63–90 years), and eligible patients were deemed unfit for intensive chemotherapy. The overall composite response rate was 54% with a median OS of 10.1 months, with impressive responses seen in de novo AML, *NPM1* or *IDH1/2* mutant patients (CR/CRi of 71%, 89% and 72% respectively). The safety profile was manageable with treatment-induced cytopenia a limiting factor in some patients endeavouring to receive further post-remission therapy.

To confirm these results, a phase 3 randomised, placebo-controlled study (VIALE-C) was undertaken, comparing LDAC + venetoclax or placebo in 211 patients with AML ≥75 years or considered unfit for intensive chemotherapy. (Wei et al. 2020a) The primary study analysis showed that median OS in the venetoclax versus placebo arm was 7.2 months versus 4.1 months, respectively (hazard ratio [HR] 0.75 [95% CI 0.52–1.07], $p = 0.11$), which did not meet the prespecified primary endpoint. Nonetheless, closer inspection revealed a high number of censored patients in the LDAC + venetoclax arm with follow-up times <6 months. An unplanned analysis with an additional 6 months of follow-up demonstrated a median OS of 8.4 months for the venetoclax arm (HR 0.70; 95% CI 0.50–0.98; $p = 0.04$). CR/CRi rates were superior for venetoclax (48 vs. 13%), as was event-free survival, patient-reported outcomes and transfusion independence. Key grade ≥ 3 adverse events were balanced between the two arms. The need for post-study therapy was lower for patients in the venetoclax arm (23 vs. 44%). In the phase 3 trial for LDAC + venetoclax early mortality was 13%, compared to 6% in the phase 2 study. This could reflect the fact that in the phase 3 study, older patients were enrolled (76 vs. 74 years). In addition, the proportion of patients with poorer performance status (ECOG 2–3) was higher (48 vs. 29%) (Table 17.2).

**Table 17.2** Comparison between phase 1b/2 and phase 3 LDAC + venetoclax studies

| Treatment | LDAC + Placebo (Ph 3) (Wei et al. 2020a) | LDAC + VEN 600 mg (Ph 3) (Wei et al. 2020a) | LDAC + VEN 600 mg (Ph 1b/2) (Wei et al. 2019c) |
|---|---|---|---|
| N | 68 | 143 | 82 |
| Median age (years) | 76 | 76 | 74 |
| ≥75 | 59% | 57% | 49% |
| ECOG 2–3 | 50% | 48% | 29% |
| Adverse cytogenetics | 29% | 33% | 32% |
| Secondary AML | 34% | 41% | 49% |
| Prior hypomethylating agent | 21% | 20% | 29% |
| 30-day treatment-related mortality | 16% | 13% | 6% |
| CR/CRi | 13% | 48% | 54% |
| CR | 7% | 27% | 26% |
| Cri | 6% | 21% | 28% |

### 17.2.1.2 Venetoclax in Combination with HMA

Venetoclax has also been combined with either a 5-day course of decitabine or a 7-day azacitidine schedule in 145 newly diagnosed treatment-naïve patients with AML ineligible for intensive chemotherapy (DiNardo et al. 2019b). There was an initial venetoclax dose escalation phase (venetoclax 400 mg, 800 mg, 1200 mg) followed by dose expansion at venetoclax 400 mg, which was the RP2D. The overall CR/CRi rate was 67% (CR 37%, CRi 30%). The median duration of response (DOR) was 11.3 months with a median OS of 17.5 months. The adverse events were similar to that of venetoclax-LDAC, with mainly cytopenia and febrile neutropenia. Early (30-day) mortality was 3%. Subgroup analysis revealed that *NPM1* mutant cases were high responders with a CR/CRi rate of 91.5% and a median OS that was not reached. *IDH1/2* cases had a CR/CRi rate of 71% and a 24.4-month median OS. Contrary to the LDAC plus venetoclax study, this trial excluded prior HMA exposure, which could account for some of the observed differences in outcome between the two treatment approaches. With increasing use of venetoclax combined with lower-intensity therapies, recommendations for practical management have been published (DiNardo and Wei 2020; Jonas and Pollyea 2019).

Based on the promising phase 1b/2 results, a phase 3 study comparing azacitidine + venetoclax/placebo (VIALE-A) was conducted with the goal of determining whether addition of venetoclax to azacitidine will lead to improved response rates and overall survival in patients with AML ≥75 years or considered unfit for intensive chemotherapy (NCT02993523). Preliminary results have been presented at the European Haematology Association (EHA) 25th Annual Congress in June 2020. A total 286 patients received venetoclax and 145 received placebo. The primary endpoint was met with a prolonged median overall survival of 14.7 months in the venetoclax group versus 9.6 months in the placebo group (HR 0.66; 95% CI 0.52–0.85, $p < 0.001$). The CR/CRi rate was 66.4 versus 28.3% in the venetoclax and placebo group respectively. Median time to CR/CRi was 1.3 months in the venetoclax arm. The CR/CRi rates in *NPM1* and *IDH1/2* mutant patients were 67% and 75% respectively. Of interest, 55% of *TP53* mutant cases achieved CR/CRi with this regimen (vs. 0% in the placebo group).

#### 17.2.1.3 More Dose Intensive Venetoclax-Based Approaches

A phase 2 study has combined venetoclax 400 mg daily with a more intensified 10-day decitabine regimen in both newly diagnosed and R/R AML, including 31% patients with prior HMA exposure.(Maiti et al. 2019a) Venetoclax was initially given daily in a 28-day cycle, but the schedule was truncated to 21, 14, 10 or 7 days for the management of myelosuppression. After achievement of clinical response, decitabine was de-escalated to a 5-day regimen. Interim results on 101 patients demonstrated the regimen was tolerable and associated with CR/CRi rates of 95% in newly diagnosed AML ($n = 40$), 67% in untreated sAML ($n = 9$), 37% in treated sAML ($n = 19$) and 27% in R/R AML ($n = 33$). The median OS was not reached for the newly diagnosed group, 6.4 months for the treated sAML group and 7.1–7.3 months for the remaining groups. 30-day mortality was 2.5%. From these initial results, it appears that the initial response rates to 10-day decitabine plus venetoclax are higher than observed with a 5-day decitabine schedule. In the absence of comparative trials, it is not certain whether these improved initial responses will translate into enhanced overall survival in the newly diagnosed AML population.

The feasibility of combining venetoclax with intensive chemotherapy in fit older patients (age ≥65 years or ≥60 years with monosomal karyotype) with newly diagnosed AML has been explored in a phase 1b study called 'CAVEAT' (Chua et al. 2019, 2020) (ANZ Clinical Trial Registry ACTRN12616000445471) Fifty-one patients have been enrolled into five dose-escalation cohorts of venetoclax ranging from 50 to 600 mg. Venetoclax was given for 14 days (instead of the 28-day schedule in the lower intensity study), with an initial 7-day pre-phase/dose ramp up of venetoclax followed by a modified intensive 5 + 2 chemotherapy schedule (infusional cytarabine 100 $mg/m^2$ days 1–5 and idarubicin 12 $mg/m^2$ IV days 2–3) due to concerns regarding increased myelosuppression. Patients who achieved at least a partial remission (PR) proceeded to have up to 4 cycles of consolidation which consisted of venetoclax 14 days combined with cytarabine (days 1–2) and idarubicin (day 1), followed by up to 7 cycles of maintenance venetoclax monotherapy. The maximum tolerated dose was not identified for venetoclax up to 600 mg. The study reported no clinically significant tumour lysis syndrome, noting that a number of measures were implemented including the venetoclax pre-phase, a requirement for white cell counts to be $<25 \times 10^9/L$ prior to commencing therapy and sequential introduction of chemotherapy. The 30-day mortality was 6%, and no unexpected adverse events were reported. The efficacy in terms of CR/CRi was 72% in the overall cohort, and significantly higher in the de novo AML group; 97 versus 44% in the sAML group. Overall response rates (ORR) were favourable in *IDH2*, *NPM1* and *SRSF2* mutant patients (100%, 82% and 80% respectively), and unfavourable in *TP53* mutant patients (ORR 33%, all CRi). Although 80% of *FLT3*-ITD mutant patients achieved CR/CRi, the DOR was short, and majority relapsed with persistent *FLT3*-ITD mutant disease.

Another ongoing phase 1b/2 trial has examined the combination of venetoclax with an intensive FLAG-IDA induction and FLAG consolidation regimen in both newly diagnosed and R/R AML adult patients (age 18+) (Aboudalle et al. 2019). FLAG-IDA consisted of fludarabine 30 $mg/m^2$ IV D2–6, cytarabine 2 $g/m^2$ IV D2–6, idarubicin 6 $mg/m^2$ IV D4–6 (8 $mg/m^2$ for newly diagnosed AML) and filgrastim. Venetoclax was initially dosed at 200 mg on D1–21 with dose escalation to 400 mg. Due to observed gram-negative sepsis in 5 out of 6 patients during induction, dose modifications were implemented, reducing cytarabine from 2 to 1.5 g/m$^2$ and the duration of venetoclax from 21 to 14 days. Preliminary results presented at ASH 2019 included 34 patients with a median age of 48 years reported an ORR (CR/CRi/PR) of 74% in R/R AML and 93% in newly diagnosed cases (Aboudalle et al. 2019). With a short median follow-up of 5.2 months, the median OS was 7.1 months in the R/R cohort and not reached in the newly diagnosed group. Notably, 5/5 MLL-rearranged AML (including 3 R/R AML) achieved a response that allowed them to proceed to allogeneic haematopoietic stem cell transplantation (HSCT).

The above studies have demonstrated dynamic synergistic potentials of combining venetoclax with various combinations of intensive and non-intensive therapies, with impressive anti-leukaemic activities. Nonetheless, treatment-induced myelosuppression remains a key consideration when optimising the dose and scheduling of venetoclax-based combinations in AML.

### 17.2.2 Mechanisms and Predictors of Sensitivity or Resistance to BCL-2 Inhibition in AML

#### 17.2.2.1 Molecular Determinants of Response and Treatment Failure

Analysis of patients treated in the phase 2 venetoclax plus HMA or LDAC trials identified higher clinical response rates in patients with *NPM1* and/or *IDH2* mutant AML. Patients with *NPM1* mutations receiving these venetoclax-based combinations had evidence of measurable residual disease (MRD) eradication with prolonged molecular remissions observed whilst on therapy (DiNardo et al. 2020a). In contrast, clones carrying kinase activating mutants, such as *FLT3*-ITD or bi-allelic *TP53* aberrations, were found to contribute to drug resistance manifesting as either primary or adaptive treatment failure. Pre-clinical CRISPR-based screens also indicated loss of p53 function as a cause of venetoclax resistance (Nechiporuk et al. 2019). In clinical studies, rapid and sometimes discordant changes in clonal architecture could be observed after a single cycle of therapy among primary refractory cases, highlighting the dynamic impact of venetoclax in AML. Preliminary data from the more intensive venetoclax-chemotherapy study CAVEAT showed similar molecular patterns of response, suggesting that chemotherapy intensity alone may not be sufficient to overcome the adverse prognostic effects of *FLT3*-ITD and *TP53* mutations in AML (Chua et al. 2019). In an attempt to overcome the *FLT3*-ITD mediated resistance associated with venetoclax-chemotherapy combinations, venetoclax has been combined with the FLT3 inhibitor gilteritinib, which has been shown pre-clinically to synergise potently with venetoclax (DiNardo et al. 2020b). In a pilot study, the venetoclax-gilteritinib combination has shown highly promising activity in a cohort of 10 patients with relapsed/refractory *FLT3* mutant AML, with an overall response rate of 90% (CR/ CRi/morphologic leukaemia free state [MLFS]) (Perl et al. 2019a). Follow-up is ongoing.

#### 17.2.2.2 Upregulation of Pro-Survival Proteins Induce Off-Target Resistance to Venetoclax Therapy

Upregulation of the pro-survival protein MCL-1 is an established mediator of AML cell survival (Glaser et al. 2012). Preclinical studies have shown strong synergy between combined BCL-2 and MCL-1 targeting resulting in a rapid and durable anti-leukaemic effect in AML cell line xenograft models as well as patient derived xenograft models across a broad spectrum of AML genotypes (Moujalled et al. 2019). Patients receiving venetoclax plus azacitidine have also been shown to select for monocytic differentiated blasts, which show enhanced expression of MCL-1 and consequently reduced sensitivity to venetoclax (Pei et al. 2020). Primary samples from chemo-resistant patients or adverse genetic risk AML exhibit sensitivity to combined BCL-2/ MCL-1 inhibition. Enhanced MCL-1 expression observed in *FLT3* mutant AML mediated by

STAT5 activation may represent a mechanism of venetoclax resistance in *FLT3*-ITD mutant cases. The addition of an MCL-1 inhibitor (Servier S63845) to venetoclax ex vivo was able to reverse the resistance (Grundy et al. 2018). The clinical efficacy and safety of BCL-2/MCL-1 co-targeting either by direct MCL-1 or indirect downregulation (e.g. CDK9 inhibitors, MEK inhibitors) are currently under investigation in several phase 1 clinical trials in AML (venetoclax plus S64315 MCL1 inhibitor, NCT03672695; venetoclax plus AMG176 MCL1 inhibitor, NCT03797261; venetoclax plus the CDK9 inhibitor dinaciclib, NCT03484520).

On-target resistance to venetoclax has been described in patients with progressive chronic lymphocytic leukaemia (CLL), whereby a BCL-2 binding site mutation Gly101Val reduces the affinity of venetoclax to BCL-2 ~ 180 fold. (Blombery et al. 2019) On-target BCL-2 mutations have so far not been reported in patients with AML receiving venetoclax. One reason may be that in patients with AML, treatment more commonly involves venetoclax in combination with chemotherapy, which may reduce the selection of BCL-2 binding domain mutations.

### 17.2.3 Targeting Hedgehog Signalling with Glasdegib

Aberrant overexpression of Hedgehog pathway components was observed in chemotherapy-resistant AML cells leading to leukaemic stem cell survival and expansion. In vivo inhibition of Hedgehog signalling has been found to enhance chemotherapy sensitivity, forming the rationale for the BRIGHT AML 1003 trial (Fukushima et al. 2016). This was an open label, non-placebo controlled randomised phase 2 trial combining glasdegib, a potent selective oral inhibitor of the Hedgehog pathway component Smoothened (SMO), with LDAC.*(*Cortes et al. 2019b*)* Glasdegib was given 100 mg daily continuously throughout each 28-day cycle. LDAC 20 mg/m$^2$/day was administered from days 1–10. A total of 116 patients were enrolled. These included patients ≥75 years or considered unfit for intensive chemotherapy. Glasdegib led to a significantly improvement in median OS (8.3 months vs. 4.3 months, $p = 0.004$), resulting in FDA approval in November 2018. Efficacy was most pronounced in the sAML group, where the CR rate was 20 versus 0% for LDAC alone and median OS 9.1 versus 4.1 months ($p < 0.0001$). In the de novo AML group, CR rates were 18.1 versus 5.6% with LDAC alone. There were no significant differences in mutation profile in responders versus non-responders. However, there was a non-significant association between mutant *CEBPA, IDH1, NPM1, RUNX1* and *TET2* and favourable outcome, in contrast to mutant *DNMT3A, IDH2* and *NRAS/KRAS,* which were associated with an unfavourable outcome. Adverse events (AE) occurring in ≥20% of patients were fatigue, musculoskeletal pain, gastrointestinal AE (including nausea, decreased appetite, dysgeusia, mucositis, constipation) and rash. Other notable treatment-related AE includes alopecia and QTc prolongation.

Although the magnitude of survival improvement with glasdegib and venetoclax in combination with LDAC in older AML populations is similar, the clinical response rate appears higher for venetoclax + LDAC (48%), compared to glasdegib + LDAC (27%). In addition, it appears to be a specific drug-related liability related to glasdegib. The ongoing phase 3 study combining azacitidine with glasdegib/placebo or intensive chemotherapy with glasdegib/placebo (BRIGHT AML 1019, NCT03416179) will provide further evidence of the role of Hedgehog pathway inhibitors in the armamentarium of AML.

## 17.3 New Therapies Aimed at Improving Outcomes for Patients with Relapsed/Refractory AML

### 17.3.1 Inhibiting Isocitrate Dehydrogenase (IDH) in AML

IDH enzymes catalyse the oxidative decarboxylation of isocitrate to alpha-ketoglutarate (α-KG). Recurrent somatic point mutations in *IDH1* and

*IDH2* were first described in 2009 and found to result in neomorphic gain of function with aberrant reduction of α-KG to an oncometabolite 2-hydroxyglutarate (2-HG) (Mardis et al. 2009). Elevated levels of 2-HG led to epigenetic dysregulation and impaired cellular differentiation. Mutations in *IDH1* and *IDH2* occur in approximately 6–10% and 8–19% of adult AML respectively, and are associated with normal/intermediate-risk karyotype and increasing age (Mardis et al. 2009; Cancer Genome Atlas Research Network et al. 2013). *IDH2* mutations most commonly affect the R140 (80%) or R172 (20%) codons (Stein 2016). Co-occurrence of mutant *IDH1* and *IDH2* is rare, occurring in approximately 2–5% of all *IDH* mutant cases. The prognosis of IDH1/2 mutations is variable and dependent on the presence of co-existing mutations such as *NPM1,* which is associated with a favourable outcome (Mardis et al. 2009).

#### 17.3.1.1 Targeting Mutant IDH2: Enasidenib

Enasidenib (AG-221) is an orally bioavailable selective *IDH2* small-molecule inhibitor that has been approved by the FDA as monotherapy for the treatment of adult patients with R/R *IDH2* mutant AML (Yen et al. 2017). In the first-in-human phase 1/2 study of single agent enasidenib, 345 patients with *IDH2* mutant myeloid malignancies were enrolled, including 214 with R/R AML (Stein et al. 2017). In the dose expansion phase, doses of enasidenib ranging from 50 to 650 mg were evaluated, with 100 mg daily selected as the RP2D. In the R/R AML subgroup, the ORR combining CR, CRi, PR and MLFS was 38.8%, with a CR rate of 19.6% (Stein et al. 2017). These responses were similar regardless of *IDH2* mutant subtype. There was an improved ORR in those who had received fewer prior lines of therapy: 46.5% for 1 prior line, 36.9% for 2 prior lines and 25.0% for those with ≥3 prior lines ($p = 0.04$) (Stein et al. 2017). The median OS was 8.8 months (22.9 months for those who attained CR), with an estimated 1-year OS of 39% (Stein et al. 2017). A randomised phase 3 study in older patients with late stage mutant IDH2 R/R AML comparing enasidenib versus conventional care regimens has completed (NCT02577406). Disappointingly, preliminary data indicated that the study did not meet its primary end point of OS, with the detailed study evaluation awaited.

The most common adverse events associated with enasidenib were unconjugated hyperbilirubinemia (10%), thrombocytopenia (7%) and differentiation syndrome (D-S) (6%) (Stein et al. 2017). Akin to all-*trans* retinoic acid (ATRA) in acute promyelocytic leukaemia, IDH inhibitors promote differentiation in *IDH* mutant leukaemia cells, which can result in a clinical differentiation syndrome (Fathi et al. 2018). The median time to onset is 30 days from commencing therapy but can start as early as 10 days or as late as 5 months after commencing therapy (Fathi et al. 2018). Key goals for managing D-S include close monitoring, early identification and prompt treatment upon suspicion. Given the long half-life of IDH inhibitors, withholding IDH therapy alone will not lead to rapid resolution, although this should be considered in severe D-S cases. A more comprehensive management guideline is listed here (Fathi et al. 2018). Thus far, the occurrence of IDH D-S has not been shown to predict response to therapy.

One important feature of enasidenib management is the slow time to response. The medium time to first response in the phase 1/2 trial was 1.9 months (range 0.5–9.4 months), with the median time to best response ~3.7 months (Stein et al. 2017). More than 50% of responding patients responded only after cycle 4, and OS of those with stable disease for >90 days was significantly better than those who with progressive disease by day 90 (Stein et al. 2019). Among the 48% of patients with stable disease, the median time on therapy was 4 months (range: 1–23 months) with haematological improvement and reduced need for transfusions observed in 36–52% (Stein et al. 2019). These data suggest that enasidenib should be continued for at least 6 months or until disease progression. Furthermore, as enasidenib is a differentiating agent, mature myeloid cells retain the *IDH2* mutation (Stein et al. 2017). Thus, mutant *IDH2* may persist at high levels despite remission and clearance of mutant *IDH2* variant allele frequency (VAF) is not a pre-requisite for response. Nonetheless, patients who achieved CR demonstrated a higher degree of VAF reduction compared to non-responders, with correspondingly enhanced survival among those with mutant *IDH2*.

Combination studies of enasidenib are ongoing. A phase 1/2 study in the newly diagnosed *IDH2* mutant patients with AML ineligible for intensive chemotherapy has randomised patients to enasidenib 100 mg daily plus azacitidine ($n = 68$) versus azacitidine alone ($n = 33$) in a 2:1 ratio (NCT02677922) (DiNardo 2019). Interim trial results reported a significantly improved ORR of 68% in the combination arm versus 42% in the monotherapy arm ($p = 0.0155$). True CR rates were 50 versus 12% respectively. The median time to CR was 5 months (range: 1–20 months). The 60-day mortality was 7% in the combination arm and 3% in the azacitidine monotherapy arm. Notable adverse events included IDH D-S which occurred in 10% of patients. Final results of this study are pending. Ongoing studies of enasidenib include enasidenib plus azacitidine in relapsed refractory AML (NCT03683433), enasidenib plus CPX-351 in relapsed refractory AML (NCT03825796) as well as enasidenib plus intensive chemotherapy in patients eligible for intensive chemotherapy (HOVON150AML, NCT03839771).

#### 17.3.1.2 Targeting Mutant IDH1: Ivosidenib, Olutasidenib

Two orally available small molecule IDH1 inhibitors are currently in advanced stages of clinical development. Ivosidenib (AG-120) has been FDA approved in both newly diagnosed and relapsed refractory *IDH1* mutant AML based on non-randomised study data (DiNardo et al. 2018b). Ivosidenib was first evaluated in a phase 1 study including 258 patients with *IDH1* mutant AML (DiNardo et al. 2018b). A dose of 500 mg daily was selected for dose expansion based on favourable safety, efficacy and pharmacokinetics data. In the R/R AML subgroup ($n = 125$), the ORR was 41.6%, including a CR rate of 21.6%. The median OS was 8.8 months, with an 18-month survival rate of 50% in those who achieved CR/CR with partial haematologic recovery (CRh). Of the patients who attained CR/CRh, 21% had undetectable *IDH1* mutations by digital droplet PCR. In newly diagnosed IDH1 mutant AML ($n = 34$), the ORR was 54.5% with a CR rate of 30.3% (Roboz et al. 2019). Importantly, among patients with prior HMA exposure, CR/CRh was achieved in 26.7% with a CR rate of 20% (Roboz et al. 2019). Median duration of response was not reached, with 61.5% remaining in remission at 1 year. Median OS was 12.6 months. Of those who achieved CR/CRh, 64% had *IDH1* mutation clearance. The key adverse events relating to ivosidenib are QTc prolongation and IDH differentiation syndrome (10.6–18%) (DiNardo et al. 2018b; Roboz et al. 2019). Prolongation of QT interval was observed in 18–24.6% of patients including Grade 3+ in 7.8–9%. These events were reported to be managed by dose interruptions and/or dose reductions without needing to discontinue treatment. The role of ivosidenib in the frontline setting in patients fit for intensive chemotherapy is also being explored, in combination with intensive chemotherapy in the HOVON150AML trial (NCT03839771). In this trial, IDH1 inhibition will be used during induction, consolidation and maintenance phases of therapy, including the post-allogeneic stem cell transplant setting.

Olutasidenib (FT-2102, FORMA Therapeutics) is another selective IDH1 inhibitor currently undergoing evaluation. The results of the phase 1 study were presented at the American Society of Hematology (ASH) 2019 annual meeting that included 32 patients treated with olutasidenib monotherapy and 46 patients treated with olutasidenib in combination with azacitidine (Watts et al. 2019). The RP2D of olutasidenib was 150 mg BD. The ORR (CR/CRh/MLFS) was 41% for olutasidenib monotherapy and 46% in combination with azacitidine. Among treatment naïve patients with IDH1 mutant AML, the ORR was 25% and 77% for olutasidenib monotherapy and combination with azacitidine, respectively, noting that the monotherapy arm only had 4 patients. Among patients responding to olutasidenib, the *IDH1* mutation VAF was reduced to <1% in 40% of cases. In terms of adverse events, IDH differentiation syndrome occurred in 13%, QT prolongation in 7% (all in the combination cohort) and grade 3+

hepatic enzyme transaminitis in 12.8% of patients, resulting in discontinuation in 2.5%. The multi-cohort phase 2 study (NCT02719574) is ongoing and will provide clinical data on olutasidenib/azacitidine in both treatment naïve and relapsed refractory AML, maintenance therapy with olutasidenib in those with detectable *IDH1* MRD and response likelihood in patients previously failing a different IDH1 inhibitor.

### Mechanism of Resistance to IDH Inhibitors

A number of studies have shed light on why some patients do not respond to these selective inhibitors despite having the target mutation, and why some do not maintain durable remissions. A clue to on-target IDH inhibition is reduction of 2-HG oncometabolite levels. In some patients, a clue to on-target treatment failure may emerge when there is evidence of failure to suppress 2-HG production due to emergence of 'second-site' mutations or acquisition of a different IDH mutation (Intlekofer et al. 2018; Quek et al. 2018). 'Second-site' mutations were discovered after analysis of serial samples from two patients with *IDH2* mutant AML who initially responded to enasidenib but later relapsed with rising 2-HG levels (Intlekofer et al. 2018). Both cases evolved new missense mutations in the *IDH2* gene affecting the interface where enasidenib binds: Q316E in the first and I319M in the second patient, with each mutation occurring in trans (i.e. affecting the normal allele without the leukaemogenic mutation). The authors proceeded to study these mutations preclinically and found that these 'second-site' mutations only confer resistance to enasidenib when co-expressed with the *IDH2* R140Q mutation. Six novel second-site mutations have also been found in 14% (10/74 with available serial samples) of patients failing ivosidenib therapy, including 2 patients with two concurrent *IDH1* second-site mutations.(Wang et al. 2019).

The second mechanism of on-target resistance is via mutant IDH isoform switching which can occur bidirectionally, that is, from a dominant mutant *IDH1* clone to dominant mutant *IDH2* clone, and vice versa (Quek et al. 2018; Wang et al. 2019; Harding et al. 2018). Although the actual incidence of isoform switching is unknown, these mechanisms have now been well described among patients relapsing on IDH inhibitors. In the phase 1/2 ivosidenib trial, 9/74 (12.1%) patients were found to acquire a new *IDH2* R140Q mutation at relapse (Wang et al. 2019). Similarly, 2/16 (12.5%) enasidenib-failure patients studied by Quek et al. acquired an *IDH1* R132C/H mutation at time of relapse (Quek et al. 2018). Harding et al. concluded that application of selective pressure targeting one mutant IDH population may result in outgrowth of other malignant IDH subclones occurring in a different subcellular compartment (Harding et al. 2018). These mutations could be either acquired in the same clone or in distinct parallel clones, with rare cases found to harbour both *IDH1* and *IDH2* mutations at baseline. Clinical trials incorporating IDH inhibitors are increasingly excluding patients with evidence of concurrent *IDH1* and *IDH2* mutations at study entry. Given the possibility of isoform switching whilst on an IDH inhibitor, serial monitoring for both IDH isoforms on therapy is warranted. Co-targeting of *IDH1* and *IDH2* in a trial setting is a future possibility to determine if this resistance mechanism can be circumvented.

A common mechanism of IDH inhibitor resistance is clonal escape. Quek et al. examined 16 *IDH2* mutant AML cases with relapsing disease on enasidenib therapy and found that 14 (87.5%) patients had persistently suppressed 2-HG levels at the time of relapse, indicating effective on-target enasidenib activity (Quek et al. 2018). Analysis of these relapsing cases revealed diverse off-target molecular mechanisms of clonal evolution, including acquisition of additional mutations or expansion of a pre-existing clone. Two patients had emergence of a new *IDH1* mutation with concurrent elevation of 2-HG. Clinical studies with enasidenib have shown that the co-mutation burden at baseline correlated with disease response, with an ORR of 54.8% in those with $\leq$3 mutations versus 31.3% in those with $\geq$6 mutations ($p = 0.06$). The co-presence of mutations such as *FLT3*-ITD and/or *FLT3*-TKD were associated with a lack of clinical response, and mutations of *NRAS* were associated with poor response rates. Clinical experience with ivosidenib also identified receptor tyrosine kinase pathway mutations to be associated with failure to respond to ivosidenib (Roboz et al. 2019; Wang et al. 2019). In a pre-clinical study of an *IDH2* R140Q *FLT3*-ITD double mutant murine model of AML, enasidenib in combination with quizartinib was found to have enhanced anti-leukaemic activity compared to either agent alone (Shih et al. 2017). These findings have not yet been recapitulated in human trials.

### 17.3.2 Novel–Novel Combinations with IDH Inhibitors

Chan et al. utilised a large-scale RNA interference screen and found that IDH1 R132H mutant AML cells were dependent on BCL-2 and BCL-W for survival (Chan et al. 2015). Further experiments demonstrated that both *IDH1* and *IDH2* mutant primary AML cells had increased sensitivity to venetoclax when compared to *IDH* wild-type cases. The increased sensitivity was shown to be due to increased 2-HG in *IDH* mutant cases, resulting in inhibition of cytochrome c oxidase in the mitochondrial electron transport chain. This led to lowering of the mitochondrial threshold for apoptosis and thus increased susceptibility to BCL-2 inhibition. A separate study also demonstrated increased HOX family gene expression in *IDH* mutant AML cases, which has also been suggested to correlate with increased sensitivity to BCL-2 inhibition in *NPM1* mutant AML (Chaturvedi et al. 2013; Chen et al. 2019). This has led to the rational combination of enasidenib and venetoclax in a phase 1b/2 trial in relapsed refractory *IDH2* mutant AML (NCT04092179), as well as ivosidenib and venetoclax ± azacitidine in *IDH1* mutant AML (NCT03471260). Preliminary results with ivosidenib and venetoclax suggests this combination is highly active. Of 9 evaluable patients, 44% had CR and 33% CRi (Dinardo et al. 2019a).

### 17.3.3 Targeting Mutant FLT3

Several small-molecule tyrosine kinase inhibitors targeting FLT3 signalling are currently in development (Table 17.3). Thus far, two FLT3 inhibitors have been approved by the FDA: midostaurin in first-line treatment of AML in combination with intensive chemotherapy (Stone et al. 2015), and gilteritinib monotherapy in the relapsed refractory setting (Perl et al. 2019b). Two other

**Table 17.3** Summary of FLT3 inhibitors under development

| Drug | Dose | Type | FLT3 receptor selectivity | Non-FLT3 targets | Half-life | Notable toxicities |
|---|---|---|---|---|---|---|
| Midostaurin | 50 mg BD | I | + (Sensitive to TKD) | PKC, SYK, FLK-1, AKT, PKA, KIT, FGR, SRC, PDGFRa/b, VEGFR1/2 | 19 h | Gastrointestinal (GI) toxicity, QTc prolonged |
| Sorafenib | 400 mg BD | II | ++ (Resistant to TKD) | RAF, VEGFR1/2/3, PDGFRB, KIT, RET | 25-48 h | Skin rash (including hand-foot syndrome), diarrhoea |
| Quizartinib | 60 mg daily | II | +++ (Resistant to TKD) | KIT, PDGFR | 1.5 days | QTc prolongation (dose dependent), myelosuppression, alopecia |
| Crenolanib | 100 mg TID | I | ++ (Sensitive to TKD) | PDGFRB | 6-8 h | GI toxicity, hepatic transaminitis, fluid retention |
| Gilteritinib | 120 mg daily | I | ++ (Sensitive to TKD) | LTK, ALK, AXL | 113 h | GI toxicity, hepatic transaminitis, myelosuppression |

inhibitors, quizartinib and crenolanib are in the late stages of development in both front-line and relapsed refractory settings.

Each of the FLT3 inhibitors are distinct with regards to selectivity, potency and mechanism of FLT3 binding. FLT3 inhibitors are classified into first- and second-generation based on their specificity for FLT3, as well as type I or II depending on their mechanism of binding to the FLT3 receptor. First generation inhibitors such as midostaurin and sorafenib lack specificity for FLT3 and have more off-target effects by inhibiting multiple other tyrosine kinase pathways. Second-generation inhibitors such as gilteritinib and quizartinib are more specific and potent against FLT3 without targeting other parallel signalling pathways, hence these agents have a greater degree of activity as monotherapy. In terms of type I and II FLT3 inhibitors, type I inhibitors bind the ATP-binding site of the FLT3 receptor in the active conformation, whereas type II inhibitors only bind when the FLT3 receptor is in an inactive conformation thereby preventing receptor activation. The important difference between both types is that type I inhibitors inhibit both ITD and TKD mutations, whereas type II inhibitors are only active against ITD mutations.

#### 17.3.3.1 Quizartinib (AC220, Daiichi Sankyo)

Quizartinib is a second-generation type II FLT3 inhibitor with increased selectivity and potency for *FLT3*-ITD (Zarrinkar et al. 2009). In contrast to gilteritinib, quizartinib is less active against FLT3-TKD mutations, and in fact, TKD mutations have been observed to evolve in patients with acquired quizartinib resistance (Zarrinkar et al. 2009). The initial development of quizartinib was limited by excess grade 3+ QTc prolongation, occurring in 12% of patients receiving doses greater than 60 mg daily (Cortes et al. 2013, 2019a) A phase IIb dose-finding study in 76 patients with relapsed refractory AML were randomised to receive a starting dose of 30 mg or 60 mg of quizartinib daily, with dose-escalation to 60 mg or 90 mg in the setting of lack or loss of response.(Cortes et al. 2018) The composite CR rate in both groups were comparable at 47%, with similar grade 3+ QTc prolongation rates at 3–5%. A phase 3 trial (QUANTUM-R) randomised 367 patients in a 2:1 ratio to quizartinib 60 mg daily (with a 30 mg lead-in for the first 15 days) versus salvage chemotherapy (LDAC, MEC or FLAG-IDA) at first relapse or in patients refractory to standard AML therapy. Quizartinib was associated with prolonged median OS; 6.2 months versus 4.6 months (hazard ratio for death 0.76, $p = 0.0188$) and a 1-year OS rate of 27 versus 20% ($p = 0.0177$) (Cortes et al. 2019c). Composite CR rates were 48 versus 27% in the quizartinib and salvage chemotherapy arms, respectively. Response duration to quizartinib was a median of 12.1 weeks. Of note, HSCT rates were significantly higher in the quizartinib arm (32 vs. 12% in salvage chemotherapy arm, $p < 0.0001$), suggesting that quizartinib was able to bridge more patients to transplant which may have contributed to the improved survival outcomes. Despite statistically significant improvements in survival, quizartinib's new drug application was declined by the FDA based on modest improvements in OS and no significant benefit observed in the event free survival.

#### 17.3.3.2 Crenolanib (AROG Pharmaceuticals)

Another FLT3 inhibitor in development is crenolanib, a type I FLT3 inhibitor with demonstrable preclinical activity against both *FLT3*-ITD and TKD mutations. In a phase I study in relapsed refractory *FLT3* mutant AML, crenolanib 100 mg tid resulted in 39% CRi and 11% partial remission in 18 patients who were FLT3-TKI naive. The ORR was 31% in a further 36 patients with prior FLT3-TKI failure (Smith et al. 2014).

### 17.3.4 FLT3 Inhibitor Combinations

#### 17.3.4.1 Frontline FLT3 Inhibitor in Combination with Intensive Chemotherapy

All the aforementioned second-generation FLT3 inhibitors are currently undergoing development as frontline therapy in younger patients with newly diagnosed FLT3 mutant AML in combination with intensive chemotherapy. QuANTUM-First (NCT02668653) trial compared quizartinib versus placebo in combination with intensive induction and consolidation chemotherapy, followed by 12 months of maintenance therapy. This study commenced prior to the approval of midostaurin, thus the results will be difficult to interpret or incorporate into the current standard of care where midostaurin is used. Notably, midostaurin will have the advantage of activity against FLT3-TKD, which is a known mechanism of resistance to quizartinib.

Other ongoing frontline studies include a phase III randomised study comparing crenolanib versus midostaurin combined with standard chemotherapy for patients with newly diagnosed FLT3-mutant AML (NCT03258931), as well as the HOVON 156 AML trial (NCT04027309) comparing comparing gilteritinib (150 mg/day on days 8–21) versus midostaurin (50 mg BD on days 8–21) in combination with intensive chemotherapy in patients with newly diagnosed FLT3 mutant AML. The chemotherapy backbone includes 2 cycles of 7 + 3 induction (with cytarabine 200 mg/m$^2$ and daunorubicin 60 mg/m$^2$; note idarubicin is not permitted), followed by either HiDAC or mitoxantrone plus etoposide consolidation, and up to 12 months of monotherapy FLT3 inhibitor maintenance. The preliminary trial data have been encouraging, however these new FLT3 inhibitors will have to show superiority over midostaurin in combination with chemotherapy in order to gain traction in this space.

#### 17.3.4.2 FLT3-HMA Combinations

In FLT3-mutant patients who are not fit for intensive chemotherapy, several FLT3 inhibitor-HMA combinations are being explored. The LACEWING (NCT02752035) study combines gilteritinib with azacitidine and compares it to gilteritinib or azacitidine alone in newly diagnosed FLT3 mutant AML. Quizartinib is also being combined with decitabine in both untreated and relapsed FLT3-ITD mutant patients with AML (NCT03661307).

#### 17.3.4.3 FLT3 Inhibitor in Maintenance

Although many studies now incorporate FLT3 inhibitor maintenance as part of their treatment schema, the actual benefit of FLT3 inhibitors in maintenance remains to be elucidated. Multiple FLT3 inhibitors are currently being explored as maintenance in first remission as well as after HSCT: gilteritinib (NCT02927262, NCT02997202), quizartinib (NCT02668652), midostaurin (NCT0188336) and crenolanib (NCT02400255). The BMT-CTN 1506/Morpho trial (NCT02997202) using gilteritinib as maintenance after HSCT will incorporate a novel and highly sensitive next-generation sequencing assay to detect *FLT3*-ITD minimal residual disease to explore whether measuring FLT3-ITD MRD can help guide future treatment decisions in this space (Levis et al. 2018).

### 17.3.5 Mechanisms of Resistance to FLT3 Inhibitors

Despite promising initial responses with FLT3 inhibitors, the DOR is often short lived due to acquisition of resistance mechanisms. Type II inhibitors such as sorafenib and quizartinib are intrinsically inactive against *FLT3*-TKD mutations. Furthermore, emergence of on-target kinase domain mutations is a common resistance mechanism observed in patients who relapse after initial response (Smith et al. 2015a, b; Baker et al. 2013; Williams et al. 2013). These point mutations directly result in impairment of drug binding, with the most common mutation occurring at the FLT3 gatekeeper F691L position, or in the kinase activation loop affecting the D835 or Y842 residues (Smith et al. 2015b). In contrast, although type I inhibitors gilteritinib and crenolanib are active against FLT3 D835 mutations, they remain vulnerable to the FLT3 gatekeeper F691L mutation, though at a lower frequency. For instance, treatment emergent F691L mutations were only identified in 5/41 (12.2%) of patients relapsing post gilteritinib and 2/18 (11.1%) in crenolanib-treated patients (Zhang et al. 2019; Smith et al. 2019). Pre-clinical studies of gilteritinib did demonstrate activity against the F691 L gatekeeper mutation, except at relatively high concentrations, suggesting a dose-dependent relationship in the acquisition of the F691L mutation prompting caution against unnecessary dose reductions of gilteritinib in clinical use (Mori et al. 2017).

In relation to off-target resistance, activating mutations in the RAS/RAF and related mitogen associated protein kinase (MAPK) pathway have been implicated in second-generation FLT3 inhibitor failures. McMahon et al. analysed paired samples from 41 patients pre- and post-gilteritinib therapy and identified newly acquired RAS pathway mutations as the most common mechanism of resistance to gilteritinib, occurring in 15/41 (36.6%) of patients (*NRAS* 13/15, *KRAS* 3/15, *PTPN11* 3/15, *CBL* 2/15, *BRAF* 1/15), including in 5/41 (12.2%) who relapsed with *FLT3*-ITD negative disease (McMahon et al. 2019a). Other new mutations include *FLT3*-F691L, *WT1, IDH2, CEBPA, RUNX1* and *TBL1XR1*. In addition, 55.2% had clonal evolution with new cytogenetic abnormalities, including 2 patients with new *BCR-ABL1* fusions. Of note F691L and RAS pathway mutations were mutually exclusive in this cohort. Through single-cell targeted DNA sequencing of serial samples in the gilteritinib-treated patients, diverse polyclonal changes were observed over time with acquisition and expansion of RAS pathway mutations occurring in *FLT3* mutant clones as well as subclones that were FLT3 wild-type. Similarly, mutations in RAS signalling pathway genes were enriched in patients with crenolanib-failure, although *NRAS* and *KRAS* mutations were found to be present predominantly in FLT3 wild-type clones (Zhang et al. 2019). Whether combining FLT3 inhibitors with RAS pathway inhibitors such as MEK inhibitors or broader cytotoxic chemotherapy will overcome these RAS-MAPK mediated resistance is unclear and warrants further investigation.

Another important mechanism of resistance is upregulation of anti-apoptotic proteins and genes. *FLT3*-ITD AML has been found to be associated with high expression of MCL-1 and BCL-2, thereby supporting the rationale to combine FLT3 and BCL-2 family inhibitors (Kasper et al. 2012). Preclinical studies have demonstrated therapeutic synergy from combining venetoclax with midostaurin or gilteritinib which may downregulate MCL-1, thereby enhancing venetoclax activity (Ma et al. 2019). The combination of venetoclax and gilteritinib is currently being investigated in a phase Ib/II study in relapsed refractory AML (Perl et al. 2019a). Venetoclax is dosed at 400 mg/day, with 2 levels of gilteritinib at 80 mg ($n$ = 6) and 120 mg ($n$ = 16). 13/18 (87%) FLT3-ITD patients achieved a leukaemia response (defined as CR, CRi, CR with incomplete platelet recovery [CRp] and MLFS) including 3 with CR, 4 with CRi/CRp and 6 with MLFS. 2/2 FLT3-TKD mutant patients achieved CRp. Eleven out of 13 (85%) patients with prior FLT3 inhibitor exposure achieved leukaemia response.

In patients with FLT3 mutant AML, several FLT3 inhibitors are now emerging into clinical use. Key questions now include, whether a promiscuous (midostaurin) or selective FLT3 inhibitor (quizartinib) is the most effective FLT3 targeting strategy in newly diagnosed patients. It also remains to be determined how effective gilteritinib will be in patients with relapsed/refractory disease, especially after prior midostaurin or quizartinib exposure. Furthermore, the positive role of FLT3 inhibitors as maintenance therapy after allogeneic stem cell transplant was recently demonstrated for sorafenib (Burchert et al. 2018). It remains to be determined whether a more potent FLT3 inhibitor (gilteritinib) will also demonstrate this effect despite the majority of patients likely to have received prior midostaurin during the initial induction and consolidation phases of therapy.

## 17.4 New Therapies Aimed at Extending Remission Duration After Intensive Chemotherapy

### 17.4.1 CC-486 (Celgene Corp)

CC-486, an oral hypomethylating agent, is the first therapy to demonstrate significant improvements in overall survival when used as maintenance therapy in first remission after intensive chemotherapy in patients aged ≥55 years (Wei et al. 2019a). Results of the phase III QUAZAR AML-001 trial, a randomised, double-blinded placebo-controlled study, was reported at the ASH meeting in 2019 (Wei et al. 2019a) and subsequently published in the New England Journal of Medicine (Wei et al. 2020b). A total of 472 patients were enrolled, with a median age of 68 years (range: 55–86 years). CC-486 was dosed at 300 mg on days 1–14 of 28-day treatment cycles. At a median follow-up of 41.2 months, the median OS was 24.7 months versus 14.8 months ($p = 0.0009$) from time of randomisation, and median relapsed free survival was 10.2 months versus 4.8 months ($p = 0.0001$) in the CC-486 and placebo arms, respectively. The 2-year OS was 51 versus 37%, and 1-year relapse rate was 53 versus 71% in the CC-486 and placebo-controlled groups. Main adverse events reported included gastrointestinal toxicities (nausea, vomiting, diarrhea) especially during the first 2 cycles, as well as on-treatment neutropenia. No treatment related deaths were reported. It is foreseeable that CC-486 will be used as maintenance therapy in AML in the future. Key future questions will be which molecular sub-groups have the greatest benefit from CC-486 maintenance therapy and which groups of patients should be referred for allogeneic SCT compared to selection for maintenance therapy.

## 17.5 New Drugs to Activate TP53 in AML

### 17.5.1 APR-246 (Aprea Therapeutics) Plus Azacitidine in TP53 Mutant AML

A new drug putatively targeting patients with *TP53* mutant myeloid neoplasms has shown some promising results in pilot studies (Ali et al. 2011). APR-246 is a PRIMA-1 analogue which is reported to covalently modify mutant forms of p53, leading to re-activation of both mutant and wild-type p53 function (Bykov et al. 2002). Currently, however, there is controversy regarding the exact mechanism of action of how this drug works. The combination of APR-246 and azacitidine is currently being evaluated in two parallel phase 1b/2 trials (Sallman 2019; Cluzeau et al. 2019). Both studies deliver APR-246 at 4500 mg/day IV on days 1–4 and azacitidine 75 mg/m$^2$ SC/IV beginning only from day 4 to day 10. The key adverse events specific to APR-246 are neurological (approximately 20–40%, all grades), with ataxia, tremor, cognitive impairment and acute confusion reported. The majority of grade 3 or greater neurological events are reported to be transient and reversible with dose cessation/reduction. In terms of preliminary efficacy, Sallman et al. presented preliminary data at ASH 2019 in 55 patients with TP53 mutations and either MDS, oligoblastic AML (≤30% bone marrow blasts) ($n = 11$) or MDS/myeloproliferative neoplasm overlap syndrome. The reported ORR was 71% (39/55) (Sallman 2019). In the AML subgroup ($n = 11$), the ORR (CR/CRi/MLFS) was 64% (7/11), of which 4 (36%) were CR's with a response duration of 7.0 months. The median OS for the entire cohort was 10.8 months. Of interest, 44% (20/55) of patients had undetectable TP53 by NGS (sensitivity of 5%) whilst on therapy. A parallel French study evaluated this combination in patients with TP53 mutant MDS or AML (including bone marrow blasts >30%) (Cluzeau et al. 2019). The ORR (CR/CRi/MLFS) was 33% in the 12 AML patients with 20–30% blasts, and relatively lower at 20% in the 5 patients with >30% blasts.

### 17.5.2 Targeting Murine Double Minute 2 (MDM2)

MDM2 protein has been identified as a key negative regulator of p53. MDM2 ubiquitinates p53, promoting its degradation. MDM2 also impairs p53 binding to target DNA repressing gene transcription.(Wu et al. 1993) Inhibition of the MDM2-p53 interaction leads to activation of wild-type p53 and its downstream tumour suppressor functions. Importantly, the presence of TP53 mutations confers resistance to MDM2 inhibitors.

Idasanutlin (RG7399, Roche) is an orally available, second-generation small molecule inhibitor of the MDM2 protein that is currently in late-phase clinical development. The initial phase 1/1b dose-escalation trial examined idasanutlin (administered twice a day on days 1–5) either as monotherapy, or in combination with intermediate dose cytarabine (1 g/m$^2$ daily on days 1 to 5) in relapsed refractory AML (NCT01773408) (Yee et al. 2014). The composite CR rate (CR/CRi/CRh) among 75 patients was reported to be 29%, with a median response duration of 6.4 months (range: 1.1–11.9 months). Idasanutlin is has been examined in a phase 3, double-blinded, randomised study 'MIRROS', comparing intermediate dose cytarabine (1 g/m$^2$ daily on days 1 to 5) with either idasanutlin 300 mg BD or placebo in patients with primary refractory or relapsed AML as first or second salvage. (NCT02545283) (Montesinos et al. 2019). Preliminary data presented at the EHA 25th annual congress on 447 patients reported a negative primary endpoint with no improvement in OS or CR (Konopleva et al. 2020). The median OS was 8.3 months in the idasanutlin arm versus 9.1 months in the placebo arm ($p = 0.58$). The most frequent side effects related to idasanutlin were gastrointestinal in nature, with diarrhoea, nausea and vomiting reported in >96% of patients, resulting in mandatory administration of anti-diarrhoeal and anti-emetic prophylaxis during treatment.

In addition, idasanutlin has also been combined with venetoclax in a phase 1b study based on the rationale that MDM2 inhibition promotes MCL-1 degradation, thus increasing sensitivity to BCL-2 inhibition (Pan et al. 2017; Daver et al. 2019). This dose-finding study is currently being conducted in patients aged ≥60 years with relapsed refractory AML. Venetoclax was given orally daily in 28-day cycles, with idasanutlin given daily on days 1–5. Preliminary results in 49 patients reported an overall response rate of 41% (CR/CRp/CRi/PR/MLFS), with a CR rate of 6% and a CRi/CRp rate of 16%, with no significant differences between de novo ($n = 24$, ORR 38%) or sAML ($n = 25$, ORR 44%) (Daver et al. 2019). The median OS was 17.1 months for those in CR/CRp/CRi and the median duration of response was 3.0 months based on short follow-up (3.8 months). The 30-day mortality was 6%, with no unexpected AEs reported. The maximum tolerated dose was reached with venetoclax 600 mg plus idasanutlin 200 mg, with the study currently expanding at venetoclax 600 mg in combination with idasanutlin at a dose level of 150 mg. An interesting observation from this study was the acquisition of new *TP53* mutations (undetected at study entry with a threshold of 1%) in 10/32 (31%) patients at treatment discontinuation, with enrichment of *TP53, RAS, FLT3* mutations and *MLL* rearrangements in non-responders.

A number of other MDM2 inhibitors are being developed in AML, including Siremadlin (HDM201, Novartis) which is being investigated in combination with venetoclax or MBG-453 (TIM-3 inhibitor) (NCT03940352).

### 17.5.3 Epigenetic Therapies

In addition to the agents mentioned above, numerous other drugs with promising mechanisms of action are undergoing early phase development in AML. Some examples include inhibitors of the epigenetic bromodomain and extraterminal proteins (BET) resulting in disruption of transcriptional programs that drive leukaemogenesis (e.g. Birabresib) (Astorgues-Xerri et al. 2019), KMT2A-menin inhibitors (e.g. KO-539) (Burrows et al. 2018), disruptors of telomeric silencing 1-like (DOT1L) (e.g. pinometostat) (Stein et al. 2018), splenic tyrosine kinase inhibitors (Bartaula-Brevik et al. 2018) or inhibition of the downstream pathways of MAPK/extracellular-signal regulated kinase (ERK) (e.g. with binimetinib, a MEK 1/2 inhibitor) (Maiti et al. 2019b). The majority of these agents have thus far yielded only modest single-agent response rates and their application to patients with wild-type of mutant *TP53* requires further delineation.

An oral version of decitabine called ASTX727 (C-DEC, Astex Pharmaceuticals Inc) has also been developed. This compound combines decitabine and cedazuridine, a cytidine deaminase inhibitor which enables oral bioavailability of decitabine. ASTX727 given orally, daily over

5 days, has been shown to result in similar drug levels to that of IV decitabine (Garcia-Manero et al. 2019). Promising preliminary study results have led to priority review designation by the FDA for untreated intermediate or high risk MDS or chronic myelomonocytic leukaemia (CMML). A randomised open-label study comparing ASTX727 versus IV decitabine in treatment naïve MDS, CMML and AML is underway (NCT03306264).

HDAC inhibitors (HDACi) have been extensively tested in the past as monotherapy and in combination with conventional cytotoxic drugs or hypomethylating agents. Pre-clinical studies have demonstrated marked synergy between the HDACi panobinostat and venetoclax, including patient samples with TP53 mutant AML (Salmon et al. 2018). The HDACi pracinostat has been demonstrated in clinical studies to be safe with modest single-agent activity in advanced haematologic malignancies. The RP2D is 60 mg per dose (Abaza et al. 2017). Pracinostat (60 mg PO 3 days/week for 21/28 days) in combination with Azacitidine (7 5 mg/m$^2$) has shown promising efficacy in a phase 2 study in elderly AML patients ($\geq$65 years) with a CR/CRi rate of 46% and a 1-year survival of 62% (Garcia Manero et al. 2016). The benefit of this combination was most prominent within the high-risk cytogenetic group ($n = 21$, 42%), with a CR of 38%, a CR/CRi/MLFS rate of 47.6% (compared with 48.1 and 59.3% respectively in intermediate cytogenetic risk group), and a median OS of 13.5 months. No unexpected toxicities were observed with this combination therapy. A phase 3 study comparing azacitidine plus pracinostat or placebo has unfortunately been discontinued due to interim futility analysis results indicating likely failure of meeting the trial's primary endpoint of OS (NCT03151408). Whether this combination was more beneficial to the high-risk cytogenetic group remains to be elucidated.

## 17.6 Future Perspectives

After decades of therapeutic inactivity, the treatment of AML is now entering a more exciting, but challenging phase. Venetoclax in combination with lower intensity therapies has led to some improvements in outcomes for older patients that were once deemed only suitable for palliative care. Mutation-directed targeted therapies are now available for *FLT3, IDH1, IDH2* mutant AML, whom account for approximately 45–50% of AML patients. Results from clinical trials combining these novel agents with intensive chemotherapy and other novel agents are producing interesting results and have the potential to radically change the therapeutic landscape. The concept of maintenance therapy has also come to the fore, with CC-486 on track to become a new standard of care for patients not proceeding to HSCT. New therapies are also being developed with promise against poor risk AML subgroups, such as TP53 mutant AML. Questions to be answered in future studies include ongoing strategies to better understand mechanisms of treatment resistance, how best to optimally sequence new therapies (such as FLT3 inhibitors), and how these new therapies will influence pre- and post-HSCT practices. Effective therapies for R/R AML without targetable mutations, treated secondary AML or de novo AML failing HMA, however, remain areas of unmet clinical need desperate for new agents. In summary, although there has been exciting progress in the field of AML, many challenges remain, in particular, how best to understand and pre-empt emerging drug resistance that is common among patients on targeted therapy treatment. Furthermore, it is possible that sequential use of novel AML therapies may afford a better and more precision-guided approach to extending patient survival, in contrast to the strategy of compiling more novel drugs together in potentially more toxic and expensive treatment combinations.

## References

Abaza YM, Kadia TM, Jabbour EJ, Konopleva MY, Borthakur G, Ferrajoli A, Estrov Z, Wierda WG, Alfonso A, Chong TH, Chuah C, Koh L-P, Goh B-C, Chang JE, Durkes DE, Foudray MC, Kantarjian HM, Dong XQ, Garcia-Manero G (2017) Phase 1 dose escalation multicenter trial of pracinostat alone and in combination with azacitidine in patients with advanced hematologic malignancies. Cancer 123(24):4851–4859. https://doi.org/10.1002/cncr.30949

Aboudalle I, Konopleva MY, Kadia TM, Naqvi K, Vaughan K, Kurt M, Cavazos A, Pierce SA, Takahashi K, Masarova L (2019) A phase Ib/II study of the BCL-2 inhibitor Venetoclax in combination with standard intensive AML induction/consolidation therapy with FLAG-IDA in patients with newly diagnosed or relapsed/refractory AML. American Society of Hematology, Washington, DC

Ali D, Jönsson-Videsäter K, Deneberg S, Bengtzén S, Nahi H, Paul C, Lehmann S (2011) APR-246 exhibits anti-leukemic activity and synergism with conventional chemotherapeutic drugs in acute myeloid leukemia cells. Eur J Haematol 86(3):206–215

Astorgues-Xerri L, Vázquez R, Odore E, Rezai K, Kahatt C, Mackenzie S, Bekradda M, Coudé M-M, Dombret H, Gardin C (2019) Insights into the cellular pharmacological properties of the BET-inhibitor OTX015/MK-8628 (birabresib), alone and in combination, in leukemia models. Leuk Lymphoma 60(12):3067–3070

Baker SD, Zimmerman EI, Wang Y-D, Orwick S, Zatechka DS, Buaboonnam J, Neale GA, Olsen SR, Enemark EJ, Shurtleff S (2013) Emergence of polyclonal FLT3 tyrosine kinase domain mutations during sequential therapy with sorafenib and sunitinib in FLT3-ITD–positive acute myeloid leukemia. Clin Cancer Res 19(20):5758–5768

Bartaula-Brevik S, Lindstad Brattås MK, Tvedt THA, Reikvam H, Bruserud Ø (2018) Splenic tyrosine kinase (SYK) inhibitors and their possible use in acute myeloid leukemia. Expert Opin Investig Drugs 27(4):377–387. https://doi.org/10.1080/13543784.2018.1459562

Blombery P, Anderson MA, Gong J-N, Thijssen R, Birkinshaw RW, Thompson ER, Teh CE, Nguyen T, Xu Z, Flensburg C (2019) Acquisition of the recurrent Gly101Val mutation in BCL2 confers resistance to venetoclax in patients with progressive chronic lymphocytic leukemia. Cancer Discov 9(3):342–353

Burchert A, Bug G, Finke J, Stelljes M, Rollig C, Wäsch R, Bornhäuser M, Berg T, Lang F, Ehninger G (2018) Sorafenib as maintenance therapy post allogeneic stem cell transplantation for FLT3-ITD positive AML: results from the randomized, double-blind, placebo-controlled multicentre sormain trial. Blood 132(Suppl 1):661

Burrows F, Wu T, Kessler L, Li S, Zhang J, Zarrinkar P, Li L, Cierpicki T, Grembecka J, Ren P (2018) Abstract LB-A27: a novel small molecule menin-MLL inhibitor for potential treatment of MLL-rearranged leukemias and NPM1/DNMT3A-mutant AML. AACR

Bykov VJ, Issaeva N, Shilov A, Hultcrantz M, Pugacheva E, Chumakov P, Bergman J, Wiman KG, Selivanova G (2002) Restoration of the tumor suppressor function to mutant p53 by a low-molecular-weight compound. Nat Med 8(3):282–288

Cancer Genome Atlas Research Network, Ley TJ, Miller C et al (2013) Genomic and epigenomic landscapes of adult de novo acute myeloid leukemia. N Engl J Med 368(22):2059–2074. https://doi.org/10.1056/NEJMoa1301689

Castaigne S, Pautas C, Terré C, Raffoux E, Bordessoule D, Bastie J-N, Legrand O, Thomas X, Turlure P, Reman O (2012) Effect of gemtuzumab ozogamicin on survival of adult patients with de-novo acute myeloid leukaemia (ALFA-0701): a randomised, open-label, phase 3 study. Lancet 379(9825):1508–1516

Chan SM, Thomas D, Corces-Zimmerman MR, Xavy S, Rastogi S, Hong W-J, Zhao F, Medeiros BC, Tyvoll DA, Majeti R (2015) Isocitrate dehydrogenase 1 and 2 mutations induce BCL-2 dependence in acute myeloid leukemia. Nat Med 21(2):178

Chaturvedi A, Cruz MMA, Jyotsana N, Sharma A, Yun H, Görlich K, Wichmann M, Schwarzer A, Preller M, Thol F (2013) Mutant IDH1 promotes leukemogenesis in vivo and can be specifically targeted in human AML. Blood 122(16):2877–2887

Chen S-L, Qin Z-Y, Hu F, Wang Y, Dai Y-J, Liang Y (2019) The role of the HOXA gene family in acute myeloid leukemia. Genes 10(8):621

Chua CC, Reynolds J, Salmon JM, Fong C, Ting SB, Tiong IS, Fleming S, MacRaild S, Moujalled DM, Pomilio G (2019) Anti-leukemic activity of single agent Venetoclax in newly diagnosed acute myeloid leukemia: a sub-set analysis of the Caveat study. American Society of Hematology, Washington, DC

Chua CC, Roberts AW, Reynolds J, Fong CY, Ting SB, Salmon JM, MacRaild S, Ivey A, Tiong IS, Fleming S, Brown FC, Loo S, Majewski IJ, Bohlander SK, Wei AH (2020) Chemotherapy and Venetoclax in elderly acute myeloid leukemia trial (CAVEAT): a phase Ib dose-escalation study of Venetoclax combined with modified intensive chemotherapy. J Clin Oncol 38(30):3506–3517. https://doi.org/10.1200/jco.20.00572

Cluzeau T, Sebert M, Rahmé R, Cuzzubbo S, Walter-Petrich A, Lehmann-che J, Peterlin P, Beve B, Attalah H, Chermat F (2019) APR-246 combined with Azacitidine (AZA) in TP53 mutated myelodysplastic syndrome (MDS) and acute myeloid leukemia (AML). A phase 2 study by the Groupe Francophone Des Myélodysplasies (GFM). American Society of Hematology, Washington, DC

Cortes JE, Kantarjian H, Foran JM, Ghirdaladze D, Zodelava M, Borthakur G, Gammon G, Trone D, Armstrong RC, James J (2013) Phase I study of quizartinib administered daily to patients with relapsed or refractory acute myeloid leukemia irrespective of FMS-like tyrosine kinase 3–internal tandem duplication status. J Clin Oncol 31(29):3681

Cortes J, Perl AE, Döhner H, Kantarjian H, Martinelli G, Kovacsovics T, Rousselot P, Steffen B, Dombret H, Estey E (2018) Quizartinib, an FLT3 inhibitor, as monotherapy in patients with relapsed or refractory acute myeloid leukaemia: an open-label, multicentre, single-arm, phase 2 trial. Lancet Oncol 19(7):889–903

Cortes JE, Ganguly S, Krämer A, Levis MJ, Martinelli G, Perl AE, Russell NH, Choi Y, Mendell J, Namuyinga R (2019a) Pooled safety analysis of Quizartinib monotherapy in patients with relapsed/refractory (R/R)

acute myeloid leukemia (AML). American Society of Hematology, Washington, DC
Cortes JE, Heidel FH, Hellmann A, Fiedler W, Smith BD, Robak T, Montesinos P, Pollyea DA, DesJardins P, Ottmann O (2019b) Randomized comparison of low dose cytarabine with or without glasdegib in patients with newly diagnosed acute myeloid leukemia or high-risk myelodysplastic syndrome. Leukemia 33(2):379
Cortes JE, Khaled S, Martinelli G, Perl AE, Ganguly S, Russell N, Krämer A, Dombret H, Hogge D, Jonas BA (2019c) Quizartinib versus salvage chemotherapy in relapsed or refractory FLT3-ITD acute myeloid leukaemia (QuANTUM-R): a multicentre, randomised, controlled, open-label, phase 3 trial. Lancet Oncol 20(7):984–997
Czabotar PE, Lessene G, Strasser A, Adams JM (2014) Control of apoptosis by the BCL-2 protein family: implications for physiology and therapy. Nat Rev Mol Cell Biol 15(1):49–63. https://doi.org/10.1038/nrm3722
Daver NG, Garcia JS, Jonas BA, Kelly KR, Assouline S, Brandwein JM, Fenaux P, Olin RL, Martinelli G, Paolini S, Pigneux A, Pollyea DA, Powell BL, Roboz GJ, Tafuri A, Vey N, Visani G, Yee KWL, Dail M, Green C, Kirschbrown WP, Hong W-J, Ott MG, Onishi M, Wang J, Konopleva MY, Andreeff M (2019) Updated results from the Venetoclax (Ven) in combination with Idasanutlin (Idasa) arm of a phase 1b trial in elderly patients (pts) with relapsed or refractory (R/R) AML ineligible for cytotoxic chemotherapy. Blood 134(Suppl_1):229. https://doi.org/10.1182/blood-2019-123711
DiNardo C (2019) Enasidenib plus azacitidine significantly improves complete remission and overall response compared with azacitidine alone in patients with newly diagnosed acute myeloid leukemia (AML) with isocitrate dehydrogenase 2 (IDH2) mutations: interim phase II results from an ongoing, randomized study. In: 61st Annual Meeting and Exposition (December 7–10, 2019), 2019. ASH
DiNardo CD, Wei AH (2020) How I treat acute myeloid leukemia in the era of new drugs. Blood 135(2):85–96
DiNardo CD, Pratz KW, Letai A, Jonas BA, Wei AH, Thirman M, Arellano M, Frattini MG, Kantarjian H, Popovic R, Chyla B, Xu T, Dunbar M, Agarwal SK, Humerickhouse R, Mabry M, Potluri J, Konopleva M, Pollyea DA (2018a) Safety and preliminary efficacy of venetoclax with decitabine or azacitidine in elderly patients with previously untreated acute myeloid leukaemia: a non-randomised, open-label, phase 1b study. Lancet Oncol 19(2):216–228. https://doi.org/10.1016/S1470-2045(18)30010-X
DiNardo CD, Stein EM, de Botton S, Roboz GJ, Altman JK, Mims AS, Swords R, Collins RH, Mannis GN, Pollyea DA (2018b) Durable remissions with ivosidenib in IDH1-mutated relapsed or refractory AML. N Engl J Med 378(25):2386–2398
DiNardo C, Takahashi K, Kadia T, Loghavi S, Naqvi K, Bose P, Daver N, Tippett GD, Borthakur G, Cortes J, Chan S, Quek L, Vyas P, Kantarjian H, Konopleva M (2019a) A phase 1b/2 clinical study of targeted IDH1 inhibition with ivosidenib, in combination with the BCL-2 inhibitor venetoclax, for patients with IDH1-mutated (mIDH1) myeloid malignancies: PF291. HemaSphere 3:97. https://doi.org/10.1097/01.Hs9.0000559376.17429.23
DiNardo CD, Pratz K, Pullarkat V, Jonas BA, Arellano M, Becker PS, Frankfurt O, Konopleva M, Wei AH, Kantarjian HM (2019b) Venetoclax combined with decitabine or azacitidine in treatment-naive, elderly patients with acute myeloid leukemia. Blood 133(1):7–17
DiNardo CD, Tiong IS, Quaglieri A, MacRaild S, Loghavi S, Brown FC, Thijssen R, Pomilio G, Ivey A, Salmon J (2020a) Molecular patterns of response and treatment failure after frontline venetoclax combinations in older patients with AML. Blood 135(11):791–803
DiNardo CD, Tiong IS, Quaglieri A, MacRaild S, Loghavi S, Brown FC, Thijssen R, Pomilio G, Ivey A, Salmon J, Glytsou C, Fleming SA, Zhang Q, Ma H, Patel KP, Kornblau SM, Xu Z, Chua CC, Chen X, Blombery P, Flensburg C, Cummings N, Aifantis I, Kantarjian H, Huang DCS, Roberts AW, Majewski IJ, Konopleva M, Wei AH (2020b) Molecular patterns of response and treatment failure after frontline venetoclax combinations in older patients with AML. Blood 135(11):791–803. https://doi.org/10.1182/blood.2019003988
Fathi AT, DiNardo CD, Kline I, Kenvin L, Gupta I, Attar EC, Stein EM, de Botton S, AG221-C-001 Study Investigators (2018) Differentiation syndrome associated with Enasidenib, a selective inhibitor of mutant isocitrate dehydrogenase 2: analysis of a phase 1/2 study. JAMA Oncol 4(8):1106–1110. https://doi.org/10.1001/jamaoncol.2017.4695
Fukushima N, Minami Y, Kakiuchi S, Kuwatsuka Y, Hayakawa F, Jamieson C, Kiyoi H, Naoe T (2016) Small-molecule hedgehog inhibitor attenuates the leukemia-initiation potential of acute myeloid leukemia cells. Cancer Sci 107(10):1422–1429
Garcia Manero G, Atallah E, Khaled SK, Arellano M, Patnaik MM, Odenike O, Sayar H, Tummala M, Patel PA, Ghalie RG, Medeiros BC (2016) A phase 2 study of Pracinostat and Azacitidine in elderly patients with acute myeloid leukemia (AML) not eligible for induction chemotherapy: response and long-term survival benefit. Blood 128(22):100
Garcia-Manero G, McCloskey J, Griffiths EA, Yee KW, Zeidan AM, Al-Kali A, Dao K-H, Deeg HJ, Patel PA, Sabloff M (2019) Pharmacokinetic exposure equivalence and preliminary efficacy and safety from a randomized cross over phase 3 study (ASCERTAIN study) of an oral hypomethylating agent ASTX727 (cedazuridine/decitabine) compared to IV decitabine. American Society of Hematology, Washington, DC
Glaser SP, Lee EF, Trounson E, Bouillet P, Wei A, Fairlie WD, Izon DJ, Zuber J, Rappaport AR, Herold MJ (2012) Anti-apoptotic Mcl-1 is essential for the development and sustained growth of acute myeloid leukemia. Genes Dev 26(2):120–125
Grundy M, Balakrishnan S, Fox M, Seedhouse CH, Russell NH (2018) Genetic biomarkers predict response to dual BCL-2 and MCL-1 targeting in acute myeloid leukaemia cells. Oncotarget 9(102):37777–37789. https://doi.org/10.18632/oncotarget.26540

Harding JJ, Lowery MA, Shih AH, Schvartzman JM, Hou S, Famulare C, Patel M, Roshal M, Do RK, Zehir A, You D, Selcuklu SD, Viale A, Tallman MS, Hyman DM, Reznik E, Finley LWS, Papaemmanuil E, Tosolini A, Frattini MG, MacBeth KJ, Liu G, Fan B, Choe S, Wu B, Janjigian YY, Mellinghoff IK, Diaz LA, Levine RL, Abou-Alfa GK, Stein EM, Intlekofer AM (2018) Isoform switching as a mechanism of acquired resistance to mutant Isocitrate dehydrogenase inhibition. Cancer Discov 8(12):1540. https://doi.org/10.1158/2159-8290.CD-18-0877

Intlekofer AM, Shih AH, Wang B, Nazir A, Rustenburg AS, Albanese SK, Patel M, Famulare C, Correa FM, Takemoto N (2018) Acquired resistance to IDH inhibition through trans or cis dimer-interface mutations. Nature 559(7712):125

Jonas BA, Pollyea DA (2019) How we use venetoclax with hypomethylating agents for the treatment of newly diagnosed patients with acute myeloid leukemia. Leukemia 33(12):2795–2804. https://doi.org/10.1038/s41375-019-0612-8

Kasper S, Breitenbuecher F, Heidel F, Hoffarth S, Markova B, Schuler M, Fischer T (2012) Targeting MCL-1 sensitizes FLT3-ITD-positive leukemias to cytotoxic therapies. Blood Cancer J 2(3):e60–e60. https://doi.org/10.1038/bcj.2012.5

Konopleva M, Letai A (2018) BCL-2 inhibition in AML: an unexpected bonus? Blood 132(10):1007–1012

Konopleva M, Contractor R, Tsao T, Samudio I, Ruvolo PP, Kitada S, Deng X, Zhai D, Shi Y-X, Sneed T, Verhaegen M, Soengas M, Ruvolo VR, McQueen T, Schober WD, Watt JC, Jiffar T, Ling X, Marini FC, Harris D, Dietrich M, Estrov Z, McCubrey J, May WS, Reed JC, Andreeff M (2006) Mechanisms of apoptosis sensitivity and resistance to the BH3 mimetic ABT-737 in acute myeloid leukemia. Cancer Cell 10(5):375–388. https://doi.org/10.1016/j.ccr.2006.10.006

Konopleva M, Pollyea DA, Potluri J, Chyla B, Hogdal L, Busman T, McKeegan E, Salem AH, Zhu M, Ricker JL (2016) Efficacy and biological correlates of response in a phase II study of venetoclax monotherapy in patients with acute myelogenous leukemia. Cancer Discov 6(10):1106–1117

Konopleva MY, Rollig C, Cavenagh J, Deeren D, Girshova L, Krauter J, Martinelli G, Montesinos P, Neubauer A, Petrini M, Pigneux A, Rambaldi A, Recher C, Rodriguez-Veiga R, Taussig D, Vey N, Yoon S-S, Ott MG, Gamel K, Monnet A, Beckermann BM, Muehlbauer S, Catalani O, Genevray M, Fenaux P, Wei AH (2020) A randomized double-blind phase 3 trial of cytarabine with MDM2 inhibitor idasanutlin or placebo in relapsed/refractory acute myeloid leukemia (R/R AML): primary analysis results of the MIRROS study. In: Paper presented at the 25th EHA annual congress, virtual edition, June 12 2020

Lancet JE, Uy GL, Cortes JE, Newell LF, Lin TL, Ritchie EK, Stuart RK, Strickland SA, Hogge D, Solomon SR, Stone RM, Bixby DL, Kolitz JE, Schiller GJ, Wieduwilt MJ, Ryan DH, Hoering A, Banerjee K, Chiarella M, Louie AC, Medeiros BC (2018) CPX-351 (cytarabine and daunorubicin) liposome for injection versus conventional Cytarabine plus Daunorubicin in older patients with newly diagnosed secondary acute myeloid leukemia. J Clin Oncol 36(26):2684–2692. https://doi.org/10.1200/jco.2017.77.6112

Levis MJ, Perl AE, Altman JK, Gocke CD, Bahceci E, Hill J, Liu C, Xie Z, Carson AR, McClain V, Stenzel TT, Miller JE (2018) A next-generation sequencing–based assay for minimal residual disease assessment in AML patients with FLT3-ITD mutations. Blood Adv 2(8):825–831. https://doi.org/10.1182/bloodadvances.2018015925

Ma J, Zhao S, Qiao X, Knight T, Edwards H, Polin L, Kushner J, Dzinic SH, White K, Wang G, Zhao L, Lin H, Wang Y, Taub JW, Ge Y (2019) Inhibition of Bcl-2 synergistically enhances the Antileukemic activity of Midostaurin and Gilteritinib in preclinical models of FLT3-mutated acute myeloid leukemia. Clin Cancer Res 25(22):6815. https://doi.org/10.1158/1078-0432.CCR-19-0832

Maiti A, DiNardo CD, Rausch CR, Cortes JE, Pemmaraju N, Daver NG, Ravandi F, Garcia-Manero G, Borthakur GM, Naqvi K (2019a) Ten-day Decitabine with Venetoclax (DEC10-VEN) in acute myeloid leukemia: updated results of a phase II trial. American Society of Hematology, Washington, DC

Maiti A, Naqvi K, Kadia TM, Borthakur G, Takahashi K, Bose P, Daver NG, Patel A, Alvarado Y, Ohanian M, DiNardo CD, Cortes JE, Jabbour EJ, Garcia-Manero G, Kantarjian HM, Ravandi F (2019b) Phase II trial of MEK inhibitor Binimetinib (MEK162) in <em>RAS</em>−mutant acute myeloid leukemia. Clin Lymphoma Myeloma Leuk 19(3):142–148.e141. https://doi.org/10.1016/j.clml.2018.12.009

Mardis ER, Ding L, Dooling DJ, Larson DE, McLellan MD, Chen K, Koboldt DC, Fulton RS, Delehaunty KD, McGrath SD (2009) Recurring mutations found by sequencing an acute myeloid leukemia genome. N Engl J Med 361(11):1058–1066

McMahon CM, Canaani J, Rea B, Sargent RL, Qualtieri JN, Watt CD, Morrissette JJD, Carroll M, Perl AE (2019a) Gilteritinib induces differentiation in relapsed and refractory FLT3-mutated acute myeloid leukemia. Blood Adv 3(10):1581–1585. https://doi.org/10.1182/bloodadvances.2018029496

McMahon CM, Ferng T, Canaani J, Wang ES, Morrissette JJ, Eastburn DJ, Pellegrino M, Durruthy-Durruthy R, Watt CD, Asthana S (2019b) Clonal selection with Ras pathway activation mediates secondary clinical resistance to selective FLT3 inhibition in acute myeloid leukemia. Cancer Discov 9(8):1050–1063

Montesinos P, Esteve J, Konopleva M, Martinelli G, Ottmann O, Rodriguez-Veiga R, Röllig C, Wei A, Vey N, Chiu I (2019) MIRROS: an ongoing randomized phase 3 trial of idasanutlin + ARA-C in patients with relapsed or refractory acute myeloid leukemia. Am Soc Clin Oncol

Mori M, Kaneko N, Ueno Y, Yamada M, Tanaka R, Saito R, Shimada I, Mori K, Kuromitsu S (2017) Gilteritinib, a FLT3/AXL inhibitor, shows antileukemic activity in mouse models of FLT3 mutated acute myeloid leukemia. Invest New Drugs 35(5):556–565. https://doi.org/10.1007/s10637-017-0470-z

Moujalled DM, Pomilio G, Ghiurau C, Ivey A, Salmon J, Rijal S, Macraild S, Zhang L, Teh T-C, Tiong I-S,

Lan P, Chanrion M, Claperon A, Rocchetti F, Zichi A, Kraus-Berthier L, Wang Y, Halilovic E, Morris E, Colland F, Segal D, Huang D, Roberts AW, Maragno AL, Lessene G, Geneste O, Wei AH (2019) Combining BH3-mimetics to target both BCL-2 and MCL1 has potent activity in pre-clinical models of acute myeloid leukemia. Leukemia 33(4):905–917. https://doi.org/10.1038/s41375-018-0261-3

Nechiporuk T, Kurtz SE, Nikolova O, Liu T, Jones CL, D'Alessandro A, Culp-Hill R, d'Almeida A, Joshi SK, Rosenberg M (2019) The TP53 apoptotic network is a primary mediator of resistance to BCL2 inhibition in AML cells. Cancer Discov 9(7):910–925

Pan R, Ruvolo V, Mu H, Leverson JD, Nichols G, Reed JC, Konopleva M, Andreeff M (2017) Synthetic lethality of combined Bcl-2 inhibition and p53 activation in AML: mechanisms and superior antileukemic efficacy. Cancer Cell 32(6):748–760.e746. https://doi.org/10.1016/j.ccell.2017.11.003

Pei S, Pollyea DA, Gustafson A, Stevens BM, Minhajuddin M, Fu R, Riemondy KA, Gillen AE, Sheridan RM, Kim J (2020) Monocytic subclones confer resistance to Venetoclax-based therapy in acute myeloid leukemia patients. Cancer Discov 10(4):536–551

Perl AE, Daver NG, Pratz KW, Maly J, Hong W-J, Bahceci E, Tong B, Tian T, Dilley K (2019a) Venetoclax in combination with Gilteritinib in patients with relapsed/refractory acute myeloid leukemia: a phase 1b study. American Society of Hematology, Washington, DC

Perl AE, Martinelli G, Cortes JE, Neubauer A, Berman E, Paolini S, Montesinos P, Baer MR, Larson RA, Ustun C (2019b) Gilteritinib or chemotherapy for relapsed or refractory FLT3-mutated AML. N Engl J Med 381(18):1728–1740

Quek L, David MD, Kennedy A, Metzner M, Amatangelo M, Shih A, Stoilova B, Quivoron C, Heiblig M, Willekens C (2018) Clonal heterogeneity of acute myeloid leukemia treated with the IDH2 inhibitor enasidenib. Nat Med 24(8):1167

Roboz GJ, DiNardo CD, Stein EM, de Botton S, Mims AS, Prince GT, Altman JK, Arellano ML, Donnellan W, Erba HP, Mannis GN, Pollyea DA, Stein AS, Uy GL, Watts JM, Fathi AT, Kantarjian HM, Tallman MS, Choe S, Dai D, Fan B, Wang H, Zhang V, Yen KE, Kapsalis SM, Hickman D, Liu H, Agresta SV, Wu B, Attar EC, Stone RM (2019) Ivosidenib induces deep durable remissions in patients with newly diagnosed IDH1-mutant acute myeloid leukemia. Blood 135(7):463–471. https://doi.org/10.1182/blood.2019002140

Sallman D (2019) Phase 2 results of APR-246 and Azacitidine (AZA) in patients with TP53 mutant myelodysplastic syndromes (MDS) and oligoblastic acute myeloid leukemia (AML). In: 61st Annual Meeting and Exposition (December 7–10, 2019), 2019. ASH

Salmon J, Pomilio G, Moujalled D, MacRaild S, Teh C, Rijal S, Ivey A, Teh T-C, Ekert P, Schoumacher M (2018) Combined BCL-2 and HDAC targeting has potent and TP53 independent activity in AML. Exp Hematol 64:S99–S100

Shih AH, Meydan C, Shank K, Garrett-Bakelman FE, Ward PS, Intlekofer AM, Nazir A, Stein EM, Knapp K, Glass J (2017) Combination targeted therapy to disrupt aberrant oncogenic signaling and reverse epigenetic dysfunction in IDH2-and TET2-mutant acute myeloid leukemia. Cancer Discov 7(5):494–505

Smith CC, Lasater EA, Lin KC, Wang Q, McCreery MQ, Stewart WK, Damon LE, Perl AE, Jeschke GR, Sugita M (2014) Crenolanib is a selective type I pan-FLT3 inhibitor. Proc Natl Acad Sci 111(14):5319–5324

Smith CC, Lin K, Stecula A, Sali A, Shah NP (2015a) FLT3 D835 mutations confer differential resistance to type II FLT3 inhibitors. Leukemia 29(12):2390–2392. https://doi.org/10.1038/leu.2015.165

Smith CC, Zhang C, Lin KC, Lasater EA, Zhang Y, Massi E, Damon LE, Pendleton M, Bashir A, Sebra R (2015b) Characterizing and overriding the structural mechanism of the quizartinib-resistant FLT3 "gatekeeper" F691L mutation with PLX3397. Cancer Discov 5(6):668–679

Smith CC, Levis MJ, Perl AE, Martinelli G, Neubauer A, Berman E, Montesinos P, Baer MR, Larson RA, Chou W-C (2019) Emerging mutations at relapse in patients with FLT3-mutated relapsed/refractory acute myeloid leukemia who received Gilteritinib therapy in the phase 3 admiral trial. Blood 134(Suppl_1):14

Stein EM (2016) Molecular pathways: IDH2 mutations-co-opting cellular metabolism for malignant transformation. Clin Cancer Res 22(1):16–19. https://doi.org/10.1158/1078-0432.CCR-15-0362

Stein EM, DiNardo CD, Pollyea DA, Fathi AT, Roboz GJ, Altman JK, Stone RM, DeAngelo DJ, Levine RL, Flinn IW (2017) Enasidenib in mutant IDH2 relapsed or refractory acute myeloid leukemia. Blood 130(6):722–731

Stein EM, Garcia-Manero G, Rizzieri DA, Tibes R, Berdeja JG, Savona MR, Jongen-Lavrenic M, Altman JK, Thomson B, Blakemore SJ, Daigle SR, Waters NJ, Suttle AB, Clawson A, Pollock R, Krivtsov A, Armstrong SA, DiMartino J, Hedrick E, Löwenberg B, Tallman MS (2018) The DOT1L inhibitor pinometostat reduces H3K79 methylation and has modest clinical activity in adult acute leukemia. Blood 131(24):2661–2669. https://doi.org/10.1182/blood-2017-12-818948

Stein EM, DiNardo CD, Fathi AT, Pollyea DA, Stone RM, Altman JK, Roboz GJ, Patel MR, Collins R, Flinn IW, Sekeres MA, Stein AS, Kantarjian HM, Levine RL, Vyas P, MacBeth KJ, Tosolini A, VanOostendorp J, Xu Q, Gupta I, Lila T, Risueno A, Yen KE, Wu B, Attar EC, Tallman MS, de Botton S (2019) Molecular remission and response patterns in patients with mutant-IDH2 acute myeloid leukemia treated with enasidenib. Blood 133(7):676–687. https://doi.org/10.1182/blood-2018-08-869008

Stone RM, Mandrekar S, Sanford BL, Geyer S, Bloomfield CD, Dohner K, Thiede C, Marcucci G, Lo-Coco F, Klisovic RB (2015) The multi-kinase inhibitor midostaurin (M) prolongs survival compared with placebo (P) in combination with daunorubicin (D)/cytarabine (C) induction (ind), high-dose

C consolidation (consol), and as maintenance (maint) therapy in newly diagnosed acute myeloid leukemia (AML) patients (pts) age 18–60 with FLT3 mutations (muts): an international prospective randomized (rand) P-controlled double-blind trial (CALGB 10603/RATIFY [Alliance]). American Society of Hematology, Washington, DC

Stone RM, Mandrekar SJ, Sanford BL, Laumann K, Geyer S, Bloomfield CD, Thiede C, Prior TW, Döhner K, Marcucci G (2017) Midostaurin plus chemotherapy for acute myeloid leukemia with a FLT3 mutation. N Engl J Med 377(5):454–464

Wang H, Choe S, DiNardo CD, Stein EM, de Botton S, Fathi AT, Tallman MS, Kantarjian HM, Stone RM, Quek L (2019) Complex polyclonal resistance mechanisms to Ivosidenib monotherapy in IDH1-mutant relapsed or refractory acute myeloid leukemia revealed by single cell sequencing analyses. American Society of Hematology, Washington, DC

Watts JM, Baer MR, Yang J, Prebet T, Lee S, Schiller GJ, Dinner S, Pigneux A, Montesinos P, Wang ES (2019) Olutasidenib (FT-2102), an IDH1m inhibitor as a single agent or in combination with Azacitidine, induces deep clinical responses with mutation clearance in patients with acute myeloid leukemia treated in a phase 1 dose escalation and expansion study. American Society of Hematology, Washington, DC

Wei A, Strickland SA, Roboz GJ, Hou J-Z, Fiedler W, Lin TL, Walter RB, Enjeti A, Chyla B, Popovic R (2017) Phase 1/2 study of venetoclax with low-dose cytarabine in treatment-naïve, elderly patients with acute myeloid leukemia unfit for intensive chemotherapy: 1-year outcomes. American Society of Hematology, Washington, DC

Wei AH, Döhner H, Pocock C, Montesinos P, Afanasyev B, Dombret H, Ravandi F, Sayar H, Jang JH, Porkka K (2019a) The QUAZAR AML-001 maintenance trial: results of a phase III international, randomized, double-blind, placebo-controlled study of CC-486 (oral formulation of azacitidine) in patients with acute myeloid leukemia (AML) in first remission. American Society of Hematology, Washington, DC

Wei AH, Strickland SA Jr, Hou J-Z, Fiedler W, Lin TL, Walter RB, Enjeti A, Tiong IS, Savona M, Lee S (2019b) Venetoclax combined with low-dose cytarabine for previously untreated patients with acute myeloid leukemia: results from a phase Ib/II study. J Clin Oncol 37(15):1277–1284

Wei AH, Strickland SA, Hou J-Z, Fiedler W, Lin TL, Walter RB, Enjeti A, Tiong IS, Savona M, Lee S, Chyla B, Popovic R, Salem AH, Agarwal S, Xu T, Fakouhi KM, Humerickhouse R, Hong W-J, Hayslip J, Roboz GJ (2019c) Venetoclax combined with low-dose Cytarabine for previously untreated patients with acute myeloid leukemia: results from a phase Ib/II study. J Clin Oncol 37(15):1277–1284. https://doi.org/10.1200/JCO.18.01600

Wei AH, Montesinos P, Ivanov V, DiNardo CD, Novak J, Laribi K, Kim I, Stevens DA, Fiedler W, Pagoni M, Samoilova O, Hu Y, Anagnostopoulos A, Bergeron J, Hou J-Z, Murthy V, Yamauchi T, McDonald A, Chyla B, Gopalakrishnan S, Jiang Q, Mendes W, Hayslip J, Panayiotidis P (2020a) Venetoclax plus LDAC for newly diagnosed AML ineligible for intensive chemotherapy: a phase 3 randomized placebo-controlled trial. Blood 135(24):2137–2145. https://doi.org/10.1182/blood.2020004856

Wei AH, Döhner H, Pocock C, Montesinos P, Afanasyev B, Dombret H, Ravandi F, Sayar H, Jang J-H, Porkka K, Selleslag D, Sandhu I, Turgut M, Giai V, Ofran Y, Kizil Çakar M, Botelho de Sousa A, Rybka J, Frairia C, Borin L, Beltrami G, Čermák J, Ossenkoppele GJ, La Torre I, Skikne B, Kumar K, Dong Q, Beach CL, Roboz GJ (2020b) Oral azacitidine maintenance therapy for acute myeloid leukemia in first remission. N Engl J Med 383(26):2526–2537. https://doi.org/10.1056/NEJMoa200444

Williams AB, Nguyen B, Li L, Brown P, Levis M, Leahy D, Small D (2013) Mutations of FLT3/ITD confer resistance to multiple tyrosine kinase inhibitors. Leukemia 27(1):48–55. https://doi.org/10.1038/leu.2012.191

Wu X, Bayle JH, Olson D, Levine AJ (1993) The p53-mdm-2 autoregulatory feedback loop. Genes Dev 7(7a):1126–1132

Yee K, Martinelli G, Vey N, Dickinson MJ, Seiter K, Assouline S, Drummond M, Yoon S-S, Kasner M, Lee J-H (2014) Phase 1/1b study of RG7388, a potent MDM2 antagonist, in acute myelogenous leukemia (AML) patients (Pts). American Society of Hematology, Washington, DC

Yen K, Travins J, Wang F, David MD, Artin E, Straley K, Padyana A, Gross S, DeLaBarre B, Tobin E, Chen Y, Nagaraja R, Choe S, Jin L, Konteatis Z, Cianchetta G, Saunders JO, Salituro FG, Quivoron C, Opolon P, Bawa O, Saada V, Paci A, Broutin S, Bernard OA, de Botton S, Marteyn BS, Pilichowska M, Xu Y, Fang C, Jiang F, Wei W, Jin S, Silverman L, Liu W, Yang H, Dang L, Dorsch M, Penard-Lacronique V, Biller SA, Su S-SM (2017) AG-221, a first-in-class therapy targeting acute myeloid leukemia harboring oncogenic *IDH2* mutations. Cancer Discov 7(5):478. https://doi.org/10.1158/2159-8290.CD-16-1034

Zarrinkar PP, Gunawardane RN, Cramer MD, Gardner MF, Brigham D, Belli B, Karaman MW, Pratz KW, Pallares G, Chao Q (2009) AC220 is a uniquely potent and selective inhibitor of FLT3 for the treatment of acute myeloid leukemia (AML). Blood 114(14):2984–2992

Zhang H, Savage S, Schultz AR, Bottomly D, White L, Segerdell E, Wilmot B, McWeeney SK, Eide CA, Nechiporuk T, Carlos A, Henson R, Lin C, Searles R, Ho H, Lam YL, Sweat R, Follit C, Jain V, Lind E, Borthakur G, Garcia-Manero G, Ravandi F, Kantarjian HM, Cortes J, Collins R, Buelow DR, Baker SD, Druker BJ, Tyner JW (2019) Clinical resistance to crenolanib in acute myeloid leukemia due to diverse molecular mechanisms. Nat Commun 10(1):244. https://doi.org/10.1038/s41467-018-08263-x

# 18 Future Developments: Measurable Residual Disease

Adriano Venditti, Peter J. M. Valk, Nigel H. Russell, and Sylvie D. Freeman

## 18.1 Introduction

The prognostic impact of MRD at different treatment time points of standard regimens has been established by numerous previous studies. Several trial groups have now tested whether MRD assessments are feasible in real time to guide treatment. Improved leukemia genomic classification combined with the clinical availability of next generation sequencing (NGS), the increasing delivery of allogeneic transplantation to high-risk patients, new therapies, and assay development all have to be incorporated into the framework of MRD testing. This presents challenges but also opportunities to extend and improve its utility in clinical practice and advancing treatment options.

A. Venditti
Hematology, Department of Biomedicine and Prevention, University Tor Vergata, Rome, Italy

P. J. M. Valk
Department of Hematology, University Medical Center, Rotterdam, the Netherlands

N. H. Russell
Haematology, Guy's and St Thomas' NHS Foundation Trust, Guy's Hospital, London, UK

S. D. Freeman (✉)
Institute of Immunology and Immunotherapy, University of Birmingham, Birmingham, UK
e-mail: s.freeman@bham.ac.uk

## 18.2 MRD-Directed Therapy: Update from Clinical Trials

The ever more expanding knowledge of the biology of acute myeloid leukemia (AML) has not only driven the discovery of novel agents with a targeted mechanism of action (Gerstung et al. 2017) but also encouraged the development of new strategies such as the "risk-adapted approach." Such a strategy is based on the assumption that the old-fashioned approach "one size fits all" should be replaced by an alternative one that counterbalances the intensity of therapeutic intervention based on the genetic characteristics of AML and its risk of relapse (Cornelissen et al. 2012). The philosophy behind this strategy consists in the attempt to preserve as much as possible a favorable cost/benefit ratio, avoiding over-treatment of patients with low-risk AML or under-treatment of those with high-risk disease. The evolving criteria of response make such a scenario even more complex. In fact, morphologic complete remission (mCR), although still representing the gold standard, provides an unfaithful picture of the quality of response (Freeman and Hourigan 2019; Schuurhuis et al. 2018). Therefore, multiparameter flow cytometry (MFC) and/or polymerase chain reaction (PCR), first applied for diagnostic purposes, have become leading techniques to explore the quality of response below the threshold of mCR, by quantifying the so-called "measurable residual disease"



C. Röllig, G. J. Ossenkoppele (eds.), *Acute Myeloid Leukemia*, Hematologic Malignancies, https://doi.org/10.1007/978-3-030-72676-8_18

(MRD) (Schuurhuis et al. 2018). Whatever the technique applied, the prognostic role of MRD is widely recognized in several retrospective studies showing that the cumulative incidence of relapse (CIR) of patients without detectable MRD is 6–40% whereas it is 50–80% in those with MRD (Freeman et al. 2018; Ivey et al. 2016; Jongen-Lavrencic et al. 2018; Terwijn et al. 2013; Guenot et al. 2019; Hoffmann et al. 2019; Hollein et al. 2018a; Buccisano et al. 2012; Rucker et al. 2019). Indeed, the frequently observed association between MRD status and clinical outcome has led the European LeukemiaNet (ELN) to include mCR-MRD negative as a new criterion of response (Dohner et al. 2017). However, unequivocal acknowledgment of MRD as a critical tool to implement the therapeutic decision-making process requires that its role is demonstrated also in prospective studies. If the role of MRD is confirmed prospectively, it may serve as a biomarker rather than as a simple prognosticator. In this view, the perfect trial is the one randomizing patients with MRD to intensified therapy (e.g., allogeneic stem cell transplant) versus conventional therapy (e.g., multiple consolidation courses or autologous stem cell transplant). It is unlikely that such a trial will ever see the light for younger patients and, as of today, MRD-based decisions still represent a difficult task in AML. In such a complicated context, efforts are being made to explore prospectively the impact of MRD assessment in patients with AML. In the following section, we discuss the current prospective MRD-driven trials in AML and the implications of their findings.

## 18.3 MRD-Guided Preemptive Treatment

Studies focusing on sequential MRD detection have shown that the persistence or re-emergence (molecular relapse) of the relevant molecular marker may be detected in advance of morphological relapse, allowing therapeutic intervention before overt hematological relapse and potentially improving long-term outcome.

The updated analysis of the RELAZA-2 trial (Platzbecker et al. 2018, 2019) now provides data for 94 patients who received MRD-driven treatment with azacitidine. In patients with AML or high-risk myelodysplastic syndrome who were in remission after appropriate treatments (including allogeneic stem cell transplant), MRD positivity was defined by either molecular MRD (quantitative PCR) or as a fall in CD34+/CD117+ cell chimerism below the threshold of 80%. In the first cohort of 198 screened patients, MRD reappeared in 53 patients and they were given pre-emptive azacitidine (Platzbecker et al. 2018). This prevented relapse in 51% of patients with MRD (median follow-up of 13 months) whereas in the remaining overt hematologic recurrence did not occur until a median of 422 days. In the subsequent cohort of 41 additional patients converting to an MRD-positive test (Platzbecker et al. 2019), the authors observed that 6 months from preemptive azacitidine initiation, 25 (61%) were still in mCR; 19 had a decline of the level of MRD below the predefined threshold. The combined 94 patients had 6 months relapse-free survival of 60%. Although not randomized, the prospective RELAZA-2 trial provides evidence that an MRD-guided intervention can prolong survival in MRD-positive patients by preventing or significantly postponing disease recurrence.

The NCRI AML17/19 trial is also evaluating whether early intervention at the time of molecular relapse improves overall survival compared to the standard of care. Patients were eligible for a monitor versus no monitoring randomization if they had an RT-qPCR molecular MRD target, that is, chimeric fusion genes generated by balanced chromosomal rearrangements or *NPM1* mutations, which collectively are present in over 50% of AML presenting in younger adults (Grimwade et al. 2016). Over 600 non-APML AML patients have entered this randomization which was made 2:1 in favor of monitoring. Patients in the monitoring arm undergo sequential BM sampling following each cycle of therapy and then 3 monthly for 2 years but can continue for longer if there is a relapse when the monitoring clock is reset. It was calculated that a total of 600 patients was sufficient to give a 90% power to detect an improvement in survival from 40 to 52.5%. The results are expected by 2022 along with analyses of Quality of Life and resource utilization.

## 18.4 MRD Risk-Adapted Strategies

In the recently reported GIMEMA AML1310 trial (Venditti et al. 2019), the investigators adopted a risk-adapted strategy by integrating pre-treatment prognosticators such as cytogenetics and molecular genetics with post-treatment MRD assessment (Fig. 18.1a). Adults aged 18–60 years, after induction and a first course of consolidation, were directed to an autologous or an allogeneic stem cell transplant if qualified as low- or high-risk, respectively. Intermediate risk patients were allocated to autologous or allogeneic stem cell transplant based on the MRD status after the first course of consolidation; MRD was assessed by MFC. The study showed, although in a non-randomized fashion, that delivering an allogeneic stem cell transplant to MRD-positive patients prolonged their OS and DFS to coincide with outcomes of patients without detectable MRD who received an autologous stem cell transplant. In the AML12 CETLAM trial, the Spanish investigators adopted a similar risk-adapted post-remission allocation based on genetic data and MRD (Sierra et al. 2019). MRD was determined by RT-qPCR when a suitable molecular marker was identified or MFC. After induction and a first consolidation course, patients with favorable genetics and negative MRD-test (FG-MRDneg) received 3 additional courses of consolidation, those with intermediate genetics and negative MRD-test (IG-MRDneg) 1 additional course of consolidation and then autologous or allogeneic stem cell transplant according to the local policy. In patients categorized as high-risk (HR), either by adverse genetics or positive MRD-test, allogeneic stem cell transplant was mandatory, after the first consolidation. By applying this strategy, 57 of 542 patients who were risk-allocated shifted from the favorable- or intermediate-risk genetic category to the HR one due to a positive MRD-test after the first consolidation and therefore were directed to allogeneic stem cell transplant. Four-year OS and event-free survival (EFS) of these 57 patients were 53 ± 8% and 45 ± 7%, respectively. Four-year OS of the whole series was 48% ± 2; EFS of FG-MRDneg, IG-MRDneg, and HR was 77% ± 3, 45% ± 6, and 34% ± 4, respectively (Sierra et al. 2019).

In the ongoing UK NCRI trial for younger adults, MRD assessment has been applied to improve prognostication, particularly in patients with intermediate-risk AML in first remission which has been an area where decision-making about the choice of post-remission therapy has been the most problematic. In patients <60 years, the AML17 trial showed that post-course 2 MRD measured either by RT-qPCR in *NPM1*-mutated disease or by MFC in patients who were *NPM1* wild-type (*NPM1*wt) could identify patients at very high risk of relapse (Freeman et al. 2018; Ivey et al. 2016). For *NPM1*-mutated disease, the 3-year overall survival (OS) was 24% in patients who were RT-qPCR positive for *NPM1*-mutated transcripts in the peripheral blood (PB) post-course 2 compared with 75% for those who tested negative. In a multivariate analysis that included clinical parameters and mutational profile, MRD status was the only factor to retain significance. These results are supported by the French ALFA0702 study, which also enrolled patients aged <60 years, and showed a >4 log reduction in transcript levels in the PB or bone marrow after one cycle of induction was associated with a 3-year OS of ~90% (Balsat et al. 2017). The ALFA0702 study has also shown that the poorer outcomes of MRD-positive *NPM1*-mutated patients can be improved by allogeneic stem cell transplant (SCT) in first remission (Balsat et al. 2017). In our ongoing NCRI AML19 trial, the approximately 30% of patients who are identified post-course 2 of induction as having high-risk *NPM1*-mutated AML are recommended for intensified salvage therapy randomizing FLAG-Ida versus CPX-351 followed by repeat MRD assessment before allogeneic SCT (Fig. 18.1b). The same approach is applied to patients with intermediate risk AML who lack an *NPM1* mutation (*NPM1*wt) using MFC-MRD detection.

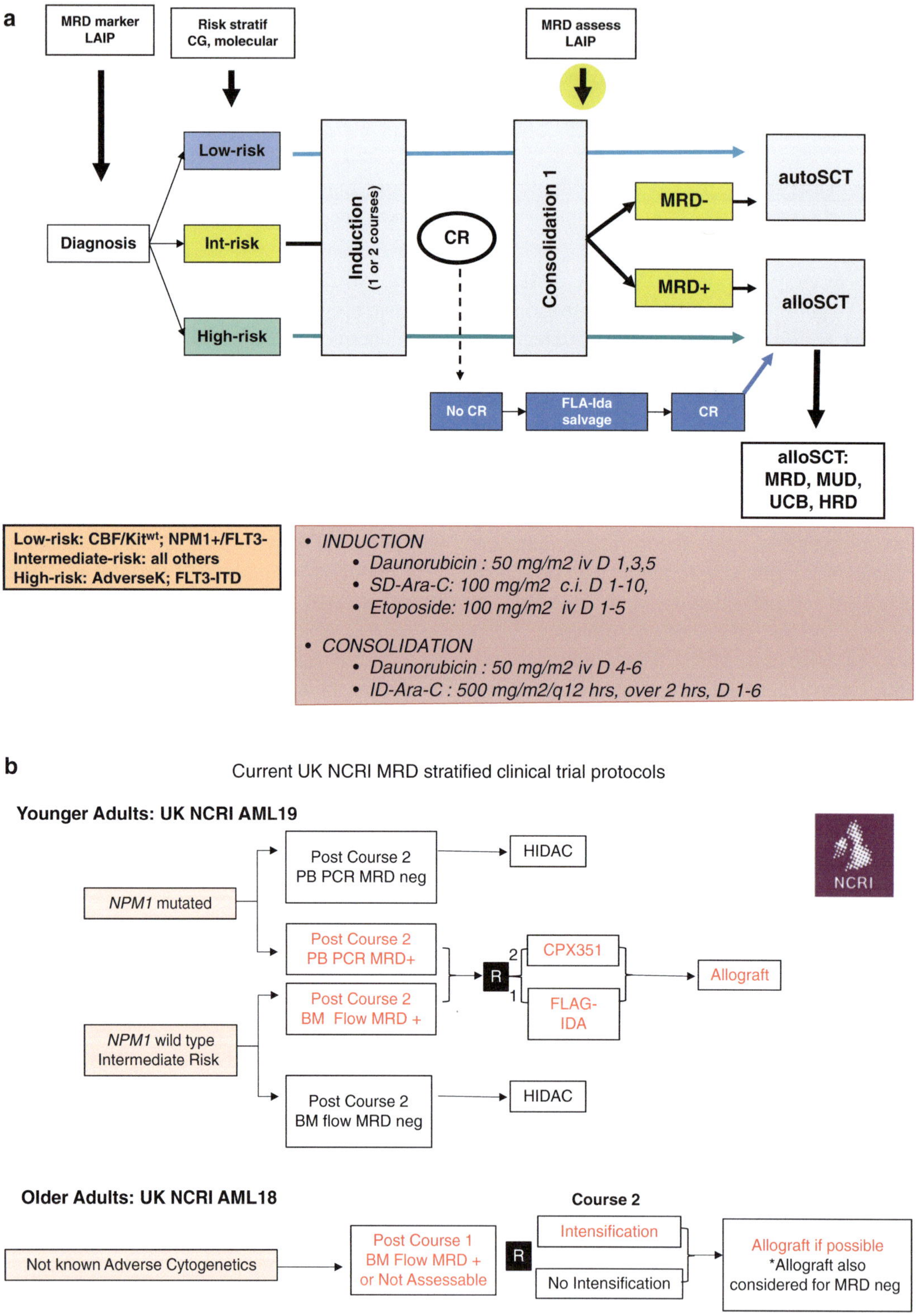


**Fig. 18.1** Examples of MRD risk-adapted strategies implemented in clinical trials. (**a**) GIMEMA AML1310 trial. *LAIP* leukemia associated phenotype, *CG* cytogenetic, *CR* complete remission, *MRD* minimal residual disease, *autoSCT* autologous stem cell transplant, *alloSCT* allogeneic stem cell transplant, *MRD* matched related donor, *MUD* matched unrelated donor, *UCB* umbilical cord blood, *HRD* haploidentical related donor, *FLA-Ida* Fludarabine-Arabinoside-Idarubicin. (**b**) NCRI (UK, Denmark, New Zealand) AML19 and AML18 Trials: role of MRD-directed intensification. (**c**) HOVON132 AML/SAKK 30/13 study: role of MRD after induction cycle II

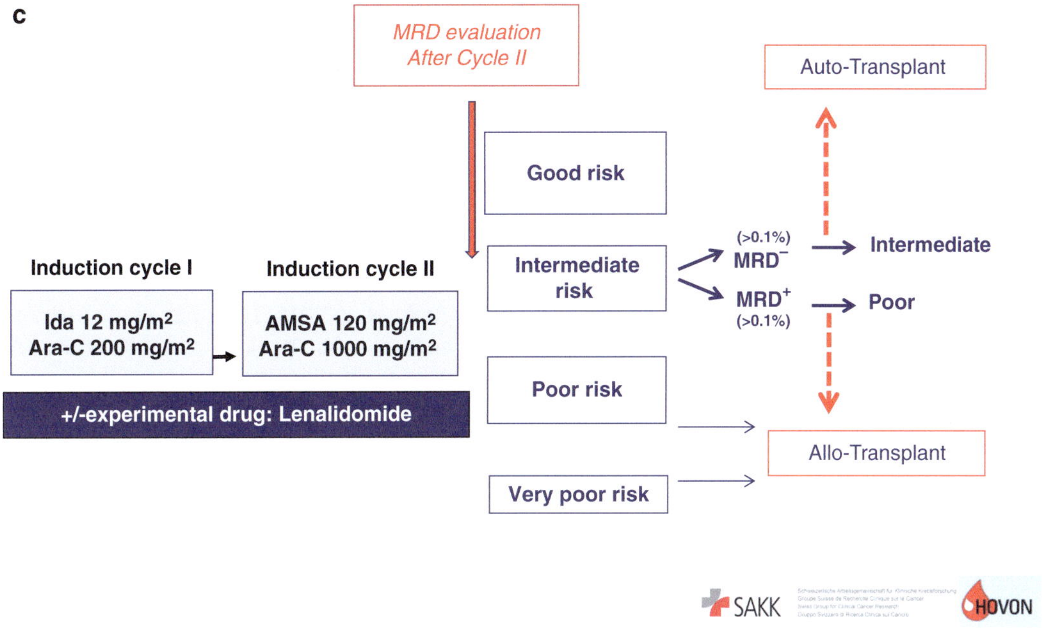


**Fig. 18.1** (continued)

In a study which globally involved 2450 NCRI AML17 trial patients, post-course 2MFC-MRD positivity, which was detected in about 30% of *NPM1*wt intermediate risk patients, predicted a significantly poorer survival (5-year OS, 33 vs. 63% for MRD– patients) and a high probability of relapse when MRD level was ≥0.1% (3-year cumulative incidence of relapse, 89%) (Freeman et al. 2018). Furthermore, transplant benefit was more apparent in patients with MRD+ (HR, 0.72; 95% CI, 0.31 to 1.69) than those with MRD– (HR, 1.68 [95% CI, 0.75–3.85]) (Freeman et al. 2018). As a consequence, MFC-MRD assessment was implemented in the NCRI AML19 trial to stratify otherwise intermediate risk *NPM1*wt patients as high risk and eligible for the same high-risk randomization as high-risk *NPM1*-mutated AML (Fig. 18.1b).

Finally, the results of the HOVON 132 AML/SAKK 30/13 clinical trial are now available (Löwenberg et al. 2021). The trial was closed to further recruitment last year, and the final analysis showed that with an MRD guided approach, MRD status after cycle 2 lost prognostic value in intermediate-risk AML in the risk-adjusted treatment context. The trial design was reminiscent of the GIMEMA study, with a post-induction-2 stratification of patients belonging to the intermediate-risk genetic category based on the level of MRD, assessed by MFC and mutant *NPM1* (Fig. 18.1c). The GIMEMA, NCRIAML17/19, and HOVON132 AML/SAKK 30/13 trials are coincident in their selection of time point for MRD assessment and subgroup deemed to benefit the most from such a determination. Their experience demonstrates the feasibility of MRD assessment after 2 courses of chemotherapy (1 Induction and 1 consolidation or 2 induction courses) to help planning tailored post-remission programs for adults belonging to the intermediate-risk category, at least in the frame of specifically designed trials. In addition, the results of the AML12 CETLAM trial point to the hypothesis that MRD status also has a role in guiding post-remission management of low-risk patients.

As discussed above, the best trial is the one that randomizes MRD-positive patients to intensified therapy against continuing conventional therapy. The current UK NCRI AML18, which is designed for patients >60 years without known adverse risk cytogenetics and fit for intensive chemotherapy, has such a design (Fig. 18.1b). Patients entering the trial have centralized testing for an MFC-MRD target (identified in over 90% of patients). Following a first induction course of DA chemotherapy plus gemtuzumab, BM samples are assessed for remission status and MFC-MRD. Patients not in remission or who are MRD positive are randomized between continuing standard chemotherapy as course 2 or intensified therapy with the addition of cladribine to DA or a FLAG-Ida regimen. In the MRD + ve arm, MRD is reassessed following count recovery. As of writing 493 patients have entered this randomization. The rationale was based on the findings of our previous NCRI AML16 trial in this age group which demonstrated that MRD negativity (inducible in 51% of patients in remission after one cycle of intensive chemotherapy) was associated with a significantly better 3-year survival (42 vs. 26% in MRD-positive patients) (Freeman et al. 2013). Of course, treatment intensification may not result in MRD negativity or improve survival as these patients have already demonstrated chemorefractoriness to standard induction therapy and intensification may adversely affect treatment-related mortality. What is desirable is a less toxic targeted approach to treat MRD and indeed such an approach using a combination Venetoclax and low dose cytarabine may be highly effective in *NPM1*-mutated older adults remaining MRD positive by RT-qPCR after intensive chemotherapy (Tiong et al. 2019).

## 18.5 Managing Pre-transplant MRD

The ELN AML working party consensus statement, by adopting a dynamic risk-assessment approach including MRD determination, recommends that allogeneic stem cell transplant should be favored when the risk of relapse exceeds 35–40% and when the projected disease-free survival is expected to improve by at least 10% (Cornelissen et al. 2012). Based on this, it appears that allogeneic stem cell transplant represents the optimal option to offer in the situation of MRD positivity since it reduces relapses (Cornelissen et al. 2012). However, some retrospective studies reported that being MRD positive before allogeneic stem cell transplant had a negative impact on post-transplant outcome, regardless of the intensity of the conditioning regimen that was delivered (Araki et al. 2016; Walter et al. 2015). Indeed, patients who were MRD positive before allogeneic stem cell transplant had outcomes comparable to those transplanted with active disease (Araki et al. 2016; Hourigan et al. 2016). A large meta-analysis (Buckley et al. 2017), including 19 retrospective studies published between 2005 and 2016, confirmed that pre-transplant MRD positivity was associated with a shorter duration of leukemia-free survival and OS and higher rates of CIR. The unfavorable effect of pre-transplant MRD positivity took place irrespective of detection method, conditioning intensity, and patient age. These experiences are sometimes used as an argument not to transplant "pre-transplant MRD positive patients." Therefore, the question is whether a consolidative allogeneic stem cell transplant remains a valid option also for this category of patients or should alternative strategies be pursued? A retrospective analysis of 547 patients enrolled in the HOVON/SAKK protocols demonstrated that all AML risk-categories benefited from allogeneic stem cell transplant; however, the absolute benefit was greater in pre-transplant MRD-positive than MRD-negative patients (Versluis et al. 2017). The authors assumed that the graft vs leukemia potential was equally effective in MRD-positive as well as MRD-negative patients. In a prospective, non-randomized trial of 137 patients with t(8;21), Zhu et al. (2013) distinguished high-risk (*RUNX1-RUNX1T1* transcript reduction <3 logs after second consolidation course) from low-risk (*RUNX1-RUNX1T1* transcript reduction >3 logs after second consolidation course) individuals. Of 69 high-risk patients, 40 received allogeneic stem cell transplant and 29 additional courses of chemotherapy or autologous stem cell transplant. Patients who received allogeneic stem cell transplant had a significantly lower CIR and superior OS and DFS as compared to those not allocated to allogeneic stem cell transplant. In spite of the non-randomized treatment allocation, the results of the trial suggest the potential survival advantage of a risk-adapted strategy, even in patients who were pre-transplant MRD positive. In fact, subjects who received treatments different from those scheduled according to their risk status did worse than patients who received the assigned treatment. Thol et al. (2018) demonstrated that error-corrected NGS-MRD can be applied in mCR before allogeneic stem cell transplant and that it is highly predictive. In competing risk analysis, CIR of pre-transplant MRD-positive patients was significantly higher than in pre-transplant MRD-negative ones. The authors suggested that NGS-MRD may be a very useful tool to help refining transplant and post-transplant management of patients with AML. A paradigmatic example of NGS potential was recently published by Hourigan and coworkers (2020). The authors investigated whether modulation of the intensity of conditioning regimen could reduce the risk of relapse in patients who were pre-transplant MRD positive. Pre-conditioning blood samples collected from adult patients in mCR were tested by NGS-MRD, looking for the 13 most commonly mutated genes in AML. Patients were randomly assigned to myeloablative conditioning (MAC) or reduced-intensity conditioning (RIC). No difference in terms of CIR and OS was observed between MAC and RIC patients, who were pre-transplant NGS-MRD negative. Among those who were pre-transplant NGS-MRD positive, 3-year CIR and OS were significantly improved in MAC versus RIC patients (19 vs. 67%, $p < 0.01$ and 61 vs. 43%, $p = 0.02$). This study provides evidence that MAC rather than RIC improves the outcome of pre-transplant MRD-positive patients, consistent with previous retrospective EBMT data (Gilleece et al. 2018). Altogether, these studies lend support to the hypothesis that the mere presence of MRD should not be an absolute obstacle to the delivery of an allogeneic stem cell transplant. In this view, a relevant question raises as to whether the burden of MRD is a critical factor influencing the post-transplant outcome. Theoretically, the higher the levels of MRD the greater the required neutralization from "graft vs leukemia" (GVL). Leung et al. (2012) observed that CIR and OS of a series of pediatric patients worsened proportionally to the increasing levels of pre-transplant MRD, with patients categorized as "high positive" (MRD > 1%) having the highest CIR and shortest OS. Buccisano et al. (2017) reported a very similar experience in a series of 81 pre-transplant MRD-positive adult patients. Allogeneic stem cell transplant conferred a statistically significant survival advantage to patients with "low burden MRD" (MRD < 1%). Moreover, in the NCRI AML17 trial only higher levels of pre-transplant *NPM1* mutant MRD had an adverse effect on post-transplant outcomes of *NPM1* mutated patients who were *FLT3*-ITD negative at diagnosis (Dillon et al. 2020). Prospective studies using comparable assays would help further address this issue. If a green light is given to the decision to transplant "pre-transplant MRD positive" patients, the question is how to potentiate the antileukemic effect of allogeneic stem cell transplant. Delivery of additional cytotoxic therapy before allogeneic stem cell transplant appears questionable. MRD persistence reflects most probably a condition of leukemia chemoresistance. Therefore, provision of cytotoxic therapy appears not the right approach and could be even detrimental. Relapses and/or toxicities can occur, interfering with the subsequent transplant procedure. However, the availability of new agents has paved the way for potential intervention on MRD status to overtake its prognostic role. The timely use of these new agents appears a critical factor for a successful control/eradication of MRD. In the RATIFY study (Stone et al. 2017), delivery of allogeneic stem cell transplant in first mCR was associated with a superior survival advantage in patients randomized in the midostaurin plus chemotherapy arm. This observation suggests that midostaurin might have induced a better quality of response before allogeneic stem cell transplant. A similar finding emerged also in the phase 3 CPX-351 clinical trial (Lancet et al. 2018). These experiences indicate that a proper use of new drugs might increase the proportion of patients who are "pre-transplant MRD negative." On the other hand, the availability of new agents has also revitalized the role of maintenance therapy (Wei et al. 2019a), suggesting that preemptive treatments are feasible even after allogeneic stem cell transplant (Platzbecker et al. 2019; Burchert et al. 2018). CC-486 (oral azacitidine) promises to be a strong candidate to investigate in clinical trials of post-transplant maintenance.

In conclusion, even though there is robust evidence of the negative prognostic role of "pre-transplant MRD positivity," we believe that it is not a valid justification to desist from a potentially curative approach such as allogeneic stem cell transplant. Such a habit appears even more convincing in an era of broad accessibility to new agents that might contribute to improving transplant outcomes. Also, the discovery of ever more sophisticated techniques promises to help to refine our therapeutic decisions in a way that they are tailored to the individual risk of recurrence. Controlled, clinical trials are needed to validate the value of these approaches, and patients should be encouraged to enter such trials.

## 18.6 MRD in the Era of Novel Therapies

MRD negativity is not yet an EMA/FDA accepted early surrogate outcome endpoint in AML but complete remission with MRD negativity (CR MRD−) is now included as a response criterion (Dohner et al. 2017) to categorize remissions that are ≥1–4 logs below the CR threshold ($10^{-3}$ to $10^{-6}$) as measured by standard MRD assessments (genetic markers by RT-qPCR or by MFC-MRD). In most published studies, CR MRD− frequencies are reported for composite mCR patients, that is, CR and CR with incomplete neutrophil or platelet recovery. Increasingly recent trials of newer AML therapies have reported rates of these deeper responses, either by standard MRD assessments or, in the case of IDH and FLT3 inhibitors, clearance of targeted mutations. In the absence of randomized studies, currently the only comparison for these data is from historical cohorts treated by chemotherapy.

Excluding gemtuzumab ozogamicin and midostaurin, novel treatments have been approved for (1) adults ≥75 years or unfit with newly diagnosed AML or (2) relapsed/refractory AML. In the setting of relapsed/refractory AML, a preliminary report suggests that about 60% of adults in remission following intermediate or high dose cytarabine salvage have a CR MRD− ($10^{-3}$ to $10^{-4}$, MFC-MRD) (Short et al. 2019). Regarding older adults in remission from standard treatments, previously published rates of CR MRD− (by MFC-MRD) ranged from 11% (Buccisano et al. 2015) to ~50% (Freeman et al. 2013) after intensive chemotherapy and 41% with HMA (hypomethylating agents) (Boddu et al. 2018). Table 18.1 shows the MRD data with frequencies of remission and CR MRD− reported so far for newer therapies. In some studies, especially for combination regimens, CR MRD− rates are certainly encouraging. However, the extent to which CR MRD− impacts on outcome compared to blast reduction below CR threshold of 5% remains uncertain. Factors that restrict determining this include the relatively small cohorts, modest, often short-lived outcome benefits and in some cases a selected MRD marker that may have lower prognostic value. Do less intensive regimens reduce the potential survival benefit of CR MRD− by limiting how much leukemia can be cleared below the MRD detection threshold? Interestingly, the prognostic advantage from CR MRD− (MFC) appears equivalent in adjusted analyses between intensive versus less intensive standard induction although more patients achieve negativity with the former (Hochman et al. 2019). It will be important to extend this evaluation to the newer combinations. A further consideration is that non-intensive novel drugs have different therapeutic activities from standard cytotoxics as they promote leukemic blast maturation; this could further alter the prognostic effect of MRD. Indeed, treatment benefit in AML may not always require leukemia clearance below $10^{-3}$ to $10^{-6}$ or even below the CR threshold as demonstrated in HMA trials (Santini and Ossenkoppele 2019; Yee et al. 2019). Moreover, any benefit from CR MRD− may be outweighed by greater treatment toxicity. A third of remission responses to HMA were CR MRD− (by MFC-MRD) (Boddu et al. 2018) (Table 18.1). Although relapse was reduced in these "best"

**Table 18.1** New drugs and MRD: MRD information generated in studies of novel therapies

| | AML status | Median age | Number of patients monitored by MRD | MRD marker | % CR[a] (overall cohort) | % MRD− (% of patients in remission) | % CR[a] MRD− (% of overall cohort) | ? Improved outcome in MRD- patients | | Comment |
|---|---|---|---|---|---|---|---|---|---|---|
| | | | | | | | | Relapse | Overall survival | |
| *Treatment* | | | | | | | | | | |
| *HMA alone* | | | | | | | | | | |
| Decitabine (Boddu et al. 2018) Gaudecitabine Azacitidine Off-trial | New diagnosis | 76 yrs | 116 | Flow cytometry | 59% | 41% (by 3 m post remission time-point) | 24% | Yes (2 yr. CIR 48% vs 86% for other CR patients) | No | HIgh non- relapse mortality in MRD- group |
| *Venetoclax* | | | | | | | | | | |
| Venetoclax with HMA (DiNardo et al. 2019c) | Treatment naive | 74 yrs | 145 | Flow cytometry | 67% | 29% | 19% | Trend for median duration of CR (not reached vs 11.3 months) | Uncertain (median OS not reached for CR) | Highest [a]CR % In *NPM1* and *IDH* mutated |
| Venetoclax with LDARAC (Wei et al. 2018, 2019b) | Treatment naïve or prior HMA | 74 yrs | 82 | Flow cytometry | 54% | 32% | 17% | Not reported | Uncertain (median OS not reached for [a]CR MRD−) | Highest [a]CR % In *NPM1* and *IDH* mutated |
| Venetoclax with Azacytidine (Winters et al. 2019) Off-trial | Treatment naïve or prior HMA | 72 yrs (off trial) | 14 (responders, off-trial) | Custom *ddPCR* assays based on diagnostic mutations | 63% | 29% | 18% | NA | NA | No relapses in MRD- responders |
| Venetoclax with CLAD/LDARAC alternating with Aza (Kadia et al. 2019) | Newly diagnosed | 69 yrs | 24 | Flow cytometry | 92% | 83% | 76% | NA | NA | |

(continued)

**Table 18.1** (continued)

| | AML status | Median age | Number of patients monitored by MRD | MRD marker | % CR[a] (overall cohort) | % MRD− (% of patients in remission) | % CR[a] MRD− (% of overall cohort) | ? Improved outcome in MRD- patients | | Comment |
|---|---|---|---|---|---|---|---|---|---|---|
| | | | | | | | | Relapse | Overall survival | |
| Venetoclax with HMA or LDARAC (Tiong et al. 2019) Off-trial | NPM1 mutated with molecular relapse or persistence | 61 yrs | 10 | *mNPM1*RT–qPCR | Not applicable | 80% | Not applicable | NA | NA | |
| DiNardo Blood 2020 | | | | | | | | | | |
| **IDH inhibitors** | | | | | | | | | | |
| *Ivosidenib* | | | | | | | | | | |
| Ivosidenib monotherapy (Roboz et al. 2020) | New diagnosis | 76.5 yrs | 30 | *IDH1 R132* mutations by ddPCR | 42% | 64% | 27% | NA | NA | RTK mutations enriched for non-responders |
| Ivosidenib with standard chemotherapy (Stein et al. 2018) | New diagnosis | 63 yrs | 31 | *IDH1* mutations by ddPCR<br>Flow cytometry<br>In some | 78% | 41% by mutation clearance<br>89% by flow cytometry (8 of 9 patients) | 32% by mutation clearance | NA | NA | |
| Ivosidenib monotherapy (DiNardo et al. 2018) | Relapsed refractory | 67 yrs | 73 | *IDH1* mutations by ddPCR | 30% | 21% | 6% | Trend for median duration of CR (11.1 vs 6.5 months) | Trend for median OS<br>But<br>MRD+ not restricted to CR | |

| | | | | | | | | | | |
|---|---|---|---|---|---|---|---|---|---|---|
| *Enasidenib* | | | | | | | | | | |
| Enasidenib with standard chemotherapy (Stein et al. 2018) | New diagnosis | 63 yrs | 60 | *IDH2* mutations by ddPCR Flow cytometry In some | 69% | 30% by mutation clearance 58% by flow cytometry (7 of 12 patients) | 21% | Not reported | Not reported | |
| Enasidenib monotherapy (Stein et al. 2019) | Relapsed refractory | 68 yrs | 101 | *IDH2* mutations by ddPCR | 29% | 28.6% | 8% | Not known | Yes for median OS <u>When</u> MRD+ not restricted to CR | No survival difference for CR MRD− vs CR MRD+ *NRAS* and *Flt3* mutations enriched for non-responders |
| *Flt3 inhibitors* | | | | | | | | | | |
| +/− FLT3 inhibitor with standard induction followed by CR1 allogeneic transplant (Levis et al. 2020) | New diagnosis *FLT3*-ITD mutated and *NPM1*-mutated | 59 yrs | 17 (8 had FLT3 inhibitor) | *FLT3*-ITD mutations by custom PCR-NGS assay plus CE-PCR | Not applicable | 7 of 8 Flt3 inhibitor patients *Flt3*-ITD VAF <0.01% | Not applicable | NA | NA | Numbers very small but MRD significantly lower in Flt3 inhibitor vs chemo alone |
| Gilteritinib (Levis et al. 2018) CHRYSALIS trial | Relapsed/ refractory | 61 yrs | 80 | *FLT3*-ITD mutations by custom PCR-NGS assay | 55% | 45% VAF $\leq 10^{-2}$ 30% VAF $\leq 10^{-4}$ | 25% VAF $\leq 10^{-2}$ 16.5% VAF $\leq 10^{-4}$ | NA | Prolonged median survival <u>But</u> not restricted to CR | Median survival similar for MRD $\leq 10^{-2}$ To $\leq 10^{-4}$ |

*LDARAC* low dose cytarabine, *CLAD* cladaribine, *NA* not assessable, m*NPM1* mutated *NPM1*, *ddPCR* droplet digital PCR, *NGS* next generation sequencing, *CE* capillary electrophoresis

[a]CR, composite complete remission i.e. CR with incomplete (CRi) or platelet recovery (CRp) and may in some studies include partial haematological recovery (CRh)

responders, this did not translate to a survival benefit due to a higher number of non-relapse deaths. However, when older patients were treated with a combination of HMA (decitabine) and vosaroxin (quinolone derivative, topoisomerase II inhibitor), MRD-negative status was associated with improved median overall survival (34.0 versus 8.3 months for other responders) (Daver et al. 2017). Currently investigated HMA plus novel agent combinations may be able to achieve deep remissions without concomitant increased toxicity. Encouragingly in the context of observed MRD-negative responses in phase 1/2 studies of IDH inhibitors and Venetoclax (as monotherapy or in HMA combinations) (Table 18.1, also (DiNardo et al. 2019a, b)), adverse events appear infrequent.

**IDH Inhibitors:** Mutations in either IDH1 or IDH2 can collectively be detected by NGS panels in up to 20% of AML patients by current technology (Bullinger et al. 2017). This prevalence increases in older AML cohorts (~25%) (Prassek et al. 2018) and in AML with normal cytogenetics (up to 30%) including NPM1 mutated AML (~30%) (Bullinger et al. 2017; Ferret et al. 2018; Ok et al. 2019). In retrospective studies, 45–60% of newly diagnosed IDH mutated AML patients attaining CR after standard chemotherapy cleared their *IDH* mutations (detection limit <0.2% VAF by standard dd PCR assay (Ferret et al. 2018) or <1% VAF by NGS (Ok et al. 2019)) and this was associated with reduced early relapse (Ferret et al. 2018; Ok et al. 2019). Some IDH inhibitor studies have monitored *IDH* mutations by a more sensitive dd PCR assay, (depth up to $10^{-4}$) to combine a read-out of on-target efficacy with MRD. On-target molecular remissions are observed in 20–28% of relapsed /refractory *IDH* mutated patients achieving CR or CR with partial hematological recovery from IDH inhibitor monotherapy (Stein et al. 2019; DiNardo et al. 2018). Higher percentages have been reported in early data from phase 1 /2 IDH inhibitor studies (including azacitidine combinations) of newly diagnosed AML (DiNardo et al. 2019a; Roboz et al. 2020; Stein et al. 2018). While such deep *IDH* molecular remissions may be an indicator for response duration (with Ivosidenib (DiNardo et al. 2018)), improvements in survival compared to mutation positive CR/CRh patients have not yet been reported (Stein et al. 2019; DiNardo et al. 2018; Roboz et al. 2020). Furthermore, response and survival were comparable between patients with *IDH2*-R140 or *IDH2*-R172 mutations, but only the former had a major reduction in mutation VAF (Stein et al. 2019). Ongoing differentiation, clonal hematopoiesis, or later mutation loss from clonal evolution may all contribute to reducing the prognostic significance of detectable *IDH* mutations. Established assays (e.g., RT-qPCR of *NPM1* mutations or MFC-MRD) are clinically recommended to assess AML MRD (Schuurhuis et al. 2018). Combining them with *IDH* mutation analysis currently represents the optimal monitoring strategy for assessing the efficacy of IDH inhibitors in trials.

**FLT3 Inhibitors:** There is a paucity of MRD data in published trials of FLT3 tyrosine kinase inhibitors. On-target molecular monitoring is available at low sensitivity ($10^{-2}$ VAF) by the established clinical test of capillary electrophoresis (CE) *FLT3* ITD detection. A more sensitive (up to $10^{-4}$ VAF) combination PCR NGS assay (propriety) demonstrated a 16% CR MRD− frequency in 80 relapsed/refractory AML adults who received gilteritinib monotherapy (CHRYSALIS phase 1 /2 study) (Levis et al. 2018). CR MRD− patients had a significantly longer median survival compared to those in an MRD-positive remission. However, lower levels of MRD ($\leq 10^{-3}$ VAF, detected in 25% of total cohort) did not impact on median survival (Levis et al. 2018), suggesting that in this setting an MRD threshold of $10^{-3}$ is most predictive. This or a similar assay has also been applied to remission samples of 17 newly diagnosed *FLT3* 1TD /*NPM1* mutated adults (Levis et al. 2020) (Table 18.1) and in the ongoing CTN 1506 (gilteritinib post-transplant maintenance) and Quantum-First (quizartinib in newly diagnosed AML) trials. Other NGS-based platforms linked with differing bioinformatics strategies can also monitor *FLT3* ITD mutations to the same ITD VAF depth in research settings (Thol et al. 2018; Hourigan et al. 2020; Blatte et al. 2019; Kim et al. 2018). The above higher sensitivity assays could be validated for routine clinical practice in the next couple of years. However, as late subclonal leukemic mutations, *FLT3* ITD mutations may be unreliable MRD markers (clinical false negatives) from instability / VAFs below MRD detection limits (Freeman and Hourigan 2019); this is particularly likely beyond early response and when monitoring FLT3 inhibitors as maintenance therapy. Therefore, independently of on-target *FLT3*-ITD mutation monitoring, clinically validated MRD assays (presently MFC if no RT qPCR target such as *NPM1* mutations) continue to be recommended for MRD assessment (Schuurhuis et al. 2018).

**Venetoclax:** Composite CR/CRi frequencies for the BCL2 inhibitor venetoclax in combination with either low dose AraC or azacitidine are high, ranging between 54 and 67% for elderly adults unfit for intensive chemotherapy (DiNardo et al. 2019c; Winters et al. 2019; Wei et al. 2019b). When measured in the overall cohorts, MRD levels were below $10^{-3}$ in up to a third of the remissions (Table 18.1) and duration of response may be prolonged in these patients (DiNardo et al. 2019c; Winters et al. 2019; Wei et al. 2018) although data are preliminary. There are early but encouraging indications that MRD-negative remissions to the depth of the sensitive *NPM1* mutant RT-qPCR assay are frequent and prolonged in *NPM1* mutated patients (Tiong et al. 2019; DiNardo et al. 2020) (discussed further below). Notably, MRD detection of *IDH2* mutations appears to be a poor predictor of relapse-free survival in venetoclax treated *IDH2* mutated elderly adults. Most tested patients had detectable persistent *IDH2* mutations by ddPCR despite high rates of durable clinical remissions (at least 24 months in one study) (Winters et al. 2019; DiNardo et al. 2020).

**Glasdegib:** Although MRD results are not yet available for glasdegib studies, CR MRD− (by centrally assessed MFC-MRD) is included as a secondary endpoint in the Phase 3 BRIGHT AML1019 trials of glasdegib with standard chemotherapy or azacitidine.

**Immunotherapies:** Immunotherapies are an active area of early phase studies in AML. As well as checkpoint inhibitors there are immune constructs targeting myeloid surface proteins (CD33, CD123, CLL-1) (Assi et al. 2018). CD33 positivity is a requirement for the approved use of gemtuzumab. Flow cytometric diagnostic screening for AML markers targeted by new constructs is likely to evolve into "on-target" flow cytometric MRD monitoring to assess response efficacy and evaluate target loss on residual leukemic blasts. Relevant to this is identifying and monitoring targets on immunophenotypic blast populations that are most likely to be reservoirs of relapse as enriched in leukemic stem cells (LSC) or relapse initiating cells (Haubner et al. 2019; Zeijlemaker et al. 2019). CD34+CD38− is the most tractable immunophenotype for flow cytometric monitoring of candidate LSC / relapse initiating populations. High frequencies of CD34+CD38− blasts in diagnostic samples are indicators of poor prognosis (Zeijlemaker et al. 2019; Khan et al. 2015), consistent with this immunophenotype as a baseline biomarker for resistant leukemic cells. An initial screen for immunotherapeutic targets on CD34+CD38− and other blast populations could be simplified by a single "LSC" tube that combines multiple aberrant "LSC" markers (Zeijlemaker et al. 2016).

**Molecular Determinants of Response:** Potential molecular determinants of benefit and response durability have been explored for several novel regimens, following the paradigm of CBF AML with gemtuzumab ozogamicin (GO). For example, mutations in receptor tyrosine kinase pathway genes such as *NRAS* may be associated with primary and adaptive resistance to IDH inhibitors (Amatangelo et al. 2017; Stein et al. 2019; DiNardo et al. 2018) and venetoclax (DiNardo et al. 2020) while mutations in *IDH2* and *NPM1* appear to be molecular determinants of more durable remissions from venetoclax (DiNardo et al. 2020). In the case of GO, however, activating signaling mutations such as *NRAS* correlated with improved event-free survival in the 2017 ELN good/favorable risk subgroups, including for NPM1 mutated patients (Fournier et al. 2020). Although signaling mutations are linked to resistance to IDH inhibitors and venetoclax, the observed higher CD33 levels on blasts with these mutations (Fournier et al. 2020) may be a mechanism for improved sensitivity to GO. *TP53* mutations confer resistance across different therapies including CPX-351 (Goldberg et al. 2018) and venetoclax (DiNardo et al. 2020). Even when *TP53* mutated patients enter remission after CPX-351, CR MRD− frequency may be lower (Goldberg et al. 2018) but this needs confirmation in ongoing randomized trials with integrated MRD (such as NCRI AML18 and AML19).

To use these newer agents to their full potential, response profiles need further investigation by superimposing MRD data to mutation screens in sufficiently large cohorts. This should uncover which genetic subgroups are most treatment sensitive, whether clinical activity correlates with deeper responses and the best combination of MRD assays and genetic subgroups for MRD status to provide an early indicator of outcome endpoints. Concerning the latter, there is a strong rationale for MRD in NPM1 mutated AML to assess and direct newer therapies.

## 18.7 Combining MRD with Molecular Determinants for Outcome Prediction: *NPM1* Mutated AML

*NPM1* mutations are AML-specific (as causative driver mutations) and in >90% of cases remain stable in the relapse initiating clone (Ivey et al. 2016; Cocciardi et al. 2019; Hollein et al. 2018b). Treatment responses in *NPM1* mutated patients can be measured to a depth of $1 \times 10^{-6}$ by RT-qPCR of *NPM1* mutant transcripts (Schuurhuis et al. 2018). MRD status by this very sensitive assay is highly prognostic in *NPM1* mutated AML after induction with standard chemotherapy as well as at later time points in younger adults (Freeman and Hourigan 2019; Schuurhuis et al. 2018). Durable responses and MRD negativity have been observed not only after standard chemotherapy but also in older and relapsed /refractory *NPM1* mutated patients following novel therapies (Tiong et al. 2019; Levis et al. 2020; DiNardo et al. 2020). From the present combination of best-standard AML MRD assay and leukemia response profile in *NPM1* mutated AML, it is plausible that MRD is most likely to be a predictive measure of treatment efficacy for newer treatments in this AML subtype as compared to others. MRD data from gemtuzumab (GO) trials support this. There is a survival benefit from the addition of gemtuzumab (GO) to standard chemotherapy induction despite no concomitant increase in response (Hills et al. 2014). Specifically for *NPM1* mutated patients, there were significantly fewer relapses with GO compared to standard induction for patients achieving a remission in the AMLSG 09-09 trial (Schlenk et al. 2020).

Response depth from gemtuzumab has been compared to standard treatment arm in two trials of older patients (NCRI AML16 (Freeman et al. 2013) and ALFA-0701 (Lambert et al. 2014)) by frequencies of CR and CR MRD− (below $10^{-3}$ to $10^{-4}$, measured by MFC-MRD in NCRI AML16 and by WT1 RT-qPCR in ALFA-0701). No significant differences between the treatment arms were observed although MRD was prognostic for survival in the overall cohorts. Notably however, a post-hoc analysis of the *NPM1* mutated subgroup in the ALFA-0701 trial, showed that improved survival from GO did correlate with CR MRD− frequency by *NPM1* mutant RT-qPCR (CR MRD−, 39% in GO arm versus 7% in control, $p = 0.006$) (Lambert et al. 2014).

*NPM1* mutations are prevalent in older as well as younger adults (Prassek et al. 2018; Buccisano et al. 2018) and were present in about 20% of the elderly adults enrolled in the venetoclax phase 2 trials. Venetoclax in combination with HMA or low dose cytarabine has striking efficacy by remission rates (~90% (DiNardo et al. 2019c, 2020)) in NPM1 mutated older adults ineligible for intensive chemotherapy. This responsiveness correlates with a favorable 2 years survival of over 70%, albeit in a small number of patients so far. This overall survival rate has not previously been achieved in historical cohorts of NPM1 mutated older adults treated with either HMA (Prata et al. 2018) or intensive chemotherapy including with GO (Fournier et al. 2020; Burnett et al. 2012), even for those in a CR MRD− by flow cytometry (Freeman et al. 2013). Is there any evidence that these encouraging outcomes are associated with increased and sustained MRD clearance? *NPM1* mutant MRD monitoring data are limited for venetoclax regimens. However, durable MRD negativity by *NPM1* mutant RT-qPCR from venetoclax combinations has been reported as common in the few patients tested (Tiong et al. 2019; DiNardo et al. 2020). These include patients treated for *NPM1* mutant molecular persistence or relapse (Tiong et al. 2019). Thus, *NPM1* mutant MRD is promising as a surrogate for clinical benefit from venetoclax but also may enable selection of patients with molecular progression following chemotherapy for pre-emptive venetoclax treatments.

A significant proportion of patients with actionable mutations will also have the highly sensitive MRD marker from RT-qPCR of *NPM1* mutant transcripts. Due to the association between *NPM1* and *IDH1* or *IDH2*R140 mutations, up to 45% of younger and 10–20% of older AML patients with IDH mutations (excluding *IDH2*R172) are *NPM1* mutated (Bullinger et al. 2017; Prassek et al. 2018).

*NPM1* mutations are also frequent in FLT3 mutated patients, as evident from relapsed/refractory as well as younger newly diagnosed FLT3 mutated trial cohorts; 47% of adults recruited to the ADMIRAL trial (Perl et al. 2019) (gilteritinib versus chemotherapy for relapsed/refractory AML) had co-mutated *NPM1* and 57% in the RATIFY trial (Stone et al. 2017) (midostaurin added to chemotherapy in younger untreated AML). Survival benefits from midostaurin and gilteritinib are independent of *NPM1* genotype risk/*FLT3* ITD allelic ratio (AR) risk groups (Perl et al. 2019; Döhner et al. 2020). However, it is unclear whether CR1 allogeneic transplantation should be deployed for 2017 ELN favorable (*NPM1* mutated / *FLT3*-ITD low AR) and intermediate risk patients whether or not they receive frontline midostaurin (Döhner et al. 2020) or in the future a second generation FLT3 inhibitor. *NPM1* MRD has the potential to both inform the early efficacy of FLT3 inhibitors in these risk groups and guide further transplant decisions. Recent evidence points to *FLT3* ITD mutated patients with pre-transplant MRD positivity having a very poor outcome after allogeneic transplantation (Hourigan et al. 2020; Dillon et al. 2020). Whether available peri-transplant strategies could alter this remains to be determined. It is anticipated that ongoing trials such as those testing post-transplant maintenance with integrated MRD assays (gilteritinib, BMT CTN 1506; MRD directed azacitidine, RELAZA2 (Platzbecker et al. 2019); oral azacitidine/CC-486, AMADEUS) should contribute important data to help address this critical question.

These initial results from MRD testing in trials of emerging therapies are preliminary due to tested cohort sizes. They are, however, already generating information about the relative utility and limitations of certain markers and assays as MRD read-outs. For instance, the promising CR MRD− responses observed in NPM1 mutated AML with venetoclax and FLT3 inhibitors suggests that the higher sensitivity of RT-qPCR MRD will be advantageous in this subtype to assess and direct treatment. On the other hand, MRD detection of persisting IDH mutations in CR, even in the setting of IDH inhibitors, does not appear to preclude a survival benefit. We would encourage the future incorporation of sequential MRD into studies to aid the selection and timing of further interventions by, for example, accruing data on the kinetics of MRD re-emergence in those patients relapsing after a CR MRD−.

## 18.8 NGS-Based MRD Detection: Advances and Challenges

MFC-based MRD detection has been the standard for MRD assessment in AML patients for many years and is applicable to the majority of patients (Schuurhuis et al. 2018; Hourigan et al. 2017). In contrast, the use of molecular enumeration of MRD has been limited to specific recurrent molecular aberrations, such as the core binding factor fusion transcripts *RUNX1*/*RUNX1T1* and *CBFB-MYH11* and mutant *NPM1* (Schuurhuis et al. 2018; Hourigan et al. 2017). NGS now enables detection of all mutations, including hotspot as well as patient-specific mutations, in AML at diagnosis and in CR after chemotherapy (Levine and Valk 2019). In fact, it has recently been shown that molecular MRD detection by applying NGS is potentially applicable to virtually every newly diagnosed AML patient because of the frequent prevalence (>90%) of multiple (on average 3) molecular aberrations among patients with AML (Levine and Valk 2019). However, MRD detection based on NGS faces several challenges before it can be reliably introduced in clinical practice.

Sensitive detection of all mutant (minor) cell populations at diagnosis and during the course of disease is a prerequisite for NGS-based MRD detection in routine analyses. Sequencing artifacts are introduced during DNA isolation, library prep and the actual NGS-procedure (0.1–1%), which makes sensitive detection of all possible mutations at low level (<0.01%) a challenge (Salk et al. 2018). The rate of sequencing artifacts can be reduced biochemically, for example, by using proof-reading polymerases, or computationally; however, these corrections are only modest and cannot entirely resolve the introduction of artifacts. Alternative strategies should be explored. For instance, error corrected NGS approaches using unique molecular barcodes have been shown to increase the specificity of low-frequency mutation detection (Salk et al. 2018). Recently, several studies addressed NGS-based MRD detection in relatively large AML cohorts from clinical trials, all demonstrating that NGS-based MRD carries profound prognostic impact for patients with AML (Jongen-Lavrencic et al. 2018; Thol et al. 2018; Hourigan et al. 2020; Klco et al. 2015; Hirsch et al. 2017; Getta et al. 2017; Morita et al. 2018; Press et al. 2019). In these studies, persisting mutations in CR were measured with gene panels (Jongen-Lavrencic et al. 2018; Hirsch et al. 2017), capture-based deep sequencing (Klco et al. 2015; Hirsch et al. 2017; Salk et al. 2018; Guenot et al. 2019), or targeted sequencing (Thol et al. 2018; Hourigan et al. 2020). Only in the latter two studies NGS-based MRD detection included error-correction using unique molecular identifiers, indicating that the other NGS-based MRD studies may not have been optimal. Another successful approach to correct for noise is the usage of site-specific error models (Jongen-Lavrencic et al. 2018). In these models the distribution of variants is determined in a reference set without mutations, for example, remission samples. MRD is subsequently defined by those mutations, that is, those present at diagnosis, which are statistically significantly different in CR to the distribution of the same variants in the reference set. A major drawback of such models is the requirement of a series of reference samples. In a routine setting MRD measurement in a single sample without the dependence of a large reference is obviously the preferred method. Nevertheless, since molecular MRD in CR has consistent prognostic value in AML (Jongen-Lavrencic et al. 2018; Thol et al. 2018; Hourigan et al. 2020; Klco et al. 2015; Hirsch et al. 2017; Getta et al. 2017; Morita et al. 2018; Press et al. 2019) technological improvements should be accomplished to increase both sensitivity and specificity of NGS-based MRD detection.

The recent NGS-based MRD studies in larger AML cohorts (Jongen-Lavrencic et al. 2018; Thol et al. 2018; Hourigan et al. 2020; Morita et al. 2018) revealed that gene mutations persisting in CR that are well-known to be associated with clonal hematopoiesis of indeterminate potential (CHIP) (Genovese et al. 2014; Jaiswal et al. 2014), such as mutations in *DNMT3A*, *TET2,* and *ASXL1* (*DTA*), do not impact on risk of relapse. After high dose chemotherapy, these AML patients are in a state of clonal hematopoiesis (CH), where AML-specific mutations occurring late in leukemogenesis are eradicated and CHIP-related mutations persist. However, the definition of true molecular MRD by the non-*DTA* mutations is not yet optimal. Besides acquired mutations in *DTA*, other well-known pathogenic mutations such as those in *TP53, PPM1D, JAK2, CBL, SRSF2,* and *SF3B1* have also been associated with CHIP in healthy individuals, however, at lower frequencies (Genovese et al. 2014; Jaiswal et al. 2014). Since these mutations appear at lower frequencies in newly diagnosed AML, it will require sufficiently large AML cohort to determine if and to what extent persisting mutations other than *DTA* represent either true residual leukemia or CH with and without increased risk of relapse, respectively. The association of the persisting mutations to relapse risk may relate to type of mutation(s) but also the time and order of mutation acquisition, the allelic burden and/or number of mutations. For instance, later events such as mutations in the RAS pathway-related mutations *FLT3, RAS, KRAS, PTPN11,* and *KIT* as well as *NPM1* are generally cleared by high dose chemotherapy and persistence of these mutations, representing the frank leukemia, has been shown to be clearly associated with a higher risk of relapse (Jongen-Lavrencic et al. 2018; Thol et al. 2018; Hourigan et al. 2020; Klco et al. 2015; Hirsch et al. 2017; Getta et al. 2017; Morita et al. 2018; Press et al. 2019). AML patients with *TP53* mutations at presentation either fail to reach a CR or can relapse quickly after induction therapy, irrespective of their molecular MRD status from data in the HOVON study (Jongen-Lavrencic et al. 2018) (personal communication, Peter Valk). Thus, certain subtypes of AML may whereas others may not benefit from NGS-based MRD testing. Altogether, the definition of true residual leukemia needs to be refined in the coming years with a focus on the persistence of AML-specific mutations with a clear association to an increased risk of relapse.

Today, only a few studies compared NGS- to MFC MRD detection in AML (Jongen-Lavrencic et al. 2018; Ok et al. 2019; Getta et al. 2017). A concordance of 70% in MRD detection between both technologies existed, where those AML patients with detectable MRD by both MFC and NGS having the highest risk of developing a relapse (Jongen-Lavrencic et al. 2018; Ok et al. 2019; Getta et al. 2017). Interestingly, however, those AML cases with MRD detected by NGS or MFC were also associated with an inferior prognosis (Jongen-Lavrencic et al. 2018; Ok et al. 2019; Getta et al. 2017). Improvement of the sensitivity as well as specificity of our NGS-based MRD assays and our understanding of the biology of CH after high dose chemotherapy will enable us to better understand the discordant cases and determine whether we require both technologies or not.

Thus, NGS-based MRD detection focusing on certain (combinations of) mutations persisting in CR carries profound prognostic value for AML patients. The major limitations of the NGS-based MRD detection methodology relate to limited sensitivity and specificity of the assay and the inability to correctly discriminate between residual leukemia and CH. Improvements should be made in all these areas before NGS-based MRD detection can successfully be implemented in routine practice. Initial studies of NGS-based MRD detection were focused on the time of CR after intensive chemotherapy; however, AML patients with a high risk of relapse can also be recognized by NGS-based MRD detection post-allogeneic transplant (Kim et al. 2018; Thol et al. 2019). In addition, NGS-based MRD data of AML patients receiving alternative treatment schedules, including the novel therapies, exist but are limited. It is therefore essential to collect this type of data during the course of disease in the current clinical trials. The ultimate goal will be to dynamically monitor all AML-specific mutations during the course of disease by NGS to adequately follow therapy responses in AML and guide treatment.

## 18.9 Conclusions

The feasibility of MRD risk-directed and preemptive strategies has been demonstrated and its utility will be informed further by reporting of key studies in 2020/2021. Experience of MRD testing to identify deep responders with novel regimens is also building and combined with genetic subtyping should provide further insights into how best to target therapies and evaluate their clinical benefit. High-quality NGS-based MRD assays could contribute to this but more data, in different treatment settings, are required to clarify the prognostic value of MRD levels of mutations that are associated with CH as well as leukemia.

## References


Amatangelo MD, Quek L, Shih A et al (2017) Enasidenib induces acute myeloid leukemia cell differentiation to promote clinical response. Blood 130:732–741

Araki D, Wood BL, Othus M et al (2016) Allogeneic hematopoietic cell transplantation for acute myeloid leukemia: time to move toward a minimal residual disease-based definition of complete remission? J Clin Oncol 34:329–336

Assi R, Kantarjian H, Ravandi F et al (2018) Immune therapies in acute myeloid leukemia: a focus on monoclonal antibodies and immune checkpoint inhibitors. Curr Opin Hematol 25:136–145

Balsat M, Renneville A, Thomas X et al (2017) Postinduction minimal residual disease predicts outcome and benefit from allogeneic stem cell transplantation in acute myeloid leukemia with NPM1 mutation: a study by the Acute Leukemia French Association Group. J Clin Oncol 35:185–193

Blatte TJ, Schmalbrock LK, Skambraks S et al (2019) getITD for FLT3-ITD-based MRD monitoring in AML. Leukemia 33(10):2535–2539

Boddu P, Jorgensen J, Kantarjian H et al (2018) Achievement of a negative minimal residual disease state after hypomethylating agent therapy in older patients with AML reduces the risk of relapse. Leukemia 32:241–244

Buccisano F, Maurillo L, Del Principe MI et al (2012) Prognostic and therapeutic implications of minimal residual disease detection in acute myeloid leukemia. Blood 119:332–341

Buccisano F, Maurillo L, Piciocchi A et al (2015) Minimal residual disease negativity in elderly patients with acute myeloid leukemia may indicate different postremission strategies than in younger patients. Ann Hematol 94:1319–1326

Buccisano F, Maurillo L, Piciocchi A et al (2017) Pretransplant persistence of minimal residual disease does not contraindicate allogeneic stem cell transplantation for adult patients with acute myeloid leukemia. Bone Marrow Transplant 52:473–475

Buccisano F, Dillon R, Freeman SD et al (2018) Role of minimal (measurable) residual disease assessment in older patients with acute myeloid leukemia. Cancers (Basel) 10:215

Buckley SA, Wood BL, Othus M et al (2017) Minimal residual disease prior to allogeneic hematopoietic cell transplantation in acute myeloid leukemia: a meta-analysis. Haematologica 102:865–873

Bullinger L, Dohner K, Dohner H (2017) Genomics of acute myeloid leukemia diagnosis and pathways. J Clin Oncol 35:934–946

Burchert A, Bug G, Finke J et al (2018) Sorafenib as maintenance therapy post allogeneic stem cell transplantation for FLT3-ITD positive AML: results from the randomized, double-blind, placebo-controlled multicentre Sormain trial. Blood 132(Suppl 1):661–661

Burnett AK, Russell NH, Hills RK et al (2012) Addition of gemtuzumab ozogamicin to induction chemotherapy improves survival in older patients with acute myeloid leukemia. J Clin Oncol 30:3924–3931

Cocciardi S, Dolnik A, Kapp-Schwoerer S et al (2019) Clonal evolution patterns in acute myeloid leukemia with NPM1 mutation. Nat Commun 10:2031

Cornelissen JJ, Gratwohl A, Schlenk RF et al (2012) The European LeukemiaNet AML working party consensus statement on allogeneic HSCT for patients with AML in remission: an integrated-risk adapted approach. Nat Rev Clin Oncol 9:579–590

Daver N, Kantarjian H, Garcia-Manero G et al (2017) Vosaroxin in combination with decitabine in newly diagnosed older patients with acute myeloid leukemia or high-risk myelodysplastic syndrome. Haematologica 102:1709–1717

Dillon R, Hills RK, Freeman SD et al (2020) Molecular MRD status and outcome after transplantation in NPM1 mutated AML: results from the UK NCRI AML17 study. Blood 135(9):680–688

DiNardo CD, Stein EM, de Botton S et al (2018) Durable remissions with Ivosidenib in IDH1-mutated relapsed or refractory AML. N Engl J Med 378:2386–2398

DiNardo CD, Stein AS, Stein EM et al (2019a) Mutant IDH1 inhibitor ivosidenib (IVO; AG-120) in combination with azacitidine (AZA) for newly diagnosed acute myeloid leukemia (ND AML). J Clin Oncol 37(15 suppl):7011–7011

DiNardo CD, Schuh AC, Stein EM et al (2019b) Enasidenib plus Azacitidine significantly improves complete remission and overall response compared with Azacitidine alone in patients with newly diagnosed acute myeloid leukemia (AML) with isocitrate dehydrogenase 2 (IDH2) mutations: interim phase II results from an ongoing, randomized study. Blood 134(Suppl 1):643–643

DiNardo CD, Pratz K, Pullarkat V et al (2019c) Venetoclax combined with decitabine or azacitidine in treatment-naive, elderly patients with acute myeloid leukemia. Blood 133:7–17

DiNardo CD, Tiong IS, Quaglieri A et al (2020) Molecular patterns of response and treatment failure after frontline venetoclax combinations in older patients with AML. Blood 135(11):791–803

Dohner H, Estey E, Grimwade D et al (2017) Diagnosis and management of AML in adults: 2017 ELN recommendations from an international expert panel. Blood 129:424–447

Döhner K, Thiede C, Jahn N et al (2020) Impact of NPM1/FLT3-ITD genotypes defined by the2017 European LeukemiaNet in patients with acute myeloid leukemia. Blood 135(5):371–380

Ferret Y, Boissel N, Helevaut N et al (2018) Clinical relevance of IDH1/2 mutant allele burden during follow-up in acute myeloid leukemia. A study by the French ALFA Group. Haematologica 103:822–829

Fournier E, Duployez N, Ducourneau B et al (2020) Mutational profile and benefit of gemtuzumab ozogamicin in acute myeloid leukemia patients treated in the ALFA0701 trial. Blood 135(8):542–546

Freeman SD, Hourigan CS (2019) MRD evaluation of AML in clinical practice: are we there yet? Hematology Am Soc Hematol Educ Program 2019:557–569

Freeman SD, Virgo P, Couzens S et al (2013) Prognostic relevance of treatment response measured by flow cytometric residual disease detection in older patients with acute myeloid leukemia. J Clin Oncol 31:4123–4131

Freeman SD, Hills RK, Virgo P et al (2018) Measurable residual disease at induction redefines partial response in acute myeloid leukemia and stratifies outcomes in patients at standard risk without NPM1 mutations. J Clin Oncol 36:1486–1497

Genovese G, Kahler AK, Handsaker RE et al (2014) Clonal hematopoiesis and blood-cancer risk inferred from blood DNA sequence. N Engl J Med 371:2477–2487

Gerstung M, Papaemmanuil E, Martincorena I et al (2017) Precision oncology for acute myeloid leukemia using a knowledge bank approach. Nat Genet 49:332–340

Getta BM, Devlin SM, Levine RL et al (2017) Multicolor flow cytometry and multigene next-generation sequencing are complementary and highly predictive for relapse in acute myeloid leukemia after allogeneic transplantation. Biol Blood Marrow Transplant 23:1064–1071

Gilleece MH, Labopin M, Yakoub-Agha I et al (2018) Measurable residual disease, conditioning regimen intensity, and age predict outcome of allogeneic hematopoietic cell transplantation for acute myeloid leukemia in first remission: a registry analysis of 2292 patients by the acute leukemia working party European Society of Blood and Marrow Transplantation. Am J Hematol 93:1142–1152

Goldberg AD, Talati C, Desai P et al (2018) TP53 mutations predict poorer responses to CPX-351 in acute myeloid leukemia. Blood 132(Suppl 1):1433–1433

Grimwade D, Ivey A, Huntly BJ (2016) Molecular landscape of acute myeloid leukemia in younger adults and its clinical relevance. Blood 127:29–41

Guenot C, Lacombe F, Allou K et al (2019) Peripheral blood minimal/measurable residual disease assessed in flow cytometry in acute myeloblastic leukemia. Leukemia 33(7):1814–1816

Haubner S, Perna F, Kohnke T et al (2019) Coexpression profile of leukemic stem cell markers for combinatorial targeted therapy in AML. Leukemia 33:64–74

Hills RK, Castaigne S, Appelbaum FR et al (2014) Addition of gemtuzumab ozogamicin to induction chemotherapy in adult patients with acute myeloid leukaemia: a meta-analysis of individual patient data from randomised controlled trials. Lancet Oncol 15:986–996

Hirsch P, Tang R, Abermil N et al (2017) Precision and prognostic value of clone-specific minimal residual disease in acute myeloid leukemia. Haematologica 102:1227–1237

Hochman MJ, Othus M, Shaw C et al (2019) Does intensity of induction chemotherapy affect the impact of measurable residual disease (MRD) on prognosis in acute myeloid leukemia (AML)? J Clin Oncol 37(15 suppl):7031–7031

Hoffmann H, Thiede C, Glauche I et al (2019) The prognostic potential of monitoring disease dynamics in NPM1-positive acute myeloid leukemia. Leukemia 33(6):1531–1534

Hollein A, Jeromin S, Meggendorfer M et al (2018a) Minimal residual disease (MRD) monitoring and mutational landscape in AML with RUNX1-RUNX1T1: a study on 134 patients. Leukemia 32:2270–2274

Hollein A, Meggendorfer M, Dicker F et al (2018b) NPM1 mutated AML can relapse with wild-type NPM1: persistent clonal hematopoiesis can drive relapse. Blood Adv 2:3118–3125

Hourigan CS, Goswami M, Battiwalla M et al (2016) When the minimal becomes measurable. J Clin Oncol 34:2557–2558

Hourigan CS, Gale RP, Gormley NJ et al (2017) Measurable residual disease testing in acute myeloid leukaemia. Leukemia 31:1482–1490

Hourigan CS, Dillon LW, Gui G et al (2020) Impact of conditioning intensity of allogeneic transplantation for acute myeloid leukemia with genomic evidence of residual disease. J Clin Oncol 38(12):1273–1283

Ivey A, Hills RK, Simpson MA et al (2016) Assessment of minimal residual disease in standard-risk AML. N Engl J Med 374:422–433

Jaiswal S, Fontanillas P, Flannick J et al (2014) Age-related clonal hematopoiesis associated with adverse outcomes. N Engl J Med 371:2488–2498

Jongen-Lavrencic M, Grob T, Hanekamp D et al (2018) Molecular minimal residual disease in acute myeloid leukemia. N Engl J Med 378:1189–1199

Kadia TM, Cortes JE, Konopleva MY et al (2019) Venetoclax combined with Cladribine + low dose AraC (LDAC) alternating with 5-Azacytidine produces high rates of minimal residual disease (MRD) negative complete remissions (CR) in older patients with newly diagnosed acute myeloid leukemia (AML). Blood 134:2647–2647

Khan N, Freeman SD, Virgo P et al (2015) An immunophenotypic pre-treatment predictor for poor response to induction chemotherapy in older acute myeloid leukaemia patients: blood frequency of CD34+ CD38 low blasts. Br J Haematol 170:80–84

Kim T, Moon JH, Ahn JS et al (2018) Next-generation sequencing-based posttransplant monitoring of acute myeloid leukemia identifies patients at high risk of relapse. Blood 132:1604–1613

Klco JM, Miller CA, Griffith M et al (2015) Association between mutation clearance after induction therapy and outcomes in acute myeloid leukemia. JAMA 314:811–822

Lambert J, Lambert J, Nibourel O et al (2014) MRD assessed by WT1 and NPM1 transcript levels identifies distinct outcomes in AML patients and is influenced by gemtuzumab ozogamicin. Oncotarget 5:6280–6288

Lancet JE, Uy GL, Cortes JE et al (2018) CPX-351 (cytarabine and daunorubicin) liposome for injection versus conventional cytarabine plus daunorubicin in older patients with newly diagnosed secondary acute myeloid leukemia. J Clin Oncol 36:2684–2692

Leung W, Pui CH, Coustan-Smith E et al (2012) Detectable minimal residual disease before hematopoietic cell transplantation is prognostic but does not preclude cure for children with very-high-risk leukemia. Blood 120:468–472

Levine RL, Valk PJM (2019) Next-generation sequencing in the diagnosis and minimal residual disease assessment of acute myeloid leukemia. Haematologica 104:868–871

Levis MJ, Perl AE, Altman JK et al (2018) A next-generation sequencing-based assay for minimal residual disease assessment in AML patients with FLT3-ITD mutations. Blood Adv 2:825–831

Levis M, Shi W, Chang K et al (2020) FLT3 inhibitors added to induction therapy induce deeper remissions. Blood 135:75–78

Löwenberg B, Pabst T, Maertens J et al (2021) Addition of lenalidomide to intensive treatment in younger and middle-aged adults with newly diagnosed AML: the HOVON-SAKK-132 trial. Blood Adv 5(4): 1110–1121

Morita K, Kantarjian HM, Wang F et al (2018) Clearance of somatic mutations at remission and the risk of relapse in acute myeloid leukemia. J Clin Oncol 36:1788–1797

Ok CY, Loghavi S, Sui D et al (2019) Persistent IDH1/2 mutations in remission can predict relapse in patients with acute myeloid leukemia. Haematologica 104:305–311

Ossenkoppele G, Schuurhuis GJ, van de Loosdrecht A et al (2019) Can we incorporate MRD assessment into clinical practice in AML? Best Pract Res Clin Haematol 32:186–191

Perl AE, Martinelli G, Cortes JE et al (2019) Gilteritinib or chemotherapy for relapsed or refractory FLT3-mutated AML. N Engl J Med 381:1728–1740

Platzbecker U, Middeke JM, Sockel K et al (2018) Measurable residual disease-guided treatment with azacitidine to prevent haematological relapse in patients with myelodysplastic syndrome and acute myeloid leukaemia (RELAZA2): an open-label, multicentre, phase 2 trial. Lancet Oncol 19:1668–1679

Platzbecker U, Middeke JM, Sockel K et al (2019) Azacitidine for pre-Emptive treatment of measurable-residual disease in MDS/AML patients at high risk of hematological relapse: results of the second cohort of the RELAZA2 trial. Blood 134(suppl 1):644–644

Prassek VV, Rothenberg-Thurley M, Sauerland MC et al (2018) Genetics of acute myeloid leukemia in the elderly: mutation spectrum and clinical impact in intensively treated patients aged 75 years or older. Haematologica 103:1853–1861

Prata PH, Bally C, Prebet T et al (2018) NPM1 mutation is not associated with prolonged complete remission in acute myeloid leukemia patients treated with hypomethylating agents. Haematologica 103:e455–e457

Press RD, Eickelberg G, Froman A et al (2019) Next-generation sequencing-defined minimal residual disease before stem cell transplantation predicts acute myeloid leukemia relapse. Am J Hematol 94:902–912

Roboz GJ, DiNardo CD, Stein EM et al (2020) Ivosidenib induces deep durable remissions in patients with newly diagnosed IDH1-mutant acute myeloid leukemia. Blood 135(7):463–471

Rucker FG, Agrawal M, Corbacioglu A et al (2019) Measurable residual disease monitoring in acute myeloid leukemia with t(8;21)(q22;q22.1): results from the AML study group. Blood 134:1608–1618

Salk JJ, Schmitt MW, Loeb LA (2018) Enhancing the accuracy of next-generation sequencing for detecting rare and subclonal mutations. Nat Rev Genet 19:269–285

Santini V, Ossenkoppele GJ (2019) Hypomethylating agents in the treatment of acute myeloid leukemia: a guide to optimal use. Crit Rev Oncol Hematol 140:1–7

Schlenk RF, Paschka P, Krzykalla J et al (2020) Gemtuzumab ozogamicin in NPM1-mutated acute myeloid leukemia: early results from the prospective randomized AMLSG 09-09 phase III study. J Clin Oncol 38(6):623–632

Schuurhuis GJ, Heuser M, Freeman S et al (2018) Minimal/measurable residual disease in AML: a consensus document from the European LeukemiaNet MRD working party. Blood 131:1275–1291

Short NJ, Rafei H, Daver NG et al (2019) Achievement of complete remission (CR) with measurable residual disease (MRD) negativity is highly prognostic in patients (pts) with relapsed or refractory (R/R) acute myeloid leukemia (AML) receiving first salvage chemotherapy. Blood 134(Suppl 1):735–735

Sierra J, Garrido A, Diaz Beya M et al (2019) Final results of the AML12 trial of the Spanish Cetlam Group in Adults with acute myeloid leukemia (AML) up to the age of 70 years: risk adapted post-remission allocation based on genetic data and minimal residual disease. Blood 134:289–289

Stein EM, DiNardo CD, Fathi AT et al (2018) Ivosidenib or Enasidenib combined with induction and consolidation chemotherapy in patients with newly diagnosed AML with an IDH1 or IDH2 mutation is safe, effective, and leads to MRD-negative complete remissions. Blood 132(Suppl 1):560–560

Stein EM, DiNardo CD, Fathi AT et al (2019) Molecular remission and response patterns in patients with mutant-IDH2 acute myeloid leukemia treated with enasidenib. Blood 133:676–687

Stone RM, Mandrekar SJ, Sanford BL et al (2017) Midostaurin plus chemotherapy for acute myeloid leukemia with a FLT3 mutation. N Engl J Med 377:454–464

Terwijn M, van Putten WL, Kelder A et al (2013) High prognostic impact of flow cytometric minimal residual disease detection in acute myeloid leukemia: data from the HOVON/SAKK AML 42A study. J Clin Oncol 31:3889–3897

Thol F, Gabdoulline R, Liebich A et al (2018) Measurable residual disease monitoring by NGS before allogeneic hematopoietic cell transplantation in AML. Blood 132:1703–1713

Thol F, Heida B, Buettner K et al (2019) Post transplantation measurable residual disease (MRD) monitoring using next-generation sequencing is highly predictive for relapse after allogeneic stem cell transplantation. Blood 134(Suppl 1):184–184

Tiong IS, Dillon R, Ivey A et al (2019) Rapid elimination of NPM1 mutant measurable residual disease (MRD) using low intensity Venetoclax-based combinations in acute myeloid leukemia (AML). Blood 134(Suppl 1):2648–2648

Venditti A, Piciocchi A, Candoni A et al (2019) GIMEMA AML1310 trial of risk-adapted, MRD-directed therapy for young adults with newly diagnosed acute myeloid leukemia. Blood 134:935–945

Versluis J, Kalin B, Zeijlemaker W et al (2017) Graft-versus-leukemia effect of allogeneic stem-cell transplantation and minimal residual disease in patients with acute myeloid leukemia in first complete remission. JCO Precis Oncol 1:1–13

Walter RB, Gyurkocza B, Storer BE et al (2015) Comparison of minimal residual disease as outcome predictor for AML patients in first complete remission undergoing myeloablative or nonmyeloablative allogeneic hematopoietic cell transplantation. Leukemia 29:137–144

Wei A, Strickland SA, Hou J-Z et al (2018) Venetoclax with low-dose Cytarabine induces rapid, deep, and durable responses in previously untreated older adults with AML ineligible for intensive chemotherapy. Blood 132(Suppl 1):284–284

Wei AH, Döhner H, Pocock C et al (2019a) The QUAZAR AML-001 maintenance trial: results of a phase III international, randomized, double-blind, placebo-controlled study of CC-486 (oral formulation of azacitidine) in patients with acute myeloid leukemia (AML) in first remission. Blood 134(Suppl 2):LBA-3

Wei AH, Strickland SA Jr, Hou JZ et al (2019b) Venetoclax combined with low-dose Cytarabine for previously untreated patients with acute myeloid leukemia: results from a phase Ib/II study. J Clin Oncol 37:1277–1284

Winters AC, Gutman JA, Purev E et al (2019) Real-world experience of venetoclax with azacitidine for untreated patients with acute myeloid leukemia. Blood Adv 3:2911–2919

Yee KWL, Roboz GJ, O'Connell CL et al (2019) Landmark response and survival analyses from 206 AML patients treated with guadecitabine in a phase 2 study demonstrate the importance of adequate treatment duration to maximize response and survival benefit. Survival benefit not restricted to patients with objective response. Blood 134(Suppl 1):3846

Zeijlemaker W, Kelder A, Oussoren-Brockhoff YJ et al (2016) A simple one-tube assay for immunophenotypical quantification of leukemic stem cells in acute myeloid leukemia. Leukemia 30:439–446

Zeijlemaker W, Grob T, Meijer R et al (2019) CD34(+) CD38(−) leukemic stem cell frequency to predict outcome in acute myeloid leukemia. Leukemia 33:1102–1112

Zhu HH, Zhang XH, Qin YZ et al (2013) MRD-directed risk stratification treatment may improve outcomes of t(8;21) AML in the first complete remission: results from the AML05 multicenter trial. Blood 121:4056–4062

# Future Developments: Immunotherapy in AML

# 19

Marion Subklewe

## Abbreviations

| | |
|---|---|
| alloSCT | Allogeneic stem cell transplantation |
| AML | Acute myeloid leukemia |
| BCP-ALL | B-cell precursor acute lymphoblastic leukemia |
| BissCAR | Bispecific and split chimeric antigen receptor |
| BiTE | Bispecific T-cell engager |
| CAR | Chimeric antigen receptor |
| cCAR | Compound chimeric antigen receptor |
| CR | Complete remission |
| CRS | Cytokine release syndrome |
| DART | Dual affinity retargeting |
| DLBCL | Diffuse large B-cell lymphoma |
| FC | Crystallizable fragments |
| GvHD | Graft-versus-host disease |
| GvL | Graft-versus-leukemia |
| HLA | Human leukocyte antigen |
| HMA | Hypomethylating agent |
| HSC | Hematopoietic stem cell |
| HSPC | Hematopoietic stem and progenitor cells |
| ICPIs | Immune checkpoint inhibitor |
| LSC | Leukemic stem cell |
| MDS | Myelodysplastic syndrome |
| MHC | Major histocompatibility complex |
| MRD | Measurable (minimal) residual disease |
| Nb | Nanobody |
| ORR | Objective response rate |
| STAR | Sequentially tumor-selected antibody and antigen retrieval |
| TCR | T-cell receptor |

M. Subklewe (✉)
Medizinische Klinik und Poliklinik III, Medizinische Fakultät Ludwig-Maximilian-Universität, Klinikum der Universität München Großhadern, Munich, Germany
e-mail: Marion.Subklewe@med.uni-muenchen.de

## 19.1 Challenges of Immunotherapy in AML

The five-year survival rate in acute myeloid leukemia (AML) remains low due to a high incidence of relapse caused by chemo-refractory residual leukemic cells. These relapse-initiating cells are the target of novel immunotherapeutic strategies (Yang et al. 2017; DiNardo and Cortes 2016). Consolidation therapy with allogeneic stem cell transplantation (alloSCT) has been shown to be the most successful anti-leukemic treatment strategy in AML (Koreth et al. 2009). Donor T-cells represent the key contributors to the success of this therapy facilitating the desired graft-versus-leukemia (GvL) effect and reactivating the power of the immune system to fight against AML blasts and precursor cells. Nevertheless, alloSCT is limited to a small subset



C. Röllig, G. J. Ossenkoppele (eds.), *Acute Myeloid Leukemia*, Hematologic Malignancies,
https://doi.org/10.1007/978-3-030-72676-8_19

of patients and is associated with severe complications including graft-versus-host disease (GvHD). The success of alloSCT is further compromised by a significant relapse rate attributed to several AML-associated immune escape mechanisms. These include reduced expression of major histocompatibility complex (MHC) molecules, enhanced expression of inhibitory ligands, reduced expression of activating ligands and receptors, and manipulation of soluble factors within the microenvironment (Khaldoyanidi et al. 2021).

Several immunomodulatory platforms were developed against hematologic malignancies to enable T-cell-based therapy outside the alloSCT setting and thereby have the potential to (1) increase therapeutical efficacy and (2) reduce T-cell cytotoxicity against healthy tissues. Immune checkpoint inhibitors (ICPIs) have evolved within the last decade as valuable tools in cancer immunotherapy by blocking inhibitory checkpoints and reactivating the immune system's abbilities to fight cancer cells. Checkpoint inhibitors rely on the reactivation of endogenous T-cell responses whereas other immunotherapy platforms rely on the recognition of AML-associated surface antigens. Bispecific T-cell engagers (BiTEs) and other T-cell recruiting antibody constructs represent a novel class of antibody constructs that bind to T-cells and cancer cells simultaneously enhancing the T-cell-mediated cytotoxic activity against the tumor cell. Chimeric antigen receptor (CAR) T-cells are genetically modified T-cells featuring an extracellular single-chain variable fragment targeting a specific tumor-associated antigen together with at least one intracellular costimulatory signaling domain. The mentioned techniques will be described and discussed in more detail in the following sections of this chapter. The chapter will not cover vaccine-based approaches that aim to induce and possibly reactivate endogenous T-cell responses against AML-associated target antigens. Albeit dendritic cell-based vaccines have shown promising data, the number of patients treated in early clinical trials is still rather small. Also omitted in this chapter are antibody–drug conjugates as this topic is integrated into other chapters addressing intense induction chemotherapy combinations.

In hematology, ICPIs have only been approved for the treatment of Hodgkin's lymphoma and primary mediastinal B-cell lymphoma. To date, bispecific antibody constructs and CAR T-cells are restricted for the treatment of B-cell neoplasia. The BiTE blinatumomab is used in B-cell precursor acute lymphoblastic leukemia (BCP-ALL) and CAR T-cells were successfully applied in heavily pretreated BCP-ALL (until the age of 26) and diffuse large B-cell lymphoma (DLBCL) patients (Kantarjian et al. 2017; Burt et al. 2019).

Although these promising results were achieved for B-cell neoplasia, the strategies cannot be easily translated to AML due to the lack of suitable target antigens.

## 19.2 Target Antigens in T-Cell-Based Immunotherapy in AML

In cancer immunotherapy, T-cells are valuable tools as they secrete cytokines and generate cytotoxic reactions against other cells that feature cancerous alterations. The efficacy and safety of such T-cell-based therapies depend on the choice of the right target antigens. Based on the current knowledge, three different groups of target antigens in AML can be classified.

### 19.2.1 Leukemia-Specific Antigens

Tumor-specific antigens, or tumor neoantigens, play a crucial role in tumor-specific T-cell-mediated anti-tumor immunity. In the case of leukemia, specific neoantigens ideally originate from leukemogenic mutations and are therefore exclusively expressed in malignant clones that make them suitable AML-specific target antigens. However, most of the leukemia-specific neoantigens are intracellularly expressed human leukocyte antigen (HLA)-restricted antigens that can only be recognized by T-cell receptors (TCRs). The benefit of leukemia-specific neoantigens is their high specificity to tumor cells and their absence in normal cells, but some limitations including the low number of protein-coding mutations in hematologic malignancies and the potential of the malignant cell to reduce HLA expression as an escape mechanism make this approach highly challenging (Biernacki and Bleakley 2020). In clinical trials, leukemia-specific neoantigen-based therapy concepts have not been introduced so far.

### 19.2.2 Lineage-Restricted Antigens

For the therapy of AML, another concept is to use lineage-restricted antigens of the myeloid lineage. Myeloid progenitor antigens like CD33 and CD123 are expressed on both AML and hematopoietic stem cells (HSCs; Fig. 19.1). Clinical trials utilizing antibody constructs or CAR T-cells in AML patients commonly target lineage-restricted antigens like CD33 and CD123. Different modifications are under evaluation to shorten observed HSC ablation and resulting myelosuppression (Lulla et al. 2019).

### 19.2.3 Leukemia-Associated Antigens

The selection of leukemia-associated antigens is based on their overexpression in AML cells compared to healthy tissue. Leukemia-associated antigens are usually not lineage-specific, which reduces undesired HSC ablation, but these antigens are also expressed in non-hematopoietic tissues, leading to on-target, off-tumor toxicities. A considerable number of AML-related antigens have been characterized within the last decades, but only a small number of leukemia-associated antigens, like WT1 and PRAME, were selected for investigation in early phase clinical trials on patients with AML so far (Tawara et al. 2017; Anguille et al. 2017; Lichtenegger et al. 2020). In current studies, alternative leukemia-associated target antigens like CD44v6 or TIM3, which are not expressed on HSCs, are also tested for their applicability in AML treatment. In one study, the expression of CD44v6 in keratinocytes did not promote CAR T-cell-induced lysis of this physiological cell type. This phenomenon might be explained by the significant co-expression of PD-L1 together with CD44v6 on the keratinocytes and demonstrated that not all target antigen-expressing tissues and cell types are comparably prone to

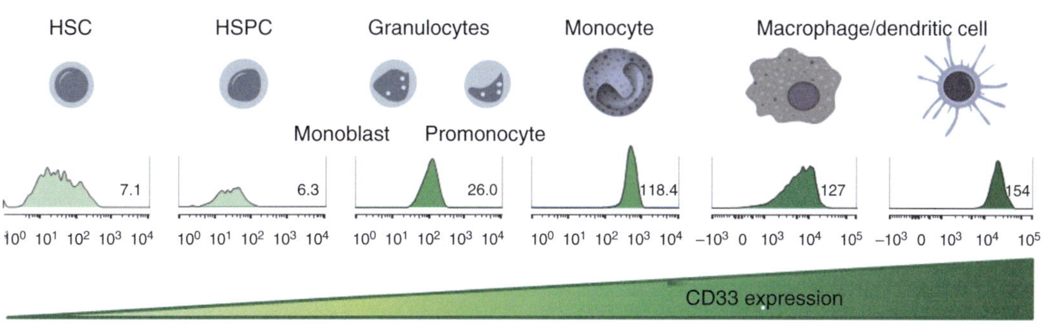


**Fig. 19.1** CD33 expression during the healthy myeloid hematopoiesis. CD33, a member of the sialic-acid-binding immunoglobulin-like lectin family, is used as both a diagnostic marker and a therapeutic target for AML. Despite its expression in AML cell populations, CD33 is also present on the surface of normal myeloid cells with increasing expression intensity during maturation. Although hematopoietic stem cells (HSC) and progenitor cells (HSPCs) feature low levels of this antigen, anti-CD33 antibodies might also target these healthy cell populations and induce fatal HSC ablation

T-cell-induced cytotoxicity (Casucci et al. 2013). Whether comparable resistance mechanisms can be adopted by AML bulk cells and leukemic stem cells (LSCs) remains unclear.

#### 19.2.3.1 Exploring New Target Antigen Candidates in AML

Several characteristics must be considered when the applicability of a target antigen in cancer immunotherapy is evaluated. The first important aspect is the cellular localization of the antigen. Intracellular antigens can only be targeted via the specific T-cell receptor while antigens expressed on the cellular surface can be directly targeted by Fab domains of bispecific antibody constructs or CAR T-cells. Secondly, the intensity of antigen expression represents a potential limiting factor as some antigens can be expressed at very low levels, which cannot be detected even by highly sensitive techniques like flow cytometry in the clinical approach. In addition to the intensity of expression, the distribution of an antigen affects its applicability as a target antigen. The expression pattern of the target antigen might influence the pharmacokinetics, efficacy, and toxicity of the targeted molecule.

## 19.3 Immune Checkpoint Inhibitors in AML

The characterization and functional utilization of blocking the immune checkpoints CTLA-4 and PD-1/PD-L1 was a hallmark of the last decade infighting cancer. More recently, checkpoint inhibitors have also received approval for treatment of relapsed/refractory Hodgkin's lymphoma. Preclinical studies and preliminary data from early clinical trials suggest their utilization in hematological malignancies including AML and myelodysplastic syndrome (MDS) (Boddu et al. 2018; Robert 2020).

An important factor related to the efficacy and safety of ICPIs as a single-agent strategy in AML is prior or subsequent alloSCT. The incidence of alloSCT-related GvHD is known to be a multivariable event, including the allograft donor source, the type of post-alloSCT GvHD prophylaxis, the history of individual GvHD, and the dosing and duration of the applied ICPI (Oran and Daver 2019).

Combinatorial therapies significantly improved response and long-term survival rates. The diversity of successful combinational therapies mirrors the complexity of both, the immunosuppressive biology of the tumor microenvironment and the heterogeneity of anti-tumor immunity (Teague and Kline 2013). Especially in AML, different ICPI monotherapies were identified to be less effective compared to the same strategies applied to solid tumors. This divergence is mainly related to the pronounced heterogeneity of AML and the relatively lower number of mutational alterations in AML bulk cells compared to solid tumor cell populations. Furthermore, the protective bone marrow microenvironment is also assumed to exert an immunosuppressive role either by preventing access of T-cells to AML blasts or potentially by secretion of immune-dampening metabolites (Teague and Kline 2013). Many targeted and non-targeted therapies have recently been approved for AML, and strategies combining ICPIs with different regimens are presented below.

## 19.4 Combinatorial Therapy of ICPIs and Chemotherapy in AML

The combination of chemotherapy with other therapeutic interventions is currently being investigated in clinical trials. The cytotoxic effects of chemotherapy vice versa might also activate the immune response against cancer cells and their specific microenvironment and make them more vulnerable to subsequent therapeutic strategies like ICIPs. In mouse models, injection of cytosine arabinoside (cytarabine) induced the expression of the costimulatory molecules CD80/CD86 and reduced the expression of PD-1 on leukemic cells, making them more susceptible to cytotoxic T-cell-mediated killing (Vereecque et al. 2004). Exposure of calreticulin on the surface of dying leukemic cells after exposure to chemotherapy has been shown to enhance cellular anti-tumor immune responses in AML patients (Wemeau et al. 2010). In a phase II clinical trial, high-dose cytarabine was followed by the anti-PD-1 ICPI pembrolizumab (Zeidner et al. 2019). The overall response rate was 46% and the complete response/complete response with incomplete blood recovery rate was 38%. This study is still ongoing and the relevance of the combination of checkpoint inhibition and chemotherapy remains unclear.

## 19.5 Combinatorial Therapy of ICPIs and Hypomethylating Agents in AML

Hypomethylating agents (HMAs) feature two different mechanisms important for AML treatment. On the one hand, HMAs promote antitumor immune response, and on the other hand, HMAs reduce the immune response by increased immune checkpoint molecule expression. The enhanced expression of immune checkpoint molecules is assumed to be responsible for the commonly observed resistance of AML cell populations against HMAs like azacytidine. Therefore, the combination of HMAs and ICPIs is supposed as a valuable tool in AML therapy and several combinations are currently under investigation in early clinical trials (Stahl and Goldberg 2019).

The combination of azacytidine with different ICPIs is based on the fact that demethylation of genomic regions called CpG islands affects gene expression of PD-1 and CTLA-4 in T-cells, and PD-L1 expression in tumor cells, resulting in an azacytidine-induced reduction of the T-cell-based anti-tumorigenic immune response. Therefore, the combination of azacytidine with ICPIs targeting these antigens features promising synergies. Nivolumab and pembrolizumab (anti-PD1 ICPIs), ipilimumab and tremelimumab (targeting CTLA-4 receptors on T-cells), and durvalumab and atezolizumab (anti-PD-L1 ICPIs) are currently under investigation for combinational therapy with azacytidine in AML patients (Daver et al. 2018).

## 19.6 CD47: A Macrophage Immune Checkpoint in AML

All previously mentioned strategies utilizing immunotherapeutic approaches to fight AML are based on stimulation of the adaptive immune system via T-cell recruitment. A different strategy is targeting the innate immune system. As macrophages are the key mediators of the innate immune response, a macrophage checkpoint protein, namely CD47, became of interest in current preclinical and early clinical studies. Activation of the CD47-SIRPα pathway induces the "do not eat me" signal of a cell, which allows tumor cells to evade phagocytosis by macrophages. CD47 expression was observed to be highly upregulated in myeloid malignancies, but blocking of CD47 resulted in engulfment of the leukemic cells by macrophages. This anti-cancer activity was tested in multiple AML and MDS clinical studies using the first-in-class anti-CD47 antibody magrolimab (Hu5F9-G4) (Chao et al. 2020). At the 2020 American Society of Hematology Meeting, an update of the phase 1b trial was given reporting on 52 AML patients that were treated with magrolimab plus azacytidine. Noteworthy, the majority of patients were of poor-risk cytogenetics including 65% of patients carrying a p53 mutation. Overall, 22 or 34 evaluable patients achieved an objective response (44% of the patients achieving a complete remission [CR]). Treatment-related adverse events were generally transient and reversible. Further data of the expansion cohort with longer follow up are expected in 2021.

### 19.6.1 Bispecific Antibodies in AML

In the 1980s, the combination of antigen recognition sites of two or more antibodies in one bispecific antibody enabled the simultaneous binding to multiple targets and introduced this technique to redirect the immune system against tumor cells (Guy and Uy 2018). Bispecific T-cell engagers (BiTEs) and other bispecific antibody constructs (e.g., dual affinity retargeting [DART]) represent a specific class of bispecific antibodies designed to harness the immune system. These recombinant proteins recruit T-cells through CD3 engagement and target tumor cells through binding to a tumor-associated antigen. Up to date, only one bispecific candidate, namely blinatumomab, was approved in the United States and Europe. This BiTE was designed to bind to CD19 on B-cells and CD3 on T-cells and was successfully applied in patients with refractory BCP-ALL and adult patients with measurable residual disease (MRD; previously termed minimal residual disease (Schuurhuis et al. 2018)). The success of this BiTE is based on the specificity of CD19 for B-cell malignancies. In AML the lineage-restricted antigens like CD33, CD123, CLL-1 (CLEC12A), and FLT3 are currently under evaluation in early clinical trials. Additionally, combination strategies of BiTEs with anti-PD-1 and anti-PD-L1 antibodies are assumed to improve the efficacy of this treatment strategy. Therefore, the combination of an anti-CD33 BiTE antibody construct with the PD-1 inhibitor pembrolizumab is currently under investigation in an early clinical trial (NCT04478695).

The toxicity profile of bispecific antibodies is dominated by cytokine release syndrome (CRS), and anti-inflammatory prophylaxis and individual dose adjustments are utilized to allow high doses of bispecific antibodies being administered to patients. Different formats of bispecific antibodies are currently evaluated in ongoing trials. Smaller-sized constructs feature shorter in vivo half-lives, which allow interrupting or adjusting doses faster, but require continuous infusion. Larger-sized constructs enable slower clearance increasing their in vivo half-lives and do not require continuous infusion. Furthermore, the implementation of crystallizable fragments (FC) in larger constructs can increase their efficacy by promoting FC-mediated cell killing (Brinkmann and Kontermann 2017; Labrijn et al. 2019).

The ubiquitous expression of a target antigen, like CD33, might also interfere with the efficacy of a BiTE construct raised against this protein. The widespread expression of CD33 on different cell types (monocytes, immature granulocytes, HSCs, and Kupffer cells) induces an increased number of BiTE molecules to bind to off-tumor targets. This failure increases the risk for on-target, off-tumor toxicity, but also reduces the presumed anti-tumorigenic effect. The reduction of efficacy by nonlinear pharmacokinetics was also observed for patients receiving the anti-CD47 antibody magrolimab. The expression of CD47 is not restricted to AML cells, and therefore the CD47 antibody was bound to several different cell types in addition to the tumor cells, which made it less effective than a highly specific antibody detecting a tumor-specific antigen. Despite this on-target, off-leukemia effect, a high objective response rate (ORR) even in p53 mutated AML was observed. Clearly, the specificity of the target antigen represents a key component for a successful introduction of antibody constructs in AML therapy.

### 19.6.2 Chimeric Antigen Receptor T-Cell Therapy in AML

In B-lineage malignancies, anti-CD19 CAR T-cell therapies were successfully introduced in clinical practice and approved in the United States and Europe (Schuster et al. 2019). In contrast to B-lineage malignancies, most of the potential AML target antigens are not restricted to the tumor cells and are additionally expressed in HSCs and different cell populations of healthy organs as mentioned before. This circumstance increases the risk of on-target, off-tumor toxicity of CAR T-cell therapies in AML and has to be strongly considered in the process of target antigen evaluation.

In 2013, the first reported clinical trial utilizing a second-generation CD28-ζ CAR directed against the Lewis Y antigen was published (Ritchie et al. 2013). Although limited efficacy was reported, that study demonstrated first-time biological activity of CAR T-cells in AML in the absence of overt hematopoietic toxicity. Current early phase clinical trials (NCT03018405, NCT02159495) applying CAR T-cells in AML are mostly targeting CLL-1, CD33, or CD123. More than 60% of AML blasts are positive for both CLL-1 and CD33, indicating that this might be a suitable target antigen combination (Ma

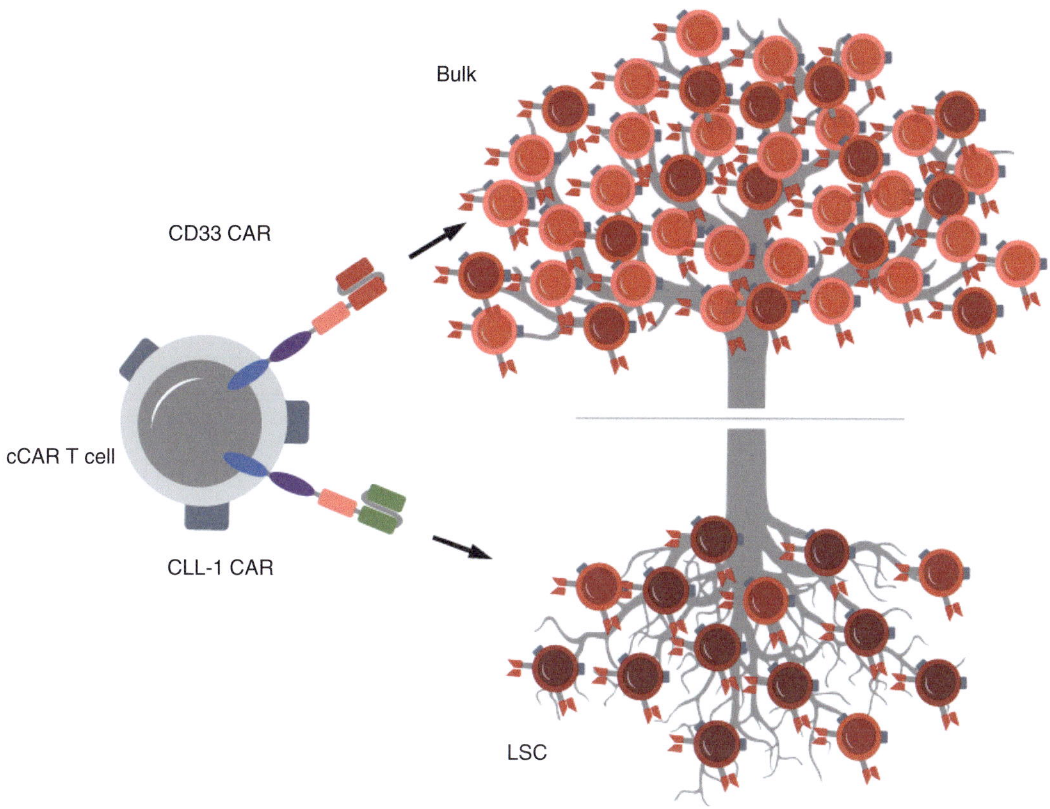


**Fig. 19.2** Advanced chimeric antigen receptor (CAR) T-cell immune therapy in AML. The development of compound CAR (cCAR) T-cells allows the combination of two different CARs expressed on one CAR T-cell. This new technology enables the targeting of leukemic stem cells (LSCs) via, e.g., CLL-1 antigen expression and CD33 positive AML cell populations. The combination of these two antigen recognition sites increases the efficacy of the CLL1-CD33 cCAR T-cells to target AML cells. Alternative CAR T-designs based on conditional recognition of two antigens might increase specificity and thereby reduce the risk of on-target, off-tumor toxicity

et al. 2019). Compound CAR (cCAR) targeting two AML-associated antigens is currently evaluated in a phase I clinical study (Fig. 19.2) (Liu et al. 2018; Sallman et al. 2018). The increase in the specificity of a CAR T-cell system will enhance the efficacy and safety of this therapeutic approach.

Another new strategy to combine different recognizing elements in one CAR T-cell in AML is based on the recent discovery of nanobodies, which represent the “third-generation” of potential therapeutic antibodies. Nanobodies are the smallest, functional monoclonal antibody fragments featuring only two heavy chains with a single variable domain of about 15 kDa as the antigen-binding element. This domain features high affinity and specificity for the respective target antigen, with low off-target accumulation reducing potential toxicity. Furthermore, their small size allows nanobodies to penetrate tumors deeply, additionally increasing their efficacy (Yang and Shah 2020). Such nanobodies were recently isolated via a sequentially tumor-selected antibody and antigen retrieval (STAR) system in AML and nanobody (Nb) 157 was identified with a high affinity for CD13 (He et al. 2020). Based on this observation, a bispecific and split CAR (BissCAR) T-cell was designed targeting CD13 via Nb 157 together with TIM3, an antigen highly expressed in LSCs. The combination of these two recognition elements redirected the BissCAR T-cells effectively against AML cells in murine models and patient-derived xenografts. Due to its increased specificity, BissCAR

T-cell-therapy induced reduced toxicity to normal HSCs, progenitors, and other organ systems in these preclinical settings (He et al. 2020). The STAR system represents a valuable tool to isolate AML-specific and CAR-compatible nanobodies that can redirect BissCAR T-cells specifically to eradicate human AML. Nanobodies feature increased affinity to bind target antigens and their structure allows binding to traditionally inaccessible cavity-like epitopes. These characteristics introduce a broader spectrum of potential AML target antigens and specific epitopes and thus make nanobodies a promising new approach for developing an effective CAR T-cell therapy for AML.

## 19.7 Conclusions and Outlook

The introduction of new technologies and the steadily increasing understanding of the immune biology of AML promote the development of novel T-cell-based and macrophage-based strategies to fight AML. The notable heterogeneity of this disease makes it difficult to find a consistent therapeutic strategy. Searching for valid biomarkers will help to identify patients most likely to respond to specific therapeutic approaches and to foster personalized therapeutic strategies. The identification and optimization of novel checkpoint proteins and AML-specific target genes, as well as the increasing awareness and improved management of therapy-induced immune toxicities and prolonged myelosuppression, will enable the evolvement of new immunotherapeutic strategies in AML in the upcoming years.

## References

Anguille S, Van de Velde AL, Smits EL, Van Tendeloo VF, Juliusson G, Cools N et al (2017) Dendritic cell vaccination as postremission treatment to prevent or delay relapse in acute myeloid leukemia. Blood 130:1713–1721

Biernacki MA, Bleakley M (2020) Neoantigens in hematologic malignancies. Front Immunol 11:121. https://doi.org/10.3389/fimmu.2020.00121. PMID: 32117272; PMCID: PMC703345

Boddu P, Kantarjian H, Garcia-Manero G, Allison J, Sharma P, Daver N (2018) The emerging role of immune checkpoint based approaches in AML and MDS. Leuk Lymphoma 59(4):790–802. https://doi.org/10.1080/10428194.2017.1344905. Epub 2017 Jul 6. PMID: 28679300; PMCID: PMC5872841

Brinkmann U, Kontermann RE (2017) The making of bispecific antibodies. MAbs 9:182–212

Burt R, Warcel D, Fielding AK (2019) Blinatumomab, a bispecific B-cell and T-cell engaging antibody, in the treatment of B-cell malignancies. Hum Vaccin Immunother 15(3):594–602. https://doi.org/10.1080/21645515.2018.1540828. Epub 2018 Nov 20. PMID: 30380973; PMCID: PMC6605719

Casucci M, Nicolis di Robilant B, Falcone L, Camisa B, Norelli M, Gentner B et al (2013) Off-tumor target expression levels do not predict CAR-T cell killing: a foundation for the safety of CD44v6-targeted T cells. Blood 122:142

Chao MP, Takimoto CH, Feng DD, McKenna K, Gip P, Liu J, Volkmer JP, Weissman IL, Majeti R (2020) Therapeutic targeting of the macrophage immune checkpoint CD47 in myeloid malignancies. Front Oncol 9:1380. https://doi.org/10.3389/fonc.2019.01380. PMID: 32038992; PMCID: PMC6990910

Daver N, Boddu P, Garcia-Manero G, Yadav SS, Sharma P, Allison J, Kantarjian H (2018) Hypomethylating agents in combination with immune checkpoint inhibitors in acute myeloid leukemia and myelodysplastic syndromes. Leukemia 32(5):1094–1105. https://doi.org/10.1038/s41375-018-0070-8. Epub 2018 Feb 22. PMID: 29487386; PMCID: PMC6916728

DiNardo CD, Cortes JE (2016) Mutations in AML: prognostic and therapeutic implications. Hematology Am Soc Hematol Educ Program 2016(1):348–355. https://doi.org/10.1182/asheducation-2016.1.348. PMID: 27913501; PMCID: PMC6142505

Guy DG, Uy GL (2018) Bispecific antibodies for the treatment of acute myeloid leukemia. Curr Hematol Malig Rep 13(6):417–425. https://doi.org/10.1007/s11899-018-0472-8. PMID: 30280288; PMCID: PMC6295344

He X, Feng Z, Ma J, Ling S, Cao Y, Gurung B, Wu Y, Katona BW, O'Dwyer KP, Siegel DL, June CH, Hua X (2020) Bispecific and split CAR T cells targeting CD13 and TIM3 eradicate acute myeloid leukemia. Blood 135(10):713–723. https://doi.org/10.1182/blood.2019002779. PMID: 31951650; PMCID: PMC7059518

Kantarjian H, Stein A, Gökbuget N, Fielding AK, Schuh AC, Ribera J-M et al (2017) Blinatumomab versus chemotherapy for advanced acute lymphoblastic leukemia. N Engl J Med 376:836–847

Khaldoyanidi S, Nagorsen D, Stein A, Ossenkoppele G, Subklewe M (2021) Immune biology of acute myeloid leukemia: implications for immunotherapy. J Clin Oncol 39(5):419–432

Koreth J, Schlenk R, Kopecky KJ et al (2009) Allogeneic stem cell transplantation for acute myeloid leukemia in first complete remission: systematic review and meta-analysis of prospective clinical trials. JAMA 301(22):2349–2361. https://doi.org/10.1001/jama.2009.813. PMID: 19509382; PMCID: PMC3163846

Labrijn AF, Janmaat ML, Reichert JM, Parren PWHI (2019) Bispecific antibodies: a mechanistic review of the pipeline. Nat Rev Drug Discov 18:585–608

Lichtenegger FS, Schnorfeil FM, Rothe M, Deiser K, Altmann T, Bücklein VL et al (2020) Toll-like receptor 7/8-matured RNA-transduced dendritic cells as post-remission therapy in acute myeloid leukaemia: results of a phase I trial. Clin Transl Immunol 9:e1117

Liu F, Cao Y, Pinz K, Ma Y, Wada M, Chen K et al (2018) First-in-human CLL1-CD33 compound CAR T cell therapy induces complete remission in patients with refractory acute myeloid leukemia: update on phase 1 clinical trial. Blood 132(Suppl 1):901

Lulla PD, Mamonkin M, Brenner MK (2019) Adoptive cell therapy for acute myeloid leukemia and T-cell acute lymphoblastic leukemia. Cancer J 25(3):199–207. https://doi.org/10.1097/PPO.0000000000000376. PMID: 31135527; PMCID: PMC6602906

Ma H, Padmanabhan IS, Parmar S, Gong Y (2019) Targeting CLL-1 for acute myeloid leukemia therapy. J Hematol Oncol 12(1):41. https://doi.org/10.1186/s13045-019-0726-5. PMID: 31014360; PMCID: PMC6480870

Oran B, Daver N (2019) Check-point inhibitors before and after allogeneic hematopoietic stem cell transplant: the double-edge sword. Biol Blood Marrow Transplant 25:e1–e2

Ritchie DS, Neeson PJ, Khot A, Peinert S, Tai T, Tainton K et al (2013) Persistence and efficacy of second generation CAR T cell against the LeY antigen in acute myeloid leukemia. Mol Ther 21:2122–2129. https://doi.org/10.1038/mt.2013.154

Robert C (2020) A decade of immune checkpoint inhibitors in cancer therapy. Nat Commun 11(1):3801. https://doi.org/10.1038/s41467-020-17670-y. PMID: 32732879; PMCID: PMC7393098

Sallman DA, Kerre T, Poire X, Havelange V, Lewalle P, Davila ML et al (2018) Remissions in relapse/refractory acute myeloid leukemia patients following treatment with NKG2D CAR-T therapy without a prior preconditioning chemotherapy. Blood 132(Suppl 1):902

Schuster SJ, Bishop MR, Tam CS, Waller EK, Borchmann P, McGuirk JP et al (2019) Tisagenlecleucel in adult relapsed or refractory diffuse large B-cell lymphoma. N Engl J Med 380:45–56

Schuurhuis GJ, Heuser M, Freeman S et al (2018) Minimal/measurable residual disease in AML: a consensus document from the European LeukemiaNet MRD working party. Blood 131(12):1275–1291. https://doi.org/10.1182/blood-2017-09-801498. Epub 2018 Jan 12. PMID: 29330221; PMCID: PMC5865231

Stahl M, Goldberg AD (2019) Immune checkpoint inhibitors in acute myeloid leukemia: novel combinations and therapeutic targets. Curr Oncol Rep 21(4):37. https://doi.org/10.1007/s11912-019-0781-7. PMID: 30904967

Tawara I, Kageyama S, Miyahara Y, Fujiwara H, Nishida T, Akatsuka Y et al (2017) Safety and persistence of WT1-specific T-cell receptor gene−transduced lymphocytes in patients with AML and MDS. Blood 130:1985–1994

Teague RM, Kline J (2013) Immune evasion in acute myeloid leukemia: current concepts and future directions. J Immunother Cancer 1:1

Vereecque R, Saudemont A, Quesnel B (2004) Cytosine arabinoside induces costimulatory molecule expression in acute myeloid leukemia cells. Leukemia 18:1223–1230

Wemeau M, Kepp O, Tesnière A, Panaretakis T, Flament C, De Botton S et al (2010) Calreticulin exposure on malignant blasts predicts a cellular anticancer immune response in patients with acute myeloid leukemia. Cell Death Dis 1:e104

Yang EY, Shah K (2020) Nanobodies: next generation of cancer diagnostics and therapeutics. Front Oncol 10:1182. https://doi.org/10.3389/fonc.2020.01182. PMID: 32793488; PMCID: PMC7390931

Yang D, Zhang X, Zhang X, Xu Y (2017) The progress and current status of immunotherapy in acute myeloid leukemia. Ann Hematol 96(12):1965–1982. https://doi.org/10.1007/s00277-017-3148-x. Epub 2017 Oct 28. PMID: 29080982

Zeidner JF, Vincent BG, Esparza S, Ivanova A, Moore DT, Foster MC et al (2019) Final clinical results of a phase II study of high dose cytarabine followed by pembrolizumab in relapsed/refractory AML. Blood 134(Suppl_1):831

# 20 Future Developments: Innovative Trial Design

Elihu Estey

For many years, clinical trials in acute myeloid leukemia (AML) and other malignancies have followed a stereotyped pattern. A phase 1 trial aims to determine the "maximum tolerated dose" (MTD), above which there is excess toxicity. The MTD, or a dose one level below, is then investigated in a phase 2 trial whose goal is to determine efficacy. Assuming enough efficacy is seen, a phase 3 trial randomly assigns patients between the new treatment and an accepted, "standard" treatment.

Here we will emphasize that the phase 1–phase 2–phase 3 paradigm outlined above does not reflect clinical reality. Numerous new clinical trial designs aimed to address these deficiencies have been described both in the statistical and the medical literature. We will describe several of these, particularly those employing a Bayesian approach, which we believe may lend itself to easier interpretation than the conventional *p*-value based ("frequentist") approach (Berry 2006; Berger and Berry 1988).

E. Estey (✉)
Hematology Division, University of Washington School of Medicine, Seattle, WA, USA

Clinical Research Division, Fred Hutchinson Cancer Research Center, Seattle, WA, USA
e-mail: eestey@seattlecca.org

## 20.1 Deficiencies of the Current Approach

### 20.1.1 Focus on a Single Outcome in Each of Phase 1 and Phase 2

It is often said the primary purpose of a phase 1 trial is to determine the MTD. Although efficacy, for example, response, is cited as a "secondary endpoint," the typical phase 1 study contains no formal mechanism to stop accrual into the trial if the response rate is too low. However, it seems likely patients enter phase 1 trials to achieve response rather than to avoid serious toxicity, providing a rationale to formally monitor response. Of course, it is possible that responses will not be seen at the initial phase 1 doses, with response rate increasing with increasing dose. However, given patients' interest in response, it seems reasonable to move a drug at a given dose from phase 1 to phase 2 only if that dose seems plausibly associated with an adequate response rate. This is not the current practice.

Because only 6–12 patients are often treated in phase 1 at the dose recommended for phase 2, knowledge of toxicity (as well as response) at that dose is incomplete. However, just as response is only informally monitored in phase 1, toxicity is only informally measured in phase 2. Given the above, we believe every phase 1 trial is also a phase 2 trial and every phase 2 trial is also a phase 1 trial. This suggests the desirability of



C. Röllig, G. J. Ossenkoppele (eds.), *Acute Myeloid Leukemia*, Hematologic Malignancies,
https://doi.org/10.1007/978-3-030-72676-8_20

simultaneously monitoring both efficacy and toxicity in early phase trials, with "adaptive" decisions regarding stopping or continuing the trial based on both endpoints. Below, we describe a design (called "eff-tox") to accomplish this purpose.

### 20.1.2 Lack of Attention to Patient Heterogeneity in Phase 1 and Phase 2

The typical phase 1 trial regards dose as the only determinant of toxicity. However, it is intuitively obvious that, for example, a 70-year-old person is more likely to have "dose-limiting toxicity" (DLT) than a 40-year-old person. Sixteen years ago, Rogatko et al. examined determinants associated with DLT and with a "toxicity index" (TI) in 459 patients treated on solid tumor phase 1 (65%) or early phase 2 trials (35%) (Rogatko et al. 2004). The TI indicates whether a DLT was observed while also possibly distinguishing between two patients who had (did not have) a DLT. Baseline renal and hepatic function was normal or minimally abnormal and performance status generally 0–1. Dose did not correlate significantly with TI or DLT for carboplatin, tomudex, or docetaxel, whereas pretreatment alkaline phosphatase or bilirubin correlated with DLT, TI, or both for all three agents. Correlations between serum bilirubin and TI occurred over the whole range of serum bilirubin values, not just values above the upper limit of normal. Performance status predicted TI, but not DLT, for paclitaxel and estramustine, while other predictors of DLT or TI were weight loss, and tobacco use. These data suggest there may be several MTDs depending on a patient's constellation of covariates. This complexity is routinely ignored in phase 1 trials.

Of course, with the introduction of "targeted" therapies the MTD is often replaced for phase 2 studies by the "optimal biologic dose" (OBD), that is, the dose that while not producing DLT, optimally inhibits or otherwise affects the drug's presumed target. However, it is plausible efficacy may also depend on the status of targets that do not lend themselves to ready assessment. Under these circumstances it might be of interest to determine both an MTD and an OBD for various drugs. Patients might then be randomized between the MTD and OBD in phase 2 studies, allowing us to test the hypothesis that our knowledge of AML biology is sufficient to replace MTD with OBD.

Patient heterogeneity is also typically disregarded in single-arm phase 2 trials. Probably the most commonly used design for such studies is the Simon 2-stage design (S2S), which considers a new agent worthy of further investigation if the response rate ("rate of interest") is sufficiently higher than that with a standard, accepting false positive and false negative rates of 10–20% (Simon 1989). Consider a trial that uses S2S to investigate a new therapy for persons aged >65 years with newly diagnosed AML. The historical control complete remission (CR) rate and rates of interest are assumed to be 40% and 60%, respectively, with false negative rate of 10% and (1-sided) false positive rate set at 10%. A "minimax" S2S (see http://cancer.unc.edu/biostatistics/program/ivanova/SimonsTwoStageDesign.aspx) calls for entry of 28 patients in the first stage with early stopping if <12 CRs are seen, otherwise continuing to treat 13 additional patients (total = 41) and declaring the drug of interest efficacious if the CR rate is at least 20/41. Say, the early stopping rule is not applicable and the final CR rate is 25/41. However, considering the drug to thus be of interest, as suggested by S2S, assumes that the historical and current groups differ only in treatment. Given the heterogeneity of newly diagnosed AML in older patients, this assumption is likely incorrect. Consequently, a truly useful drug may be considered not useful and vice versa depending on the entry, by chance, of patients with particularly poor or particularly better prognoses. A simple means to address this problem is via multivariate analysis accounting for prognostic covariates as well as historical vs. new treatment. A problem here however is *C*-statistic values suggest that our ability to predict outcomes (CR, event-free survival [EFS], relapse-free survival [RFS], survival) using even multiple pretreatment prognostic variables is at best intermediate between certainty and a coin flip. This suggests the need to begin randomization much earlier than is done today. Below, we describe phase 2–phase 3 design that begins randomization in phase 2 and, depending on results, "seamlessly" and with no/minimal delay transitions to phase 3.

### 20.1.3 Problems with Conventional Randomized Trials

1. *They are insufficiently adaptive*: Randomization is thus essential to balance, as much as possible, unknown prognostic factors among enrollees in different arms of a trial since only known prognostic factors can be dealt with via multivariable analyses. However, randomization raises problems when the control arm of the randomized trial is known to provide unsatisfactory efficacy. For example, it is highly likely many patients with AML and TP53 mutations would much prefer to receive APR-246 in combination with azacytidine or 7 + 3 than to receive the latter drugs + placebo given the well-established highly unfavorable effect of TP53 mutations on survival in patients receiving azacytidine or 7 + 3. Assuming randomization to the standard arm is necessary, as we argued above, one possibility is 2:1 or 3:1 randomization. However, this results in an increased probability of a false negative result ("loss of power"). A more versatile approach entails "adaptive randomization" (ARAN) such that, depending on results, initial randomization probabilities might change, including one arm being discontinued, as the results of the trial are known. ARAN too is not ideal from the standard statistical view point. The latter, aiming to preserve a final false positive probability of 0.05 ($p = 0.05$), allows interim closure of an arm only if at one of very few interim analyses, the $p$-value is much less than 0.05, with the exact value depending on which of several "group sequential designs" is employed, the existence of these various designs suggesting subjectivity in the decision-making process. Regardless of which sequential group design is used, patients may continue to be treated when there is often 90% probability that the new treatment is superior to a standard, a circumstance likely incompatible with patients' expectations. As noted below, we believe the Bayesian approach is appealing in this situation, leading us to describe a Bayesian ARAN design.
2. *Typical false positive and false negative rates seem inappropriate for AML*: When reading the medical literature, it is difficult not to be struck with the pervasiveness of $p = 0.05$ and power = 0.80–0.90 in trials of therapies in widely different situations. This appears counterintuitive. For example, many more successful therapies are available for hypertension than for poor-prognosis AML. Hence, the consequences of a false positive is much greater in a trial of a new anti-hypertensive than in a trial of a new AML drug; likewise avoiding a false negative appears more important in AML. Under these circumstances it seems that while $p = 0.05$ is reasonable for an anti-hypertensive drug trial, $p = 0.15$–$0.20$ might be appropriate for an AML trial, with powers of 0.80 and 0.90 for the former and latter, respectively.
3. *Desired rates of improvement may be too low for AML*: Randomized trials are often criticized because they take too long to complete. Higher rates of acceptable improvement require smaller sample sizes and thus can be completed sooner. Here it is important to distinguish relative and absolute improvement. For example, achieving a 50% improvement in survival (hazard ratio = 0.5) may translate into an improvement in median survival of only several months, which is important to bear in mind when considering that the life expectancy for the average 75-year-old man is 11 years and 13 years for the average 75-year-old woman. This suggests it is important not only to measure the relative improvement (as measured by the hazard ratio) but also the absolute improvement, as quantified by the number needed to treat (NNT) to prevent one death or one relapse. Of course, setting the minimal rate of acceptable improvement too

high would result in rejection of many drugs that are in fact improvements. However, we believe the issues of minimal acceptable improvement rates, false positive and false negative rates, and lack of adaptation in randomized trials are worthy of more discussion than they have received.

## 20.2 Bayesian Approach (Berry 2006; Berger and Berry 1988)

Bayes' theorem states:

$$P(A|B) = \frac{P(B|A)P(A)}{P(B|A)P(A) + P(B|\text{not } A)P(\text{not } A)}$$

where P(A) is the prior probability of a hypothesis (often referred to as the "prior"), P(B|A) is the probability of data given the hypothesis (often referred to as the "likelihood"), and P(A|B) is the probability of the hypothesis given the observed data. The denominator is the probability of the observed data.

More simply put, one begins with a prior probability (for example the CR rate with a new drug is 20%). Data are then observed with Bayes theorem used to update the prior, that is, to generate a posterior. The posterior becomes the new prior and the process is repeated iteratively, as shown in Fig. 20.1.

The values on the vertical axis represent the weight assigned to each CR probability. Prior to treatment, the prior probability distribution (dotted line) is such that, although the average CR rate is thought to be 20%, some credence is assigned to each probability of CR. After observing five of ten CRs (dashed line), the average CR rate is close to 50% and no credence is given to CR rates less than 10% or more than 90%, reflecting the impact of the observed data on the prior. This dashed line now becomes the new prior. After observing 7 CRs in the next 30 patients, for an overall CR rate of 12 of 40, the average CR rate is approximately 30% and no credence is given to a CR rate more than 60% (solid line).

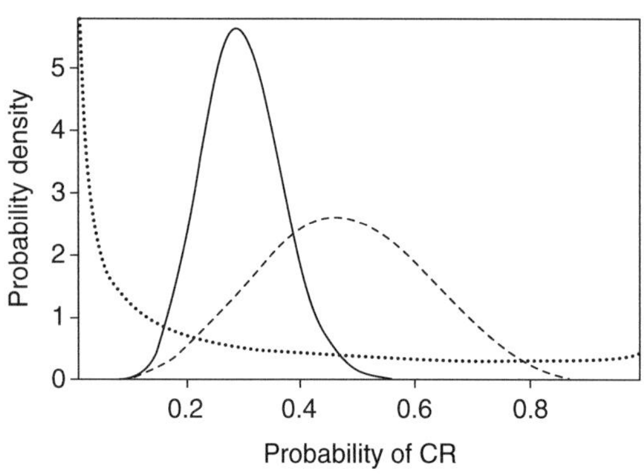


**Fig. 20.1** Bayesian Probability Distributions

An important issue is the derivation of the prior distribution. For example, the average CR rate with prior therapies for relapsed AML has been about 20%, making this a sensible average for the prior. But how "disperse" (i.e., wide) should the prior be? The wider it is the more weight is given to the observed data and the tighter it is the less weight will be given to the observed data. An extreme would be a person with a very strictly held religious belief that was felt to be impervious to data; such a person might be said to have a completely non-disperse prior, which graphically would take the form of a spike.

The influence of the prior on the posterior is a major criticism of the Bayesian approach. In practice, the prior's width might be based on the totality of historical data. But, as we noted above, the historical patients can be very heterogeneous. Another, perhaps preferable, approach is to test the influence of several different priors, together with the data observed in the trial, on the posterior.

Bayesian and *p*-valued ("frequentist") approaches should lead to similar conclusions. However, to this author, the Bayesian approach lends itself to easier interpretation. The interpretation of $p = 0.04$ (for example) would be that under the null hypothesis of no difference between two treatments, the probability of the observed result or a more extreme result is 0.04, suggesting one treatment is better than another. Although $p < 0.05$ is widely taken to note statistical significance, there is of course nothing sacrosanct about 0.05. Furthermore, without knowing how many tests of statistical significance were performed, it is impossible to interpret a $p$-value for any given comparison. In contrast, a Bayesian interpretation might be as follows: with a specific prior probability distribution, the posterior probability that a new treatment is better than a standard is 0.60, the posterior probability that it is at least 10% better is 0.30, and the posterior probability that it is at least 30% better is 0.10. Results would be as follows if a different prior were used. This framework lends itself simple stopping rules for clinical trials: for example, stop the trial if the posterior probability that the new treatment is at least 10% better than the standard is <0.30. With any design, $p$-value based or Bayesian, the importance of examining the "operating characteristics" of these rules and whether they are appropriate to the medical situation at hand cannot be overstated. Operating characteristics refer to the performance of the design using various values for the criterion probability (below which a drug would be judged unsuccessful and a trial stopped), the minimum acceptable improvement, the maximum number of patients, and the number of patients per cohort. Particularly important metrics for performance are the probability of correctly (incorrectly) selecting a drug whose success rate "truly" (in a practically infinite number of patients) meets (does not meet) the minimum acceptable improvement. These are evaluated by computer simulation (usually at least 10,000 simulations) of each of various scenarios (e.g., a new drug truly has the same success rate as an older drug, it is 10%, 20%, etc. better, 10%, 20%, etc. worse).

What follows are examples of Bayesian designs intended to address some of the deficiencies of current designs noted in the first section. It should be emphasized that frequentist approaches could also be employed, although as noted Bayesian methodology may allow easier interpretation (Berry 2006; Berger and Berry 1988).

## 20.3 Bayesian Designs

### 20.3.1 Simultaneously Examining Efficacy and Toxicity (Thall et al. 1999; Thall et al. 1996): "Eff-Tox" Design for Multiply Relapsed AML

Here we will examine four dose levels (D1, D2, D3, D4). At each dose, we will define priors separately for response (R) and for toxicity (T). Patients can have response (e.g., CR), toxicity (e.g., grade 3–4 non-hematologic), or neither. The design does not allow for a patient to have both efficacy and toxicity since it is assumed that toxicity will be defined such that its occurrence renders response irrelevant, the most extreme case being where toxicity is death. We will enter patients in cohorts of 3, beginning at D1, and enrolling a maximum of 45 patients. After each cohort we compute posteriors for response and toxicity, and we determine which doses remain "acceptable." A dose will be considered unacceptable if the posterior probability is >90% that the dose is associated with a response rate < 12% or if the posterior probability is >95% that the dose is associated with a toxicity rate > 30%, more formally: $\Pr([\theta(R,D)] < 0.12|\text{data}) > 0.90$ and $\Pr([\theta(T,D)] > 0.30\ |\text{data}) > 0.95$. The minimum 12% CR rate is based on data showing that the historical response rate in such patients is 5%. The maximum 30% toxicity rate is based on the standard 3 + 3 design's consideration of a toxicity rate of 17% (1/6) acceptable but a toxicity rate of 33% (2/6) unacceptable. If more than one dose is found acceptable, we will choose the one with the highest response rate for the next cohort.

To examine the operating characteristics (hereafter OCs) of these rules, we will examine three dose–outcome scenarios:

| Scenario | D1 | | D2 | | D3 | | D4 | |
|---|---|---|---|---|---|---|---|---|
| | θ(R) | θ(T) | θ(R) | θ(T) | θ(R) | θ(T) | θ(R) | θ(T) |
| 1 | .02 | .10 | .05 | .15 | .15 | .25 | .20 | .30 |
| 2 | .01 | .05 | .05 | .10 | .10 | .15 | .20 | .25 |
| 3 | .01 | .05 | .02 | .10 | .05 | .15 | .02 | .25 |

In scenario 1, dose levels D3 and D4 are each acceptable (at least 12% response rate and toxicity not >30%). In scenario 2, only D4 is acceptable, while in scenario 3 no dose levels are acceptable. Thus, the OCs of the design should indicate a high probability of accepting for future study only D3 and D4 in scenario 1 and only D4 in scenario 2. These OCs based on 10,000 computer simulations are shown below in comparison to those using the standard 3 + 3 design:

| Scenario | "Correct" Dose(s) | Probability Correct Selection | | Mean Number Patients | |
|---|---|---|---|---|---|
| | | With Eff-Tox | With 3+3 | With Eff-Tox | With 3+3 |
| 1 | 3,4 | 0.89 | 0.35 | 44 | 14 |
| 2 | 4 | 0.83 | 0.12 | 43 | 14 |
| 3 | None | 0.86 | 0.01 | 29 | 14 |

Similar simulations and clinicians' satisfaction with OCs underlie determinations of maximum sample size (here 45), cohort size (here 3), and criterion probabilities (here 0.90 and 0.95).

Eff-tox's ability to outperform 3 + 3 reflects its monitoring of response as well as toxicity. The advantage of 3 + 3 is it requires fewer patients. However, this advantage is largely lost when one considers after completion of 3 + 3 a separate phase 2 trial is needed to assess response. To address this problem, the possibility of "dose-expansion cohorts" is frequently included in the phase 1 design, but the OCs of these are infrequently provided.

It is also instructive to compare decisions made by eff-tox and 3 + 3 for cohort 2 after the first cohort of three patients have been enrolled and evaluated:

| # Resp | # Tox | # Neither | Decision for cohort 2: 3+3 | Decision for cohort 2: Eff-Tox |
|---|---|---|---|---|
| 0 | 2 | 1 | ↓ dose | same dose |
| 1 | 2 | 0 | ↓ dose | same dose |
| 2 | 0 | 1 | ↓ dose | same dose |
| 3 | 0 | 0 | ↓ dose | same dose |

If two of the first three have toxicity, the 3 + 3 routinely decreases the dose for the next cohort (or stops enrollment if there is no lower dose contemplated). In contrast, eff-tox retains the same dose because the true probability that the toxicity rate is greater than the maximum acceptable 30% is 81% if two of the first three have toxicity, which is lower than the 95% criterion probability specified above. If this is considered clinically unacceptable a priori, the criterion probability could be lowered to 80%. While this seems sensible, it ignores the possibility referred to above that the two patients may have had toxicity because of for example older age, etc., rather than dose. Retaining the same dose allows this possibility to be investigated further, recalling that in 3 + 3 a dose once deemed too toxic is never revisited. Likewise, because eff-tox monitors response as well as toxicity it retains the same in the event that two to three of the first three patients have a response, even though none has toxicity. Although it might be contended that increasing the dose might increase the response rate, eff-tox allows more patients to be evaluated at the initial dose, thus providing a more accurate guide to the response rate at that dose. Both these examples illustrate a general weakness of conventional designs: too few patients are often treated to gain enough information.

Eff-tox illustrates how multiple outcome designs allow consideration of clinically realistic trade-offs. Other examples might be: (Berry 2006) a design for a lower-intensity therapy that seeks to improve median survival without decreasing rate of measurable residual disease (MRD) negative CR by >10%, on the grounds that long-term survivors will likely be derived from this group; or (Berger and Berry 1988) a design for a higher-intensity therapy that aims to improve MRD negative CR rate without increasing the proportion of patients who do not receive treatment because of fear of toxicity.

### 20.3.2 Selection Designs (Thall and Estey 1993, 2002)

The need to avoid confounding between effect of a treatment and effects of covariates is explicit in phase 3 trials. Paradoxically however, this need is ignored in the usual phase 2 trial, which determines if a phase 3 trial will be conducted. This has led to the use of phase 2 Bayesian "selection designs." Prior probability distributions (see Fig. 20.1) are established for each of three to four generally new treatments; the priors are generally the same for each treatment. Patients are randomized among the treatments, and after each response is known the prior is updated (see Fig. 20.1). The resultant posteriors for each treatment are referred to an early stopping criterion, for example stop if the posterior indicates the probability of a response rate >20% is <10%. If early stopping does not occur, fixed numbers of patients are treated and the treatment with the highest posterior mean is selected for further treatment, for example in a phase 3 trial compared to a standard treatment.

As usual, the operating characteristics of the design, adjusted to be satisfactory to the clinicians involved in the trial, are critical. Of particular importance is the probability of correct selection (PCS) of a treatment if it meets a prespecified response rate and of incorrectly selecting a treatment if it does not. Typical PCS values with selection designs involving four drugs are 60%. It is natural to contrast such PCS with the power of 80–90% to which many are accustomed and thus consider a selection design as an "underpowered" phase 3 trial. However, it is critical to realize the 80% power figure is nominal and ignores how a new treatment to compare with a standard in phase 3 is selected. Specifically, it is important to recognize the role of empiricism in clinical research in AML. Drugs such as all-transretinoic acid and arsenic trioxide in acute promyelocytic leukemia, fludarabine in chronic lymphocytic leukemia, and thalidomide (which begat lenalidomide) in multiple myeloma are examples of the role of empiricism. Conversely, seemingly rational drugs have often produced only transient responses. Examination of the National Cancer Institute's (NCRI's) website (https://clinicaltrials.gov/) indicates there are many new drugs being investigated in newly diagnosed or relapsed AML, suggesting uncertainty as to which is best in the absence of clinical data. Assume for example there are four new inhibitors of a molecular "target." In the absence of clinical data, the probability of correctly selecting the best one is in principle 25%. A phase 3 trial comparing one of the new therapies with a standard may be noted to have 80% power. But this figure is nominal, ignoring the process by which the new drug was selected; accounting for this, the true power of the study is 80% × 25%, which compares unfavorably with the 60% PCS of a selection design. Simply put, the worst false negative may result if a new treatment is not studied at all. This problem may become more acute as, especially, the potential number of combinations of new therapies increases.

### 20.3.3 Seemless Phase 2–3 Design

The NCRI group in the United Kingdom popularized the use of selection designs, which they call "pick-a-winner" designs (Hills and Burnett 2011). A relatively small number of patients is randomized between a standard and a newer therapy. Provided the new therapy "wins," it is advanced to larger randomized study. If it does not, another new therapy takes its place. Formal "seemless" phase 2–3 designs have been proposed, which randomize between a standard (S) and an experimental (E) treatment throughout (Inoue et al. 2002). The study begins at a few centers, with repeated interim decisions based on response and relapse-free survival. Possible decisions are (1) stop and conclude declare E is better, (2) stop and conclude E is no better in which case a new E is introduced, (3) continue the trial, and (4) conclude more centers will be needed to answer the question at which time the phase 3 trial begins. The seemless phase 2–3 design avoids the waste of information attendant on the inability to use single-arm phase 2 data in phase 3; even with randomization in phase 2 the decision to proceed to phase 3 is typically based only on response rather than response and relapse-free survival. Use of the seemless phase 2–3 design also avoids the need to write separate phase 2 and phase 3 protocols. A drawback is the need for interim analyses with its requirements for timely documentation.

It is of course important that the study's endpoint can be observed relatively quickly to prevent patients from presenting for treatment before the outcomes in the previous cohort can be observed. For the same reason the more rapid is accrual, the more difficult these designs are to implement.

### 20.3.4 Adaptive Randomization

Randomization is essential to be as sure as possible that a standard and an experimental treatment are balanced with respect to covariates that, although unknown, have an important role in determining outcome. The effect of such unknown covariates on our ability to predict outcomes such as CR, survival, or event-free survival and be quantified by use of *C*-statistics or areas under receiver operating characteristic curves (AUC). If a prognostic model incorporating known covariates such as mutations or measurable residual disease (MRD in the case of survival or event-free survival) forecasts patient A will do better than patient B, B will do better than C, C better than D, etc.; and if each of these forecasts proves correct, AUC = 1.0 (perfect prediction). If, in contrast, only half the predictions are correct, AUC = 0.5, the equivalent of a coin toss (no prediction). AUC values for most prognostic models are typically around 0.70, that is, approximately intermediate between the value associated with perfect prognostication (1.0) and the value associated with no prognostication (Estey and Gale 2017). Many would conclude a value of 0.7 is too low to permit a conclusion that a new treatment is better than an older treatment even after performance of multivariate analyses including multiple prognostic factors as well as treatment (new vs. old). The purpose of randomization is to attempt to achieve balance with respect to unknown covariates. Indeed, if all prognostic factors were known and none were unknown, comparisons between experimental and standard would require only a multivariable analysis incorporating the known prognostic factors rather than randomization.

However, the scientific need for randomization must be balanced against patients' perspectives. Thus, a patient fully informed of the results of a standard therapy, for example, for TP53-mutated AML ("informed consent" forms often do not suffice, as recently noted by Schiffer (1999)), might be reluctant to be randomized to the standard; after all AUC values for TP53 are not 0.5. This dilemma has led to frequent use of 2:1 randomization in favor of the experimental arm, as for example in a recent trial of azacytidine + venetoclax or + placebo in newly diagnosed patients with AML judged "unfit" for intensive induction (DiNardo et al. 2020).

Another approach involves adaptive randomization (ARAN) (Berry 2006). ARAN begins with 1:1 randomization between S and E. Subsequent patients are randomized proportionate to updated posterior probabilities, with this process repeated. An arm is dropped when probability of randomization to it becomes suitably low. However, a closed arm can reopen should results in the open arms deteriorate.

Giles et al. described a trial using ARAN in patients aged ≥50 years with newly diagnosed adverse-karyotype AML (Glles et al. 2003). The three arms were idarubicin + cytosine arabinoside (IA, the standard), troxacitabine + cytosine arabinoside (TA, experimental), and troxacitabine + idarubicin (TI, experimental). The endpoint was CR within 50 days or not. We chose this endpoint, rather than simply CR, because data suggested CRs occurring after one course but only after this time was associated with a probability of relapse (Estey et al. 2000). A maximum of 75 patients were to be randomized. Initial randomization was 1:1:1, and relatively non-informative priors were used allowing the posterior probability distributions, and thus the updated randomization probabilities, to be heavily influenced by the incoming data. If at any time these posteriors indicated there was at least 85% probability that response rate was higher with TA or TI than IA, accrual to IA would be suspended with patients randomized adaptatively between TA and TI. Analogous rules were used with TI and TA. An arm that dropped out could be reopened if information (i.e., three additional CRs in a dropped arm) became available from patients previously randomly assigned to that arm or if the other arms performed sufficiently poorly, subsequent to closure of the arm in question.

After response had been observed in 19 patients, the TI arm was closed, given probability of randomization to this arm had become zero in light of response rates of TI 0/5, TA 3/7, and IA 5/9. At this time the probability of randomization to IA became 0.87 and 0.13 to TI. After response had been observed in 34 patients, response rates were 3/11 TA and 10/18 IA (remaining 0/5 for TI) and since the probability of randomization to TA was now <5%, the TA arm was dropped. Subsequent information in people who had been randomized, but in whom information was initially incomplete did not change these conclusions.

As always, crucial to the design was preliminary examination of its operating characteristics; some of these are shown in the table below:

| True "success" rates (CR by day 50) | | | Probability Selection | | | Mean Sample Size | | |
|---|---|---|---|---|---|---|---|---|
| IA | TA | TI | IA | TA | TI | IA | TA | TI |
| 30% | 30% | 50% | 0.03 | 0.18 | 0.80 | 11 | 12 | 17 |
| 40% | 20% | 20% | 0.54 | 0.24 | 0.24 | 25 | 19 | 19 |
| 30% | 30% | 30% | 0.10 | 0.45. | 0.45 | 16 | 18 | 18 |

Thus, if TA were "truly" (i.e., in extremely large number of patients) superior to the standard IA, the ARAN design would have correctly selected it with 80% probability, even with a relatively small number of patients; the same would apply with TI. However, if IA were truly superior by the same amount, it would have been selected in only 54% of 10,000 simulations. Furthermore, if all three arms produced the same response rate, the standard would have been selected in only 10% of cases. Thus, the design provided much greater protection against a false negative than a false positive. Having a larger maximum sample size than 75 would have partially addressed this problem. However, the investigators also viewed a false negative as much worse than a false positive in a patient group where prognosis with the standard (IA) is very poor. This would not be the case in a disease such as hypertension where standard therapy is typically successful, and thus the medical consequence of replacing it with a new (falsely positive) therapy is much greater. Of course, it could be argued that, even in the AML case, the time spent in discovering the false positive prevents other new therapies from being investigated.

It is also instructive to contrast the consequences of ARAN with those of the more typical 1:1:1 randomization. In this trial, 34 patients were ultimately randomized (Giles et al. 2003). With 1:1:1 randomization, 11–12 of the 34 would have received IA with 22–23 receiving the seemingly inferior TA or TI. With ARAN, 18 received IA and 16 TA or TI.

## 20.4 Conclusions

The standard phase 1 followed by phase 2 followed by phase 3 approach has been used for at least 40–50 years. Nonetheless, it is not difficult to identify its problems. Almost certainly patients enter phase 1 studies with the primary goal of achieving a "response," not "no toxicity."

However, current phase 1 studies move a dose from phase 1 to phase 2 regardless of response rate, presumably under the assumption that, not necessarily validated in AML, responses are unlikely in phase 1. Likewise, although only a small number of patients are treated in phase 1, at the eventual phase 2 dose toxicity is typically not formally examined in phase 2. Just as toxicity is assumed solely determined by dose, response is assumed solely determined by receipt of drug X rather than drug Y, although in both cases other covariates play a major role in determining toxicity and response. Despite the existence of many often equally plausibly effective drugs, little attention is given to the process by which drugs are selected to compete with standard treatments in large randomized trials; hence the nominal power of the latter is often exaggerated. Insufficient attention is given to the dilemma between the need for randomization and truly informed patients' desires to avoid randomization to a therapy highly unlikely to be successful based on prior experience.

In this chapter, the author has described alternative designs ("eff-tox," "selection," "seamless phase 2–3," "adaptive randomization") to address these problems. The designs are Bayesian, if only because I believe thinking in terms of Bayesian posterior probabilities is more natural than thinking in terms of *p*-values. However, regardless of whether a Bayesian or "frequentist" (*p*-value-based) approach is taken, the designs are more complicated than current designs. If account were to be made of covariates in phase 1 or phase 2, they would be particularly time consuming. The author believes that this price is worth paying. Our knowledge of AML has increased greatly in recent years, and this is reflected in treatment. Despite promulgation of new designs in the statistical (and at times medical) literature, it seems curious that we are largely using the same designs we did 40–50 years ago.

Perhaps most importantly the author believes clinicians have become too deferential to statisticians. The critical feature of any design is its operating characteristics. Determining satisfactory operating characteristics is fundamentally a clinical exercise, heavily dependent on the disease under investigation. It follows that trial design requires extremely close collaboration between clinician and statistician.

## References


Berger J, Berry D (1988) Statistical analysis and the illusion of objectivity. Am Sci 76(2):159–165

Berry D (2006) Bayesian clinical trials. Nat Rev Drug Discov 5:27–36

DiNardo CD, Jonas BA, Pullarkat V et al (2020) Azacitidine and venetoclax in previously untreated acute myeloid leukemia. N Engl J Med 383:617–629

Estey E, Gale R (2017) How good are we at predicting the fate of someone with acute myeloid leukemia. Leukemia 31:1255–1258

Estey E, Shen Y, Thall P (2000) Effect of time to complete remission on subsequent survival and disease-free survival time in AML, RAEB-t, and RAEB. Blood 95:72–77

Glles F, Kantarjian H, Cortes J et al (2003) Adaptive randomized study of idarubicin and cytarabine versus troxacitabine and cytarabine versus troxacitabine and idarubicin in untreated patients 50 years or older with adverse karyotype acute myeloid leukemia. J Clin Oncol 21:1722–1727

Hills R, Burnett A (2011) Applicability of a "pick a winner" trial design to acute myeloid leukemia. Blood 118:2389–2394

Inoue L, Thall P, Berry D (2002) Seamlessly expanding a phase 2 randomized trial to phase 3. Biometrics 58:823–831

Rogatko A, Babb H, Wang H et al (2004) Patient characteristics compete with dose as predictors of acute treatment toxicity in early phase clinical trials. Clin Cancer Res 10:4645–4651

Schiffer C (1999) An important gap in informed consent documents for oncology clinical trials: lack of quantitative details about expected treatment outcomes. JAMA Oncol, 1399–1400

Simon R (1989) Optimal two-stage designs for phase 2 clinical trials. Control Clin Trials 10:1–10

Thall P, Estey E (1993) A Bayesian strategy for screening cancer treatments prior to phase II clinical evaluation. Stat Med 12:1197–1211

Thall P, Estey E (2002) New designs for phase 2 clinical trials. Blood 102:442–448

Thall P, Simon R, Estey E (1996) New statistical strategy for monitoring safety and efficacy in single-arm clinical trials. J Clin Oncol 14:296–303

Thall P, Estey E, Sung H (1999) A new statistical method for dose-finding based on efficacy and toxicity in early phase clinical trials. Invest New Drugs 17:155–167

MIX
Papier aus verantwortungsvollen Quellen
Paper from responsible sources
FSC® C105338

If you have any concerns about our products,
you can contact us on
**ProductSafety@springernature.com**

In case Publisher is established outside the EU,
the EU authorized representative is:
**Springer Nature Customer Service Center GmbH**
**Europaplatz 3, 69115 Heidelberg, Germany**

Printed by Libri Plureos GmbH
in Hamburg, Germany